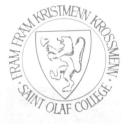

A publication of the
American Medical Association

The Health of Adolescents

William R. Hendee
Editor

The Health of Adolescents

Understanding and Facilitating Biological, Behavioral, and Social Development

Jossey-Bass Publishers

San Francisco • Oxford • 1991

THE HEALTH OF ADOLESCENTS
Understanding and Facilitating Biological, Behavioral, and Social Development
by William R. Hendee, Editor

Copyright © 1991 by: American Medical Association
515 North State Street
Chicago, Illinois 60610

Library of Congress Cataloging-in-Publication Data

The Health of adolescents : understanding and facilitating biological,
   behavioral, and social development / William R. Hendee, editor. —
   1st ed.
       p.   cm. — (A joint publication in the Jossey-Bass health
series and the Jossey-Bass social and behavioral science series)
   "A publication of the American Medical Association" — Prelim. p.
   Includes bibliographical references.
   Includes index.
   ISBN 1-55542-308-6 (alk. paper)
   1. Teenagers — Health and hygiene.   2. Adolescence.   I. Hendee,
William R.   II. American Medical Association.   III. Series:
Jossey-Bass health series.   IV. Series: Jossey-Bass social and behavioral science series.
   [DNLM: 1. Adolescent Behavior.   2. Adolescent Medicine.
3. Adolescent Psychology.   4. Disease — in adolescence.   WS 460
H4348]
RJ141.H43   1991
613'.0443 — dc20
DNLM/DLC
for Library of Congress   90-15627
                                                                      CIP

Manufactured in the United States of America

The paper in this book meets the guidelines for
permanence and durability of the Committee on
Production Guidelines for Book Lengevity of the
Council on Library Resources.

JACKET DESIGN BY WILLI BAUM

FIRST EDITION

Code 9108

A joint publication in
The Jossey-Bass Health Series
and
*The Jossey-Bass
Social and Behavioral Science Series*

Contents

Tables, Figures, and Exhibits

Figures

Exhibit

Preface

Adolescence is the developmental period between childhood and adulthood, characterized by physical, sexual, and psychological maturation. Adolescence traditionally has been thought of as a period of personal growth and opportunity, an interval of physical, emotional, and intellectual development beyond the immediate dominance of parents and yet unhampered by the daily struggles and cares of adulthood. For many young people today, however, adolescence is a time of confusion, trouble, and danger. Recognition of the many challenges to the well-being of adolescents is important to all who work with or are concerned about adolescents. This book is intended as a guide and resource for such people.

Until recently, the age group fifteen to twenty-four was the only one in which the death rate was increasing. In 1960, the annual mortality rate for this group was 106 deaths per 100,000 in the United States; by 1969, the rate had risen to 129 deaths per 100,000, higher than in any other developed nation. The rate declined over the 1970s to a level of 96 per 100,000 by 1983; this rate is still high compared to those in most other cultures. In addition, the rate has remained extraordinarily high for certain subgroups, especially black males.

Premature death is only one indicator of the problems of adolescence in our society. Substance abuse is a major national challenge. Sexuality and pregnancy pose multiple problems, which reflect in part the inexperience of adolescents and in part the naiveté of a society that exploits sexual attractiveness and activity in its media and yet expects young people to behave in a sexually responsible manner. Teens are frequent victims of physical, sexual, and mental abuse and other forms of exploitation, including prostitution and pornography. Emotional disorders of young people, including suicide and inordinate risk taking, are gaining recognition as national problems. Less well recognized but equally troubling are the poor self-esteem, academic difficulties, and tendency to depression of many young people. Other difficulties, including sexually transmitted diseases, traumatic injury, and misunderstanding of basic health information, contribute to premature morbidity and mortality. All of these problems are addressed in this text by authors well-known for their experience and understanding in dealing with young people and the challenges they face in today's society.

The problems of adolescence result in part from the internal conflicts of young people as they attempt to interpret and comply with the often contradictory messages of their culture and society. These conflicts are exacerbated by temptations and directives posed by celebrities, the public media, and, not infrequently, the home environment. In many ways, the values and behaviors of young people are a reflection of the values of adults in a society, at least insofar as those values are interpreted by youth. In examining adolescent characteristics and their manifestations in physical and emotional problems in young people, we must always recognize that they are a mirror image of our own characteristics, filtered perhaps by the adolescent peer group as a substitute for the extended family and neighborhood community of previous generations. Young people today are intrinsically not much different from the youth of past decades. The fact that their physical and emotional health and well-being may be increasingly fragile is more a reflection of a harsher, less-nurturing society and world than an indication of a change in the fundamental character of young people. This text emphasizes the impact of our cultural values on today's youth as well as ways to mediate the influence of these values on children who are experiencing difficulties in coping.

No socioeconomic or racial group is immune to the troubles of adolescents. Both the underprivileged and the affluent have their share of problems and casualties. Nevertheless, poverty is the most profound and pervasive factor exacerbating the problems of adolescents. Poverty puts children at greater risk through the direct physical consequences of deprivation, the indirect consequences of severe stress on parent-child relationships, and the insidious influence of diminished status in the social environment. Although poverty is not confined to particular racial or ethnic groups, it is more widespread in the black and Hispanic populations of our society. It is these populations that continue to show the highest birthrates.

Almost every form of childhood trauma is more prevalent among the poor. Children raised in poverty, regardless of their ethnic backgrounds, are at greater risk for illness, disability, injury, or death than are children who are not poor. Furthermore, the number of children raised in poverty is increasing. In 1973, 14 percent of America's children under age eighteen lived in poverty. By 1983, the proportion had increased to 22 percent. Of all poor people in the United States in 1983, 40 percent were below the age of eighteen.

Adequate income and high social status improve the likelihood of, but certainly do not guarantee, healthy growth and development. Alcohol and drug abuse, accidents, suicides, sexually transmitted diseases, pregnancy, eating disorders, violent behavior, and other health and social problems are plentiful in middle-class and highly privileged populations. These problems are somewhat less visible in these populations, because troubled adolescents in them are more likely to benefit from effective intervention and treatment programs and because the problems may be sheltered from view through parental and societal action. Nevertheless, problems do exist, as can be attested to by adults working with adolescents from various social, ethnic, and economic subgroups within our culture.

Because of adolescents' problems and their portrayal in the public media, it is tempting to assume that many, maybe even most, adolescents are experiencing severe difficulties. Such an assumption is an exaggeration of the issue; most adolescents are coping successfully, if not altogether painlessly, with their lives. However, it is probably true that no previous period of our history has presented young people with so many obstacles to a supportive self-identity and a productive life-style.

Essential to effective counseling and guidance of young people is an understanding of the obstacles young people face in achieving self-identity and self-fulfillment. A distinguishing feature of our culture is its exploitation of young people as a mass market for consumer goods and the entertainment media. There is intense pressure to conform and to suppress the individual personality in favor of the psyche of the peer group. Under pressure, young people sometimes lose direction and need effective guidance. Helping those who wish to provide such guidance is a major objective of this book.

Fortunately, adolescence is also a time of plasticity and responsiveness to challenge. Not infrequently, young people recover from periods of prob-lem behaviors and emotional disorders and mature into responsible and functional young adults. Adolescence presents an exceptional opportunity for prevention of casualties and remediation when they occur. Interventional strategies that help guide individuals toward productive and rewarding life-styles are at least as likely, and probably more likely, to work with adolescents than with any other age group. The identification of these strategies is one of the major purposes of this text.

The opportunity to contribute to the health of forty million adoles-cents in the United States offers a major challenge to all of us in critical positions of counseling, advising, and directing young people. Gaining and maintaining their confidence and helping them through the turbulent pe-riod of adolescence are not easy objectives. They are, however, essential if teen health and self-identity are to be improved in our society. We can all contrib-ute to healthier and happier adolescents by respecting them as individuals living in the tumult of the present rather than by viewing them as birds of passage in flight from the nest to the mountaintop.

Intended Audience

This book is intended as a resource for all professionals who work with adolescents, including physicians, nurses, teachers, social workers, coun-selors, volunteers in community programs for young people, and many others. As individuals, we can help guide selected adolescents along the precarious journey on their way to adulthood. By working in groups, we can extend our influence and assistance, and improve the likelihood that more young people will survive the journey without permanent scarring. This book will have succeeded if it proves useful to any or all of the groups working to improve the health of adolescents in the United States and around the world.

Overview of the Contents

The introductory chapter describes the present demographics and trends of adolescent health and offers projections as to what the future will hold if new initiatives are not introduced into society to offset the trends. These projections aid in the identification of major health issues affecting adolescents today and over the next few years if the trends continue.

Part One focuses on the development of the "normal" adolescent, defined as one without major health or psychological problems. This portrayal, while allowing for a wide variation in developmental progress, provides a guide for the definition of abnormal health and psychosocial development.

Part Two considers family and social factors that influence adolescent development and its direction toward normal or deviant behaviors. Emphasized in this part is the need for much more research and understanding of the societal issues underlying adolescent development if we hope to deal successfully with the health problems of adolescents.

Part Three is devoted to detailed discussions of the present status of selected adolescent health problems in our society. These problems should be interpreted as reflections of fundamental shortcomings in the cultural environment of our young people. Attempting to treat these problems without addressing the fundamental societal shortcomings that give rise to them is like treating the symptoms of a disease without trying to resolve the underlying disease itself.

There are several obstacles to the recognition of adolescent health problems and to the initiation of successful interventions. Among these obstacles is the diffusion of responsibility for the health care of adolescents, with the result that often no one assumes responsibility—not the parents, not the health care providers, and not the young people themselves. As a consequence, adolescents constitute the age group in our society with the poorest utilization of health services and the poorest compliance with these services when they are initiated. Furthermore, there are many obstacles to access to health care for those adolescents who desire it. These obstacles and their consequences are considered in Part Four.

The fifth and final part considers the responsibilities of various sectors of society in moving toward our goal of improving the health and well-being of adolescents. Of particular significance in working toward this goal are the many people who interact with adolescents as part of their daily activities, including counselors, teachers, health care providers, volunteers, and parents. Being knowledgeable about and alert to developing problems among adolescents is an essential first step to successful intervention in the problems. Knowing where to seek assistance is another essential step.

Background

Contributors were selected for this book not only because they have written scholarly articles but also, and more important, because they have accumulated considerable experience in working with, guiding, and caring for young people. Capturing this experience and expressing it in the book were major goals of the editorial team. To this end, the contributors were given the freedom to express ideas and opinions unencumbered by the need to provide annotated references. This freedom also makes the chapters easier and more interesting to read. As a guide to further study and insight, a list of suggested readings is provided at the end of each chapter.

Acknowledgments

Many individuals have contributed to the development of this book. The section editors and chapter authors have responded magnificently to a number of deadlines and to the editor's several revisions and comments— some of which may have been a bit provocative. It has become obvious that the contributors are committed personally as well as professionally to improvement of the health of adolescents. During the early stages of planning this undertaking, several useful suggestions were provided by Bonnie Wilford of the AMA staff. Vickie Grosso of the AMA has kept track of the entire project since its inception; without her it is doubtful that the text could have been completed. Two of my secretaries, Charmaine Price and Diane Reuter, have assisted in admirable fashion when asked. This undertaking has enjoyed the support of three very important individuals at the AMA—M. Roy Schwarz, M.D., James H. Sammons, M.D., and James S. Todd, M.D. Their encouragement and endorsement have been important to the authors and editors.

Chicago, Illinois   William R. Hendee
January 1991

The Editor

William R. Hendee is vice-president of science and technology at the American Medical Association. He is also adjunct professor at the Northwestern University School of Medicine and clinical professor of radiology and biophysics at the Medical College of Wisconsin. He received his B.S. degree (1959) from Millsaps College in physics and his Ph.D. degree (1962) from the University of Texas in radiological physics. He holds an honorary doctorate from Millsaps College.

Hendee's major research efforts have been directed to the development and improvement of medical imaging systems and to the exploration of human visual perception. In the area of adolescent health, he has focused principally on the subject of the exploitation of youth by marketing tactics in American culture. His awards include the Coolidge Award for Scientific Achievement (American Association of Physicists in Medicine); the Elda Anderson Award for Scientific Achievement (Health Physics Society); the Robert Landauer Award (Midwest Medical Physics Society); and the Benedict Cassen Research Pioneer Award (Southern California Nuclear Medicine Society). He has authored more than three hundred scientific papers and written or edited more than twenty books, including *Medical Radiation Physics* (1991, 3rd edition) and *Perception of Visual Information* (forthcoming). He has served as president of the Society of Nuclear Medicine and of the American Association of Physicists in Medicine.

Contributors

Paul L. Adams, a physician in private practice in Louisville, Kentucky, is professor emeritus at the University of Texas, Galveston, where he was Kempner Professor of Child Psychiatry until 1989. He has also taught at the University of Florida, the University of Miami, and the University of Louisville. Adams is now engaged in research, writing, editing, clinical practice, and forensic consultations. Author of seven psychiatric texts, he received his B.A. degree (1943) from Centre College of Kentucky in sociology and philosophy and both his M.A. degree (1948) in social psychology and his M.D. degree (1955) from Columbia University. His sociopsychiatric interest is in the delivery of psychiatric services to poor people and particularly to the mother-only family.

Jeffrey C. Bauer is president of a health care consulting firm, The Bauer Group, in Hillrose, Colorado, that specializes in the development of creative strategic plans emphasizing the importance of clinical science, medical technology, and consumer marketing. He received his B.A. degree (1969) from Colorado College, Colorado Springs, in economics and his Ph.D. degree (1975) from the University of Colorado in economics. Bauer was a Boettcher Scholar (1965–1969), a Ford Foundation Independent Scholar (1966–1969), a Fulbright Scholar (Switzerland, 1971–1972), and a Kellogg Foundation National Fellow (1980–1983). He was a full-time teacher and administrator at the University of Colorado Health Sciences Center in Denver from 1973 to 1984.

Judith S. Bensinger has established a multidisciplinary medical practice, Northshore Adolescent Medicine Associates, for adolescents and young adults ages ten through twenty-five and is on staff at Highland Park Hospital, Highland Park, Illinois. She is trained in family practice and handles the general medical and gynecological needs of this age group. Bensinger received her M.D. degree (1968) from Northwestern University Medical School and began her medical career as a field physician for the Head Start Program in Chicago; she served in this capacity for six years and also trained the program's nurse practitioners. In 1970 she also established a primary care clinic for the mentally retarded at Goodwill Industries in Springfield, Illinois. She served as medical director of this facility for four years. In 1974 she received the Ten Outstanding Women Award and in 1975 the Marshall Bynum Award, Chicago, for Humanitarian Vision.

Robert W. Blum is professor of pediatrics at the University of Minnesota School of Medicine and chief of the Division of General Pediatrics and Adolescent Medicine. Blum received his M.D. degree (1973) from Howard University. He received both his M.P.H. degree (1977) in maternal and child health and his Ph.D. degree (1978) in hospital and health care administration from the School of Public Health at the University of Minnesota. He has written and edited two volumes on adolescent health services, has served on the editorial board of three pediatric journals (*Pediatrician, Journal of Adolescent Health Care,* and *Pediatric Annals*), and is a consultant to the World Health Organization.

Claire D. Brindis is codirector of the Center for Reproductive Health Policy Research at the Institute for Health Policy Studies, University of California, San Francisco (UCSF), and assistant adjunct professor in the Department of Pediatrics, Division of Adolescent Medicine, UCSF. She received her B.A. degree (1972) from the University of California, Los Angeles (UCLA), in sociology and her M.P.H. degree (1973) in the Division of Maternal and Child Health, Family Planning, and International Health at UCLA in maternal and child health, family planning, and international health. Her D.P.H. (1982) was received from the University of California, Berkeley. Brindis's research interests are in the areas of reproductive health policy, adolescent pregnancy and pregnancy prevention, and at-risk adolescents. She has recently completed a book entitled *Adolescent Pregnancy Prevention: A Guidebook for Communities for the Stanford University Health Promotion Center*. Previous books include *Adolescent Pregnancy and Parenting in California: A Strategic Plan for Action* (1988); *Evaluating Your Information and Education Project* (1987); and *Evaluation Guidebook for Family Planning Information and Education Projects* (1986).

William A. Daniel, Jr., is professor emeritus of pediatrics and chief of the Division of Adolescent Medicine in the Department of Pediatrics, University of Alabama School of Medicine at Birmingham. He received his B.S. (1936) and M.D. (1940) degrees from Northwestern University. He is a past president of the Society for Adolescent Medicine and recipient of the Jacobi Award of the American Medical Association and the American Academy of Pediatrics.

Robert H. DuRant is assistant professor of pediatrics at the Medical College of Georgia and director of the Children and Youth Project of Georgia. He received his B.A. degree (1974) from Appalachian State University in Boone, North Carolina, in sociology and his M.A. (1976) and Ph.D. (1987) degrees from Emory University in sociology. DuRant is currently a member of the Executive Council of the Society for Adolescent Medicine and is one of two members of the society with Ph.D. degrees to be elected fellows in the Society for Adolescent Medicine. He also serves as the representative of the Society for Research on Adolescence in the American Medical Association's National Coalition on Adolescent Health.

Elias J. Duryea is associate professor of health promotion, health education faculty, Department of Health Promotion, University of New Mexico. He received his B.S. degree (1977) from San Diego State University in health science, his M.S. degree (1979) from the University of Utah in health education, and his Ph.D. degree (1982) from the University of Nebraska in psychological studies. Duryea was Presidential Lecturer at the University of New Mexico during the 1985–86 academic year and was awarded the College of Education's Research Award (1987–88).

Gayle Geber is program director of the National Center for Youth with Disabilities. She received her B.A. degree (1977) in early childhood development and family studies and her M.P.H. (1987) in maternal and child health, both from the University of Minnesota.

Elizabeth A. Gerken currently is a research associate with the Southern California Injury Prevention Research Center and was formerly a program consultant with the Injury Control Section of the North Carolina Department of Environment, Health, and Natural Resources. She received her A.B. degree (1984) from Davidson College in religion and her M.S.P.H. degree (1987) from the University of North Carolina, Chapel Hill, in health policy and administration.

David A. Hamburg has been president of the Carnegie Corporation of New York since 1983. He received his A.B. degree (1944) in anatomy and physiology and his M.D. degree (1947) from Indiana University. He was chief of the Adult Psychiatry Branch of the National Institute of Mental Health from 1958 to 1961; professor and chair of the Department of Psychiatry and Behavioral Sciences from 1961 to 1972, and professor of human biology from 1972 to 1976, at Stanford University; president of the Institute of Medicine, National Academy of Sciences, from 1975 to 1980; and director of the Division of Health Policy Research and Education at Harvard University from 1980 to 1982. He served as president and then chairman of the board of the American Association for the Advancement of Science from 1984 to 1986.

Janet B. Hardy is professor emerita of pediatrics at Johns Hopkins University, where she directed the Adolescent Pregnancy and Parenting Programs and their evaluation from 1975 to 1985, and the research and demonstration intervention program directed at preventing pregnancy among students in two inner-city schools from 1981 to 1985. She received her M.D.C.M. degree (1942) from McGill University, Montreal, Quebec, in medicine. She is the author of many papers concerned with aspects of child development and is the senior author of a forthcoming book describing adolescent pregnancy in an urban environment—*Adolescent Pregnancy in an Urban Environment: Issues, Programs & Evaluations* (with J. Hardy and L. Zabin).

Kenneth I. Howard is professor of psychology and director of the Graduate Program in Clinical Psychology at Northwestern University and professor in the Department of Psychiatry and Behavioral Sciences at the Northwestern University Medical School. He received his B.A. degree (1954) from the University of California, Berkeley, in psychology and his Ph.D. degree (1959) from the University of Chicago in clinical psychology. Howard's main research activities have been in psychotherapy and in adolescence. He has been president of the Society for Psychotherapy Research and has received the Distinguished Research Career Award of that society. His books include *Varieties of Psychotherapeutic Experience* (1975, with D. E. Orlinsky); *The Adolescent: A Psychological Self-Portrait* (1981, with D. Offer and E. Ostrov); and *The Teenage World: Adolescents' Self-Image in Ten Countries* (1988, with D. Offer, E. Ostrov, and R. Atkinson).

Charles E. Irwin, Jr., is professor of pediatrics and director of the Division of Adolescent Medicine at the University of California, San Francisco (UCSF). He received his B.S. degree (1967) from Hobart College in biology/chemistry and his M.D. degree (1971) from UCSF. Upon completion of his pediatric residency (1973) at UCSF, he completed a Robert Wood Johnson Foundation Clinical Scholars Fellowship (1977), studying adolescent health behavior. In 1977, he founded the Division of Adolescent Medicine at UCSF. Irwin's main research activities have focused on risk-taking behavior in adolescents.

M. Susan Jay is associate professor of pediatrics and director of adolescent medicine at the Loyola University Medical Center. She is currently executive secretary-treasurer of the Society for Adolescent Medicine. She received her B.S. degree (1972) from Loyola University in biology and her M.D. degree (1976) from the University of Illinois.

William M. Kane is a consultant in disease prevention and health promotion. He was for eight years the executive director of the American College of Preventive Medicine in Washington, D.C. Prior to that, he was the executive director of the Association for the Advancement of Health Education. He received his B.S. degree (1969) from Northwest Missouri State University in secondary education (health and safety), his M.S. degree (1970) from the University of Utah in health education, and his Ph.D. degree (1977) from the University of Oregon in educational policy and management. He has several years' experience as a public school teacher of health education and is the lead author of a high school health education textbook.

Richard E. Kreipe is associate professor of pediatrics, associate chair (academic affairs), and director of adolescent services at the University of Rochester School of Medicine within the Division of Adolescent Medicine. He received his B.A. degree (1971) from LaSalle College, Philadelphia, in biology and his M.D. degree (1975) from Temple University School of Medicine.

Elizabeth R. McAnarney is professor of pediatrics, associate chair (academic affairs), and chief of the Division of Adolescent Medicine at the University of Rochester Medical Center. She received her B.A. degree (1962) from Vassar College in child study and her M.D. degree (1966) from the State University of New York Upstate Medical Center in Syracuse. She completed fellowship training (1970) at the University of Rochester in behavioral pediatrics. She is a member of the Society for Pediatric Research, the American Pediatric Society, the American Academy of Pediatrics, and the Society for Adolescent Medicine. She is a member of the editorial board of the *American Journal of Diseases of Children.*

Richard G. MacKenzie is director of the Division of Adolescent Medicine at Childrens Hospital of Los Angeles. He is also associate professor of pediatrics and medicine at the University of Southern California. He received his B.Sc. degree (1962) from Mount Allison University, New Brunswick, Canada, in biology and his M.D. degree (1966) from McGill University. MacKenzie was named Outstanding Young Canadian in 1969. He completed his residency training in internal medicine at Royal Victoria Hospital, Montreal, and a fellowship in adolescent medicine (1971) at Childrens Hospital of Los Angeles. He assumed the directorship in 1974. He was president of the Society for Adolescent Medicine in 1979 and Wyeth Visiting Professor in Adolescent Medicine in 1988. He has provided international lectureships in Australia, China, Hong Kong, the Philippines, and Greece. He has participated in the design of communitywide systems of health care for at-risk youth. MacKenzie's research interests include substance abuse, high-risk behaviors, HIV infection in adolescents, gynecological endocrinology, and medical education.

Frank B. Miller has served as attending adult and child psychiatrist and clinical consultant and director of adolescent psychiatric services at Scottsdale Camelback Hospital, Arizona; attending adolescent psychiatrist and family therapy consulting supervisor at the Wendy Paine O'Brien Adolescent Treatment Center, Scottsdale; attending adult and child psychiatrist at Phoenix Camelback Hospital; attending physician at Scottsdale Memorial Hospital; and chairperson of the Committee on HIV Issues at the American Academy of Child and Adolescent Psychiatry. Miller received both his B.A. degree (1970) in physiological psychology and his M.D. degree (1974) from the University of Michigan, Ann Arbor.

Kimball Austin Miller is associate professor of internal medicine and pediatrics at the University of Oklahoma College of Medicine, Tulsa, where he is director of the Section of Health Care Design and the Section of Adolescent Health Care. He received his B.S. degree (1971) from Cornell University in genetics, his M.S. degree (1987) from the University of Colorado Graduate School of Business Administration in health administration, and his M.D. degree (1975) from the University of Michigan. He is a fellow of the Society for Adolescent Medicine, a fellow of the American College of Physician Executives, and a faculty associate of the American College of Healthcare Executives.

Susan G. Millstein is associate professor of pediatrics, University of California, San Francisco (UCSF). She received her B.A. degree (1974) from Northwestern University in psychology, her M.S. degree (1976) from the University of Illinois Medical Center in medical psychology, and her Ph.D. degree (1983) from UCSF in psychology. Her research has focused on health and risk-taking behaviors in adolescents. From 1987 to 1989, she served as associate director for the Carnegie Council on Adolescent Development and director of its adolescent health program.

Marilyn Moon is a senior research associate in the health policy center of the Urban Institute. She received her B.A. degree (1969) from Colorado College in economics and her M.S. (1972) and Ph.D. (1974) degrees from the University of Wisconsin, also in economics. Moon's research interests include health care financing and reimbursement reform, Medicare, and income security issues. She has also been a senior analyst at the Congressional Budget Office and the first director of the Public Policy Institute of the American Association of Retired Persons.

Allyn M. Mortimer is a program associate at the Carnegie Corporation of New York. She received her B.S. degree (1981) from the University of Maryland in geography and her M.A. degree (1984) from the Maxwell School of Citizenship and Public Affairs, Syracuse University, also in geography.

Anna-Barbara Moscicki is assistant professor of pediatrics at the University of California, San Francisco (UCSF). She received her B.S. degree (1977) from Northwestern University in medical science and her M.D. degree (1979) from Northwestern University Medical School. She finished her pediatric training at Vanderbilt Children's Hospital, Nashville, Tennessee, and an adolescent medicine fellowship at UCSF. In addition, she completed training in molecular virology at Stanford University. Moscicki's main research activities have included epidemiological work and studies in *Chlamydia trachomatis* infection and both epidemiological and basic science work in human papillomavirus infections. In 1989, Moscicki was awarded the Young Investigators Award by the Society for Adolescent Medicine for her work on the human papillomavirus.

Abigail H. Natenshon is a psychotherapist in private practice and is on the staff of Highland Park Hospital, Highland Park, Illinois. Formerly on the teaching faculty of Loyola University School of Social Work, she works with groups, families, and individuals, specializing in the treatment of eating disorders. She received her B.A. degree (1968) from Simmons College in humanities and her M.A. degree (1970) from the University of Chicago School of Social Service Administration in community organizations and clinical social work. A diplomate in social work and a member of the Academy of Certified Social Workers, she is affiliated with the National Association of Social Workers. She is a corporate consultant, has lectured widely in the Chicago area, and has published articles in local newspapers.

Lawrence S. Neinstein is associate professor of pediatrics and medicine at the University of Southern California School of Medicine and associate director of the Division of Adolescent Medicine at Childrens Hospital of Los Angeles. He received both his B.S. degree (1971) in premedical studies and his M.D. degree (1974) from the University of California, Los Angeles. Neinstein was board certified in internal medicine in 1978 and became a fellow of the American College of Physicians in 1985. His major activities have been in clinical, educational, and research areas of adolescent health care. His research interests have been mainly in the areas of reproductive health, resident education, and sexually transmitted diseases in adolescents. Neinstein has published extensively on adolescent health issues, including two books, *Adolescent Health Care: A Practical Guide* (1991, 2nd edition) and *Contraception in Chronic Illness: A Clinician's Sourcebook* (1986).

Elena O. Nightingale is special adviser to the president of the Carnegie Corporation of New York, senior program officer at the corporation, and adjunct professor of pediatrics at Georgetown University. She received her B.A. degree (1954) from Barnard College, Columbia University, in zoology, her Ph.D. degree (1961) from Rockefeller University in microbial genetics, and her M.D. degree (1964) from the New York University School of Medicine. Nightingale is a member of the Institute of Medicine, National Academy of Sciences, and is a fellow of both the American Association for the Advancement of Science and the New York Academy of Sciences.

Daniel Offer is professor of psychiatry at the Northwestern University Medical School. Offer is also the editor-in-chief of the *Journal of Youth and Adolescence*. He received his B.S. degree (1953) from the University of Rochester in general sciences and his M.D. degree (1957) from the University of Chicago. He is the 1989 recipient of the Adele Hofmann Award of the American Academy of Pediatrics.

Nancy A. Okinow is executive director of the National Center for Youth with Disabilities, a collaborative program of the Society for Adolescent Medicine and the Adolescent Health Program at the University of Minnesota. She received both her B.A. degree (1963) in sociology and her M.S.W. degree (1976) in social work administration from the University of Minnesota. Okinow's professional work has been in the area of program planning and policy development for children and youth with disabilities.

Joanne Oreskovich is a doctoral candidate in sociology at the University of Minnesota, where she is an instructor in the Sociology Department. She has done research with the Conflict and Change Center and with the Crime Control Institute in Minneapolis (1988–1990) and was a faculty member in sociology at Dawson Community College in eastern Montana (1984–1986). Oreskovich received two B.A. degrees (1980), in cell and molecular biology/premedical sciences and in sociology, and her M.A. degree (1984) in sociology from the University of Montana. Her main research interests are in the areas of crime, law, and public health and policy issues.

Eric Ostrov is a forensic psychologist in private practice and director of public safety evaluation at Isaac Ray, Inc. He was formerly a research psychologist at Michael Reese Hospital and Medical Center. He received his B.A. degree (1961) from Brooklyn College in physics, his Ph.D. degree (1974) from the University of Chicago in human development (clinical psychology), and his J.D. degree (1980) from the University of Chicago School of Law.

Carol W. Runyan is a faculty member in the School of Public Health at the University of North Carolina, Chapel Hill, where she is also director of the Injury Prevention Research Center. She received her B.A. degree (1972) from Macalester College in biology; her M.P.H. degree (1975) from the University of Minnesota in public health; and her Ph.D. degree (1983) from the University of North Carolina, Chapel Hill, School of Public Health in public health. She received postdoctoral training (1985) at the Johns Hopkins University School of Hygiene and Public Health. Runyan is an injury epidemiologist interested in the epidemiology and prevention of injuries affecting children and adolescents.

Olle Jane Z. Sahler is associate professor of pediatrics, psychiatry, medical humanities, and medical informatics at the University of Rochester School of Medicine and Dentistry. She received her B.A. degree (1966) from Radcliffe College in biochemical sciences and her M.D. degree with distinction in research (1971) from the University of Rochester. Sahler is a behavioral pediatrician with a special interest in children and adolescents with chronic and fatal illnesses. She is the editor of *The Child and Death* (1978) and the author of *The Child from Three to Eighteen* (1981, with E. R. McAnarney).

Carolyn Seymore is assistant professor of pediatrics at the Medical College of Georgia. She received her B.S. degree (1977) from the University of Georgia in biochemistry and her M.D. degree (1981) from the Medical College of Georgia. She completed her pediatric residency as well as a chief resident year at the Medical College of Georgia, and then went to Duke University Medical Center for a Robert Wood Johnson General Academic Pediatric Fellowship. Seymore's main research activities have been in adolescent health beliefs and adolescent mothers.

Mary-Ann B. Shafer is associate professor of pediatrics and associate director of the Division of Adolescent Medicine at the University of California, San Francisco (UCSF). Shafer received her B.S. degree (1969) from the University of California, Davis, in biological sciences. She received her M.D. degree (1973) from Yale University; received her pediatric training at the University of California, San Diego, and at UCSF from 1973 to 1976; and completed fellowships in adolescent medicine and the Robert Wood Johnson Clinical Scholar Program at UCSF from 1976 to 1978. She is former chair of the Section on Adolescent Health and current editor of the *Adolescent Health Update* of the American Academy of Pediatrics. Her research interests include sexually transmitted diseases of adolescents, with a specific focus on chlamydial infections and development of school-based AIDS intervention for teenagers.

Robert W. ten Bensel is professor of public health, pediatrics, and social work at the University of Minnesota. He is currently in the School of Public Health's maternal and child health major and chairs the Child Abuse Committee of the University of Minnesota Hospitals and Clinics. He received his B.A. degree (1958) from Dartmouth College in history, his M.D. degree (1961) from Harvard Medical School, and his M.P.H. degree (1974) from the University of Minnesota.

Mary E. L. Vernon is assistant professor of pediatrics at Duke University Medical Center and director of adolescent health care at Lincoln Community

Health Center in Durham, North Carolina. She received her B.S. degree
(1972) from South Carolina State College in biology and her M.D. degree
(1976) from Columbia College of Physicians and Surgeons in New York City.
She received her first residency training in pediatrics (1976–1979) and was a
Robert Wood Johnson General Academic Pediatric Fellow (1979–1981) at
Duke University Medical Center. Vernon's main research activities have been
in adolescent health issues, especially teenage pregnancy prevention. Her
experience also includes the evaluation of a health promotion program for
at-risk youth.

The Health of Adolescents

1

Sociodemographic Trends and Projections in the Adolescent Population

Susan G. Millstein, Ph.D.
Charles E. Irwin, Jr., M.D.
Claire D. Brindis, D.P.H.

Planning for adequate health services requires an understanding of the sociodemographic composition of the population to be served. Through the use of population descriptions and analyses of population trends, policy makers, planners, and health care providers have the opportunity to plan services to meet future population needs.

During the next decade and beyond, the size, composition, living conditions, and location of the adolescent population will be undergoing major changes. These changes will have a significant effect on the health status of youth and on the range and quantity of services that will be required to serve them.

In tracking sociodemographic changes in the population, we rely on a variety of indicators that are generated by both public and private sources of data. The ability of these indicators to adequately describe specific populations varies considerably. In the case of the adolescent population, currently available statistics are generally inadequate. The most significant and pervasive problem with available data sources is that they do not even consider adolescents as a separate group. In most national surveys, respondents are

Note: Susan G. Millstein was supported by the Carnegie Council on Adolescent Development during preparation of this chapter. The research was supported in part by funds from the Bureau of Maternal and Child Health and Resources Development, MCJ000978, Charles E. Irwin, principal investigator. The authors thank Elaine Vaughan and Susan Brodt for their assistance in data analysis and Paul Newacheck for his comments on the manuscript.

classified into age groups of zero to fourteen years and fifteen to twenty-four years. Thus, trends pertaining to adolescents cannot be separated from those pertaining to children and young adults. In surveys that do classify adolescents separately, there is inconsistency in the age ranges used to define adolescence. For example, some surveys define adolescence as encompassing ages ten to nineteen years, while others use the range of thirteen to nineteen years. These inconsistencies make meaningful comparisons of different data sources impossible. Unless noted otherwise, the term *adolescent* as used throughout this chapter will refer to youth from ages ten to nineteen years.

The most meaningful data sources currently available are those that separate adolescence into two periods: (1) early adolescence, ages ten to fourteen, and (2) late adolescence, ages fifteen to nineteen. These data sources provide a much richer and more accurate view of the adolescent period, since they recognize the vast developmental differences between younger and older adolescents. Although this approach is superior to others, an age classification based on biological and psychosocial development would be of even greater use. Using these parameters, adolescents might be classified into three groups: early (ages ten to thirteen), middle (ages fourteen to sixteen), and late (ages seventeen to nineteen).

Despite these limitations, there are enough data on the adolescent population to allow us to make some predictions about its present and future composition. The remainder of this chapter examines these population trends and the implications of the anticipated changes.

The Current and Future Adolescent Population

Population Overview

In 1985, there were more than 35 million adolescents between the ages of ten and nineteen years in the United States, representing approximately 14.8 percent of the U.S. population. As shown in Figure 1.1, the adolescent population is currently undergoing a decline in size, with the number of adolescents expected to hit a low of 33.8 million in 1990. By 1995, this trend is expected to reverse itself, and the adolescent population will begin to increase in size, reaching 38.5 million by the year 2000.

If we examine the anticipated changes in the adolescent population in relation to changes in other age groups, a slightly different picture emerges. While the absolute number of adolescents will increase in the early 1990s, they will represent a smaller proportion of the total U.S. population. In 1980, adolescents represented 17.3 percent of the total U.S. population; by 2000, they will represent 14.4 percent.

The reasons for these shifts in the size and proportion of the adolescent population are best understood through a description of the impact of the "baby boom" generation. Between 1945 and 1960, fertility in the United States reached an all-time high, resulting in a sizable cohort referred to as the

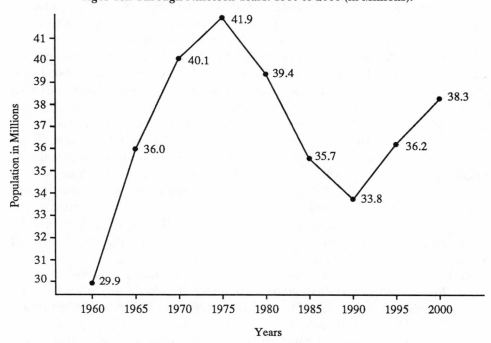

**Figure 1.1. Actual and Projected Adolescent Population,
Ages Ten Through Nineteen Years: 1960 to 2000 (in Millions).**

Note: Data from 1960 to 1985 are enumerated; data after 1985 are estimated.

baby boom generation. From a birthrate in 1940 of 2.5 million, births during
this period grew to 3.6 million in 1950, reaching a high of 4.3 million in 1957.
As this large cohort works its way through the life cycle, it creates a bulge in
the population.

Around 1958, the first of the baby boomers entered adolescence. In
1960, the number of children between the ages of ten and nineteen years
totaled 29.9 million (Figure 1.1). The adolescent population continued to
grow dramatically, reaching a high in 1975 of 41.9 million. As the last of the
baby boomers completed adolescence in the late 1970s, the population in
the ten- to nineteen-year-old group began a steady decline.

Projections for the 1990s suggest that the adolescent population will
have xit a low of 33.8 million in 1990. In the decade of 1980 to 1990, the
overall adolescent population will have decreased by 14.3 percent. By 1995,
this trend is expected to reverse itself. The adolescent population is expected
to increase by 7.3 percent, followed by an additional 5.7 percent increase
between 1995 and 2000, for a total 13.5 percent increase in the adolescent
population between 1990 and 2000. The greatest increase (16.2 percent) is
expected to occur among younger adolescents (ages ten to fourteen years).
Overall, by the year 2000, the adolescent population is expected to reach 38.5
million.

Beginning around 2010, the first of the baby boomers will reach the age of sixty-five, creating what is expected to be the largest elderly population ever. A significant proportion of the work force needed to support this large elderly population will consist of individuals now in their teens.

Age and Gender Description. Table 1.1 shows the current and expected age and gender distribution of adolescents through the year 2000. Little change is expected in the sex distribution of adolescents; decreases and increases in the size of the population will be relatively similar for both males and females. Age differences are expected, however. Expected decreases in the adolescent population between 1980 and 1990 will be much larger among older adolescents (ages fifteen to nineteen) than among younger adolescents. The older adolescent population is expected to decline by 19.8 percent, compared to a 7.9 percent decrease among younger adolescents. This shift toward a younger adolescent population will be compounded when population increases take place during the following decade. While the older adolescent population will grow at a rate of 10.8 percent, the number of younger adolescents will increase by 16.2 percent. As a result, the adolescent population in the year 2000 will be a younger one than it is today.

Racial and Ethnic Distribution. Adolescent population trends are reflective of the increasing racial and ethnic diversity in the general population of the United States, with increasing proportions of adolescents belonging to racial and ethnic minority groups (black, Asian, Hispanic, Native American). The size of the minority population (Table 1.2) is often underestimated, however, given the manner in which the U.S. Bureau of the Census (BOC) considers race and ethnicity. The BOC, which uses separate classifications

Table 1.1. Actual and Projected Age and Gender Distribution of Adolescents Ages Ten Through Nineteen Years: 1980 to 2000 (in Thousands).

	Year				
	1980	*1985*	*1990*	*1995*	*2000*
Males					
Ages 10–14	9,316	8,762	8,586	9,602	9,986
Ages 15–19	10,755	9,477	8,670	9,170	9,532
Total	20,071	18,239	17,256	18,772	19,519
Females					
Ages 10–14	8,926	8,340	8,207	9,170	9,532
Ages 15–19	10,413	9,110	8,299	8,300	9,262
Total	19,339	17,450	16,506	17,470	18,794
Both sexes					
Ages 10–14	18,242	17,102	16,793	18,772	19,518
Ages 15–19	21,168	18,587	16,969	17,470	18,794
Total	39,410	35,689	33,762	36,242	38,312

Note: Data for 1980 are enumerated; data after 1980 are projected. The data slightly underestimate the adolescent population, since members of the armed forces serving overseas are not included.

**Table 1.2. Racial and Ethnic Distribution of Adolescents
Ages Ten Through Nineteen: 1980 to 2000 (in Thousands).**

			Year		
Race-Ethnicity	*1980*	*1985*	*1990*	*1995*	*2000*
White	32,776	29,051	27,528	28,803	30,701
Black	5,698	5,442	5,055	5,625	6,361
Hispanic [a]	3,081	3,217	3,449	3,945	4,566

[a] Hispanics may be of any race.

for race and ethnicity, classifies individuals as belonging to one of three racial groups: black, white, or other. People of Hispanic origin may be classified in any one of the three racial groups but are usually classified as white. Estimates based on these classifications thus fail to disaggregate Hispanics and overestimate the size of the white population. However, because the percentage of Hispanics classified in each of the three racial groups is known, it is possible to adjust the estimates so that they more accurately represent the size of the minority population.

Using these adjusted figures, it is estimated that by the year 2000, 30.9 percent of the adolescent population will belong to a racial or ethnic minority group (Figure 1.2). Approximately 11.9 percent of the adolescent population will be of Hispanic origin by the year 2000. Between 1985 and 2000, this group will increase by 41.9 percent, making it the most rapidly increasing ethnic group. Larger increases will occur in geographical areas that currently have a high concentration of Hispanics. In states such as California, it is expected that Hispanic children will represent 35 percent of the school-age population by the year 2000.

Another rapidly growing minority group is Asians, primarily because of high net immigration rates. Asians currently represent 44 percent of the immigration into the United States. Between 1970 and 1980, the proportion of Asian and Pacific Island adolescents in the U.S. population doubled, to 1.5 percent. As with the Hispanic population, a large proportion of Asian youth will reside in western states. By the year 2000, it is estimated that 11 percent of all school-age children will be of Asian or Pacific Island descent.

In contrast to the steady growth of the Hispanic and Asian adolescent populations, whites and blacks will show alternating periods of growth and decline. Population declines will have taken place in both groups between 1985 and 1990, shifting to growth periods from 1990 to 2000. Although the absolute number of black adolescents will increase by 16.9 percent during this period, their rates of growth will be smaller than those of Hispanic and Asian youth. Blacks will thus represent a slightly smaller proportion of the adolescent minority population, declining from 55 percent in 1985 to 52 percent in 2000.

Figure 1.2. Racial and Ethnic Distribution of Adolescents: 1985 and 2000.

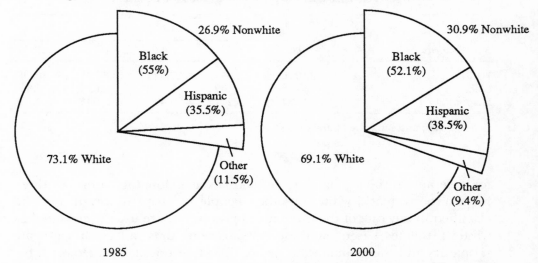

1985   2000

Note: Percentages in parentheses represent proportions within the nonwhite population.

Location of the Future Adolescent Population

Geographical Region. Increases in the adolescent population will not occur equally across all geographical areas. As shown in Table 1.3, portions of the South and West will experience population increases, while other regions, primarily the East, will experience decreases. Three Public Health Regions will experience population growth of 20 percent or more between 1980 and 2000: Region VI (Arkansas, Louisiana, New Mexico, Oklahoma, Texas); Region IX (California, Arizona, Hawaii, Nevada); and Region X (Alaska, Idaho, Oregon, Washington). Regions that will experience declines of more than 20 percent in their adolescent population between 1980 and 2000 include Region I (Connecticut, Maine, Massachusetts, New Hampshire, Rhode Island, Vermont) and Region III (Delaware, District of Columbia, Maryland, Pennsylvania, Virginia, West Virginia).

These data show shifts in the overall proportion of adolescents in different geographical areas but do not highlight how population changes in different racial and ethnic groups will affect growth in selected parts of the country. In California, for example, the proportion of school-age children who belong to minority groups rose from 27 percent in 1970 to about 43 percent in 1980. By 1990, minority students represent the majority in California schools.

Among Hispanics, the largest growth in the adolescent population is expected to occur in a few states, including California, New York, and Texas. Approximately two-thirds of Hispanic youth will reside in these three states. Asian youth will show less geographical concentration than Hispanic youth;

Table 1.3. Geographic Distribution of Adolescents Ages Ten Through Nineteen by Public Health Regions: 1980 and 2000 (in Thousands).

Public Health Region	Year		Percentage Change
	1980	2000	
I	2,178.5	1,650.5	− 24.2
II	3,744.7	3,045.7	− 18.7
III	4,251.5	3,357.1	− 21.0
IV	6,772.7	7,074.5	+ 4.5
V	8,157.3	6,794.3	− 16.7
VI	4,485.0	5,509.2	+ 22.8
VII	2,014.0	1,845.4	− 8.4
VIII	1,214.2	1,765.0	+ 4.5
IX	4,691.1	5,647.2	+ 20.4
X	1,290.7	1,604.6	+ 24.3

Note: The Public Health Regions are as follows: 1—Connecticut, Maine, Massachusetts, New Hampshire, Rhode Island, Vermont; II—New Jersey, New York; III—Delaware, District of Columbia, Maryland, Pennsylvania, Virginia, West Virginia; IV—Alabama, Florida, Georgia, Kentucky, Mississippi, North Carolina, South Carolina, Tennessee; V—Illinois, Indiana, Michigan, Minnesota, Ohio, Wisconsin; VI—Arkansas, Louisiana, New Mexico, Oklahoma, Texas; VII—Iowa, Kansas, Missouri, Nebraska; VIII—Colorado, Montana, North Dakota, South Dakota, Utah, Wyoming; IX—Arizona, California, Hawaii, Nevada; X—Alaska, Idaho, Oregon, Washington.

however, more than 50 percent of Asian youth will live in western states, primarily California and Hawaii.

Metropolitan and Nonmetropolitan Areas. In 1980, more than two-thirds of American youth (ages fifteen to twenty-four years) were residing in metropolitan areas. A geographic area is considered a Metropolitan Statistical Area (MSA) if it includes a city of at least fifty thousand population, or if it includes a Census Bureau–defined urbanized area of at least fifty thousand with a total population area of at least one hundred thousand (seventy-five thousand in New England). Twenty-eight percent were living in large central cities. (A central city is the largest city within any given Metropolitan Statistical Area.) The trend toward living in metropolitan areas is especially evident among youth belonging to racial and ethnic minority groups. In large cities such as Los Angeles, Chicago, Baltimore, and Detroit, more than 75 percent of the adolescents are of minority backgrounds. Black adolescents are most likely to be living in these high-population-density areas. In 1980, 56 percent of black youth (ages fifteen to twenty-four) lived in central cities, compared with 23 percent of white youth.

The number of adolescents living in large central cities is expected to grow during the next decade, especially among minority youth. It is estimated that approximately two-thirds of Hispanic youth will reside in large central cities in California, Texas, and New York. More than half of Asian youth will reside in large central cities as well.

Table 1.4. Percentage of Children Ages Eighteen Years
and Younger Living Below Poverty Level: 1975 and 1985.

	Year		Percentage Change
	1975	1985	
Overall	16.8	20.1	+ 19.6
Black	41.4	43.1	+ 4.1
White[a]	12.5	15.6	+ 24.8
Hispanic	33.1	39.6	+ 19.6
Other[b]	20.0	26.0	+ 30.0

Note: The poverty level in 1975 for a family of four was a yearly income of $5,500 or less. In 1985, the poverty level was $10,989.

[a] Includes Hispanics. If Hispanics are excluded, the percentage for whites in 1985 is closer to 12.1 percent.

[b] Includes Native Americans and Asian/Pacific Islanders.

Economic Status

The proportion of children and adolescents who are being raised in poverty is increasing, especially within the Hispanic population (Table 1.4). In 1975, 16.8 percent of all children under the age of eighteen years were living in households that reported income below the poverty level. By 1985, the percentage of children living in poverty grew to 20.1 percent, with the highest rates among blacks and Hispanics. It is estimated that there will be more than twenty million children living in poverty by the year 2020, an increase of about 37 percent since 1985.

Clearly, not all of the nation's poor children are adolescents. It is estimated that among the approximately seven million children receiving benefits from Aid to Families with Dependent Children (AFDC), 34 percent are adolescents (Table 1.5). A comparison of AFDC recipients shows higher rates among younger children: 11.4 percent of all children (age eighteen and younger) receive benefits, compared with 6.7 percent of adolescents. This difference may reflect the greater likelihood of labor force participation among mothers of older children.

The increasing overall number of poor children can be attributed in part to the significant increase in the percentage of Hispanic children who are living in poverty, from 33 percent in 1975 to almost 40 percent in 1985. Poverty in the Hispanic population varies as a function of specific national origin: 42 percent of Hispanics from Puerto Rico were living in poverty in 1985, compared to 24 percent of Mexicans and Central and South Americans, and 13 percent of Cubans. This increase in poverty is taking place among the fastest-growing population group and will therefore be associated with greater overall levels of poverty among youth in the future.

Family Structure and Living Conditions

Youth in Single-Parent Households. At one time, it was the norm for children to be raised in homes in which both parents were present. However,

Table 1.5. Children and Adolescents Receiving Aid to Families with Dependent Children (AFDC): 1985 (in Thousands).

	Number Receiving AFDC
All children (ages 0–17)	7,050
Black	2,954
White	2,439
Hispanic	1,022
Asian	204
Native American	78
Unknown	353
All adolescents (ages 10–18)	2,404
Younger (ages 10–14)	1,593
Older (ages 15–18)	811

with significant increases in the divorce rate (115 percent increase between 1965 and 1980) and in the number of children born to unmarried women (11 percent in 1970; 17 percent in 1985), this family constellation represents a much smaller percentage of American families today. Between 1970 and 1980, the percentage of family groups with children under the age of eighteen years that were characterized as single-parent families nearly doubled, to 19.5 percent. By 1985, the percentage grew to 26.1 percent.

Although decreases in the proportion of families classified as intact have occurred equally across racial and ethnic groups, the actual proportions differ significantly (Figure 1.3). In 1985, 80 percent of white children were living with both parents, compared with 67.8 percent of Hispanic children and 39.5 percent of black children. Among black children, the intact, two-parent family has become the exception; a majority of black children are raised by mothers alone.

One of the most significant consequences of being raised in a single-parent household is the economic impact. Children from these families are far more likely to be raised in poverty than are children from homes in which both parents are present. In 1985, for example, 20.1 percent of children (eighteen years of age or younger) were raised in poverty. Among children from single-parent, female-headed households, the percentage was 53.6 percent, more than twice the overall rate.

The negative economic consequences of single-parent families are particularly severe for minorities (Table 1.6). Among children being raised in single-parent families headed by Hispanic females, 72.5 percent were living in poverty; among those with black female heads of household, the percentage was 66.9 percent; and among those headed by non-Hispanic whites, it was 37.0 percent. Blacks living in nonmetropolitan areas fare even worse. Seventy-five percent of black single-parent families residing in nonmetropolitan areas live below the poverty line.

"Latchkey Children." In 1955, about 60 percent of the households in the

Figure 1.3. Percentage of White, Black, and Hispanic Children Under Eighteen Years of Age Living in Intact and Single-Parent Families.

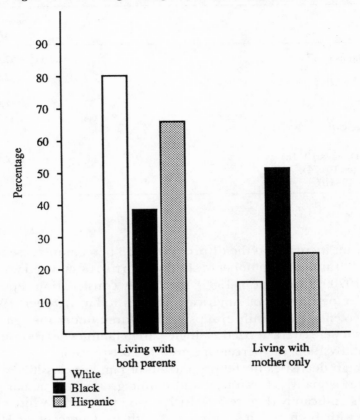

Table 1.6. Percentage of Children Ages Seventeen Years and Younger in Single-Parent Families Living Below Poverty Level, by Race and Ethnicity: 1985.

	Percentage Below Poverty Level
All single-parent families (female head)	53.6
Black	66.9
White	45.2
Hispanic[a]	72.5
Non-Hispanic white	37.0
Other	52.4

Note: The poverty level in 1975 for a family of four was a yearly income of $5,500 or less. In 1985, the poverty level was $10,989.

[a] Hispanics may be of any race.

United States consisted of a working father, a housewife mother, and two or more school-age children. In 1980, that description fit 11 percent of U.S. homes, and in 1985 only 7 percent. By mid 1985, nearly 70 percent of mothers with children between the ages of six and seventeen years were in the labor force, leaving three-quarters of the thirteen- to fourteen-year-old children in the United States in self-care or with a younger sibling for more than ten hours a week. Given the expected increase in the number of single-parent families, we can also expect the number of latchkey children to increase as these single parents enter the labor force.

Youth in Independent Living Situations. While most adolescents live in related family units, some do not. In 1985, 3.2 percent of adolescents between the ages of fifteen and nineteen years were married and living with their spouses, 2.8 percent were living with unrelated individuals, and 0.7 percent were living alone. Two important categories of youth who do not live in related family units are those who are incarcerated and those in the military.

Approximately 500,000 youth under the age of twenty-two are placed in correctional institutions each year. On any given day, almost 50,000 youth are in detention. Almost 13,500 nonoffenders are held in juvenile custody facilities. Most juveniles held in custody are male (87 percent), white (57 percent), and between the ages of fourteen and seventeen years (81 percent). Racial and ethnic minorities are overrepresented. Black youth between the ages of fifteen and nineteen years are four times as likely as white youth to be placed in correctional institutions. The proportion of juveniles placed in custody has been rising, from a rate of 167 per 100,000 juveniles in 1979 to a rate of 185 per 100,000 in 1985. It is likely that these rates will continue to increase, given the large numbers of adolescents who will live in poor, metropolitan areas who have limited educational and employment opportunities.

Military service among youth is primarily a male experience: 90 percent of the youth who serve in the armed forces are males. The military is also young; 55 percent are between the ages of sixteen and twenty-four. Black youth are more likely to serve than white youth; among sixteen- to twenty-four-year-old males, 6.8 percent of blacks and 4.9 percent of whites are in military service.

Educational Patterns

Nationally, 30 percent of primary and secondary school students in the United States are considered to be educationally at risk. Educationally at-risk students include those youth who are members of ethnic and racial minority groups, immigrants, non-English-speaking, and economically disadvantaged. In some major cities, the percentage of educationally at-risk youth exceeds 80 percent.

Enrollment Patterns. Nationally, almost three out of ten students who enter high school leave before graduation. Each year, approximately 700,000 students drop out of school. Youth who drop out of school severely limit their chances for success in the labor market, experience higher rates of unemployment, have lower earnings, and often require public assistance. School dropouts also experience poorer health than individuals who finish school.

A variety of methods of calculating the dropout rate exists. The Bureau of the Census computes the dropout rate as the proportion of a given age cohort that is not enrolled in school and has not completed high school. In contrast, the High School and Beyond Survey, conducted by the United States Department of Education, considers the dropout rate to be the proportion of high school sophomores who fail to graduate within the following two-year period.

Irrespective of how one defines dropouts, the highest rates are among minority youth, poor youth, and youth residing in inner cities, western states, and southern states. Conservative estimates of the dropout rate, according to data from the High School and Beyond Survey, are 29 percent among Native Americans, 18 percent among blacks, 17 percent among Hispanics, 12 percent among whites, and 3 percent among Asians. Analyses of the dropout rate that consider wider time spans show the rate to be 35 percent among Hispanic youth, 24 percent among blacks, and 18 percent among whites. Differences exist within subgroups of the Hispanic population; there are higher dropout rates in the Cuban and Mexican American subgroups.

Regardless of race or ethnicity, students from poor families are more likely to drop out of school than are youth from more affluent backgrounds. Poverty appears to be a more significant predictor of school dropout than race or ethnicity. A 1985 comparison of dropout rates among poor eighteen- to twenty-one-year-olds showed that 56 percent of the poor black youth and 53 percent of the poor white youth failed to graduate.

Educational Achievement. Children who do poorly in school are most likely to drop out, and it has been estimated that 1.4 million students are enrolled two or more years below their expected grade level. Poor children and those from minority backgrounds enter school with significantly lower achievement scores than their more advantaged peers. This gap widens as they progress through school. School delay among Hispanics is especially high: 10 percent of Hispanic children between the ages of eight and thirteen and 25 percent of those between fourteen and twenty are held back in school. Language difficulties among non-English-speaking Hispanics are a likely contributor to these delays.

At the same time, the number of youth enrolling in college has never been higher. In 1985, 58 percent of high school graduates enrolled in postsecondary programs. Hispanics enroll at approximately half the rates for whites. Blacks fall in between. While rates of college enrollment for black and white high school graduates were nearly equal in 1977, the gap is widening, and blacks are currently enrolling at lower rates than whites.

Youth Employment

Youth unemployment has risen over the past thirty-five years. Between 1950 and 1980, the unemployment rate for sixteen- to nineteen-year-olds increased from 12.2 percent to 17.8 percent, compared to rates among adults of 4.4 percent to 5.1 percent. Black adolescent unemployment is highest, almost 40 percent in 1984. It is anticipated that unemployment rates will rise as the proportion of available jobs for unskilled labor decreases.

Discussion and Projections

Over the next decade and beyond, the size, composition, location, living conditions, and skills of the adolescent population will undergo major changes. Compared with adolescents of today, the youth of tomorrow will include greater numbers of poorly educated, non-English-speaking adolescents living in impoverished metropolitan areas. There will be greater numbers of youth who belong to racial and ethnic minority groups, and more of them will have been raised in poverty by a single parent. Overall, more than 25 percent of adolescents over the next decade will have been raised by a single parent, usually the mother. Fewer than 10 percent of adolescents will have been raised in households that were once considered the norm, with a working father, a housewife mother, and two or more school-age children.

These changes in the characteristics of the adolescent population have significant implications for a variety of societal institutions and for how society will function in general. Among the most serious implications are those that deal with projections for the work force. The work force that will bring us into the twenty-first century will be largely composed of today's youth, who will be expected to support the largest elderly population ever. By 2030, the proportion of Americans over the age of sixty-five years will have doubled, and each worker in the labor pool will be supporting three retirees. There are legitimate concerns regarding the ability of tomorrow's youth to contribute this support.

Although the jobs of the future will require more skill than those of today, the population entering the labor market will be less educated. The U.S. Bureau of Labor Statistics estimates that for the most skilled occupations (executive, professional, and technical jobs), the next decade will bring an increase of 6.2 million jobs. In comparison, unskilled jobs are expected to rise by only 1.2 million. Clearly, the pool of jobs for the most disadvantaged is shrinking at the same time as their numbers are increasing.

This picture of increasing numbers of unskilled individuals in a highly skilled labor market will have a major impact on the quality of the labor force. Employers will suffer diminished productivity, higher training costs, and competitive disadvantages in comparison with other nations. A decline in the functional work force will erode tax revenues and place greater pressures on the middle class to pay for welfare, as well as generating rising costs in the criminal justice system as young people take their business from the workplace to the streets. Further friction in the form of intergenerational conflict may also emerge as a result of diminished resources for youth compared to the large aging population.

The changing sociodemographic profile of youth also has significant implications for the health care systems, including differences in the health status of adolescents, the type of health problems that they experience, and the services that are available to meet their needs.

Although the number of adolescents will diminish, it is likely that their health care needs will actually increase, primarily as a result of the changes in their economic conditions. The well-documented association between poverty and health status suggests that these youth are likely to have high rates of unmet medical needs, poorer general health status, and more chronic limitations on activity levels. Limitations in the services available to adolescents may even exceed those of today, if earlier decreases in population result in decreases in available services. Alternatively, if we take seriously these projections, we have a real opportunity to address the health problems of youth, since their absolute numbers are decreasing.

Changes in the causes of morbidity and mortality may also occur. The large numbers of adolescents living in large metropolitan cities are likely to result in increasing rates of violence against and between youth. Suicide rates, which are associated with poverty, may also increase. The higher rates of poverty may also generate higher rates of alcoholism, other forms of substance abuse, and premature sexuality.

The changing sociodemographic composition of the adolescent population clearly has crucial implications for future generations and for American society. The discouraging nature of these projections should not, however, lead one to believe that they are inevitable. To the degree that we take these population projections seriously, we have an opportunity to plan now for the future and to develop and implement policies and programs to address the problems that are likely to occur. An investment in youth is the first step toward these solutions.

Suggested Readings

Commission on Minority Participation in Education and American Life. *One-Third of a Nation.* Washington, D.C.: American Council on Education, Education Commission of the States, 1988.

Irwin, C. E. Jr., Brindis, C. D., Brodt, S. E., Bennett, T. A., and Rodriguez, R. Q. *The Health of America's Youth: A Prelude to Action.* Rockville, MD: Bureau of Maternal and Child Health and Resources Development, Public Health Service, in press.

U.S. Congress, House Select Committee on Children, Youth, and Families. *U.S. Children and Their Families: Current Conditions and Recent Trends.* 100th Congress, 1st Sess., 1987.

U.S. Department of Commerce, Bureau of the Census. *Statistical Abstract of the United States*. Washington, D.C.: U.S. Government Printing Office, 1986.

Wagenaar, T. C. "What Do We Know About Dropping Out of High School?" *Research in the Sociology of Education and Socialization*, 1987, 7, 161–190.

Wetzel, J. R. *American Youth: A Statistical Snapshot*. Washington, D.C.: William T. Grant Foundation Commission on Work, Family, and Citizenship, 1987.

Part One

Normal Adolescent Growth and Development

PART EDITOR
Elizabeth R. McAnarney, M.D.

Introduction

Elizabeth R. McAnarney, M.D.

The second decade of life brings rapid physical and psychological growth and development. Major physical changes include both somatic and sexual growth. Rapid physical growth occurs under the influence of hormonal regulatory systems in the hypothalamus, pituitary gland, gonads, and adrenal glands. Despite identification of these specific hormonal changes, we still do not understand the exact signals that trigger puberty in individuals. There are also wide variations in the time of onset, time of completion, magnitude, and velocity of pubertal changes.

Chapter Two reviews the development of endocrine regulatory mechanisms related to puberty and includes the newest information on the hypothalamic control of physical development. The authors discuss the maturation of the gonads and adrenal glands as target endocrine organs and also focus on somatic growth. The sequence of pubertal growth and the orderly appearance of sexual changes in both females and males are then reviewed. Finally, questions are raised for future research.

In Chapter Three, the authors discuss psychosocial development during adolescence, a topic equally as dramatic as adolescent physical development. Most young people acquire formal operational thinking (the ability to use abstract thinking) during adolescence. Their understanding of themselves and others deepens so that their world moves beyond a narcissistic adolescent focus to other people, at both a personal and a societal level.

No single psychological theory provides a sufficient construct for considering adolescence; hence, the authors of Chapter Three review psychosexual theory (Sigmund Freud), psychosocial theory (Erik Erikson), cognitive intellectual theory (Jean Piaget), and learning theory. These theories provide a broad view of the dramatic psychological changes that occur during adolescence. The authors then discuss the three substages of adolescence: early, middle, and late adolescence. These substages help clinicians to evaluate whether individual adolescents are functioning at a developmentally age-appropriate level.

Chapter Three closes with a discussion of clinical considerations in the application of psychological developmental theory. The example of risk taking as a clinical problem is timely, as many problem adolescent behaviors, such as experimentation with cigarette smoking, alcohol ingestion, drug use, sexuality, and driving, have common origins in the risk-taking behavior of young people.

In the future, we expect to know more about the relationships of biology and behavior during the adolescent years. New studies are focusing on hormonal changes and adolescent sexual behavior; new technologies, particularly in neurobiology, will provide unprecedented opportunities to study brain function and cognitive change during adolescence. We look forward to improved understanding of the relationships of rapid biological and psychosocial changes during adolescence.

2

Physical Growth and Development in Normal Adolescents

Richard E. Kreipe, M.D.
Olle Jane Z. Sahler, M.D.

Although they are often used synonymously, there is a distinction between the terms *adolescence* and *puberty*. *Adolescence* refers to the psychosocial transition from childhood to adulthood. The maturational process is influenced by cultural views, ethnic background, religious beliefs, moral values, familial organization, geographical location, political climate, and economic status. The nature of adolescence changes from one historical era to the next. Like puberty, it is a dynamic process, but, unlike puberty, it is highly contextual. Adolescence tends to be determined by a number of factors extrinsic to the individual; the way it is expressed cannot be as easily predicted as can be puberty. Chapter Three addresses specific psychosocial issues related to adolescence.

Puberty, on the other hand, is the dynamic biological process that ultimately results in manhood or womanhood. Determined by highly ordered mechanisms that are intrinsic to each human organism, puberty proceeds with predictable regularity in every normal boy and girl. Many chronic illnesses are associated with delayed puberty, and a few medical conditions are associated with precocious puberty. Related primarily to the acquisition of reproductive function, puberty results in numerous changes in physical appearance, body composition, and biochemical regulation. This chapter focuses on the physical changes of puberty that constitute the normal changes of adolescent physical growth and development.

Several features characterize the physical growth and development of puberty. First, change is the most constant trait of this process. Hormonal regulatory systems in the hypothalamus, pituitary, gonads, and adrenal glands undergo major qualitative and quantitative transformations from their prepubertal state. The maturation of these systems results in an internal milieu that is different from that of either the child or the adult. These changes ultimately result in the production of viable eggs and sperm (primary sex characteristics). In addition, the rapid growth in height and weight as well as the acquisition of secondary sex characteristics result in the metamorphosis of a boy into a man and a girl into a woman.

Second, timing of onset and completion, velocity, and magnitude of the expected physical changes of puberty vary widely between females and males and from person to person. Tanner notes that "the one generalization about puberty that one can make without fear of contradiction is that it is variable in every possible manner between individuals." Such variability makes it difficult to define the limits of normality for various pubertal events. Even models describing "normal" populations cannot define these limits with certainty; many adolescents who fall above or below the third percentile for a given characteristic are, in all respects, normal.

Third, "sequencing" is a characteristic of growth and development that emphasizes the orderliness of the pubertal process. Although the timing of the various events of puberty varies greatly among individuals, the sequence of the events themselves is serially ordered. So predictable is the order of events that deviation from the expected sequence often raises the possibility of unrecognized pathology. In males, for example, penile enlargement and peak height velocity are responses to androgens (male hormones) rising from the developing testes; testicular enlargement precedes these two events by one year and two-and-a-half years, respectively. If an adolescent male undergoes peak height velocity and penile enlargement before enlargement of the testes, another source of androgen, such as the adrenal gland or exogenous anabolic steroids, must be sought.

Fourth, the emergence of the secondary sex characteristics can be grouped into a series of stages and rated. Such rating of sexual maturation has been most extensively described by Tanner, and the five stages of physical development from prepubertal (sexual maturity rating [SMR1]) to adult (SMR 5) have been aptly termed the "Tanner stages." Because they relate to pubertal development, sexual maturity ratings correlate more closely with physical maturity than with chronological age. Sexual maturity ratings also relate to the appearance of medical conditions such as acne, gynecomastia, scoliosis, and slipped capital femoral epiphysis, as well as elevation of serum alkaline phosphatase in both sexes and hemoglobin in males (Table 2.1). Thus, the SMR is a more clinically relevant variable than is chronological age.

A fifth important feature of adolescent growth and development is the change that has occurred over the last century in the age and size of individuals undergoing puberty. Youth now attain greater stature and body weight and experience puberty earlier than they did before the Industrial Revolution (Figure 2.1). This "secular trend" toward earlier and greater growth has occurred worldwide in industrialized countries and has recently

Table 2.1. Relationships Between Clinical Conditions and Sexual Maturity Ratings.

Clinical Condition	SMR
Hematocrit rise (male)	2–5
Alkaline phosphatase peak (male)	3
Alkaline phosphatase peak (female)	2
Adolescent hormonal levels (rise in estrogen for females, testosterone for males)	2–5
Peak height velocity (male)	3–4
Peak height velocity (female)	2–3
Short male with growth potential	2
Short male with limited growth potential	4–5
Usual timing of menarche	Late 3 or early 4
Appearance of menarche	1 to 3.6 years post-stage 2
Slipped capital femoral epiphysis	(obese) 2 or 3
Acute worsening of idiopathic adolescent scoliosis (time for close monitoring)	2–4
Osgood-Sclatter disease	3
Oral contraceptive prescription	4
Diaphragm prescription	4–5
Observe for worsening of straight-back syndrome	2–4
Appearance of "normal" gynecomastia	2 or 3
Usual appearance of acne vulgaris	2 or 3
Gonococcal vaginitis	1
Gonococcal cervicitis (with or without pelvic inflammatory disease)	2 +
Timing of orchiopexy	1
Decreased incidence in serous otitis media	2 or 3
Mild regression with virginal hypertrophy	5
Timing of breast reduction	5
Timing of rhinoplasty	5
Strong suspicion for organic disease	2–5 (abnormal progression or regression)
Counseling for further breast growth	2
Increase levels of serum uric acid in males	2–5

Prepared by D. E. Greydanus, M.D.

Source: Reproduced with permission from W. A. Daniel, "Growth at Adolescence: Clinical Correlates." *Seminars in Adolescent Medicine*, 1985, *1*, 15–24.

become evident in some developing countries as well. It is generally believed that this trend is the result of improved nutrition and living conditions. Over the last two decades, this trend has plateaued in most of North America and Europe. However, because the real cause of this trend is unknown, it is impossible to determine whether the recent leveling will be permanent.

Because normal puberty depends on a series of finely controlled changes directed toward gonadal development, the maturation of the endocrine regulatory systems that are related to puberty is addressed first in this chapter. Analysis of the mechanisms that control gonadal and adrenal function and growth in height and weight requires attention to the distinct contributions made by the hypothalamus, the anterior pituitary, the target organs, and the end organs.

Figure 2.1. Secular Trend in Stature, Weight, and Age at Menarche.

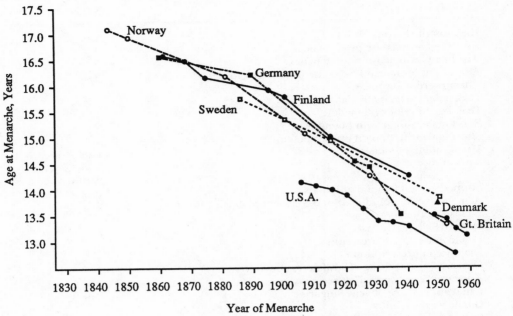

Source: Adapted with permission from J. M. Tanner and F. Falkner, *Human Growth: A Comprehensive Treatise.* (2nd ed.) New York: Plenum, 1986, p. 196.

There are certain characteristics of the biological changes (such as growth of the skeleton, muscles, and fat, gain in weight, and biochemical alterations) occurring during puberty that are common to females and males. Common concerns of pubertal adolescents and normal variants also are addressed. The chapter closes with a discussion of unanswered questions.

Development of Endocrine Regulatory Mechanisms Related to Puberty

Hypothalamus

Hypothalamic Control of Gonadal Development. Control over the majority of events constituting puberty resides primarily in the hypothalamus. Although the signal that initiates puberty has yet to be identified definitively, much has been learned in the last two decades about the role that the hypothalamus plays in the overall orchestration of this complex process. The hypothalamus exerts control by secreting substances that either promote or inhibit the release of hormones from the pituitary gland.

Hypothalamic control over gonadal function during fetal life and early infancy is similar to that during adulthood, with the hypothalamus producing relatively large amounts of gonadotropin releasing hormone (GnRH)—also known as luteinizing hormone releasing hormone (LHRH), luteinizing hormone releasing factor (LHRF), or luteinizing releasing factor (LRF)—as a result of relative insensitivity to negative feedback from sex steroids. However, at about six months of age in the male and one to two years of age in the female, the concentration of GnRH decreases to a low level and remains there throughout childhood. Hypothalamic secretion of GnRH during childhood is restrained by an exquisitely sensitive negative feedback mechanism in which there is a reciprocal relationship between the levels of sex steroid and GnRH. In the prepubertal period, minute amounts of estrogen or testosterone are able to inhibit GnRH release from the hypothalamus by inhibiting the "gonadostat" that controls GnRH release.

In addition to hypothalamic control, extrahypothalamic central nervous system (CNS) centers also inhibit GnRH secretion. Dopaminergic, catecholaminergic, and opioid neuronal networks and nonsteroidal regulators of secretion of follicle stimulating hormone (FSH) produced by germinal tissue ("inhibins") also appear to inhibit the tonic release of GnRH. Thus, suppression of gonadotropin levels during mid-childhood occurs even in individuals without gonads (for example, those with Turner's syndrome). As a result of these two separate inhibitory mechanisms—one mediated by sex steroid negative feedback and one mediated by intrinsic CNS control—levels of both gonadotropins and sex steroids remain low, and the individual remains sexually immature during childhood.

As puberty begins, the hypothalamic gonadostat (Figure 2.2) becomes decreasingly sensitive to negative feedback, resulting in a reactivation of GnRH release. In response to neural signals that initiate puberty, the terminal axons of neurosecretory peptidergic neurons in the arcuate nucleus of the medial basal hypothalamus synthesize and release increasing amounts of GnRH into the primary plexus of the hypothalamic-hypophyseal portal circulation. GnRH is then carried directly to the gonadotroph cells in the lateral portion of the anterior pituitary, which respond by releasing glycoprotein hormones—luteinizing hormone (LH) and follicle stimulating hormone.

In addition to the increased tonic secretion permitted by a weakening negative feedback system that is estimated to be six to fifteen times less sensitive in late adolescence than in prepuberty, there are also positive feedback impulses, mediated by CNS influences, that stimulate the intermittent release of pulses of GnRH in a periodic fashion. The response of the anterior pituitary to these pulsations depends on their amplitude as well as their frequency. Evidence of these pulses of GnRH release must be inferred from measurements of LH and FSH levels rather than from direct measurement of GnRH itself, because GnRH has an extremely short half-life and does not enter the peripheral circulation; therefore, it cannot be measured in the urine or peripheral blood. LH and FSH, on the other hand, have half-lives of approximately one and six hours, respectively, and must be released into the peripheral circulation in order to act on the gonads. Thus, serum levels of LH

Figure 2.2. Changes in Sensitivity of the Hypothalamic Gonadostat.

Gonadal steroids	— Low —	— Unchanged —	— Adult level
Feedback	Operative and sensitive	Decreasing in sensitivity	Operative at adult level
Gonadotropins	— Low —	— Increasing —	— Adult level

Pre Puberty   Initiation of Puberty   Adult

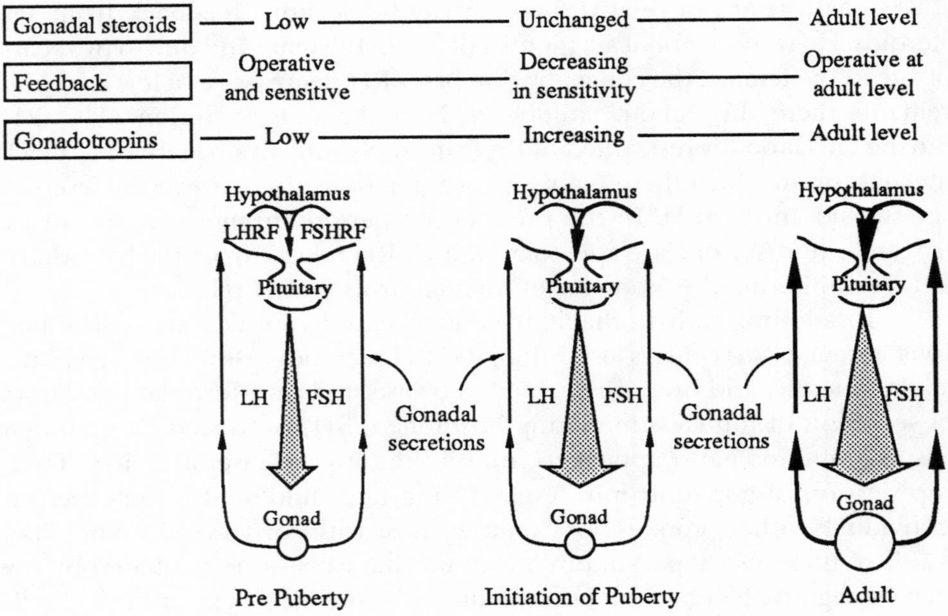

Note: A schematic diagram of the changes in sensitivity of the hypothalamic gonadostat. In the prepubertal state the concentration of sex steroids and gonadotropins is low; the hypothalamic "gonadostat" is functional but highly sensitive to low levels of sex steroids. With the onset of puberty there are decreased sensitivity of the hypothalamus to negative feedback by sex steroids, increased release of LRF, and enhanced secretion of gonadotropins. In the negative feedback mechanism the hypothalamus is less sensitive to feedback by sex steroids (adult set point) and adult levels of gonadotropins and sex steroids are present.

Source: Reproduced with permission from M. M. Grumbach, J. C. Roth, S. L. Kaplan, and R. P. Kelch, "Hypothalamic-Pituitary Regulation of Puberty in Man: Evidence and Concepts Derived from Clinical Research." In M. M. Grumbach, G. D. Grave, and F. F. Mayer (eds.), *Control of the Onset of Puberty.* New York: Wiley, 1974, p. 128. ·

and FSH can be measured, and from these data, inferences can be made about GnRH pulsation.

By measuring LH levels every twenty minutes over a twenty-four-hour period, Boyar and colleagues found that once sexual maturation has been initiated, a definite and progressive pattern of pulsatile GnRH release occurs over the course of puberty for both boys and girls (Figure 2.3). FSH levels do not show such episodic variation. Whereas prepubertal children have relatively static, low levels of LH, the mean LH level in early puberty remains low during wakefulness but becomes moderately elevated during sleep; wide variations indicate the beginning of pulsatile GnRH release. Such augmentation of LH is truly related to sleep rather than to the time of day or night; in fact, it is most closely related to non-random-eye-movement sleep and disappears on awakening. Sleep augmentation of LH is considered an early marker of pubertal maturation.

Figure 2.3. Sleep Augmentation of LH Secretion During Early Puberty.

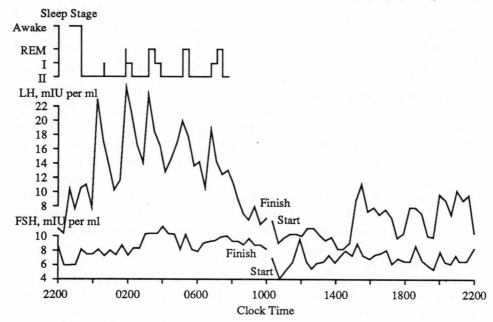

Note: Plasma LH and FSH concentrations sampled every twenty minutes for twenty-four hours in a normal thirteen-year-old pubertal girl.

A sleep histogram is shown above the period of nocturnal sleep. Sleep stages are awake, and REM (rapid eye movement) = ————, stages 1–4 by the depth of line graph.

Source: Reproduced with permission from R. Boyar and others, "Twenty-Four Hour Patterns of Plasma Luteinizing Hormone Secretion with Sleep During Puberty." *New England Journal of Medicine*, 1972, *289*, 282–286.

In mid-puberty, the mean waking LH concentration rises and the frequency and amplitude of LH pulses during sleep become more marked. Later in puberty, the pulsatile pattern, which had been present only during sleep, also occurs while awake. As hypothalamic maturation approaches completion (SMR 3–4), a pattern of intermittent LH secretion without sleep augmentation becomes apparent. Because these pulses of LH occur every 90 to 120 minutes throughout the day and night, there is no recognizable baseline level of LH by late puberty. There can be a twofold difference between the nadir and apex of normal LH concentrations in a given individual (from 100 picograms [pg] per milliliter to more than 200 picograms per milliliter). This results in a mean concentration of LH that is several times higher than that found in prepuberty.

A third pattern of GnRH secretion, related to the menstrual cycle, occurs in females from mid-puberty to the menopause. This cyclical pattern of positive feedback involves estrogenic stimulation of GnRH release, with a subsequent surge of LH and FSH, during the latter part of each follicular phase. For this pattern to develop, females must possess ovarian follicles capable of sustaining blood concentrations of estradiol at 200 to 300 picograms per milliliter for at least twelve hours, as well as pituitary gonadotropin secreting cells that are sensitive to GnRH. Before mid-puberty, most adolescents cannot meet these requirements; thus, this pattern of GnRH secretion and menstruation occurs as a relatively late feature of female development.

Hypothalamic Control of Growth. Two hypothalamic peptides — somatocrinin, also known as growth hormone releasing hormone (GHRH), growth hormone releasing factor (GHRF), or growth releasing factor (GRF), and somatostatin, an inhibitor of GHRH-induced GH release — regulate secretion of somatotropin from the eosinophilic somatotroph cells of the anterior pituitary. The inhibitory effect of somatostatin on the pituitary is quite transient and lasts only a few minutes; it is followed by a rebound release of GH. In addition to the hypothalamus, somatostatin is also normally found elsewhere in the CNS, where it functions as a neurotransmitter; in the delta cells of the pancreatic islets; and in the antrum of the stomach and the duodenum.

Somatotropin, better known as growth hormone (GH), is released in a pulsatile fashion during sleep stages 3 and 4 in early puberty. The bursts of GH secretion are irregular and do not show the predictable periodicity of LH secretion, but they do exhibit an increased overall amplitude as puberty progresses, reaching a maximum during the height spurt (SMR 3).

Hypothalamic Control of Adrenal Androgen Development. Prior to any of the recognizable physical changes that occur during puberty, the adrenal glands of both females and males begin producing androgens (male hormones). Both the trigger and the effector mechanisms for this process remain unknown. A distinct pituitary adrenal androgen stimulating hormone (AASH) has been postulated to exist by Grumbach and colleagues and Parker and Odell, but it has not been identified. It is unlikely to be LH, FSH, or GH. Rich and colleagues have proposed that a combination of changes leads to an altered response to ACTH in the androgenic zone of the adrenal cortex, so that ACTH might act in modulating the process. Likewise, Higuchi and colleagues suggest that prolactin has a direct synergistic effect with ACTH on adrenal cells to increase adrenal androgen release. Whatever the stimulus, the process is complex and plays an as yet undetermined role in puberty. It may be that adrenal androgens affect the maturation of the neuroendocrine system by increasing gonadotropin bioactivity or selectively promoting prepubertal or pubertal growth.

Anterior Pituitary

Anterior Pituitary Control of Gonadal Development. By responding to hypothalamic controls and, in turn, bringing about responses in various endocrine target organs, the anterior pituitary is an intermediate transmitter of chemical messages related to puberty. Changes in the pattern of secretion

Figure 2.4. FSH Responsivity in Prepubertal, Pubertal, and Adult Subjects.

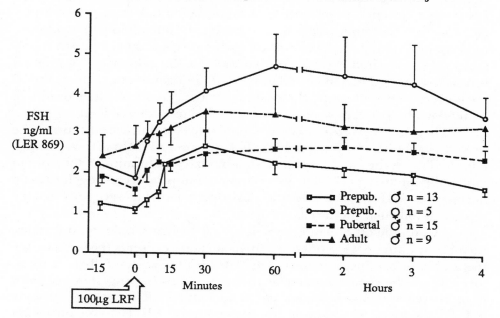

Source: Reproduced with permission from M. M. Grumbach, J. C. Roth, S. L. Kaplan, and R. P. Kelch, "Hypothalamic-Pituitary Regulation of Puberty in Man: Evidence and Concepts Derived from Clinical Research." In M. M. Grumbach, G. D. Grave, and F. F. Mayer (eds.), *Control of the Onset of Puberty.* New York: Wiley, 1974, p. 137.

of hypothalamic factors are reflected in changes in pituitary gonadotropins, whose target organ is the gonad.

Although GnRH is the releasing factor for both FSH and LH, their function and pattern of secretion are different during puberty both within and between the sexes. FSH responsivity to GnRH is comparable in prepubertal, pubertal, and adult individuals, showing no increasing sensitivity (Figure 2.4). However, females show a responsivity of FSH to GnRH that is greater than that of males at all stages of sexual development.

In contrast, prepubertal LH response to GnRH is sluggish, apparently as a result of lack of previous exposure to adequate amounts of GnRH. Prior to puberty, there is only a small pool of readily releasable LH, but with continued GnRH stimulation, the LH release mechanism is "primed." As puberty progresses, proportionately greater amounts of LH are secreted (Figure 2.5). In addition, LH bioactivity increases fivefold during puberty. Eventually, the adult pattern of LH response emerges, and the serum concentration of LH exceeds that of FSH.

In addition to previous exposure to GnRH, normal pubertal LH release also requires pauses between bursts of GnRH secretion. That is, GnRH levels must rise and fall every 90 to 120 minutes in order for normal puberty to proceed. Adolescent females who lose a great deal of weight, such as in anorexia nervosa, experience a drop in LH levels and loss of pulsative LH release; cessation of menstrual cycles and even failure of pubertal progression can occur until weight is restored. On the other hand, in precocious puberty, normal puberty occurs at an early age. Cessation of pubertal progression is a desired therapeutic outcome in this situation. Continuous infusion of exogenous GnRH obliterates the endogenous pattern of cyclical release and not only stops the pubertal progression but often results in regression of secondary sex characteristics to a prepubertal level.

There are differences in gonadotropin release and action between the sexes. In females undergoing puberty, FSH rises quickly at first, then plateaus after SMR 3. As the name implies, FSH stimulates maturation of the ovarian follicles by inducing follicular granulosa cells to produce estrogen (female hormones). FSH also induces the development of LH receptors on the surface of follicular theca cells.

LH, on the other hand, rises slowly during early puberty in females, then rapidly after SMR 3 (Figure 2.6). Its primary action is to stimulate the theca cells to produce progesterone. After ovulation, the follicle is transformed into the corpus luteum, a structure so rich in progesterone that it becomes yellow (hence its name: *lutea* is the Latin word for "yellow"). In early puberty, the theca cells respond relatively poorly to LH. However, once FSH

Figure 2.5. LH Responsivity in Prepubertal, Pubertal, and Adult Subjects.

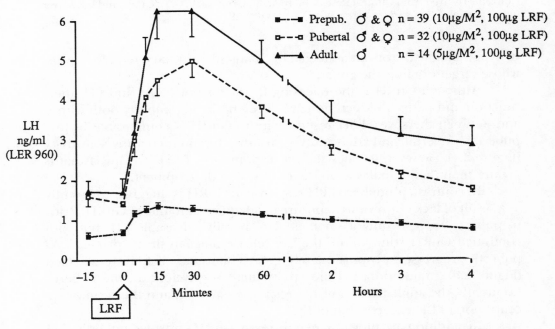

Source: Reproduced with permission from M. M. Grumbach, J. C. Roth, S. L. Kaplan, and R. P. Kelch, "Hypothalamic-Pituitary Regulation of Puberty in Man: Evidence and Concepts Derived from Clinical Research." In M. M. Grumbach, G. D. Grave, and F. F. Mayer (eds.), *Control of the Onset of Puberty.* New York: Wiley, 1974, p. 136.

Figure 2.6. Mean Plasma FSH, LH, and Estradiol Concentrations in Females by Sexual Maturity Rating.

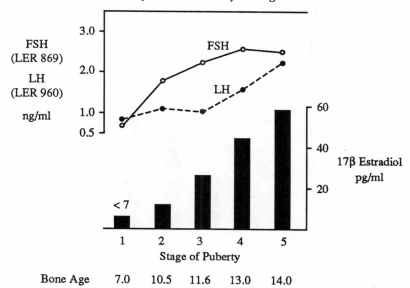

Source: Reproduced with permission from M. M. Grumbach, "Onset of Puberty." In S. R. Berenberg (ed.), *Puberty: Biologic and Psychosocial Components.* Leiden, Netherlands: Stenfert-Kroese, 1975, p. 3.

induces the development of adequate surface receptors, LH is able to effect its full action in regulating the menstrual cycle.

For males, FSH rises relatively uniformly throughout puberty (Figure 2.7). It has three main actions. First, it induces germinal cells in the seminiferous tubules to undergo spermatogenesis. Second, it stimulates the aromatization of testosterone into estradiol in the Sertoli cells of the testes. Third, it causes the development of gonadal LH receptors in males.

The testicular LH receptors are on the surface of the interstitial cells of Leydig; before the chemical structure of the hormone was known, LH was called interstitial cell stimulating hormone (ICSH). LH stimulates Leydig cells to produce androgens, most notably testosterone. Its effect is weak in early puberty because there are few LH receptors then. As puberty progresses, the number of androgen-producing cells, the number of receptors per cell, and the overall levels of LH increase; as a result, during puberty a thirtyfold increase in testosterone occurs.

Anterior Pituitary Control of Growth. Unlike pituitary hormones that have their effect on puberty by stimulating endocrine organs, the anabolic activity of GH is mediated through a polypeptide hormone produced in the liver (somatomedin-C) that promotes the cell multiplication required for growth in the skeleton, connective tissue, muscles, and viscera. GH is controlled by a self-regulatory negative feedback system. It acts on the hypothalamus by stimulating somatostatin secretion and on the pituitary itself by inhibiting GHRF-stimulated GH secretion.

Figure 2.7. Mean Plasma FSH, LH, and Estradiol Concentrations in Males by Sexual Maturity Rating.

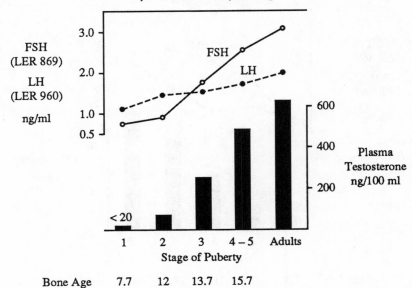

Source: Reproduced with permission from M. M. Grumbach, "Onset of Puberty." In S. R. Berenberg (ed.), *Puberty: Biologic and Psychosocial Components.* Leiden, Netherlands: Stenfert-Kroese, 1975, p. 4.

Anterior Pituitary Control of Adrenal Androgen Production. The activation of 17-ketosteroid biosynthetic pathways in the adrenal cortex results in the production of androgenic substances that have an action similar to that of testosterone. As mentioned previously, the hypothalamic adrenal androgen stimulating factor is not well defined, but its production initiates this process at approximately seven years of age for females and eight years of age for males. It represents a distinctly different pattern of adrenal secretion from that seen in earlier childhood; there is no concomitant increase in glucocorticoid or mineralocorticoid levels.

Until recently, it was thought that adrenal maturation was linked to gonadal maturation. Relatively insensitive methods used in the past to measure twenty-four-hour urinary excretion of 17-ketosteroids were unable to detect the small increases in adrenal androgen production that occur in the few years prior to puberty. However, although there now are known to be measurable increases in adrenal androgenic substances at age seven or eight, these increases are too small to result in observable physical changes, and development of pubic hair usually coincides with gonadal androgenic development.

Thus, the physical changes attributable to adrenal androgens tend to appear at about the same time as the gonads begin to mature, but the relationship is temporal rather than dependent on gonadal maturation. This relationship was clarified by Sklar and colleagues, who demonstrated that patients with precocious puberty before age six exhibit gonadal development in the absence of adrenal maturation and that patients with absent gonadal function had normal onset of adrenal maturation. Furthermore, they showed that patients with constitutionally delayed growth often exhibit a delay in both adrenal and gonadal maturation.

Maturation of Target Endocrine Organs in Puberty

Adrenal Glands

Increased activity in the zona reticularis of the adrenal cortex produces a disproportionate increase in plasma levels of androgens, most notably dehydroepiandrosterone (DHEA) and DHEA-sulfate, which continue to rise severalfold during puberty to attain adult levels by mid-puberty. In females, DHEA and DHEA-sulfate of adrenal origin are the most important androgens. Although the ovaries do possess enzymatic pathways to produce androgens, their role is secondary to that of the adrenals. Male adrenals produce these same substances, but they merely add to the massive effects of virilization resulting from testosterone released from the testes.

The development of pubic hair is the most noticeable physical change attributed to adrenal androgens, but several years often elapse between the time when adrenal androgenic activity actually begins and the time when it becomes sufficiently powerful to induce pubic hair growth. *Adrenarche* (or *pubarche*) refers to the first appearance of pubic hair.

Gonads: Primary Sex Characteristics

Ovaries. The primary female sex characteristic is the development and release of eggs from ovarian follicles approximately every twenty-eight days. Early in puberty, FSH causes maturation of many follicles, each contributing to the overall increasing concentration of estradiol. However, the contained eggs fail to mature to the extent of ovulation.

Late in mid-puberty, estrogens are produced in sufficient amounts to result in endometrial proliferation and menstruation. The onset of menstruation is termed *menarche*. At the menarche, eggs still do not generally mature to the point of being released, because adequate concentrations of estrogens and progesterone cannot be sustained.

As puberty progresses, one follicle becomes dominant during each cycle and produces increasing amounts of estradiol during the follicular phase of the menstrual cycle. At mid-cycle, there is a surge of LH and FSH that results in ovulation. After ovulation, the follicle involutes into a corpus luteum, which does not require continued high levels of LH to be maintained. Instead, the corpus luteum autonomously produces increasing concentrations of progesterone, which result in the secretory changes in the endometrium that occur in the second half of each menstrual cycle. After about fourteen days, the corpus luteum begins to degenerate, levels of estradiol and progesterone begin to fall, and the endometrial lining is shed in menstruation. As the levels of sex steroids decline, negative feedback on gonadotropin release declines, and the concentration of FSH again begins to rise in preparation for the next ovulatory cycle.

From this greatly simplified overview of ovarian maturation during puberty, it is obvious that menarche is a relatively late occurrence in the series of physical changes noted in females. Furthermore, although a few females ovulate in their first menstrual cycle, the first six to twelve months of menses are generally anovulatory and irregular.

Testes. The primary male sex characteristic is the development of viable sperm (spermatogenesis). In this process, males do not experience a discrete event analogous to ovulation or menstruation. The first release of spermatozoa outside of the body (*spermarche*) generally first occurs during masturbation or in nocturnal emissions ("wet dreams"). Hirsch and colleagues devised an unobtrusive means of detecting spermarche, examining multiple first voided morning urine samples for sperm. By this relatively insensitive method, they determined that the mean time of spermarche is around the thirteenth birthday and that it is significantly associated with maturation of the secondary sex characteristics.

In addition to not being readily identifiable clinically, spermatogenesis also lacks the periodicity of the ovulatory cycle; the release of spermatozoa occurs without a recognizable pattern. The development of sperm within the seminiferous tubules is initiated by FSH and sustained by testosterone. Testosterone levels in boys increase dramatically after SMR 3, even though the mean concentration of LH increases only slightly.

Effects of Sex Hormones on End Organs

The actions of the various sex hormones in both males and females are summarized in Table 2.2.

Estrogenic Pubertal Changes. Estrogenic activity is shared by a great number of chemical compounds; as a group, these substances account for many of the physical attributes of femininity. By direct action, they cause growth and development of the vagina, uterus, and Fallopian tubes. Breast enlargement occurs because of ductal growth and stromal development; the skin of the nipples and areolae also darkens in response to estrogen. At low levels, estrogens tend to stimulate growth, but at higher levels, they inhibit growth and cause closure of the epiphyses. Estrogen also promotes growth of pubic and axillary hair, pigmentation of the genital skin, and widening of the pelvic inlet and the hips.

Androgenic Pubertal Changes. Androgenic activity is also shared by different compounds; as a group, these substances produce masculinization. Most notably, they produce growth of the penis, scrotum, prostate, and seminal vesicles. Their tremendous growth-promoting properties result in

Table 2.2. Primary Action of Major Hormones of Puberty.

Hormone	Sex	Action
FSH (Follicle-Stimulating Hormone)	Male	Stimulates gametogenesis.
	Female	Stimulates development of primary ovarian follicles.
		Stimulates activation of enzymes in ovarian granulosa cells to increase estrogen production.
LH (Luteinizing Hormone)	Male	Stimulates testicular Leydig cells to produce testosterone.
	Female	Stimulates ovarian theca cells to produce androgens and the corpus luteum to synthesize progesterone.
		Midcycle surge induces ovulation.
Estradiol (E$_2$)	Male	Increases rate of epiphyseal fusion.
	Female	Stimulates breast development.
		Low level enhances linear growth while a high level increases the rate of epiphyseal fusion.
		Triggers midcycle surge of LH.
		Stimulates development of labia, vagina, uterus, and ducts of the breasts.
		Stimulates development of a proliferative endometrium in the uterus.
		Increases fat mass of the body.
Testosterone	Male	Accelerates linear growth.
		Increases rate of epiphyseal fusion.
		Stimulates development of the penis, scrotum, prostate, and the seminal vesicles.
		Stimulates growth of pubic, facial, and axillary hair.
		Increases larynx size and thus deepens the voice.
		Stimulates sebaceous gland secretion of oil.
		Increases libido.
		Increases muscle mass.
		Increases red blood cell mass.
	Female	Accelerates linear growth.
		Stimulates growth of pubic and axillary hair.
Progesterone	Female	Converts a proliferative uterine endometrium to a secretory endometrium.
		Stimulates lobuloalveolar breast development.
Adrenal Androgens	Male and Female	Stimulates pubic hair and linear growth.

Source: Reproduced with permission from *Adolescent Health Care* by Lawrence S. Neinstein, M.D., copyright 1984, Urban & Schwarzenberg, Baltimore-Munich.

rapid increases in muscle mass, skeletal growth, and bone age and density. The bones of the shoulders and vertebral column, the cartilage in the larynx, and the red blood cell precursors are especially sensitive to androgenic growth promotion. In both sexes, the skin becomes thicker (while sub-cutaneous fat is lost in males) and hair follicles produce more sebum. Pubic, axillary, and eventually facial and body hair develops. Clinically, increased androgenic activity is associated with such varied conditions as acne, body odor, deepening of the voice, and, for males, broadening of the shoulders, the height spurt, and elevation of hemoglobin levels.

Physical Growth During Puberty

Growth Tempo

Because adolescents grow at varying tempos, they exhibit a variation of size and shape not seen during childhood. Ultimate size is not related to growth tempo, however. The average early developer and the average late developer each arrive at the same average adult height. Similarly, the average rapid developer (who also tends to be early) and the average slow developer (who also tends to be late) each usually arrive at the same average adult height. Such statements cannot be made for youngsters with pathological growth patterns such as true precocious puberty; these individuals have short adult stature. But it is clear from normal height and weight charts that an adolescent's growth tempo determines only when he or she completes growth, without an independent influence on ultimate adult size.

This finding is, in part, explained by the fact that there is a great deal of overlap between the tempos of early and late developers. For example, there are early developers who grow at slow rates and late developers who grow at rapid rates. Genetic endowment is clearly the strongest predictor of stature. But all else being equal, early developers who grow at a slow rate tend to reach adulthood being quite short, while late developers who grow at a fast rate can become tall.

In a similar vein, Reynolds and Wines demonstrated that the timing of the onset of breast development in females has no relationship to breast size at the completion of puberty. From their longitudinal study of forty-nine girls, they found that breasts that were eventually small began developing at about the same time as breasts that eventually became large. Interestingly, they noted that adolescents with large breasts experienced menarche about 1.1 years later than those who had small breasts.

Another generalization that can be made about growth tempo is that most of the events of puberty have a Gaussian distribution in the population and a standard deviation of approximately one year. This means that about 95 percent of the members of a normal population will experience a given event within two years of the mean. The mean age of menarche is 12.8 years, but about 2.5 percent of normal females will begin to menstruate before age

10.8, and about 2.5 percent of normal females will not begin to menstruate until after age 14.8. Tanner points out that 3 in 1,000 normal females do not have their first menstrual period until age 15.5, and the same number of males do not have their peak height velocity until age 16.5 years. Being outside of the normal curve does not necessarily means that one suffers a pathological condition.

All estimates of growth tempo are indirect. Bone age (BA) is the measure that best assesses the tempo of growth. Standard BA tables (Greulich and Pyle; Bayley and Pinneau) make use of the fact that the epiphyses of various bones close in a highly predictable sequence in response to sex steroids. The degree of physical maturity can be determined by the pattern of epiphyseal closure found on x-ray; BA can then be compared to chronological age. Individuals with BA in advance of their chronological age are considered early developers, while those with BA less than their chronological age are considered late developers. The velocity at which SMR levels are achieved is the best clinical (and most inexpensive) estimate of tempo, because the physical changes occurring in both males and females are, like BA, the result of sex steroid activity.

Skeletal Growth

"Growing up" is one of the outstanding features of puberty. Immediately prior to puberty, linear growth (height velocity) is at its nadir; during puberty, it is at its apex. Pubertal linear growth must therefore accelerate, resulting in a burst of growth called the height spurt. When linear growth is occurring at maximal speed, adolescents are said to be experiencing their peak height velocity. Plotting an adolescent's yearly increase in height against age reveals a slightly skewed curve with an ascending limb of about two years' duration and a descending limb of about three or more years' duration.

All else being equal, tall children tend to grow into tall adults, and short children tend to grow into short adults. Only about 30 percent of the variability in adult height can be accounted for on the basis of pubertal growth patterns. The correlation between height before the height spurt and final adult height is about 0.8. Early maturers have a peak that is about one centimeter per year higher and two years earlier than average. Late maturers have a peak that is about one centimeter per year lower and two years later than average.

Close inspection of the height curves published by Tanner and Davis point out a subtle feature of adolescent growth that is often unappreciated: Normal individual adolescents undergoing puberty often do not follow normal population height curves. Those who develop early may cross from below the seventy-fifth percentile to above the ninety-fifth percentile, with an early plateau, while those who develop late may fall from above the twenty-fifth percentile to below the fifth percentile, followed by a late spurt. These effects are even more dramatic for boys than for girls. Such an occurrence is of great concern during childhood, since moving out of one's growth "channel" is often associated with a pathological condition. However, this is merely another example in which adolescents are different from either children or adults. Care must be taken in that merely applying an individual's growth curve to a population standard curve may lead to the erroneous conclusion that a given adolescent is growing abnormally.

The pubertal increase in linear growth follows a caudo-rostral progression. The peak velocity of leg lengthening precedes growth of the trunk by about six to nine months and that of the shoulders and chest by about one year. Even though boys have longer legs than girls, the height spurt during puberty in both sexes is related more to increased trunk length than to leg length. However, it is interesting to note that the secular trend toward greater stature mentioned at the beginning of this chapter is due almost entirely to changes that have occurred over time in leg length and not sitting height.

Even though that portion of skeletal growth (long bones and trunk) that contributes to stature receives the most attention in analyses of puberty, it is important to recognize that all bones undergo qualitative and quantitative changes during this time. The density of the skeleton increases (more so for males than for females). The bones of the face undergo marked transformation; differential growth rates result most notably in a greater prominence of the nose. In addition, characteristics of shape emerge that are considered as feminine or masculine.

Female Skeletal Growth. Prior to the onset of the growth spurt, females are growing at a rate slightly more than 5.5 centimeters per year, with a lower and upper range of about 4 and 7.5 centimeters per year, respectively. The growth spurt occurs during SMR 2 or 3. About two years after the initiation of the growth spurt, females reach their peak height velocity of slightly more than 8 centimeters per year (range of 6 to 10.5). This maximal growth rate is reached about six to twelve months before menarche. After the peak is reached, females begin to decelerate in linear growth over the next two years, reflected in a leveling off of the height curve as adult stature is approached (SMR 4). By menarche, more than 98 percent of a female's final height has been achieved. After menarche, height usually increases by less than 5 centimeters.

The most outstanding feature of female skeletal growth is the large spurt that occurs in hip width during puberty. The growth of the pelvis and hips (measured as the bi-iliac diameter) is quantitatively as great as for boys. However, females grow less in nearly all other dimensions, so that their hip width appears disproportionately large in comparison to that of males. Also, because this change tends to occur relatively early for girls, they may be distressed that they are getting "fat."

Male Skeletal Growth. Prior to the onset of their growth spurt, boys are growing at a rate of about 5 centimeters per year, with a lower and upper range of about 3.5 and 6.5 centimeters per year, respectively. They continue to increase in height at this velocity while girls are experiencing their growth spurt. Then, as their female age mates are decelerating, males begin to accelerate in growth, reaching a peak height velocity of more than 9 centimeters per year (range of 7 to 12). The mean peak height velocity for early-maturing boys is more than 10 centimeters per year (range of 8 to 12.5), compared to about 8.5 centimeters per year (range of 6.5 to 10.5) for late maturers. Thus, during their respective growth spurts, some early-maturing males may grow at a rate of only 8 centimeters per year, while some late-maturing males may grow at more than 10 centimeters per year. Individuals do not grow at their peak height velocity for long. On the average, boys grow about 7 centimeters in the first year of their spurt, 9 centimeters in the second year, 7 centimeters in the third, 3 centimeters in the fourth, and about 2 centimeters thereafter for as long as they continue to grow.

Broader shoulders, narrower hips, longer legs, and relatively still longer arms (particularly forearms) characterize the sexual dimorphism of male skeletal growth. The cartilage of those bones that demonstrate disproportionately greater growth appear to have a heightened responsiveness to androgens. The final height differential between males and females is about 13 centimeters.

Growth of Muscle

All muscles, including the heart, grow during puberty. However, skeletal muscles receive the most attention because of their role in shaping external physical appearance, especially in males. Androgens are potent stimulators of skeletal muscle hypertrophy, as is evidenced by the large increase in bulk realized by athletes taking anabolic steroids. Thus, the peak velocity for muscle growth is much greater for males than for females.

The spurt in muscle strength lags behind the spurt in muscle mass by about one year. Muscles first grow in size, increasing the volume of each fiber; later, increase in strength occurs as a result of the effects of androgens on protein structure and enzymatic activity. Muscular strength, as measured by hand grip, arm pull, or arm thrust, does not increase appreciably after menarche for females. After puberty, males continuously increase in muscular strength, especially with exercise training, reaching a maximum in the twenty-five- to thirty-five-year-old age group.

Because androgens play such an important role in determining strength, increases in strength are closely related to an adolescent's SMR. Kreipe and Gewanter demonstrated that grip strength predicted sexual maturity rating with a high degree of accuracy in boys undergoing routine physical examinations for participation in sports. However, the degree of sexual maturity was not the only determinant of strength. Early-developing boys were stronger than their chronological peers who were less physically mature but weaker than boys of similar sexual maturity who were older. Likewise, late-developing boys were weaker than their chronological peers

Table 2.3. Triceps Skinfold Thickness for Males and Females.

Age Group	n	5	10	25	50	75	90	95	n	5	10	25	50	75	90	95
				Males								Females				
1–1.9	228	6	7	8	10	12	14	16	204	6	7	8	10	12	14	16
2–2.9	223	6	7	8	10	12	14	15	208	6	8	9	10	12	15	16
3–3.9	220	6	7	8	10	11	14	15	208	7	8	9	11	12	14	15
4–4.9	230	6	6	8	9	11	12	14	208	7	8	8	10	12	14	16
5–5.9	214	6	6	8	9	11	14	15	219	6	7	8	10	12	15	18
6–6.9	117	5	6	7	8	10	13	16	118	6	6	8	10	12	14	16
7–7.9	122	5	6	7	9	12	15	17	126	6	7	9	11	13	16	18
8–8.9	117	5	6	7	8	10	13	16	118	6	8	9	12	15	18	24
9–9.9	121	6	6	7	10	13	17	18	125	8	8	10	13	16	20	22
10–10.9	146	6	6	8	10	14	18	21	152	7	8	10	12	17	23	27
11–11.9	122	6	6	8	11	16	20	24	117	7	8	10	13	18	24	28
12–12.9	153	6	6	8	11	14	22	28	129	8	9	11	14	18	23	27
13–13.9	134	5	5	7	10	14	22	26	151	8	8	12	15	21	26	30
14–14.9	131	4	5	7	9	14	21	24	141	9	10	13	16	21	26	28
15–15.9	128	4	5	6	8	11	18	24	117	8	10	12	17	21	25	32
16–16.9	131	4	5	6	8	12	16	22	142	10	12	15	18	22	26	31
17–17.9	133	5	5	6	8	12	16	19	114	10	12	13	19	24	30	37
18–18.9	91	4	5	6	9	13	20	24	109	10	12	15	18	22	26	30
19–24.9	531	4	5	7	10	15	20	22	1060	10	11	14	18	24	30	34
25–34.9	971	5	6	8	12	16	20	24	1987	10	12	16	21	27	34	37
35–44.9	806	5	6	8	12	16	20	23	1614	12	14	18	23	29	35	38
45–54.9	898	6	6	8	12	15	20	25	1047	12	16	20	25	30	36	40
55–64.9	734	5	6	8	11	14	19	22	809	12	16	20	25	31	36	38
65–74.9	1503	4	6	8	11	15	19	22	1670	12	14	18	24	29	34	36

Column header (spanning): *Triceps skinfold percentiles (mm²)*

Source: Reproduced with permission from A. R. Frisancho, "New Norms of Upper Limb Fat and Muscle Areas for Assessment of Nutritional Status." *American Journal of Clinical Nutrition,* 1981, *34,* 2540–2545. © *American Journal of Clinical Nutrition,* American Society for Clinical Nutrition.

who were more physically mature but stronger than boys of similar sexual maturity who were younger.

Growth of Fat

Subcutaneous fat in the limbs (measured as triceps, biceps, and calf skinfold thickness) continues to accumulate, but at a decreased velocity, in both boys and girls in the year immediately prior to the peak height velocity (Table 2.3). Thus, although the accumulation of truncal fat (measured as subscapular skinfold thickness) is relatively constant in that period, total body fat increases during early puberty for both boys and girls.

Boys actually lose fat, especially in the limbs, during their height spurt at SMR 4. Fat in the trunk, however, decreases little, if at all, during the male height spurt and is relatively quickly reaccumulated to prepubertal levels. Fat that is lost in the limbs of boys is much slower to reaccumulate and may never increase to prepubertal levels. Overall body fat increases in boys after the height spurt, adding to the weight gain that occurs relatively late in puberty. Fat normally accounts for about 12 percent of body weight in males by late puberty.

In contrast to boys, girls have a continuous increase in body fat during puberty, interrupted only by a short-lived slowing down of fat accumulation prior to their height spurt. At no time during puberty do females normally lose fat. After their height spurt, females lay down fat more rapidly than males, resulting in more than a quarter of their weight being fat.

Frisch has noted that pubertal females experience a 44 percent increase in lean body mass and a 120 percent increase in body fat. More to the point, the ratio of lean body mass to fat changes from 5:1 at the initiation of the growth spurt to 3:1 at menarche. She suggests that body fat is an important mediator in the initiation of menstruation and regular ovulatory cycles because it is one of the most important components of the weight spurt for females. Although arguments have been made against this theory, it is known that fat cells can affect the levels of sex steroids and that significant loss of fat, as in anorexia nervosa, is regularly associated with loss of menstrual periods.

Weight Spurt

Tanner points out that because weight is easy to measure, it has an undeserved importance as a measure of growth. Weight, however, represents the sum of many different tissue masses, and any given weight is therefore very difficult to interpret clinically. Thus, changes in height or SMR are much more likely than weight to reflect substantive changes in growth, except in instances of acute illness or starvation. In addition, the modern emphasis on thinness, especially for females, often leads to a restriction in normal weight gain.

Female Weight Spurt. The female weight spurt follows the height spurt by about three to six months and precedes the spurt in muscle mass by about the same interval. The average weight velocity at peak growth is about 8 kilograms per year, with 95 percent of normal girls gaining weight at a rate between 5.5 and 10.5 kilograms per year. Interestingly, there is no difference in the rate at which early- and late-maturing females put on weight. This is distinctly different from the case of height, in which early maturers grow at a rate about 20 percent greater than late maturers.

Male Weight Spurt. The male weight spurt coincides with both the height and muscle spurts. Thus, while females experience a sequence of peak height followed by peak weight followed by peak muscle velocity, males experience these peaks simultaneously (Figure 2.8). The average weight velocity at peak growth is about 9 kilograms per year, with 95 percent of average-maturing normal boys gaining between 6 and 12.5 kilograms per

Figure 2.8. Relationships Between Spurt in Height, Weight, Muscle, and Fat, Sex Steroid Levels, Sexual Maturity Rating, and Chronological Age.

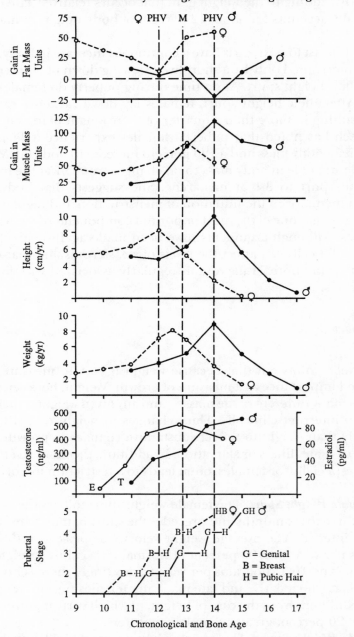

Source: Adapted and reproduced with permission from H. V. Barnes, "Adolescent Medicine." In A. M. Harvey, R. J. Johns, A. H. Owens, and R. S. Ross (eds.), *Principles and Practices of Medicine*. (19th ed.) East Norwalk, Conn.: Appleton-Century-Crofts, 1976, p. 1752.

year. In contrast to females, early-maturing males do differ from late-maturing males in the rate at which they gain weight. Boys who develop early gain an average of 9.5 kilograms per year at peak, with a range of 7 to 13 kilograms per year; late-developing boys put on only about 8.5 kilograms per year, with a range of 6 to 12 kilograms per year.

Physiological Changes of Puberty

The secondary sex characteristics of puberty that have been discussed are anatomical changes that occur in response to variations in hormonal, receptor, and enzymatic activity. During the height spurt, for example, alkaline phosphatase (an enzyme associated with bone growth) is elevated. Likewise, hemoglobin levels in males rise about 12 percent from the initiation to completion of puberty as a result of testosterone stimulation of red blood cell production.

Endocrine measures are also closely related to sexual maturation. However, for a given stage of puberty or even for a given individual, blood levels of endocrine secretions tend to have a wide range of normal values. Because of fluctuations in secretion and complex neuroendocrine interactions, timed urine collections, serial blood samples, or responses to stimulation tests tend to provide more useful clinical information than a single serum determination of an endocrine substance. Tables 2.4 through 2.7 list normal values for various substances in females and males with respect to sexual maturity rating.

The Sequence of Female Pubertal Maturation

Early Puberty (SMR 2–3)

Breast Development. The onset of breast development (*thelarche*) is one of the earliest manifestations of puberty and the first readily visible change of puberty in 85 percent of females. The tissue immediately beneath the areola enlarges in response to estrogen produced in the ovaries, marking entry into SMR 2 ("breast budding"). The mean age of occurrence for thelarche is approximately eleven years, with 95 percent of normal girls initiating breast development between ages nine and thirteen years. The rate of progression to more advanced stages varies widely, but the interval between SMR 2 and 3 of breast development averages slightly less than one year.

Growth of the breasts may not be symmetrical. Although breast asymmetry is normal, it can be quite marked and disturbing to the individual. Most adolescent females can be reassured that their breasts will become approximately the same size within two years.

Sexual Hair. The first sexual hair to develop grows along the edges of the labia majora and is fine, long, silky, dark, sparse, and generally straight. Although its appearance is due to adrenal androgens and therefore not

Table 2.4. Normal Values for Endocrinological Variables in Females During Puberty.

	Tanner Stage					Adult
	1	2	3	4	5	
Somatomedin-C[9] (U/mL)*	0.8 to 1.8	0.6 to 2.6	2.0 to 4.2	2.0 to 4.2	2.0 to 4.2	
Thyroxine (RIA)[10] (µg/dL)†	10.1	10.3	10.2	8.9	10.8	
Thyroid-stimulating hormone (RIA)[10] (µU/mL)†	10.5	9.8	7.4	8.3	8.9	
Follicle-stimulating hormone (mIU/mL)*						
mean[11]	4.2	5.5	8.0	8.0	12.3	
range[11-17]	0.5 to 8.1	0.7 to 10.0	0.8 to 15.0	1.2 to 20.0	1.3 to 20.0	4.0 to 20.0
Luteinizing hormone (mIU/mL)*						
mean[11]	2.9	3.9	8.4	11.3	18.9	
range[11-17]	0.2 to 7.5	0.4 to 11.5	0.5 to 15.0	0.6 to 34.0	0.5 to 80.0	4.0 to 25.0
Follicle-stimulating hormone (IU/24 hr)‡						
mean[18]	1.5	4.0	6.0	3.8	2.3	
range[18]	0.1 to 7.0	0.1 to 16.3	0.1 to 16.1	0.3 to 14.7	0.3 to 22.0	
Luteinizing hormone (IU/24 hr)‡						
mean[18]	1.9	5.0	13.7	14.9	16.6	
range[18]	0.1 to 15.1	0.4 to 25.7	1.5 to 43.5	3.8 to 51.0	4.9 to 42.8	
Prolactin[16] (mIU/mL)†	3.8 to 13.5	3.1 to 11.7	3.8 to 19.2	4.2 to 16.8	5.0 to 18.0	

Estrone (ng/dL)*						
mean[12]	4	5	7	12	3	
range[11-19]	1.4 to 8.0	1.0 to 9.0	1.5 to 11.0	1.6 to 19.0	2.0 to 7.7	2.0 to 18.2
Estradiol (ng/dL)*						
mean[12]	2	3	13	16	8	
range[11-19]	0.8 to 3.0	0.5 to 6.2	0.9 to 27.0	1.0 to 30.0	1.5 to 40.0	1.5 to 40.0
Progesterone[11] (ng/dL)*	10 to 13	16	16 to 23	30 to 161	29 to 758	20 to 2000
17-Hydroxyprogesterone[11] (ng/dL)*	32 to 38	38 to 52	55 to 69	101 to 127	11 to 808§	11 to 300
Testosterone (ng/dL)*						
mean[12]	11	19	28	48	38	
range[11-19]	2 to 18	14 to 65	19 to 80	20 to 85	20 to 85	15 to 85
Dihydrotestosterone[12] (ng/dL)*	2 to 16	3 to 24	9 to 25	9 to 32	—	10 to 32
Androstenedione (ng/dL)*						
mean[12]	35	72	103	176	141	
range[11-19]	10 to 100	38 to 106	40 to 150	40 to 210	58 to 224	40 to 300
Dehydroepiandrosterone (ng/dL)*						
mean[12]	133	326	427	498	741	
range[11-19]	19 to 300	45 to 1600	125 to 1700	153 to 1620	389 to 1093	200 to 1500
Dehydroepiandrosterone sulfate (μg/dL)*						
mean[20]	43	49	71	86	120	
range[20]	24 to 86	20 to 145	17 to 189	38 to 223	78 to 163	125 to 300

* plasma   † serum   ‡ urine   § follicular phase

Source: Reprinted with permission of Ross Laboratories, Columbus, OH 43216, from *Assessment of Pubertal Development*, p. 16, © 1986 Ross Laboratories.

Table 2.5. Normal Values for Physiological Variables in Females During Puberty.

	Tanner Stage				
	1	*2*	*3*	*4*	*5*
Hematocrit[3] (%)					
White *mean*	39.1	39.2	39.6	39.2	39.2
range	36.1 to 42.1	37.1 to 41.3	37.0 to 42.2	36.9 to 41.6	36.2 to 42.2
Black *mean*	37.3	38.9	39.0	38.4	38.7
range	34.6 to 39.9	35.7 to 42.1	35.2 to 42.6	34.9 to 42.8	35.9 to 41.5
Alkaline phosphatase[4] (IU/L)*					
White *mean*	70	89	76	33	38
range	51 to 90	49 to 134	36 to 108	16 to 60	23 to 76
Black *mean*	84	95	86	44	31
range	69 to 108	65 to 138	26 to 148	18 to 144	13 to 70
Cholesterol[5-7] (mmol/L)†	3.5 to 6.7	3.4 to 6.9	2.9 to 5.6	3.2 to 6.6	3.1 to 6.4
Urates[8] (μmol/L)†	183 to 361	161 to 389	167 to 380	166 to 397	163 to 376
Phosphorus[5] (mmol/L)†	1.0 to 1.5	1.0 to 1.6	1.0 to 1.4	0.9 to 1.4	0.9 to 1.3
Creatinine[8] (μmol/L)†	42 to 58	36 to 70	39 to 78	44 to 76	48 to 76

* serum   † plasma

Source: Reprinted with permission of Ross Laboratories, Columbus, OH 43216, from *Assessment of Pubertal Development*, pp. 13, 14, © 1986 Ross Laboratories.

causally related to thelarche, it generally coincides with or closely follows thelarche. However, about one-third of girls experience adrenarche before thelarche.

Internal Genitalia. Prior to puberty, the cervix is about twice the size of the body of the uterus. During early puberty, the body of the uterus enlarges so that it becomes about the same length as the cervix. The ovaries and other internal genital structures also grow in size. Changes attributable to estrogen are direct evidence that ovarian maturation is occurring. One important sign of such maturation is cornification of the vaginal epithelium.

Skeletal Growth. The height spurt is a relatively early occurrence in the female pubertal sequence, generally beginning soon after thelarche and reaching its peak about a year later, at SMR 3 breast development. Prior to the height spurt, there is widening of the hips that is often not recognized, except by the adolescent herself. Peak height velocity is typically reached between ages eleven and twelve. Early developers may have their height spurt between ages nine and ten, while late developers may not have their height spurt until between thirteen and fourteen years of age.

Some girls who have an early growth spurt are concerned because they are taller than boys their age and believe that they will continue to grow at their peak velocity, becoming unusually tall women. Using growth curves that take into account the SMR, such as those published by Tanner and Davis, one can predict the approximate final height of the individual and reassure her about such concerns. This obviates the use of x-rays to determine bone age.

Middle Puberty (SMR 3–4)

Breast Development. While the change from SMR 2 to 3 is mainly quantitative (breast "buds" to "mounds"), the change between SMR 3 and 4 is qualitative as well as quantitative and marked primarily by changes in the areolae. In SMR 4 breast development, the areolae are noticeably darker, larger, and elevated above the contour of the surrounding breast tissue, the so-called "double-mound" effect. The progression from SMR 3 to 4 occurs on average in slightly less than one year. A few normal females never progress in their breast development beyond SMR 4 or may advance to SMR 5 only during pregnancy.

Sexual Hair. Although pubic hair generally appears somewhat later than breast development, its progression proceeds more rapidly. The two processes show considerable independence, however. Among females at SMR 3 breast development, 25 percent have no pubic hair (SMR 1) and 10 percent have completely adult (SMR 5) hair. The time for progression from SMR 2 to 4 in pubic hair averages only slightly longer than one year.

Pubic hair in SMR 3 is thicker, coarser, and less straight than in the previous stage and spreads up onto the pubis. Just as in breast development, the change in pubic hair between SMR 3 and 4 is qualitative as well as quantitative and marked by the appearance of dense, curled, adult-type hair

Table 2.6. Normal Values for Endocrinological Variables in Males During Puberty.

	Tanner Stage					
	1	2	3	4	5	Adult
Somatomedin-C[9] (U/mL)*	0.7 to 1.1	0.8 to 2.2	1.4 to 2.4	1.4 to 2.4	2.0 to 3.2	
Thyroxine (RIA)[10] (μg/dL)†	10.7	9.4	8.9	8.5	8.4	
Thyroid-stimulating hormone (RIA)[10] (μU/mL)†	8.5	8.7	10.8	12.5	15.7	
Follicle-stimulating hormone (mIU/mL)*						
mean[11]	4.5	5.9	8.1	8.5	8.0	
range[11-17]	0.5 to 10.2	0.5 to 10.0	1.0 to 18.0	1.0 to 20.0	1.0 to 20.0	5.0 to 20.0
Luteinizing hormone (mIU/mL)*						
mean[11]	3.9	6.8	8.5	9.5	11.5	
range[11-17]	0.2 to 10.3	0.5 to 12.0	0.5 to 15.0	0.6 to 20.0	0.5 to 25.0	5.0 to 25.0
Follicle-stimulating hormone (IU/24 hr)‡						
mean[18]	1.6	3.2	3.7	4.7	2.8	
range[18]	0.1 to 8.0	0.1 to 12.1	0.1 to 12.8	0.5 to 15.9	0.5 to 15.1	
Luteinizing hormone (IU/24 hr)‡						
mean[18]	2.0	5.9	13.5	17.0	21.6	
range[18]	0.2 to 14.3	0.3 to 32.6	1.5 to 29.9	2.4 to 37.7	8.6 to 39.4	
Prolactin[16] (mIU/mL)†	3.6 to 10.3	2.4 to 18.9	3.0 to 15.2	4.3 to 18.1	3.1 to 15.7	

Estrone (ng/dL)*					
mean[12]	2	3	3	4	3
range[11-18]	1.1 to 5.8	1.0 to 7.1	1.1 to 6.6	2.3 to 7.3	1.0 to 6.9	2.0 to 6.0
Estradiol (ng/dL)*					
mean[12]	2	1	2	4	3
range[11-18]	0.2 to 3.5	0.2 to 4.0	0.8 to 3.2	1.1 to 6.0	1.4 to 4.9	1.5 to 5.0
Progesterone[11] (ng/dL)*	30	36	40	40	35	16 to 60
17-Hydroxyprogesterone[11] (ng/dL)*	30 to 36	34 to 40	52 to 62	78 to 93	97	38 to 200
Testosterone (ng/dL)*					
mean[12]	10	18	52	170	350
range[11-18]	3 to 110	2 to 300	27 to 910	92 to 840	200 to 1000	300 to 800
Dihydrotestosterone (ng/dL)*					
mean[12]	3	4	13	26	13
range[11-18]	2 to 20	2 to 28	6 to 36	5 to 51	1 to 76	30 to 80
Androstenedione (ng/dL)*					
mean[12]	54	49	85	69	90
range[11-18]	13 to 79	17 to 81	48 to 122	40 to 111	50 to 200	100 to 180
Dehydroepiandrosterone (ng/dL)*					
mean[12]	192	300	396	396	450
range[11-18]	2 to 326	50 to 558	119 to 592	178 to 645	180 to 700	200 to 700
Dehydroepiandrosterone sulfate (µg/dL)*					
mean[20]	42	63	73	103	123
range[20]	10 to 126	27 to 171	24 to 221	47 to 249	75 to 255	125 to 300

* plasma   † serum   ‡ urine

Source: Reprinted with permission of Ross Laboratories, Columbus, OH 43216, from *Assessment of Pubertal Development*, p. 15, © 1986 Ross Laboratories.

Table 2.7. Normal Values for Physiological Variables in Males During Puberty.

	Tanner Stage				
	1	2	3	4	5
Hematocrit[3] (%)					
White *mean*	39.5	39.8	40.9	42.3	43.8
range	37.1 to 41.8	36.7 to 42.8	38.2 to 43.5	39.7 to 44.8	41.1 to 46.4
Black *mean*	37.7	38.4	39.7	41.1	42.7
range	35.2 to 40.2	36.0 to 40.9	37.3 to 42.0	38.3 to 43.8	39.6 to 45.9
Alkaline phosphatase[4] (IU/L)*					
White *mean*	72	77	101	75	58
range	54 to 110	42 to 106	53 to 141	41 to 158	21 to 120
Black *mean*	77	94	122	116	75
range	43 to 130	53 to 204	46 to 240	32 to 228	23 to 228
Cholesterol[5-7] (mmol/L)†	3.1 to 5.9	3.0 to 6.3	2.9 to 5.2	3.1 to 5.1	3.0 to 5.1
Urates[8] (μmol/L)†	121 to 384	123 to 390	165 to 428	224 to 429	218 to 454
Phosphorus[5] (mmol/L)†	1.1 to 1.5	1.0 to 1.5	1.2 to 1.5	1.0 to 1.5	0.9 to 1.3
Creatinine[8] (μmol/L)†	39 to 63	46 to 73	44 to 80	33 to 90	44 to 90

* serum   † plasma

Source: Reprinted with permission of Ross Laboratories, Columbus, OH 43216, from *Assessment of Pubertal Development*, p. 13, © 1986 Ross Laboratories.

covering the outer surface of the labia and mons veneris in the characteristic triangular "female escutcheon." Axillary, facial, and adult-type body hair appears relatively late in the pubertal sequence, usually not before SMR 4 pubic hair has been established. There is considerable variability in sexual hair characteristics that are largely determined by the ethnic background of the individual adolescent.

Internal Genitalia. The uterus continues to enlarge, becoming twice the height of the cervix during mid-puberty, and the genital organs come to lie relatively lower in the pelvis. Cells lining the uterus also begin to develop, in preparation for later menstruation. The vagina begins to elongate to about 8 centimeters, and its secretions become acidic. The Fallopian tubes increase in diameter, and complex folds appear in the ciliated mucosa. In addition to these internal changes, the labia majora become thin, more heavily pigmented, and redundant to provide complete coverage of the introitus.

As the mucus-secreting cells lining the uterus develop, many adolescent females have a scant amount of vaginal discharge in the months preceding menarche. This is typically thin, clear or milky, and without odor. However, some girls or their mothers may be concerned about infection. They can be reassured that this normal discharge, called "physiological leukorrhea," is a sign that the uterus is preparing for menstruation. Hygienic measures can be suggested, but no treatment is necessary.

Skeletal Growth. The growth velocity begins to slow down after SMR 3 breast development is attained. Rarely, a girl may have her peak height velocity prior to any breast development, but this is not the usual sequence for the vast majority of females. Although growth in height tends to slow down after the peak height velocity, growth in both fat and muscle begins to accelerate, resulting in a weight peak.

Late Puberty (SMR 4–5)

Breast Development. Females enter SMR 5 breast development when the contour of the areola recedes to the level of the surrounding breast tissue. The papilla (nipple) is generally elevated above the contour of the surrounding areola, however. The enlargement and changes in the areola in SMR 4 are attributed to the effect of progesterone, so that most adolescents at this stage are menstruating or very near menarche.

There is often a long lag between SMR 4 and 5 breast development. The average interval between these two stages is almost two years, but it may be as short as one and a half or as long as nine years. For this reason, many clinicians consider SMR 4 to be an "adult" level of development.

Sexual Hair. When adult-type pubic hair extends down the medial aspect of the thighs, the adolescent has reached SMR 5. As with breast development, there is often a lag between SMR 4 and 5 pubic hair development. This lag is generally about sixteen months but can extend from only six to as long as twenty-eight months. This period is longer than the interval between the appearance of SMR 2 and 4 pubic hair.

Internal Genitalia. Although in late puberty the body of the uterus becomes three times the height of the cervix and the vagina lengthens to fifteen centimeters (adult), the outstanding feature of the latter part of puberty is menstruation. Menarche generally follows the growth spurt (either in late middle puberty or early late puberty), actually occurring during the phase of maximal growth deceleration; on extremely rare occasions, it may not be preceded by a growth spurt or significant breast development.

Marshall and Tanner found that only 26 percent of the normal girls whom they followed longitudinally had experienced menarche when they reached SMR 3 but that 62 percent of girls were menstruating by the time they reached SMR 4 breast development. The mean age of menarche is highly variable, depending on the ethnic, socioeconomic, and possibly athletic background of the individual. On the average, menarche occurs between 12.8 and 13.3 years, with about 95 percent of normal females beginning menstruation between 11 and 15 years of age.

Menarche occurs about two and a half years after breast development begins, about nine months after peak height velocity, about three months after peak weight velocity, and coincident with peak muscle and fat velocity. An average of 17 percent of body fat, attained at approximately 48 kilograms, seems to be needed for menarche, while about 22 percent is needed to initiate and maintain regular ovulatory cycles.

Although they are a normal feature of early menstrual cycles, many adolescents have concerns about their irregular menstrual periods soon after menarche. The average female has about twelve menstrual periods in the eighteen months following menarche and can be reassured about the eventual likelihood of regular periods. However, reassurance should not be provided without an adequate history and physical examination to rule out underlying organic pathology.

Another concern is that of delayed puberty. Most often, delay is constitutional: Normal pubertal maturation eventually occurs, but at an older than average chronological age. There is often a family history of late puberty in instances of constitutional delay. If a female has not menstruated by age sixteen, or within three years of the onset of breast development, factors other than constitutional delay should be considered. The history and physical examination are the most important first steps to take in the evaluation of such individuals.

Skeletal Growth. Growth in height slows dramatically after menarche. Although stature typically increases by no more than five centimeters, on rare occasions females may grow as much as 10 centimeters taller after beginning to menstruate. All other compartments of the body also show a decreased velocity in growth, except for fat, which continues to be added, though at a much slower rate than prior to the initiation of menstruation.

The Sequence of Male Pubertal Maturation

Early Puberty (SMR 2–3)

Testicular Development. Each prepubertal testis is less than four cubic centimeters in volume and less than two centimeters in greatest diameter. The beginning of puberty, SMR 2, is indicated by testicular growth. A testis at SMR 3 is generally eight to ten cubic centimeters in volume. Most of this increase is caused by an increase in size of the seminiferous tubules. The mean age for the initiation of male puberty is 11.5 years, only slightly later than that for the female. Normally boys may enter SMR 2 as early as 9.5 or as late as 13.5 years of age. The subsequent transition from SMR 2 to SMR 3 testicular development requires about one year.

Gonadal growth in males can be directly assessed by palpation of the testes in the scrotum and comparing their size to a testis-shaped model called an orchidometer, or Prader beads. Adolescents have demonstrated that they are able to determine their own level of development if given standards against which to compare themselves. Self-assessment is, therefore, a generally reliable method of determining sexual maturation. Enlargement of the epididymis, seminal vesicles, and prostate occurs concurrently with testicular growth but is not appreciable externally.

The size of the testicles may be difficult to appreciate by mere visual inspection, because testosterone causes wrinkling, thinning, and increased pigmentation of the scrotal skin and the testes do not fill the scrotum fully, as in childhood. The left testis generally hangs lower than the right testis once puberty begins.

Penis. The penis does not usually begin to enlarge until the testes have reached SMR 3 size, at about age 12.5 years. Growth of the penis can begin normally as early as 10.5 or as late as 14.5 years of age. The response to testosterone is initially an increase in length from its six centimeters (stretched) prepubertal size and deepened pigmentation of the scrotum.

At the time that boys are experiencing enlargement of the penis, they may also have breast development, or gynecomastia. Although the areolae normally widen from 12.5 millimeters in boys to more than 25 millimeters in men, *gynecomastia* refers to the actual growth of breast tissue in response to estrogen in the male. The amount of breast tissue usually regresses in one to two years, but its presence during that time can cause a great deal of concern for affected boys.

Sexual Hair. Pubic hair most often appears between 12 and 12.5 years of age, after puberty has begun but before significant penile enlargement has occurred. As in females, the hair is initially long, silky, dark, lightly pigmented, and straight. In early puberty, it is sparsely distributed, primarily at the base of the penis. As puberty progresses and SMR 3 pubic hair is attained, hair that is thicker and slightly curled extends across the pubis in a more dense patch. In addition, hair can be found on the scrotum.

Skeletal Growth. During early puberty, boys grow at their prepubertal rate. At the same chronological age, girls are in their growth spurt. Therefore, in the fifth and sixth grades in school, boys are often shorter than girls. It is this two-year discrepancy in growth spurt timing that accounts for the popular idea that boys lag two years behind girls in puberty. Skeletal and total body growth, including fat, occurs during early puberty, but not at an accelerated pace.

Middle Puberty (SMR 3–4)

Testicular Development. The size of each testis shows a steady enlargement during mid-puberty, reaching a volume of ten to fifteen cubic centimeters. Seminal fluid is produced in small amounts. The scrotal skin becomes thinner and the sac larger, so that the testes hang some distance from the body. Normal spermatogenesis requires a relatively constant temperature so that the ability to raise or lower the testes is an important factor in fertility. Sperm are first released during mid-puberty, generally between twelve and fourteen years of age.

Penis. During mid-puberty, the penis continues to grow in length, but more noticeably in width. Erections occur more frequently and are especially prominent on awakening. Growth of the penis tends to occur relatively rapidly and is essentially complete before either full testicular or full pubic hair development has occurred.

Sexual Hair. As in females, there is both a qualitative and quantitative difference between pubic hair at SMR 3 and 4. The latter is defined by adult-type hair that covers the entire pubic area but does not extend down the medial thigh or up the midline. The timing of the mid-pubertal changes is highly variable but generally occurs between 12.5 and 14.5 years of age. However, in the Harpenden Growth Study, up to 15 percent of normal males at SMR 4 testicular development had pubic hair at SMR 1. Rarely is the converse true.

Also as in females, axillary hair in the male generally does not appear before SMR 4 pubic hair. Facial hair appears only after SMR 4 pubic hair, and does so in an ordered sequence: the outer corners of the upper lip; the whole upper lip; the upper cheeks and middle of the lower lip; followed finally by hair along the sides and lower border of the chin. Body hair develops gradually after facial hair. The extent of body hair is determined to a large degree by ethnic and familial factors.

Skeletal Growth. Although the velocity of skeletal growth begins to increase noticeably when the penis starts to enlarge (about 12.5 years), the peak height velocity tends to occur late in middle puberty or early in late puberty (about 13.5 years). Boys can begin their growth spurt as early as 10.5 or as late as 16 years of age, lagging behind girls by about two years. The larynx also undergoes a growth spurt, associated with a "cracking" and deepening of the voice characteristic of growing boys.

Simultaneously with the height spurt, males experience a peak in muscle mass and in weight, despite actually losing total body fat. Boys who are delayed in this development are usually normal but often are concerned about being smaller than their peers. If the history and physical examination suggest constitutional delay of puberty, they should be reassured that they will experience normal puberty, but at a later age than their peers.

Late Puberty (SMR 4–5)

Testicular Development. The growth of the testes is considered complete (adult, SMR 5) when they attain a volume of approximately twenty cubic centimeters each. From initiation to completion, pubertal growth of the testes occurs over a period of about four years, with most adolescents attaining SMR 5 testicular development between 13.5 and 17 years of age. However, the timing of the onset has little relationship to the velocity of change. Thus, a class of seventh-grade boys could be expected to have representatives from every SMR, from prepuberty to adulthood.

Penis. The average penis length at completion of growth is about fifteen centimeters. From initiation to completion, penile growth takes less than three years. The normal ages for beginning and completing penile growth are about 12.5 and 14.5 years of age, respectively. The age range for initiation is 10.5 to 14.5 years of age; the range for completion is 12.5 to 16.5 years of age.

Sexual Hair. When adult-type pubic hair extends onto the medial thigh, SMR 5 (adult) pubic hair development has been attained. Some clinicians have suggested that hair extending up the midline of the abdomen in the typical diamond-shaped "male escutcheon" be designated SMR 6, but there is no evidence that this pattern represents a more mature stage of development than SMR 5. Pubic hair at this stage tends to blend in with body hair over the lower abdomen and legs. Although a mustache may be present at SMR 4, a beard indicates the SMR 5 level of maturation.

Skeletal Growth. Although the growth spurt tends to be a relatively late event for males, it tends to continue for a prolonged period of time after attaining peak velocity. Males can continue to grow, albeit minimally, beyond their teenage years.

Questions for Future Research

Although much has been learned about adolescent pubertal growth and development, there are key areas of research that continue to have unanswered questions. For example, in the area of neuroendocrine maturation, what are the regulators of hypothalamic, pituitary, and gonadal function that inhibit GnRH production during childhood? How are these regulators affected when pulsatile exogenous GnRH is administered? What causes the onset of puberty, with the reactivation of GnRH release in a pulsatile fashion? Why is there a discordance in the potency of gonadotropins measured by bioassay compared to immunoassay? What are the biological mechanisms by which varied steroid levels, malnutrition, excessive exercise, and psychological stress affect GnRH synthesis or secretion? How are control mechanisms affected by GnRH agonists and antagonists? Definitive answers to these questions may require the development of new animal models or technology capable of exploring the molecular and histological bases of puberty.

Somatic growth also deserves further investigation. Much remains to be learned regarding the role of growth factors (somatomedins) in somatic and organ growth. What are the signals for the activation or suppression of tissue somatomedins? Does the pubertal increase in somatomedin concentrations merely reflect an increase in binding proteins, or do circulating somatomedins have some biological activity? How do somatomedins affect gonadal growth and maturation? Do cartilage- and bone-derived growth factors have a specific role in the regulation of skeletal growth at puberty? What is the mechanism of GH and androgen synergism in regulating somatic growth?

Chronic illness can affect growth and maturation. How are GH, somatomedins, insulin, and insulin-like growth factor perturbed by specific chronic illnesses, and how are they affected by treatment? Likewise, how does chronic illness disturb neuroendocrine maturation? Illnesses that are first identified during puberty, that have their antecedents during puberty but that are not discovered until later in life, and that have their highest prevalence during puberty deserve particular attention.

Finally, a key area of research involves the impact of the pubertal process on behavior and psychosocial development. How do variations in tempo of pubertal maturation affect behavior and health? Are there biological causes or markers for those risk-taking behaviors so characteristic of pubertal individuals? If a specific hormone or biological marker is found, can it be modified or manipulated to attenuate risk-taking behavior? These and many other questions relating to the interface between biology and behavior will be answered only through collaborative efforts of researchers in the fields of adolescent medicine, endocrinology, neurobiology, child psychiatry, and developmental psychology. Cooperative research efforts have been initiated and must be maintained.

Suggested Readings

Blethen, S. L., and Shenker, I. R. "Delayed Puberty and Short Stature." *Seminars in Adolescent Medicine*, 1985, *1*, 67–77.

Frish, R. E. "Fatness, Puberty, and Fertility: The Effects of Nutrition and Physical Training on Menarche and Ovulation." In J. Brooks-Gunn and

A. C. Petersen (eds.), *Girls at Puberty: Biological and Psychosocial Perspectives.* New York: Plenum, 1983.

Odell, W. D. "Physiology of Sexual Maturation and Primary Amenorrhea." *Western Journal of Medicine,* 1979, *131*, 401–416.

Penny, R., Olambiwonnu, N. O., and Frasier, S. D. "Episodic Fluctuations of Serum Gonadotropins in Pre- and Post-Pubertal Girls and Boys." *Journal of Clinical Endocrinology and Metabolism,* 1977, *45*, 307–311.

Reiter, E. O. "Neuroendocrine Control Processes: Pubertal Onset and Progression." *Journal of Adolescent Health Care,* 1987, *8*, 479–491.

Tanner, J. M. *Growth at Adolescence.* (2nd ed.) Oxford, England: Blackwell Scientific, 1962.

Tanner, J. M. "Issues and Advances in Adolescent Growth and Development." *Journal of Adolescent Health Care,* 1987, *8*, 470–478.

Tanner, J. M., and Falkner, F. *Human Growth: A Comprehensive Treatise.* (2nd ed.) New York: Plenum, 1986.

Vaughan, V. C., and Litt, I. F. *Child and Adolescent Development: Clinical Implications.* Philadelphia: Saunders, 1990.

3

Psychological Development in Normal Adolescents

Olle Jane Z. Sahler, M.D.
Richard E. Kreipe, M.D.

> I confess to pride in this coming generation. You are working out your own salvation; you are more in love with life; you play with fire openly, where we did in secret, and few of you are burned!
> — *Franklin D. Roosevelt*
> (in "Whither Bound," address at Milton Academy, 1926)

It may be difficult to believe that Roosevelt was addressing his words to our fathers or grandfathers—those staid gentlemen who decry the wanton frivolity of today's youth, wondering aloud "What's the next generation coming to?" Yet, age after age from earliest time, the young of the next generation have been seen by those who have passed to adulthood as somehow freer, less encumbered, more daring, and, possibly because of their still unbridled willingness to risk, achieving greater heights than the preceding generation. What rites of passage have the mere children of yesterday endured that permit them a place in civilized society where they have a right to be heard as well as seen?

The answer to this question lies in that intriguing space in time, habit, and disposition of the individual that is known as youth or adolescence. It is looked forward to longingly by the young as a time of freedom for experimentation with life; it is looked back on wistfully by the old as a time of carefree, exuberant seeking; it is looked on directly by the adolescent as a time of deep tragedies and soaring triumphs.

In considering the discussion that follows, it is essential to recognize that the developmental process as it occurs throughout life is complex, highly variable, and dynamic. Indeed, the dynamism inherent in development is underscored by the current notion among developmental theorists that the individual is integral to rather than separate from the environment. That is, change in the individual leads to change in the environment and vice versa through a series of successive alternating adjustments. This interactional model presupposes that individuals of all ages, even in infancy, actively contribute to rather than merely passively experience events and activities around them.

Factors That Influence Psychological Development

An individual's psychological development is determined by both biogenetic makeup (intrinsic physiological traits such as sex, race, and innate intelligence and psychological characteristics such as temperament) and environmental factors (cultural and religious attitudes, standard of living, and characteristics of the family of origin and the peer group). Although these factors are easily listed as discrete entities, interrelationships are immediately obvious: Biogenetic disposition influences both physiological pattern and psychological makeup. Similarly, peoples of specific biogenetic types are indigenous to particular areas of the world and may share certain cultural mores that have developed over time in response to certain environmental demands; these mores, in turn, determine acceptable and unacceptable responses to various situational stresses.

The factors that influence adolescent development are not unique to the stage itself; each is a potent force that shapes human behavior throughout life. Rather, the uniqueness of adolescence lies in the rapidity with which change occurs, especially along two particular dimensions of psychological development: identity formation and attainment of autonomy.

Identity can be thought of as having three component parts: the physical being, the sexual being, and the vocational being. Autonomy is the capacity for self-determination. Whereas many writers have used the term *independence* (freedom from the influence or control of another) to designate self-determination, we would argue that the disconnectedness of the individual from the needs and desires of others implied by this term does not accurately describe either the real or the desired outcome of the developmental process. Instead, the attainment of true personal autonomy (the ability to govern one's own decisions and actions through reason) means that individuals are free to enter into independent, interdependent, or even dependent relationships with others and to make decisions for themselves that will attain whatever goals they feel are important within each of these roles.

Thus, formation of a stable, although modifiable, identity and assumption of the responsibility for self-governance are the essential features of successful negotiation through adolescence. Because these dramatic changes are accomplished over a relatively short period of time, they are accompanied by variable periods of turbulence and disequilibrium in some—but by no means all—adolescents. It is these qualities of turmoil and disquiet—sometimes arising from nowhere over seemingly minor issues—that can make adolescence such a troubling and troublesome period for both teenagers and those who care for them.

Psychological Theories of Development

No single psychological theory provides sufficient perspective to explain adequately the multidimensional nature of human development. Of the many developmental theories available, three will be used here to help explain and illustrate psychological maturation: the psychoanalytical theory, which encompasses psychosexual development as embodied in the writings of Sigmund Freud and psychosocial development as interpreted by Erik Erikson; the cognitive-intellectual theory as formulated by Jean Piaget; and learning theory, a behavioristic approach to development based on stimulus-response psychology (see Figure 3.1).

Psychoanalytical theory provides a conceptual framework for understanding the development of intrinsic personality structure (Freud) and the process of integrating the individual into society (Erikson). It is a particularly useful tool for explaining the person's underlying motivations (which are often unconscious) for certain behaviors.

The cognitive-intellectual theory provides a framework for conceptualizing how children and adolescents think and therefore how they understand objects and events in the world. The work of Lawrence Kohlberg will serve as an example of the application of cognitive-intellectual theory to one aspect of human thinking: the development of moral reasoning. Clinically, cognitive-intellectual theory permits the structuring of interventions that can be comprehended and acted on appropriately by patients of various ages.

Learning theory, especially the pioneering work of Robert Sears, one of the earliest social learning theorists to integrate behavior with development in the framework of Freudian psychology, is a rich source of intervention strategies. At first glance, manipulation of behavior may appear to be a superficial approach to management of stressful situations. However, truly effective management techniques, even though based on a behavioral model, actually involve a combination of approaches that takes into account cognitive level and basic personality needs as well.

In the following discussion of these various developmental theories, several principles will emerge:

1. Development is a stepwise process.
2. The various elements of the maturational process develop in parallel.
3. Experiences in each stage influence how the individual will pass through succeeding stages.

Figure 3.1. Physiological and Psychological Growth and Development.

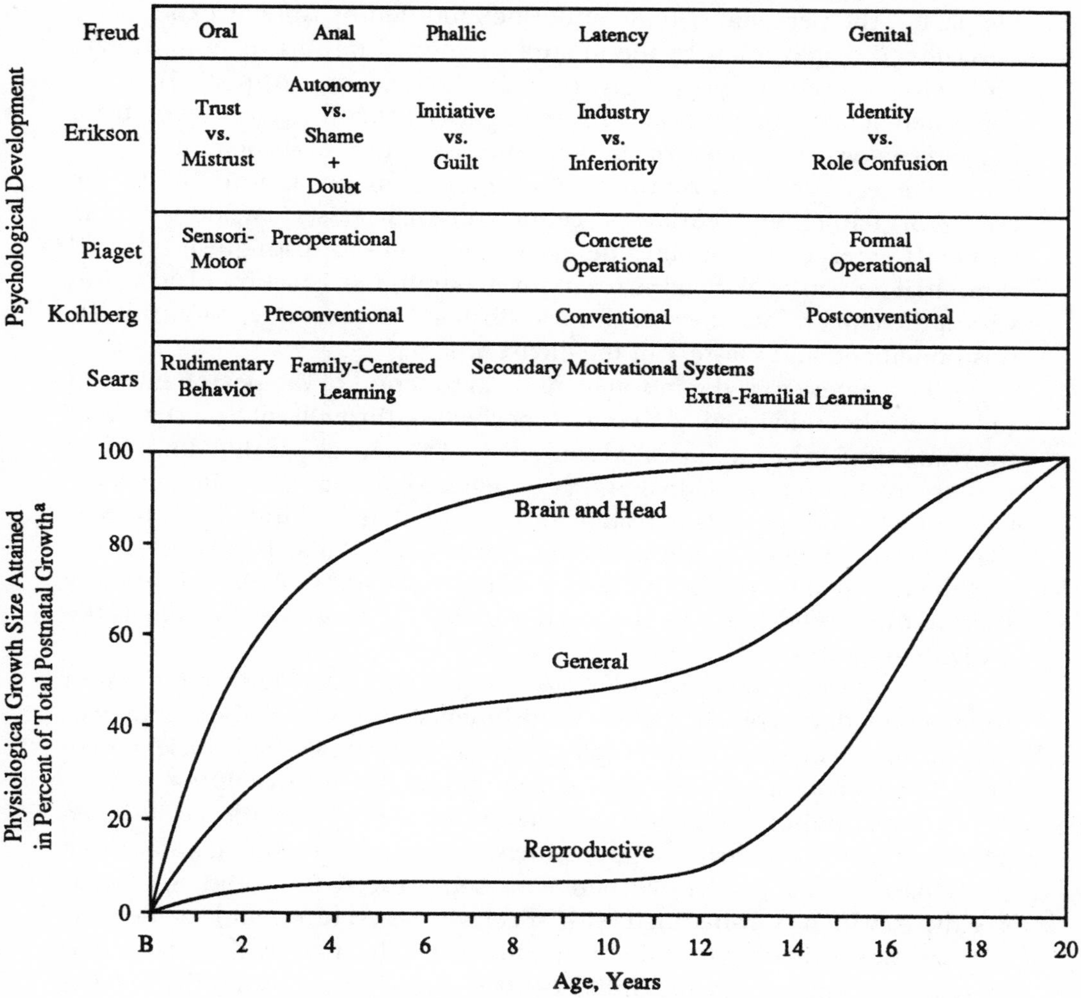
Psychological Development
Freud
Oral
Anal
Phallic
Latency
Genital
Erikson
Trust vs. Mistrust
Autonomy vs. Shame + Doubt
Initiative vs. Guilt
Industry vs. Inferiority
Identity vs. Role Confusion
Piaget
Sensori-Motor
Preoperational
Concrete Operational
Formal Operational
Kohlberg
Preconventional
Conventional
Postconventional
Sears
Rudimentary Behavior
Family-Centered Learning
Secondary Motivational Systems
Extra-Familial Learning
Physiological Growth Size Attained in Percent of Total Postnatal Growth[a]
100
80
60
40
20
0
Brain and Head
General
Reproductive
B
2
4
6
8
10
12
14
16
18
20
Age, Years

[a]Bottom figure modified from Tanner, J. M., 1962, *Growth at Adolescence.* (2nd ed.) Oxford, England: Blackwell Scientific Publications Ltd.

Source: Reproduced by permission from Sahler, Olle Jane Z., and McAnarney, Elizabeth R.: *The Child from Three to Eighteen,* St. Louis, 1981, The C. V. Mosby Co.

4. Development is multifaceted, and physiological, affective, and cognitive elements help determine and explain observable behavior.

Psychoanalytical Theory

Organization of Personality. The total personality, as envisioned by Freud, consists of three major systems: the id, the ego, and the superego. The id, or basic foundation of personality, functions to avoid pain and attain satisfaction or pleasure. According to Freud, the id represents the inaccessible part of the personality that cannot be modified by time or experience. Behaviors directed solely by the id are demanding, impulsive, nonrational, and self-centered. Interestingly, in seeking pleasure, unrestrained id-motivated behavior may actually increase pain by eliciting punishment from the external world because of the self-centered nature of its demands.

The ego, or executive function of the personality, is governed by the reality principle, an accurate perception of what exists outside the individual. It emerges as the child develops the ability to distinguish self and nonself. The aim of the ego is to attain maximum satisfaction of id drives within the constraints of the real world through, for example, compromise, postponement, and mastery of the environment.

The superego is the moral or judicial function of the personality and represents the individual's striving for perfection through internalization of the traditional ideals, values, and standards of society as handed down from parents to children. Ego-ideal and conscience represent the child's conceptions of what the parents consider morally good and morally bad, respectively. These judgments represent another set of standards (like pleasure-seeking and reality) to which the individual must adapt. Although initially rigid in the young child, the superego usually becomes more flexible as the individual matures.

According to Freud, feelings of guilt or satisfaction represent superego-mediated psychological "punishments" or "rewards." Consequences may be either physical (for example, psychosomatic illness or a sense of well-being) or psychological (for example, emotional distress or euphoria).

Other important elements of Freudian theory include (1) the two groups of instinctual drives (ego-instincts, such as hunger, thirst, and escape from pain, which are concerned with self-preservation; and libido, or sex drive, which is concerned with species preservation), and (2) defense mechanisms, which protect the individual from the anxiety that is aroused by real or imagined threats. Unlike controls, which tame or modify a drive, defense mechanisms distort reality. Examples of defense mechanisms include repression, denial, regression, projection, intellectualization, and rationalization.

Psychosexual Development. Freud conceptualized human development in terms of the sexual instinct, which includes drives for pleasurable activities involving both genital and nongenital stimulation of various body parts or erogenous zones (Table 3.1). The three primary erogenous zones are each associated with a vital need: the mouth with eating, the anus with elimination, and the genitalia with reproduction. The sequential ordering of the primacy of each erogenous zone gives rise to the five psychosexual stages of development: oral (infancy), anal (toddlerhood), phallic or oedipal (preschool), latent (school age), and genital (adolescence and beyond). Actions to reduce tension or promote pleasure in each erogenous zone can bring the child into conflict with the parents. The resulting frustrations and

Table 3.1. Freud: Psychosexual Development.

Life-Span Period	Erogenous Zone	Stage	Source of Libidinal Pleasure	Conflict	Resolution
Infancy	Mouth	Oral	Touch; incorporation; biting	Weaning	Independence; emergence of ego
Toddlerhood	Anus	Anal	Expulsion; retention	Toilet training	Self-control
Preschool/ kindergarten	Genitalia	Phallic	Masturbation	Oedipus complex	Identification with same-sexed parent; emergence of superego
School age	—	Latency	—	—	—
Adolescence/ adulthood	Genitalia	Genital	Sexual stimulation	Incest taboo: frustration of genital impulses	Selection of heterosexual partner

Source: Reproduced by permission from Sahler, Olle Jane Z., and McAnarney, Elizabeth R.: *The Child from Three to Eighteen*, St. Louis, 1981, The C. V. Mosby Co.

anxieties lead to the development of both adaptive responses and defense mechanisms.

Psychosocial Development. Erikson's "eight ages of man" represent a reformulation and extension of Freud's five psychosexual stages. At each age, a basic conflict must be resolved before the individual can move on to the next maturational age. Although there are many similarities between the theories of Freud and those of Erikson, Erikson is concerned less with the effects of child-rearing practices on intrinsic personality development and more with the effects of the contextual social milieu on the maturing individual; that is, he replaces the child-mother-father triad with the historical-cultural-social reality of the family. Erikson also focuses optimistically on an individual's potential for successful resolution of developmental crises rather than pessimistically on the potential for psychological dysfunction.

Erikson postulates that at each stage in the process of socialization (the steps by which a child becomes an adult), the individual is presented with the task of integrating him- or herself into society by confronting opposing forces that influence interactions with the environment. The goal is to establish a dynamic equilibrium among these forces in which, ideally, there is greater prominence of the positive attribute. However, whatever equilibrium the person establishes produces a new set of forces as the basis for the next maturational age. As shown in Table 3.2, the first five ages of Erikson's psychosocial scheme are closely correlated with Freud's five stages of psychosexual development but are recast in terms of trust, autonomy, initiative, industry, and identity.

Table 3.2. Erikson: Psychosocial Development—Eight Ages of Man.

Life-Span Period[a]	Psychosexual Stage	"Age"	Description
Infancy	Oral	I. Basic trust vs. basic mistrust	"The general state of trust...implies not only that one has learned to rely on the sameness and continuity of the outer providers, but also that one may trust oneself..." (p. 248)
Toddlerhood	Anal	II. Autonomy vs. shame and doubt	"From a sense of self-control without loss of self-esteem comes a lasting sense of good will and pride..." (p. 254)
Preschool and kindergarten	Phallic	III. Initiative vs. guilt	"...the child is...ready...to become bigger in a sense of sharing obligation and performance...(he moves) toward the possible and the tangible which permits the dreams of early childhood to be attached to the goals of an active adult life." (p. 258)
School age	Latency	IV. Industry vs. inferiority	"...he now learns to win recognition by producing things." (p. 259)
Adolescence	Genital	V. Identity vs. role confusion	"The sense of ego identity, then, is the accrued confidence that the inner sameness and continuity prepared in the past are matched by the sameness and continuity of one's meaning for others, as evidenced in the tangible promise of a 'career.'" (pp. 261–262)
Young adulthood	Genital	VI. Intimacy vs. isolation	"...the young adult, emerging from the search for and the insistence on identity, is eager and willing to fuse his identity with that of others. He is ready for intimacy..." (p. 263)
Middle age	Genital	VII. Generativity vs. stagnation	"Generativity, then, is primarily the concern in establishing and guiding the next generation..." (p. 267)
Old age	Genital	VIII. Ego integrity vs. despair	"Only in him who in some way has taken care of things and people and has adapted himself to the triumphs and disappointments adherent to being, the originator of others or the generator of products and ideas—only in him may gradually ripen the fruit of these seven stages." (p. 268)

Note: Based on data from Erikson, E. H. 1950. *Childhood and Society.* New York: W. W. Norton & Co., Inc.

[a] Like the stages of psychosexual development, the psychosocial developmental stages are dependent upon the attainment of characteristics that are not easily quantifiable. The designated life-span periods identify the times of life when the concerns of a particular "age" are most prominent.

Source: Reproduced by permission from Sahler, Olle Jane Z., and McAnarney, Elizabeth R.: *The Child from Three to Eighteen,* St. Louis, 1981, The C. V. Mosby Co.

Cognitive Theory

Cognitive Development. Piaget's work centered on the development of cognition, the process of acquiring and using knowledge. Cognition includes elements of both awareness and judgment and develops in parallel with emotional and social growth. Although Piaget held the premise that emotions represent the motivational force behind intellectual activity, his work focuses almost exclusively on how, rather than why, children learn. Factors that are identified as major influences on cognitive development include neurological maturation, social environment, experience, and capability for internal reorganization. Heredity sets broad limits on intellectual functioning. Primitive neurological reflexes determine most early functioning; thereafter, experience modifies or reorganizes reflexes into purposeful physical and mental activity.

The two major principles of Piaget's theory are (1) that all species tend to organize (or hierarchically order) their activities and (2) that they tend to adapt by assimilation (using already available activities) and accommodation (developing new activities in response to environmental demands). Piaget further argues that knowledge about reality is attributable both to experience (the action of things upon us) and to reason (our mental actions upon things) and that the reasoning of children is distinctly different from that of adults.

Piaget (Table 3.3) defined four sequential periods of cognitive development: the sensorimotor (preverbal; birth to two years), the preoperational (prelogical; two to seven years), the concrete operational (logical; seven to twelve years), and the formal operational (abstractive; adolescence and beyond).

Moral Development. The judgment or opinion-forming facet of cognition has been studied in the context of moral development. The work of Lawrence Kohlberg on experimental honesty in children four to fourteen years of age has revealed that, although there appears to be no consistent relationship between maturational level and ability to resist temptation, the morality of adults is qualitatively different from that of children. To explain these differences, Kohlberg attempted to apply cognitive-intellectual principles to the study of the development of moral judgment. Kohlberg's theory describes moral thought processes rather than actual behavior, thus providing some explanation for how and why a child may arrive at a particular moral decision; the theory does not, however, provide a basis for altering behavior.

Kohlberg has elaborated six stages of moral development grouped into a three-level progression from an egocentric understanding of fairness based on individual need (preconventional-premoral judgments) to a conception of fairness based on shared conventions about agreement (conventional-moral judgments) and culminating in an understanding of fairness that rests on the freestanding logic of equality and reciprocity (postconventional-principled judgments) (Table 3.4).

Table 3.3. Piaget: Cognitive Development.

Age (Approximate Years)	Stage	Distinguishing Characteristics of Cognitive Function
0 to 2	Sensorimotor	*Preverbal* Reflexive activity leading to purposeful activity Development of object permanence, rudimentary thought
2 to 7	Preoperational	*Prelogical* Inability to deal with several aspects of a problem simultaneously Development of semiotic function (use of symbols, representational language)
7 to 12	Concrete operational	*Logical* Problem solving restricted to physically present or real objects and/or imagery Development of logical operations (e.g., classification, conservation, reversibility)
12 +	Formal operational	*Abstract* Comprehension of purely abstract or symbolic content Development of advanced logical operations (e.g., complex analogy, induction, deduction, higher mathematics)

Source: Reproduced by permission from Sahler, Olle Jane Z., and McAnarney, Elizabeth R.: *The Child from Three to Eighteen*, St. Louis, 1981, The C. V. Mosby Co.

Learning Theory

The basic principles of learning theory are similar to those of strict stimulus-response (S-R) psychology and include the following:

1. Behavior is learned.
2. All varieties, combinations, and patterns of non-mutually exclusive behaviors can be learned.
3. Behavior is learned through reinforcement.
4. Behavior can be conditioned.
5. Behavior can be shaped.
6. Behavior can be learned through observation and imitation.

Of the various research approaches constituting the broad school of behaviorism, that of Robert Sears, in particular, attempted to explain the early development of the child as it can be observed and studied objectively in the laboratory setting, in the context of psychoanalytical theory. Thus, the developmental system that he devised is based on data derived from overt behavior (observable social interactions) rather than from the retrospective analysis of experiences that characterizes Freudian psychology.

Table 3.4. Kohlberg: Moral Development.

Age (Approximate Years)	Level	Basis of Moral Judgment	Developmental Stage	Characteristics
0 to 1	I. Preconventional (premoral)	Consequences (including punishment), conformity to rules	1. Punishment-obedience	Egocentric, no moral concepts
1 to 2			2. Instrumental-relativistic	Satisfaction of own needs
2 to 6	II. Conventional (moral)	Good and right roles	3. "Good boy"–"nice girl"	Desire to please others
6 to 12			4. "Law and order"	Obligation to duty, respect for authority
12 +	III. Postconventional (principled)	Principles, rights, values	5. Social contract, legalistic 6. Universal-ethical-principled	Relativism of personal values and opinions Conscience dictates action in accord with self-chosen principles

Source: Reproduced by permission from Sahler, Olle Jane Z., and McAnarney, Elizabeth R.: *The Child from Three to Eighteen*, St. Louis, 1981, The C. V. Mosby Co.

The S-R cycle is basic to Sears's behavioral formulation. The stimulus activating a response also determines when, where, and how the individual will respond. The degree or type of reinforcement associated with a response determines whether that particular action cycle will be fleeting (because it is reinforced little or not at all) or become fixed (because it is reinforced to a substantial degree). Although in classic studies of behavior in animals, food and pain are the most commonly used reinforcers, in human beings, reinforcement may be either tangible (food, money) or intangible (praise, fulfillment of a desire to be like some admired person who serves as a model). Thus, overt human behavior, to the social learning theorist, has both affective and cognitive as well as purely physiological components.

In any S-R cycle, the response of one person can act as a stimulus for a behavior in another (for example, crying in a child elicits a comforting response in the care giver). Indeed, almost all human actions are interactions; that is, a person is responding as well as socially corresponding.

In Sears's formulation (Table 3.5), behavioral development proceeds through three primary phases:

Phase I: Rudimentary (reflexive) behavior based on innate needs that is modified by family-centered learning (infancy). The child learns (imitates) behaviors modeled and reinforced by the parents or other primary care givers with whom the child identifies.
Phase II: Extended-family-centered learning (toddlerhood-preschool).

Table 3.5. Sears: A Social Learning Theory of Development.

Life-Span Period	Phase	Description
Infancy	I. Rudimentary behavior: initial behavioral learning	Basic need requirements met within intimate parental environment Positive reinforcement is primary socializing agent
Toddlerhood/ preschool	II. Secondary motivational systems: family-centered learning	Socialization within larger family environment Negative reinforcement introduced as socializing agent
School age/ adulthood	III. Secondary motivational systems: extrafamilial learning	Social penetration into neighborhood and beyond Controls universally defined and strictly enforced

Source: Reproduced by permission from Sahler, Olle Jane Z., and McAnarney, Elizabeth R.: *The Child from Three to Eighteen*, St. Louis, 1981, The C. V. Mosby Co.

The pool of models and reinforcers of behavior extends beyond the limits of the immediate nuclear family.

Phase III: Extrafamilial learning (school age and beyond). The individual learns from models derived from a variety of social groups, including teachers, peers, and serendipitous acquaintances. Imitation does not, however, preclude the development of unique individual standards and views, because the specific person is the sum of his or her own personal experiences.

In essence, social learning theory postulates that behavior is the product of the immediate social experiences that a person has while being reared; that is, behavioral development is a consequence of learning. The first teachers are the parents; later, the extended family and, finally, the social group also serve as teachers.

Infancy and Childhood: The Antecedents of Adolescence

To understand adolescence, it is important to understand the developmental processes that occur previously to bring the child to the point at which identity formation and assumption of responsibility for self-governance become the major issues of conflict and resolution. That is, adolescence marks the end of the infancy-childhood continuum; the child enters into adolescence with a long history of human experience that has already molded a certain character structure and style of coping that will influence adaptation to the physiological and psychological stresses that lie ahead. Indeed, past coping behavior is the best predictor of future coping behavior. Thus, analysis of how the child and family have met developmental challenges throughout earlier life stages provides key information about (1) how they are likely to approach the stresses of adolescence and (2) what adjustments in their usual style of functioning will be necessary to optimize the child's growth potential during this next developmental stage.

Development During Infancy

The earliest interaction of the infant is with the parents. According to Freudian developmental theory, the mouth is the major source of pleasure and tension for the infant. Because the infant is dependent on another for fulfillment of oral pleasure and relief from oral stress, giving and withholding of food become equated with love and rejection, respectively. If an infant becomes anxious when threatened by the loss of oral satisfaction, that anxiety may interfere with its learning how to satisfy its own needs and lead to overdependency on others.

In parallel with Freudian theory, the earliest stage in Erikson's theory is the "age of basic trust versus mistrust." However, rather than focusing only on issues of eating or orality, Erikson views the infant as seeking satisfaction for all bodily and emotional needs. By learning that others can be relied on and trusted to provide for these needs, children learn how to rely on and trust themselves. However, if important figures (parents) do not predictably give nurturance, the infant may never learn to trust; eventually, it may become wary of (mistrust) all relationships. Mistrust in others may ultimately result in development of an "affectionless" character style in which lasting relationships are impossible. That is, the individual can never really believe that someone could be truly committed to him or her and vice versa.

According to Piaget's cognitive theory, the distinguishing characteristic of this earliest, or sensorimotor, period is the preverbal nature of the infant's interactions with the environment. The infant uses sensory input to gain information and increasing motor capabilities to seek out new experiences and modify the environment. Important cognitive milestones during this stage include imitative, then novel, and finally purposive actions and initial understanding of object permanence. The development of language marks the end of this developmental phase.

Social learning theory, as applied by Sears to the concept of dependency, helps to explain why certain behaviors occur. The child is physiologically dependent from the moment of conception and physically dependent from the moment of birth. Psychological dependence develops during early infancy and can be directed toward the parents or others. The earliest manifestation of dependency is through innate or reflexive behavior that attracts the notice of care givers. As care givers repeatedly and consistently meet the infant's physical or psychological need as signaled by, for example, crying, the attention itself acts to reinforce the infant's behavior. Later, the child learns to recognize signs of approval (laughing) or disapproval (scolding voice) and, further, what behaviors bring approval (that is, are positively reinforced). Because, generally, behaviors that bring approval are socially conforming actions, nonconforming behaviors are extinguished or inhibited as this first stage of the socialization process proceeds.

The composite view of development during infancy, then, is that (1) innate primitive reflexes form the basis for all initial human interactions, of which nurturing through feeding is the most prominent; (2) although the parent-child dyad forms the most important interpersonal relationship, others who provide nurturing also become distinguishable to the infant and are incorporated into its world of care-giving others; and (3) through repeated, consistent, positive interactions that meet the infant's basic physical needs, the infant becomes psychologically attached in trusting relationships. The earliest nonreflexive behaviors occur as a result of spontaneous imitation. Through learning about what actions elicit approval, the infant adopts desired (socially conforming) behaviors, thereby further increasing the likelihood of positive interactions in the future.

Development During Young Childhood

Toddlerhood. The second, or anal, stage of Freudian psychosexual development typically occurs during the second to fourth years of life. Pleasure and tension are focused in the anal zone. Expulsion of fecal material that exerts pressure on the lower gastrointestinal tract brings relief. Explosive expulsion is considered by analytical theorists to be prototypical for such behaviors as emotional outbursts, temper, and rages.

Toilet training is usually the first crucial experience that a child has with discipline and external authority. It represents a conflict between instinctual drive and prescribed social behavior. A wide variety of parent-child interactions around toilet training and their possible consequences have been described; for example, strict, punitive training may result in intentional soiling.

Erikson has termed this stage "autonomy versus shame and doubt." As children learn that personal behavior can be self-determined, they constantly seek to exercise autonomy. Indeed, "me do it" is a favorite phrase of the two-year-old. The person to whom the child is most likely to reveal any limitations or from whom help might be sought is a trusted person. The child who mistrusts can never show vulnerability for fear of being ridiculed or abandoned. That is, children who never feel loved just for themselves and who believe, therefore, that they have no intrinsic self-worth that binds others to them feel compelled to always present some idealized facade of themselves to the world: "I am never wrong"; "There is nothing I can't do."

The Preschool Period. During the third psychoanalytical stage, the phallic stage, which occurs between the fourth and seventh years of life, children are actively dealing with two interrelated issues: identification with the same-sexed parent and the development of the superego.

Identification is the process, hypothesized by Freud, through which an individual comes to think, feel, and behave as though the characteristics of another person (or model) belonged to that individual. Although identification may involve imitation (acting like the model), the two terms are not synonymous. Identification is far more complex than imitation and involves acting as if one were the other person rather than merely acting like the other person. That is, the boy acts as if he were his father and the girl acts as if she were her mother. In so doing, the child adopts his or her conception of those values, standards, beliefs, and attitudes held by the parent.

Erikson's formulation of the preschool period is entitled "initiative versus guilt." As children become participants in ever widening social and spatial spheres, they are challenged to new activity and purpose. As they desire to do things as autonomous individuals, their desires may conflict with the desires of others. The role of society is to help the child learn self-modulation or self-restraint so that desires can be met, but within the limits of what is acceptable as defined by the family or social group.

According to Piaget, the child's thought processes in this second, or preoperational, stage of cognitive development are best described as pre-logical. Salient characteristics include centration (the inability to consider several aspects of a situation simultaneously); syncretism (a tendency to group several apparently unrelated objects or events together into a confused whole); juxtaposition (a tendency to connect objects or events without understanding their true connection, if any); and an inability to understand part-whole or ordinal relations. Preoperational thought also lacks reversibility (appreciation of the bidirectionality of successive changes or transformations) and is limited by egocentricism (seeing the world from one point of view, usually with the child as origin of all actions) and magical thinking (the equation of thought or fantasy with action; that is, the feeling that mere wishing can cause some external event).

Concepts of right and wrong during this stage are heavily influenced by the child's inherent and inescapable cognitive limitations. Work by Kohlberg with children at the preoperational stage has shown that the child's judgment about good and bad behavior potentially can move through as many as three levels of moral reasoning: first, a "punishment-obedience" orientation (rules are absolute; motives are not considered); then an "instrumental-relativistic" orientation (right behavior is that which satisfies the individual's own needs and, only by chance, the needs of others; there is little understanding of loyalty and gratitude; and fairness, reciprocity, and sharing are pragmatic—"I help you, you help me"); and finally a "good boy"–"nice girl" orientation (good behavior is that which pleases and helps others and is approved by them).

It is during the young childhood stage that discipline becomes a major part of the repertoire of adult-child interaction. By late in the second year, intention (the conscious desire to do some act) develops. Thus, although children have little or no understanding of the consequences of various actions, intent (sometimes misunderstood by the parent as desire to disobey rather than merely as desire to do the act) becomes a focal point for parent-child conflict and for the emergence of the concept of discipline.

Discipline is defined as training that corrects, molds, strengthens, or perfects. Discipline can occur retrospectively in the form of punishment for undesirable past behaviors or prospectively through modeling of desirable future behaviors. The potential effects of these two methods on the as yet fragile self-concept of the child are perhaps most pronounced during young childhood, the stage during which conscience (and, therefore, also guilt) is hypothesized to develop. Thus, the style of discipline that the parents choose can have major effects on how the child learns, the child's preparation for independent participation in novel experiences, and the child's self-confidence.

In the punishment mode of discipline, physical or emotional discomfort (negative reinforcement) is used to deter performance of a particular action. A major drawback to the punishment method is that, except by negative inference, little information is given to the child about appropriate and desirable future behavior. In contrast, in the modeling mode of discipline, appropriate and desirable behavior is demonstrated to the child before the occasion arises to use that behavior. Positive, rather than negative, reinforcement is used whenever the child's behavior approaches what is expected, and additional instruction is given to help the child improve the behavior even further in the future. This process is called "shaping"; it not only points out to the child what is incorrect but also gives the child some idea of what is correct so that this information can be used later.

In sum, then, young children are struggling with issues of self-determination and incorporation of standards of behavior and values that reflect those of their society as exemplified by their parents. The struggle is intensified by a number of cognitive idiosyncrasies unique to this developmental stage that prevent children from accurately understanding the world and events in it. Such limitations can fuel parent-child conflicts when parents try to use principles of logic—which the child truly cannot comprehend—to resolve differences between them. During the earliest stages of young childhood, power, whether exerted by the parent or by the child, becomes the driving force of actions. As the child matures in the context of Erikson's "initiative versus guilt," it is society's obligation to allow the child to take the lead under selected circumstances and to help the child feel good about his or her decision making even if the result is not wholly on target. This is done by identifying the positive attributes of the child's initiative while demonstrating modifications in behavior that will achieve the child's goal more effectively or with greater social desirability, without inducing feelings of guilt for having done something incorrectly.

Development During School Age

The school-age child has been described by Freud as being in a state of psychosexual latency. That is, sexual drives play a relatively minor role in motivating behavior. During this sexually quiescent period, other, nonsexual drives predominate and serve to stimulate activity. It is important to note that consolidation of gender identity (begun during the oedipal stage through identification with the same-sex parent) continues throughout this period and is assisted by almost exclusive association with same-sex playmates. Interest in sex and sex roles, although diminished, is not, however, absent. Instead, it tends to be channeled into preoccupation with physical aggressiveness in boys and fantasy play about families in girls.

In Erikson's formulation, the school-age period is known as "industry versus inferiority." Mastery of tasks and a sense of doing well with and among peers are the most important elements of this stage. Children strive to increase and improve their skills through use of tools and their knowledge of the world through systematic instruction. Both pleasure and a sense of self-worth are attained through successful completion of work. Attentiveness, application, diligence, and a desire to please are hallmarks of this period. Because children equate degree of self-worth with the quality of their work, the danger to children at this stage is that they may feel inferior if their work is seen as inadequate or if the natural strength of their skills is not equal to that of peers. As a consequence, it is crucial to help the child understand that intrinsic worth is not measured solely by performance ability.

Cognitively, school-age children are in the concrete operational stage, which is distinguished by the development of logical thinking about concrete (physically present) problems. During this period, children learn how to classify objects, the concept of inclusion, and the principle of constancy, or, in Piaget's terminology, conservation (the ability to understand that physical properties such as quantity, substance, weight, and volume are not changed by mere movement or rearrangement in space). Like all cognitive skills, the ability to conserve, for example, follows a predictable pattern. Although most children understand equality as early as four or five years of age, the ability to conserve volume, the last concept mastered in this category, does not appear until as late as eleven or twelve years of age. Such sequencing has important implications not only for appropriate developmentally based temporal structuring of school curricula but also for helping parents understand the apparently nonsensical arguments that punctuate dinner table conversations among siblings of this and earlier cognitive stages.

Moral judgment of the school-age child is tied to performance of good or right roles, maintenance of conventional order, and fulfillment of the expectations of others. The "good boy"–"nice girl" orientation gradually gives way to a "law and order" orientation, in which children focus on authority and fixed rules in their moral decision making. Right behavior consists of doing what is expected and showing respect for authority. Because of concretism, fixed laws of conduct, such as abiding by the rules and fair play, govern all aspects of the child's life. Although it is possible for children of this age to take into account intent (doing harm while trying to do good versus while breaking a rule), rules are rarely bent, because they have little understanding of the guiding principle behind a particular rule. Thus, children at this age are often very intolerant of deviation from the norm in either themselves or others.

With entry into school, children are exposed to and begin to absorb learning beyond the bounds of the family. Children seek admiration or approval (positive reinforcement) through such socially desirable behaviors as compliance with expectations. Negative attention-seeking behaviors (teasing, exhibitionism, practical joking) also persist; if not checked, they can remain integral to the child's personality. Negative reinforcement of such behaviors is only part of the solution; it is also necessary to provide positive reinforcement for more acceptable behaviors, even if they only approximate what is desired. It is essential to remember that it is as easy to destroy as it is to promote the tenuous self-concept of the school-age child.

It is, thus, these children who are psychosexually latent, industrious, curious about the world around them, strictly rule abiding, and somewhat intolerant of deviation who enter into the world of adolescence. In the best of all possible worlds, they are even-tempered, trust others, tolerate frustration, act independently but with a sense of responsibility to the whole, are comfortable with their gifts and talents, and have formed reciprocal relationships based on mutual respect for the rights of others. They have grown, slowly but steadily, and acquired many skills, almost thoughtlessly, merely by living.

Adolescence: The Search for Identity and Autonomy

Both physiologically and psychologically, adolescence is most conveniently thought of as a three-stage process. If observable physical markers are used, sexual maturity ratings (SMR) provide criteria to differentiate the stages. Early adolescence (SMR 2–3) is characterized by initial breast development, appearance of sexual hair, and the height spurt in girls and testicular development, initial penile enlargement, and the appearance of sexual hair in boys. Middle adolescence (SMR 3–4) is characterized by continued breast and sexual hair development, menarche, and slowed growth velocity in girls and seminal fluid production, more frequent erections, continued sexual hair development, and the growth spurt in boys. Late adolescence (SMR 4–5) is characterized by continued but less dramatic changes in breast contour and sexual hair distribution, establishment of a regular menstrual pattern with ovulation, and little skeletal growth in girls and by minor growth in testicular volume and penile length, completion of sexual hair development, and persistent but markedly decelerated skeletal growth in boys.

Many investigators have attempted to correlate the hormonal changes of puberty with behavior. For various reasons, some of which are discussed in Chapter Two, the methodological inadequacies of current hormone research continue to impede substantive progress in our understanding of these relationships. However, regardless of the precise mechanisms of action, the physical (hormonal, somatic) changes associated with pubescence clearly have an effect on the emotional, behavioral, and personality organization of the individual, which can result in major mood swings that often occur unexpectedly and out of proportion to the apparent provocation.

Anna Freud described adolescence as a period of increased anxiety, heightened conflict over expression of impulses, greater affective lability, and psychologically regressive behavior. It came to be assumed that a high degree of psychological conflict and stress invariably occurred. More recently, it has been found that probably only a minority of adolescents exhibit the degree of anxiety, depression, distrust, extreme mood swing, and lack of self-confidence once thought to be characteristic of this stage. However, even though only some adolescents experience true turmoil or chaos, most do experience at least periodic disequilibrium in their relationships with themselves and others.

Because of their increased ability to consider hypothetical possibilities and to "think about thinking," adolescents become cognitively more introspective and analytical as they move further away from childhood. Preoccupation with thought itself is characteristic of the early stages of the formal operational period. Similarly, fantasy, expressed at this age as "If I were" (to distinguish it from the "I am" fantasy of the preoperational period of toddlerhood), consumes a great deal of time and energy as the adolescent daydreams about the infinite variety of hypothetical roles that might be assumed or situations that might arise during life. This cognitive capacity permits contemplation of the ideal, an extraordinary yardstick against which to measure reality.

The ability to conceive both of principles that have validity apart from social authority and convention and of the ideal has a profound effect on moral reasoning. In the "social contract–legalistic" orientation characteristic of this stage, the individual defines right action in terms of general individual rights and standards, with an awareness of the relativism of personal values and opinions. Procedural rules for reaching consensus are emphasized, and laws are recognized as changeable through rational consideration of social utility. That is, adolescents come to understand that laws are made for a purpose and can be changed if they do not serve that purpose well. A possibly higher level of moral reasoning is embodied in the "universal-ethical-principled" orientation. In this orientation, right behavior is defined as a decision of conscience in accord with self-chosen ethical principles that are abstract (for example, the Golden Rule) rather than concrete (for example, the Ten Commandments); and universal principles of justice, reciprocity, equality of human rights, and respect for the dignity of human beings as individual persons are applied.

The world of the adolescent extends well beyond the boundaries of family and school, and each social system influences notions of acceptable and unacceptable behavior. Consistencies that transcend systems teach adolescents about the universality of certain acceptable behaviors: thus, they become free to move into novel situations guided by their sense of the constancy of much of human interaction.

Early Adolescence: "Who Am I as a Physical Being?" and the Pull of Peer Relationships

The hallmark of early adolescence, especially for girls, is rapid change in physical appearance. The many conspicuous biological changes occurring during this time focus the attention of the individual on the self and dramatically heighten self-awareness.

The timing of the onset of puberty and the first appearance of secondary sex characteristics defines the child as an early, average, or late developer within his or her chronological peer group. Research on the psychosocial effects of the timing of maturation has revealed that the desirability of early maturation differs for boys and for girls. In general, investigators have found that early-maturing boys appear more relaxed and attractive to adults and more attractive and popular to peers; during high school, early-maturing boys are more likely to be chosen as leaders in group activities. Greater physical prowess at an earlier age also increases the likelihood that early-maturing boys will be leaders in sports. On tests of personality, however, early maturers have been found to be more somber, anxious, and submissive as well as less exploratory and intellectually curious than late maturers. Although at first glance there may appear to be major discrepancies between how early-maturing boys are viewed by others (attractive leaders) and their intrapsychic characteristics (somber, less exploratory), the juxtaposition of the two in the same individual attests to the fact that attributes in a teenage boy that are socially desirable to adults and thus aid him in attaining positions of leadership are exactly those attributes that enhance conformity with adult authority.

Although the findings for girls are somewhat inconsistent and may depend on factors other than maturational age, most studies have revealed that early-maturing girls are more likely to feel conspicuous, be submissive and indifferent in social situations, lack poise, and display loss of control, unrest, explosive temper, introversion, and whiny behavior. Late-maturing girls, in contrast, have been found to be more outgoing, confident, and assured and have greater leadership qualities than their early-maturing counterparts.

Because of the rapid physical changes occurring during early adolescence, young adolescents are constantly evaluating and reevaluating their views of their own bodies in the context both of how they compare to their peers and of how they compare to some imaginary desired outcome. A number of intervening variables appear to be particularly important in mediating the adolescent's emotional evaluation of and adaptation to changing physique. These include (1) the evaluations, reactions, and impressions imparted by others; (2) certain personality characteristics (such as self-esteem, gender identity); and (3) sociocultural factors, such as prevailing standards of attractiveness. With regard to this last factor, it has been found that by the time children are in the fifth grade, they have already adopted society's criteria for evaluating attractiveness and can apply them consistently to body type, mode of dress, and behavior. This is not surprising given that social conformity, compliance with rules, and the belief that they are what they produce and that they are good only if others deem them so are major characteristics of the emerging adolescent.

Young adolescents are frequently self-critical, yet they also can be self-admiring. Boorishness, loudness, and faddish dress may, in part, be explained by the adolescents' failure to differentiate what they believe to be attractive and what others find so. Indeed, the perception that others are constantly evaluating them and the anticipation that the reactions of others will be as critical or as admiring of them as they are of themselves lead adolescents to continually construct or react to an "imaginary audience." It is an audience because adolescents believe that they are the focus of attention and imaginary because this is usually not the case unless they contrive to make it so. The concept of the imaginary audience helps explain the marked self-consciousness, wish for privacy, and reluctance to reveal themselves typical of many adolescents. It also helps explain their fear of critical scrutiny and the fact that shame rather than guilt is a predominant concern of the young teenager.

Perhaps because of the belief that they are so important to so many people (the imaginary audience), adolescents believe that they and their feelings are special and unique. From this belief in uniqueness emerges the "personal fable," a story that adolescents tell themselves that is not true. An example of the personal fable is the unshakable belief of a sexually active young teenage girl that although unwanted pregnancy may happen to others, it will never happen to her, and, therefore, she does not need to use contraception.

The egocentrism (obsessive belief that others are as preoccupied with their appearance and behavior as they are) of young adolescents contributes to a sense that all eyes are fastened on them, that every blemish is immediately obvious, and that any way in which they are different from others is a sign not of (desirable) uniqueness but of some (highly undesirable) failing. In attempting to hide or diminish differences among themselves that are beyond their control, adolescents form tight peer groups that promote superficial similarities by enforcing strict dress and behavior codes. Interestingly, in analyzing the behaviors of peer groups, we find that what appears to be excessive conformity to observing adults is seen as rugged individualism by adolescents. This discrepancy arises because the adults' attention focuses on the similarities of the adolescents' behavior among themselves; in contrast, the adolescent views individualism in relation to the behavior of adults. That is, neither children nor adults, adolescents form an interim culture that, to serve its purpose, must be clearly different from that of either of these two other groups. Although the need to conform with peers may vary with sex, socioeconomic background, relationship with parents, academic achievement, and personality, such variations are thought to influence only the extent of or age at which conformity occurs, rather than the developmental pattern itself. Actually, the role of the peer group in helping young adolescents define identity is particularly important, because at no other developmental stage is the sense of identity so fluid. But peer-group conformity serves another purpose as well: By achieving the semblance of a group identity of their own, adolescents also are able to satisfy some of their needs to be different from parents in more fundamental ways. Thus, as the adolescent is beginning to move away from the family of origin, both physically and emotionally, in preparation for independent living as an adult, the peer group provides a transitional support network of generationally bonded individuals with similar professed dissatisfactions with the past and present and hopes and aspirations for the future.

Even the most understanding parents are limited in their role of helping adolescents struggle to achieve their own adult status. Just by virtue of already being adults, they are regarded by adolescents as separate from them. However, conformity to the peer group does not necessarily imply total disregard of parents or parental values. Indeed, the weight given to either parental or peer opinion depends to a great extent on the adolescents' appraisal of relative merit in a specific situation. Thus, such external issues as dress, taste in music, language, and sexual behavior are more likely to be determined by the peer group, while underlying moral and social values are more likely to be determined by parental influence — although this may not become obvious to either the parents or the child until late adolescence.

Middle Adolescence: "Who Am I as a Sexual Being?" and the Process of Alienation

Middle adolescence is marked by menarche in girls and increased frequency of erections and ejaculations in boys. These pubertal changes produce unpredictable surges in the sexual drive, which are accompanied by unavoidable sexual fantasies and impulses. Just as body image is the major preoccupation of the young adolescent, sexuality is the major preoccupation of the middle adolescent.

During early adolescence, many young people, especially boys, express their sexuality through masturbation. Same-gender sexual encounters are also relatively common, perhaps because they are seen as less threatening than heterosexual behaviors. Indeed, same-gender encounters occur frequently enough to be considered a variant of normal sexual development rather than a sign of fixed homosexual orientation. In some instances, however, such behaviors may be truly indicative of homosexuality. Consequently, any questions that the adolescent may have about erotic feelings or behaviors toward persons of the same sex need to be addressed directly and explored fully; reflexive reassurance that the behavior is merely a passing stage of sexual development is not helpful to the adolescent who is troubled by such behaviors, is struggling with issues of sexual identity, and is seeking confirmation of personal worth and acceptance regardless of final sexual orientation.

Once heterosexual encounters begin, they follow a fairly predictable pattern. The first phase is group dating, with little or no actual boy-girl pairing. This is followed by a transitional phase of double dating, which leads to the final phase, individual couple dating. The earliest sexual activity is holding hands, followed by, usually in order, kissing, petting, and coitus.

Typically, sexual activity occurs more frequently among boys than among girls. Although the reasons for these differences are unclear, several hypotheses have been suggested: (1) females are less likely to discover sexual responses spontaneously, because their sexual organs are less prominent and thus less subject to manipulation learned by chance; (2) because, under experimental conditions, testosterone increases sexual and aggressive behavior in both males and females, the vastly higher levels of testosterone present in adolescent males result in greater sexual aggressiveness and more purely physical drives and gratifications; and (3) girls tend to view sexual gratification as secondary to fulfillment of other needs, such as love, affection, self-esteem, and reassurance, and thus are more likely than boys to abstain from sex in relationships that do not fill such needs. Thus, the motivation to participate in sexual activity can arise for two reasons: to gratify true sexual impulses or to gratify nonsexual needs (for example, to achieve a sense of closeness to someone, to bolster self-esteem, to consolidate gender identity, or, in some instances, to act out against authority).

Among young women, participation in sexual behavior appears to be influenced more by peer values (which tend to be permissive) than by parental values. Behavior is usually consonant with attitude. Thus, about 80 percent of those who believe that premarital sex is acceptable but fewer than 25 percent of those who believe that it is unacceptable will actually participate in coitus before marriage. Furthermore, those whose negative views on premarital sex are most like those of their parents are least likely to have such experiences or, if they do, are more likely to have intercourse only once or with only one partner during the premarital period.

Some sexually active adolescents are serial monogamists who date and have intercourse with one individual exclusively for a period of time; after such a relationship terminates, it is then succeeded by another. Others are so-called sexual adventurers who move freely between and among several sexual partners during a discrete period of time and feel no obligation for faithfulness to any. These two groups of sexually active adolescents differ in their attitudes toward and the meaning that they ascribe to sexual behavior. Most monogamists believe that they and their partner are in love, that they are open and honest with each other, and that sex is only a part of the total relationship. Although they feel that personal freedom is important and thus are not ready to commit themselves to marriage, the majority believe that they will or may marry their partner at some time in the future. In contrast, sexual adventurers report enjoying sex for its own sake, they do not believe that love is a necessary part of sexual relationships, and, although they do not believe in hurting their partners, neither do they feel any personal responsibility or commitment to them. As a group, monogamists express greater satisfaction with themselves, get along better with their parents, and are more socially, politically, and religiously conventional than sexual adventurers.

Why a particular person or persons are chosen for expression of the sexual drive and the manner in which that expression is fulfilled can be explained, in some measure, in psychoanalytical terms. In brief, Freud postulated that during adolescence there is a rebellion against the infantile superego (conscience), which, although adequate for the needs of the child, is not adequate for the adolescent. That is, the values, standards, and beliefs learned during early childhood are too simplistic or not comprehensive enough to deal with the contradictions and contingencies that adolescents actually encounter or are capable of hypothesizing through formal operational thought.

Rejection of the perceived parental value system adopted earlier through the process of identification leads to a partial recrudescence of the oedipal conflict; that is, the son or daughter no longer wants to be (like) the same-sex parent, because that person is now seen as inadequate as the ultimate role model.

It should be noted that while the parental values themselves were not necessarily simplistic, the young child's cognitive limitations required that they be presented in simplistic terms so that they could be understood. As children mature, the ability to use logic and extrapolation allows them to conjecture about dilemmas not easily solved by the yes-no answers that were sufficient previously. Typically, rather than exploring the nuances and transcendent values of their parents' belief system, adolescents reject the entire system as flawed and inadequate to meet the specific needs of their generation. Indeed, this rejection also stems from another cognitive limitation that will not be overcome until formal operational thought fully matures in late adolescence or adulthood: the inability to understand that specific situational differences do not necessarily change basic value systems.

When viewed in this light, reemergence of the oedipal conflict is actually a helpful concept for explaining some of the selective anger, competitiveness, and emotional distancing between daughters and mothers and between sons and fathers, and the alliances between children and parents of the opposite sex that peak during mid-adolescence. The adolescent knows, however, that emotional closeness to the parent of the opposite sex is impossible and, furthermore, that real competition with the same-sex parent is also impossible. Eventually, both the boy and the girl seek independence from both parents through the process of alienation—loss of affection or interest and a diversion of that affection or interest to another.

Although often painful, alienation serves to force redirection of affection toward people with whom mature genital relationships ultimately are possible. The roots of the alienation process are anchored in the young adolescents' submergence in their peer group. As adolescence progresses, ties to parents become progressively looser as greater independence is gained. In addition, intrafamily relations become strained as the adolescent deals with conflicting emotions: dependent yearnings vying with independent strivings, hostility mixed with love, conflicts over cultural values and social behavior. As a result, many areas of an adolescent's inner life and social behavior cannot be shared comfortably with parents. In addition, a frequently overlooked element is that parents, having managed to repress many of the emotional upheavals of their own adolescence, may have difficulty understanding and sharing their child's problems because of the painful memories evoked, even though they may sincerely wish they could do so.

The product of the alienation process is preparation of the adolescent for movement away from the family of origin psychologically as well as physically. Dependency needs are met elsewhere as the adolescent becomes able to establish intimate, although not necessarily genital, relationships outside the family. The boy chooses a heterosexual partner to replace his mother; similarly, the girl chooses a heterosexual partner to replace her father. According to Freud, full heterosexual maturity, or genital primacy, is attained when feelings directed toward the parent of the opposite sex are successfully transferred to a love object that is not taboo. With such successful transference, the child also completes and solidifies identification with the same-sexed parent. Reintegration into the family, when it occurs, takes place between a more mature and independent adolescent and a family that acknowledges and accommodates to the child as an adult member.

Late Adolescence: "Who Am I as a Vocational Being?" and Reintegration into the Family

The last stage of adolescence, and the one with the least definite end point, encompasses the search for a vocation and a defined role within society. The answer to the question "Who am I as a vocational being?" provides the potential for emancipation from the home, economic self-sufficiency, social recognition as an equal member of society, and the establishment of an independent family unit. As the individual approaches late adolescence, the unwavering preeminence of concern with vocational choice offers proof that, despite preoccupation with the immediate that characterizes membership in the interim peer group, the adolescent's primary goals really are directed toward inclusion in the adult world.

Before the period of real and practical experience in the working world, vocational goals tend to have a theoretical quality. As such experience is obtained, however, adolescents begin to learn whether they can, in fact, achieve a state of resolution that balances the conflicts that they feel between ideals, values, and goals and the realities of adult life. Within this process, they reassess the adult world as well as their own strengths and weaknesses and become more accepting of both.

A significant change in the sex-role stereotyping of vocational opportunities available for both men and women has occurred over the last several decades with the emergence of the two-career family. Prior to World War II, the fundamental basis of a family's status tended to reside in the occupational position of the husband and father, who, as the principal if not sole source of family income, determined the manner and standard of living of the family. During the war, family economic and national manpower considerations made it essential for women to be recruited into the work force. Once there, many stayed, either because they now found themselves sole breadwinner, because they desired the additional income, or because they enjoyed employment. Indeed, recent writing on the subject of vocational choice emphasizes the major contribution that employment outside the home can make to the level of satisfaction, self-worth, and sense of challenge experienced by women and the positive effects (increasing independence and self-reliance of children) that it can have on the family. It has been found, however, that the movement toward equal opportunity in employment is not without drawbacks. Some women who subscribe to more traditional role concepts feel that they are undervalued; women who attempt to fulfill full roles at home as well as in the workplace may suffer from excessive strain, which may be disruptive for other family members as well as for themselves.

Regardless of the potentially negative effects of maternal employment, the trend is clear. While only one-third of women over age sixteen were employed outside the home in 1947, it is estimated that two-thirds of married women, including three-quarters of married women with children living at home, were working outside the home in 1990. Both economic necessity and personal choice may raise that percentage even higher in the future.

Although a majority of the women currently employed still hold traditionally female occupations, the number of young women seeking and gaining employment in traditionally male occupations is growing. While the converse is also true, changes in employment patterns among men have been less extensive. Such changes in employment opportunities and the growing number of role models in a variety of alternative job situations have important implications for today's adolescents struggling with the issue of vocational identity. Although apparently limitless choice may be helpful by broadening horizons for some adolescents, for others it can contribute to role confusion or diffusion.

Vocational choice is actually the result of an orderly developmental process. In the earliest stage, the young child views vocation as a source of imaginative and exciting play; thus, the perceived glamour of being, for example, a firefighter who continually rescues people from burning buildings holds much appeal for the six-year-old, who has no knowledge of the more mundane aspects of that or any other career. However, as the child matures and enters adolescence, both the individual and society respond to the phenomenon of maturation by expecting that the adolescent will earn status realistically by appropriately utilizing both natural and learned skills.

Opportunities to work during middle and late adolescence allow exploration of tentative career choices through experimentation with different vocational possibilities. They also allow individuals to attain a sense of purpose and responsibility, participate in the broader society, learn to communicate more effectively with adults, develop their interests, and enhance and test their skills against real-world criteria. As choice of vocation crystallizes, it reinforces the adolescent's self-concept and becomes an important part of overall identity formation. Satisfactorily doing a job that society values enhances self-esteem and feelings of purpose. Conversely, not engaging in meaningful employment can foster self-doubt, resentment, and poor self-esteem and result in identity confusion.

Factors that influence vocational choice include not only sex but also family values, social class, and socioeconomic conditions; individual differences such as intelligence, special abilities, and aptitudes; and other personality traits, such as motivation, need for prestige, volitional independence, frustration tolerance, sense of responsibility, and degree of executive independence or decision-making capacity. Discrepancy or discord among these factors can lead to major vocational indecision or instability. The two forces that are most likely to come in conflict are family influence (which is particularly strong in adolescents who score high on personality measures of authoritarianism and conformity) and the individual's interests.

Among potential family influences, the father's occupation appears to exert a particularly significant influence on sons. These findings are thought to be related, at least in part, to (1) greater opportunity to become familiar with the father's occupation; (2) greater likelihood of access to the occupation; (3) strong parental motivation, or even pressure, for the son to enter the occupation; and (4) communication of values. Interestingly, it has been found that by age twenty-five, the use of fathers as role models is less important than it was at earlier ages. Possible reasons for this shift include greater autonomy, giving up of the internalized parent, and the increasingly significant importance of nonparental models. This may help explain the finding that career plans of twelfth-grade boys tend to be very unstable; five years after high school graduation, only a small percentage still plan the career they had chosen at the end of high school. The students' scores on interest scales, however, continue to be fairly good predictors of the careers that they will enter as adults. Thus, of the two major influences on male career choice, expressed or perceived family desires and personal interest, the latter is likely to be stronger and more lasting, at least among boys.

Among girls, those whose mothers are employed outside the home are more likely to perceive work as something that they, themselves, will do when they become adults. The vocational attitudes, aspirations, and accomplishments of girls are influenced by the mother's attitude toward employment, degree of satisfaction, sense of accomplishment, and ability to combine employment outside the home with responsibilities in the home.

If the end of adolescence is defined as the point at which the individual becomes psychosocially (emotionally and financially) independent of the family of origin, the increased specialization and prolonged periods of training necessary for career preparation in many fields often extend the last stage of adolescence well into the early to mid twenties and, occasionally, even into the thirties. This delay in becoming a "real person" who has a "real job" has been termed the "psychosocial moratorium," a time of suspended activity in movement toward adult commitments and the next developmental stage.

Erikson describes the psychosocial moratorium as a period of selective permissiveness on the part of society that allows the late adolescent the freedom and opportunity for sustained dependence and/or experimentation without pressure to move on to adulthood. During this time, youth may make deep commitments (both to people and to causes), but these are often transitory and do not become a significant part of adult identity. For the most part, such moratoriums coincide with apprenticeships, college, and even graduate school; for some adolescents, they provide the opportunity for the kinds of adventures (sailing around the world as a deckhand) that become impossible once a commitment is made to a job or spouse. After the turbulence of continuous change during adolescence, such a period of consolidation can serve a useful purpose by allowing adjustment and amendment of what has gone before and adequate preparation for subsequent stages of the adult maturational process.

Toward the end of this period, clearer goal direction emerges, and the late adolescent–young adult begins to take a distinguishable place in society. Identity within a particular vocation is assumed and becomes an integral part of the characteristics by which individuals are defined both by others and by themselves. Armed with the status of an independent contributing member of society, those who have been alienated from the family become reintegrated by negotiating a new role. This role, while necessarily preserving the parent-child relationship, also allows for communication and activity that acknowledges the independence, self-sufficiency, and self-direction of which the adult child is capable. It is of interest that adult children, regardless of the depth of their alienation, are more like their parents in terms of underlying standards and morals than they are unlike them. The evidence of countless generations, each of which has experienced both adolescent upheaval and preservation of the culture, provides strong, recurring proof of this continuity from parent to child.

Once the individual has a sense of identity as a physical, sexual, and vocational being, movement toward the next stage of psychosocial maturity, intimacy, in which the individual has sufficient sense of self to merge with another in a lasting relationship, can proceed.

Special Considerations, Limitations, and Future Directions

"Insight, of course, is an integral part of a clinician's work; when spelled out, however, it must include (rather than pass by) whatever verifiable knowledge, consistent theory, and therapeutic methods are at the clinician's disposal," said Erik H. Erikson in the preface to *Identity and the Life Cycle* (1959).

The Case for Individual Assessment and Flexibility

Just as no single theory of psychological development adequately explains all the multiple facets and determinants of human development, no two individuals grow and develop in exactly the same way. However, there are predictable patterns and interrelationships that allow for both broad generalizations about and specific interpretations of developmental level, expected behavior, and appropriate intervention strategies. In applying developmental theory to a specific problem behavior in a given individual, the practitioner must develop a differential diagnosis similar to that appropriate for any problem in clinical medicine. That is, it is important to determine the most likely etiology of a particular problem and whatever elements of the developmental process may be contributing factors. For example, risk-taking behavior, such as drug overuse, may result from the cognitive limitations characteristic of the personal fable ("I can experiment with drugs because I'll never get addicted"), may represent a desire for greater identification with the peer group in an adolescent struggling with self-identity ("Everybody else does it, so I should, too"), or may be a part of the alienation process ("You don't want me to do it, so I will"). Thus, risk taking (in whatever form) may represent a response to immaturity, curiosity, resentment of authority, anxiety, feelings of isolation, emotional lability, sense of inadequacy, or poor self-esteem. Only through careful interview and observation will the specific motivator eventually become clear and provide the basis for appropriate intervention. The least helpful basis for constructing an intervention is to assume that the motivating force is the same for all adolescents without adequately investigating each individual situation.

Flexibility is key to the treatment process. Unanticipated findings during the course of management alter the practitioner's initial diagnosis of any condition; similarly new information may shed a different perspective on psychosocial issues requiring modification or expansion of the therapeutic plan. Although sometimes discouraging, such events arise from the uncertainty of the clinical process rather than from the innate inadequacy of the clinician. But perhaps the most crucial element of all is helping the adolescent—as well as the family—to become willing partners in the treatment process. Too often, parents want to contract with the clinician to "fix" their child. Helping the family to understand that no single part of the system can be fixed until the entire system changes supports the adolescent by relieving him or her of sole responsibility for familial dysfunction and serves to distribute the burden of change among all the involved and responsible parties. If we truly believe in the interactional model of development, "It's not all your fault" is absolutely true and can be one of the most therapeutically helpful concepts we can impart to a patient of any age.

Insights into Women

A limitation of classical theories about psychological development, as pointed out by Carol Gilligan and others involved in the psychology of women, is that much of the work presented in the foregoing discussion is based on theoretical models derived primarily from experiential and experimental data obtained from boys and men. This has resulted in perhaps undue attention to issues of impulse control, rebelliousness, superego struggles, and achievement and neglect of such issues as intimacy, nurturance, and affiliation. Thus, it can be argued that only to the extent that masculine thought process is also a female trait are the theories valid for girls. Although much of Gilligan's work in considering this issue is focused on conceptions of self, morality, conflict, and choice, her findings have broader implications regarding gender differences that deserve attention in other contexts as well.

One striking difference between boys and girls that has particular relevance to understanding adolescent development is that, in most societies, the feminine personality tends to define itself in relation to and by connection to other people more than the masculine personality does. One potential explanation for this, as derived from the psychoanalytical literature, is that girls, parented during their earliest years primarily by women, tend to fuse the experience of attachment to the mother with the process of identification. Therefore, they tend to see themselves as continuous with and related to the external world. Conversely, boys, also parented primarily by women during their earliest years, need to differentiate themselves and become separate and distinct from their mothers as part of their identification process. Carrying this hypothesis further, some suggest that because masculinity is defined through separation and femininity is defined through attachment, male gender identity is threatened by intimacy, and female gender identity is threatened by separation.

Support for such a notion is provided by the social patterns of boys and girls. Whereas boys tend to fit the "law and order" orientation model described by Kohlberg, in which rules and regulations dominate fair play, girls tend to be more cooperative and will give up a game in order to preserve a friendship. That is, girls seem more capable of feeling empathy and sensitivity to others but are less able to view human relationships as generalized or abstracted. Although the apparent diffusion of judgment that results from taking the points of view of others into account might be a moral weakness, it is inseparable from girls' moral strength (overriding concern with relationships). Thus, moral dilemmas for girls arise from conflicts of interpersonal responsibility; for boys, such dilemmas arise from competing rights. Resolution for girls requires a mode of thinking that is contextual; for boys, resolution requires abstraction.

Such differences in how relationships are viewed help to explain the perceived conflict that women feel between femininity and success. At least part of the problem resides with the prevalent notion that success must be defined in terms of a competitive process: "I am successful by virtue of being better than others." This need to beat the competition, although instilled in boys from an early age, traditionally has not been fostered in girls. This does not mean that girls do not derive satisfaction from success when it is defined, as *Webster's* puts it, as "the favorable termination of a venture." Indeed, success, when defined this way, is a primary motivating force for much of human behavior. What this broader definition of success implies, however, for men as well as women, is that by appropriately valuing cooperation while not overvaluing competition, intrinsic self-worth can be fostered when mutual endeavor to achieve a common objective, rather than supremacy, is the final goal.

In the context of adolescent development and the striving for identity and independence, the connectedness of women leads to end points that are different from those usually described for men. For women, identity is *relational* (the sense of self in close connection with another), and independence often takes the form of *interdependence* (acting responsively toward both self and others in order to sustain the connection). At the most mature stage of autonomous ego development, the woman learns to modulate an excessive sense of responsibility for or to a relationship by recognizing that others are genuinely accountable for their own destinies and must be allowed to assume and exercise that accountability.

Although these special features and extensions of classic developmental theories are presented in the context of girls and women, they are neither unique to feminine identity nor applicable to all females. As the movement toward a unisexual orientation in child rearing has grown over the past several decades, the overlap between what is acceptable behavior and social orientation for both boys and girls has grown as well. Competitive success for girls and interrelatedness in boys are now both better accepted and, indeed, encouraged by society at large. What influence this will ultimately have on the continuing developmental process of adult generations to come is, of course, unknown, but it may well result in greater blending of issues and outcomes for both sexes. Regardless, the intrapsychic growth process is an evolutionary one that is both independent of and yet inseparable from the individual's sociocultural milieu. It is essential to remember that the milieu itself is in constant flux. Although certain principles of growth and development may transcend time, specific issues and interpretations are highly variable and contextual. Interpretation of behavior, in particular, reflects prevailing social values: Such interpretations can be growth promoting for a given individual in some instances and growth inhibiting in other instances. Unfortunately, it is usually only in retrospect that we say of someone that she was a person before her time or that he was a victim of his time.

The Need for Models in Future Research

Future research will be best served by the construction, dispassionate testing, and appropriate modification of hypothetical models. Much of the population-based research done to date has resulted in the accumulation of vast arrays of disparate data that, because of a statistically defined relationship, are assumed to have a relationship in fact. The fallacy of such reasoning has been proved innumerable times and underscores the need to apply logic and common sense to investigations of the already innately complex issues of human development.

Although general principles will emerge, such models will not necessarily be applicable to all individuals. Indeed, deviations deserve special attention, because they will help to both uncover limitations in our thinking and provide new insight into factors that are important, but as yet unrecognized, determinants of human behavior.

Suggested Readings

Adelson, J. *Handbook of Adolescent Psychology*. New York: Wiley, 1980.

Bandura, A. *Social Learning Theory*. Englewood Cliffs, N.J.: Prentice-Hall, 1977.

Conger, J. J., and Petersen, A. C. *Adolescence and Youth: Psychological Development in a Changing World*. (3rd ed.) New York: Harper & Row, 1984.

Elkind, D. *Children and Adolescents: Interpretive Essays on Jean Piaget*. New York: Oxford University Press, 1974.

Erikson, E. H. *Identity: Youth and Crisis*. New York: Norton, 1968.

Gilligan, C. *In a Different Voice: Psychological Theory and Women's Development*. Cambridge, Mass.: Harvard University Press, 1982.

Hall, C. S. *A Primer of Freudian Psychology*. New York: World, 1954.

Hall, C. S., and Lindzey, G. *Theories of Personality*. (3rd ed.) New York: Wiley, 1978.

Maier, H. W. *Three Theories of Child Development*. (3rd ed.) New York: Harper & Row, 1978.

Mussen, P. H., Conger, J. J., and Kagan, J. *Child Development and Personality*. (6th ed.) New York: Harper & Row, 1984.

Sears, R. R., Rau, L., and Alpert, R. *Identification and Child Rearing*. Stanford, Calif.: Stanford University Press, 1965.

Part Two

Precursors of
Adolescent Health Problems

PART EDITOR
Frank B. Miller, M.D., F.A.P.A.

Introduction

William R. Hendee, Ph.D.

Adolescence is a period of physical development, social change, and emotional turmoil. It has long been characterized as a time of special vulnerability, especially for young people who lack an appropriate social support structure to help them through adolescence. Very often, the difficulties experienced by individual adolescents can be traced directly to shortcomings in this support structure. More general relationships have been shown in a wide spectrum of studies linking higher rates of adolescent problems to fractured family relationships, poverty, and community attitudes, especially those within adolescent peer groups in the community. However, not all adolescents reared in difficult circumstances manifest the more acute problems of adolescence. And not all young people with problems have an unsatisfactory home or community life. Although the relationships are true in general, they are not causally related in an absolute sense. Much more research is needed to recognize and understand the factors that cause one young person to develop problems while another reared in the same environment does not.

The relationships between adolescent problems and their possible precursors are examined in this part. An understanding of them is essential for individuals hoping to intervene successfully in adolescent problems. Otherwise, one can deal only with the problems as they occur rather than with the causes that underlie the problems.

In most cultures, the family has been thought of as the principle bastion of security and protection for young people as they enter the tumultuous period of adolescence. However, the family has changed dramatically in the United States over the past few decades. It was not so long ago in our country that the extended family of parents, grandparents, uncles, aunts, and cousins formed the social milieu of the average adolescent. Even the community of individuals outside the extended family had its influence, as many young people grew up in the same environment as their parents and, often, even their grandparents. After World War II, however, our society rapidly became more mobile, and the concepts of extended family and community were replaced by the so-called nuclear family and, more recently, often the single-parent or, in effect, no-parent family, with both parents working to maintain a desired level of income. These changes in the fabric of family and community support of young people have greatly increased their vulnerability to the many problems of adolescence. These changes and their impact on youth are explained by Frank B. Miller in Chapter Four.

The hazards of adolescence are not confined to any one or a few of the many ethnic, social, and economic groups composing our society. A young person living in the affluent Northshore area of metropolitan Chicago is exposed to many temptations and risks, just as is an adolescent in a ghetto area of south Chicago. Nevertheless, poverty is without question the greatest risk factor in the health of adolescents and the ways in which their health can be compromised. This conclusion is alarming in light of the growing number of young people in this country who are reared in an impoverished environment. This issue and its implications for our efforts to improve the health of adolescents are explored by Paul L. Adams in Chapter Five. Adams offers some thought-provoking recommendations at the conclusion of his chapter that merit consideration by us all, especially by our political leaders.

Much of the time of most adolescents is spent in school, and the educational process is a national resource for providing ways to facilitate the transition of young people toward adulthood. Enhancement of self-image and recognition of the intellectual, artistic, and athletic abilities of young people are acknowledged contributions of our educational systems. Extracurricular activities are also important to achieving these objectives and to providing young people with a sense of place and contribution. Sometimes, however, opposite effects of these positive contributions occur within the educational system. These effects include denigration of the worth of an individual, exclusion of the individual from events and select groups, and denial of the contributions of an individual to school and peer-group activities. These effects can lead to loneliness, rolelessness, and a degraded sense of self-worth. An even greater problem is the lack of opportunity for those young people who drop out of school or who do poorly in it. The educational and extracurricular processes of our society are very important to the welfare and well-being of young people. These processes are discussed by William M. Kane and Elias J. Duryea in Chapter Six.

Young people learn and grow in part by taking risks and pursuing a life-style of overcoming challenges and developing commitments. Yet risk taking can become a goal in itself and a major threat to the well-being of the individual if not moderated in some fashion. In the past, the family and community often provided this control. Today, individuals such as teachers, counselors, and friends (including those of the same age) are frequently able to exert a tempering influence on what otherwise might become out-of-control behavior. This influence is examined in Chapter Seven by Mary E. L. Vernon, who provides some examples of community programs developed to help young people get their bearings during their transit through adolescence.

The chapters in this part are crucial to an improved understanding of the many factors that underlie the ability of young people to traverse success-fully the extended period of adolescence prevalent in our society today.

4

The Influence of the Family and Social Environment

Frank B. Miller, M.D., F.A.P.A.

The adolescent has become a source of concern and worry for parents and American society during the past several decades. As Adelson wrote years ago, "adolescence has come to weigh oppressively on the American conscience." The adolescent represents one major segment of American society registering tumultuous social change and sociobehavioral distress in recent times. The rate of adolescent suicide has dramatically risen in the past two decades, to more than 12 successful suicides per 100,000 people. This statistic highlights the turmoil of the adolescent cohort.

The family has become an increasingly important focus of study to understand many of the sources of unhealthy and maladaptive functioning in troubled adolescents. As early as the 1950s, Spiegel wrote of the importance of the relationships within the family, portending the growing clinical and theoretical attention directed to the family and its modes of functioning. In modern-day society, the family must be defined not just as the traditional nuclear unit of married heterosexual parents and children but as a system of interlocking and interdependent relationships that structure the life experience of each family member, irrespective of age or role.

The family has undergone major change since traditional nuclear family definitions dominated popular and academic views. Therein are contained both the inherent strength of the family as the building block of society and also its contradictions and dilemmas. The family has been a much maligned entity in the last twenty-five years. This has been especially true in the United States, the country whose standard of living has permitted educational access and role evolution on a larger scale than any other. In the late 1960s and early 1970s, it was not unusual to read in the popular media that the age-old institution of the family not only was under criticism and attack but was dying and facing extinction. Perhaps those prognostications would have been more correct if they had included the qualification that "the family as we have known it" was rapidly changing. Ideas such as unisexual role definition and fears that preschool education and role modeling were somehow brainwashing the very young into antiquated roles were much in vogue. The dissolution of the family by nontraditional societies such as the communal groupings of the Shakers and the Kibbutz movement in Israel was suggested as a solution to the rising problems of divorce, delinquency, unwanted offspring, drug abuse, and other growing social issues.

Statistical-Demographic Portrait of the Family

The family has reasserted itself in the past quarter century and demonstrated its resiliency and the inherent need for its functions. The need for family is reflected in the reemergence of the trend toward long-term monogamous relationships following the patterns of serial relationships of the last one-and-a-half decades. Birthrates in young marriages are increasing after a decade and a half of decline, even though in some socioeconomic groups the age of becoming a parent has increased.

In the 1984 census survey, 85.4 million households were identified in the United States. A household is defined as two or more related persons, one of whom is the householder, who own or rent the living quarters that are shared. Three main types of households were found in the survey. The vast majority, some 50.1 million, were married-couple households; families with female-run households with no husband present numbered 9.9 million; and households with male household head but with no wife present numbered 2.0 million.

Trends over the last two decades give more telling information regarding the family. Since 1970, the number of families has increased on the average by 1.2 to 1.6 million per year. However, 25 percent of the households added since 1980 have been headed by women with no husbands. This proportion is higher than the previous 18 percent increase in the number of female-headed households between 1970 and 1980.

One other major type of household is the nonfamily household, made up of householders who live alone or with others to whom they are not related. About 23.4 million or 27 percent of all households were the nonfamily type. This type of household has grown rapidly since 1980, constituting 47 percent of all households added to the population since 1980. Most of these are single persons living alone, including elderly widowed, divorced, and young adults.

The size of the family has undergone dramatic change in the last two decades. The average size of the family has decreased significantly. The average number of persons per household reached a new low of 2.71 in 1984, declining from 3.58 persons per household in 1970. The decrease is attributable almost exclusively to the drop in the average number of people under the age of eighteen in the family or household (0.99 in 1984, compared to 1.34 in 1970).

The number of marriages is expected to continue to decrease in relation to the population through the 1990s. Younger people are delaying marriage in greater numbers than thirty years ago. They are doing so to complete career training and perhaps as a result of the cumulative effects of changing societal attitudes toward marriage, which regarded it as both more valued and more fragile. The last several generations, it must be remembered, are those that have experienced the greatest number of divorces in their formative years.

Further projections of household trends bear some watching. The Bureau of the Census projects that the number of households will continue to grow at a strong rate, reaching between 102.4 and 110.2 million by the year 2000. Households that include married couples will continue to make up the majority of households, at or above 59 percent by the year 2000.

The Family in Distress

The need for the stabilizing function of the family in people's lives is demonstrated by the lack of character development in adolescents and young adults who are deprived of reasonably stable familial experiences during their developmental years. The effects of abuse, increased rates of adolescent pregnancies and illegitimate births, earlier onset of sexual activity in adolescents, and increases in sexually transmitted diseases and delinquency in the young are in large part caused by the poorer functioning of the family.

It is no surprise that the mental health profession began to see the family as the next great frontier of study and intervention some three decades ago. The discipline of family therapy came to be routinely imparted to trainees in the major study centers of psychiatry, psychology, and psychiatric social work. Fifty years ago, human service workers at all levels were beginning to be charged with the care, rehabilitation, and maintenance of families in trouble through the emergence of child guidance clinics and court-based family agencies. A body of knowledge began to emerge in the mental health professions that recognized not only that the family was the essential building block of society but also that it was in serious difficulty. This view of the family as an integral unit whose traditional existence was neither an accident nor a political contrivance began to be shared by other professions as more medical caretakers of children (for example, pediatricians and public health nurses) came to recognize the importance of the family either through the loss of early child-care capabilities or through the emergence of developmental pathologies, such as failure to thrive, that were due not to a specific pathogen but to the lack of healthy functioning of the family system.

Functional Characteristics of the Family

Forces operating within the family arise out of the earliest and most basic psychobiological attachments of which the human being is capable. Lidz has written extensively of the family's importance as a unit in forming the earliest and most persistent bond and influence in an individual's life. Parental and family ways are the only way of life that a child knows. All subsequent experiences are perceived, understood, reacted to, and integrated into the growing personality of the child or adolescent within the context provided by the parents and family. Lidz describes the family as a body composed of at least two generations, with each generation expressing different needs, prerogatives, and obligations. While the parents may be dependent on each other, they should not be dependent on the children. In Lidz's traditional definition, the family consists of two genders with different but complementary functions and roles. The relationships between family members are held firm by erotic and affectional ties.

Family therapists have long known that, clinically and interpersonally, any and all action and reaction patterns between any two family members resonate throughout the entire family. A primary assumption of family therapists is that symptomatic behavior of a family member demonstrates an area of faulty functioning of the family that the family member is "acting out." This assumption is the fundamental concept that spans the causal link between failure of the family, whether intact or fragmented, and the disturbed individual, including acting-out adolescents who come to be labeled "high-risk," antisocial, or psychologically disturbed. The dynamic communication among family members is demonstrated even in pathological families that harbor "family secrets," which usually are not "secret." Even in such toxic exigencies as incest, the unacknowledged behaviors are often known among the members.

This interdependence is the basis of all strength within the family and also of its problems, frictions, and strife. The nature of emotional ties, the roles of the members, and the duties of the members to each other form the matrices that define the boundaries and functions of the family.

Family Boundaries

Boundaries define the family as a separate system by placing distance between itself and other social systems, such as clubs, groups of employees, people caught in a traffic jam, and so on. Behaviors are prescribed that do not occur outside the family and serve to formalize the relationships as special and different from all other relationships. Overt and covert "rules" exist within the family that serve to maintain the system in balance. The function of such rules is to maintain stability within the system by encouraging redundant behavior and self-perpetuation of the system. These rules determine how relationships within the family are conducted. Under ideal circumstances, they preserve unity within the family while permitting the family and its members to grow and change. On the other hand, the family can be resistant to external change in order to buffer, monitor, and control the type and pace of change that is permitted within the family. This resistance serves largely to restrict change that would destroy the established emotional balance of forces within the family.

The family is one of the few social institutions that continue to serve the individual over time. The family remains available to the fortunate individual over all of his or her developmental epochs. Schools, even such seemingly complete systems as residential universities, do not perform this function for the individual. Most outside institutions exist for the benefit of the person only so long as the person is affiliated with them in an economic way. This relationship is time-limited. Companies decrease their relationships with a worker to a minimum level after retirement and do not provide support other than a monetary pension. Churches are perhaps the only institutions that come close to the properties of the family. Even age-related cohorts such as fraternity brothers, sorority sisters, armed services chums, and so on do not sustain the strength of ties that the family does. In these cohorts, members eventually die and the group atrophies, since there is no means of replenishing members so that the newer members of the social organization can care for the older members, as is the case with families. Families are the only social organisms that serve the needs of the individual from cradle to grave in a personal way. Families generate new members to care for elders in a way not duplicated by any other social agency or body. Families perpetuate emotionally meaningful relationships that provide what is needed psychologically. These internalized forces and needs account for the enduring nature of the family.

The Purpose of the Family

The ultimate goal of the family is to care for its members and to enable the dependent members to "graduate" from the setting of the family, taking their place autonomously and productively within the outside society and forming families of their own. To accomplish this, the family must support the developmental needs of its members at each stage of life. The family therefore must meet concomitantly the needs of the infant or child-adolescent, the needs of the parents or spouses, and the needs of society to produce socialized and productive citizens.

From the dependence of the infant or preschooler, through the independence-seeking phases of childhood and adolescence, to the affectional needs of the maturing adolescent and adult, only the family tailors its functioning to the evolving emotional needs of the ever-changing person throughout the life cycle. Most other agencies of society serve only certain ages and restrict their sphere of influence with age-related or role-determined boundaries.

Myths in America Regarding the Family

The family has been viewed for years through a sort of cultural mythology that extends even into academic views and literature. Only as the family underwent undeniable and vast changes in its form did its definitions come to be altered so that they would parallel what was being observed in the real world. The more complex viewpoint of the family goes beyond the simplistic view of the normal family structure as the "nuclear family" and has helped to provide a rubric that allows for the different forms of the family to be understood. The myth of the nuclear family came to its zenith of influence in the post–World War II era, when the popular consciousness of America, as mirrored in the media, came to consistently portray the family as a nuclear family composed of parents and children, with little more than passing reference to grandparents. Only in the past few years have grandparents come to be seen regularly on the television screen. As a corollary to this narrow view of the family, each generation was seen as entirely self-sufficient after attaining adulthood and relative autonomy from the previous generation. This view reflected the increasing geographical isolation of the basic family unit in the modern era, caused by economic forces that moved family units away from ancestral homes, grandparents, and siblings.

Several writers have enlarged our conceptualization of the dyadic relationship. The concept of the dyad between child and caretaker had been intensively studied by traditional psychiatry and psychoanalysis, to the exclusion of its impact upon and within the larger family unit. Formerly, it could be said in psychiatric theory that there was an ideology that looked upon the dyadic relationship, whether between spouses or between parent and child, as more mutually exclusive than it really is. This early view reflected the emphasis in clinical work on two-person relationships, such as in the work about the overprotected child, the borderline individual and his or her parents, and so on. The family was given short theoretical shrift in that it was viewed primarily as a collection of dyadic relationships, as units of two in the family, whether the marital pair or the parent-child unit, that were supposed to meet *all* the needs of the pair, resulting in a potentially deadening and isolating dyad.

Out of these dyadically based views came support for other myths about the family and its functioning: the myth of male superiority, related to economically determined roles until the most recent past; the primacy of ties relating to rearing children; the myth of the family as a closed system with relatively impermeable social boundaries; the view of the family as a static unit resistant to change, an immutable entity immune to social forces; the family as a homeostatic unit; the family as an entity in danger of extinction, of breaking up in the face of social and internal change; and dyadic relationships as the most stable overall force in the family. Writers and clinicians in family therapy came to consider alternate views of the triangular and more complex family relationships among more than two members as additive and stabilizing, as conflict-reducing forces. This was a move away from the earlier views of dyadic relationships as shown in the extreme overemphasis on the oedipal model as a divisive force in the family. This view was centered in the more individualistically oriented psychological theories.

Forces Affecting the Family

As society has grown ever more complex, it must be acknowledged that many nonpsychological forces outside the family have achieved greater importance. The media are a relatively new creature in the modern world. We have come a long way from the days when news from newspapers or telegraphed reports was always outdated by days or weeks. Even war journalism in World War II magazines and movie reels was delayed in reaching its audience. In the modern era, information and news are virtually instantaneous. The family is bombarded by a multiplicity of sources of information, no longer under the strict control of guardianship of the parents or church such as in Puritan times. Witness the controversy surrounding the ethics of unrestricted access to "adult material" by minors through magazines, videotapes, and cable television. Even the educational system has largely gone beyond the control and supervision of parents as local schools are asked more and more to educate the young on behalf of parents. The young are exposed to views of the world differing from those of their parents. Transgenerational change, once greatly feared in the premodern era, is now inexorable.

Changes in the types of information presented to adults and children have enormous implications for the family. Change is much more rapid than previously and is now viewed as beyond the control of parents. Parents are somewhat less important as sources of role modeling than in times past. Witness the much more widespread copying of counterculture personalities that has become almost the norm among the young since the World War II years. Indeed, some of the most momentous forces impinging on the family in the modern era have been nonpsychological and economic. The family has had to adapt to forces that strive both to support and to alter its functioning as never before.

If indeed there have been eras in which the family has been primarily an extended system of generations that lived in close proximity with little cultural or social change, then those eras have largely passed. Indeed, the family now must strive to prepare its members for change at a pace undreamed of only three to four generations ago. Historical analysis will set the stage for consideration of these forces. Until the modern era, families functioned as did much of the rest of the biological world. Primary goals were to procreate and generate new members in excess numbers, since before the introduction of antibiotics, every family lost children to infectious diseases at early ages. The value of children was more related to economic survival than it is in modern times. The agricultural family, whether of the Middle Ages of Europe, of the American Plains Indians, or even of the early industrial era, needed large numbers of children to help the family earn a livelihood. Child labor was the norm.

The changing forces of agricultural and industrial technology and the mass production of goods began to remove the pressure on the family to provide for itself. Goods began to be produced in a specialized manner. Children were no longer needed for their labor value except among the enslaved segments of society in which parents were denied the opportunity to develop a sufficient economic base for the family—the blacks of the plantation era, the Native Americans of the reservations, and the emancipated but poor whites and blacks of the sharecropper system and the modern underclass.

With the segmentation and specialization of the production of goods that began in the middle 1800s, children began to be less needed in the family economy. These changes made possible the realization of universal child education, which revolutionized the face of the family. Within a few generations, the coda of the family came to embrace a changing view of each generation as one that would exceed the achievements of its parents. This view was aided by the aspirations of the immigrant populations of emerging America. The extreme of this trend has been the educational push that sees each generation striving for the fullest educational and vocational development of the child, adolescent, and young adult, with attendant extension of adolescence into the twenties and thirties, until education is terminated in the professions.

During the Great Depression, the family endured economic insults that came to shape the economic fears and aspirations of the post–World War II generation. These aspirations formed the psychological impetus for the unprecedented consumerism of recent eras. The Depression caused the family to suffer separations in some quarters, with exit from home and school of children and adults in large numbers and migratory patterns to large cities that fractionated the family. This force was compounded by the advent of World War II, which sent large numbers of fathers, sons, and brothers away for perhaps several years. Women were thrust into economic positions of command and responsibility outside the home. The role of women changed irrevocably during the war years. Although women returned to the home after the war, they more recently reentered the world of work with the advent of the women's movement and the economic forces of worldwide inflation.

The stereotypical family with the mother in the home survived for a relatively brief period in the post–World War II era, until the costs of modern warfare and welfare combined in the 1960s in America to prompt unprecedented peacetime national inflation and hamper the earning power of the single-income family. The resulting economic influences forced the American family to change rapidly. The women's liberation movement was as much a result of these forces as an initiator of them. Generations of post–high school education had changed vast numbers of women and their aspirations.

The percentage of women who work outside the home, long a disputed indicator of changes in the American family, has changed dramatically over the last three decades. In 1960, 30.5 percent of all women worked outside the home. By 1985, nearly 55 percent of women did so. That is, by the 1980s, more than half of American families were supported by the incomes of both parents. The relative intactness of the American family was beset by the needs of the family to separate its members at much earlier junctures than ever before, except perhaps in the days of the American slaves. Mothers, formerly the main child caretakers, entered the workplace as soon as feasible after the birth of their children. Many children entered institutional child-care settings earlier than the traditional kindergarten years. Child care became one of the fastest-growing industries of the modern era, since the percentage of working mothers with children under age six increased from 18.6 percent in 1960 to 53.4 percent in 1985.

The policies of the government reflected ambivalence toward catching up with social changes besetting the family. In large measure, the families of the undereducated, the underprivileged, and the victims of society-wide discrimination were supported by welfare only if they were abandoned by the fathers in the family. This requirement perpetuated the breakdown of the family in the growing underclass. The costs of raising children were not subsidized by tax credits or deductions to the same extent as were the growth of industries or the expenses of business. Today, tax policies actually penalize couples who marry, and for a period during the radical era of the 1960s, 1970s, and early 1980s, they furnished a rationale for young adults to forgo the rites of marriage.

Finally, employment policies of the governments of most modern industrial societies came full circle with regard to isolating the young from the character-building influences of the workplace. Child labor laws were enacted in the industrial era to protect children from exploitation, especially the children of families making the transition to the modern economic era with insufficient wage-earning abilities. These laws, along with the minimum wage laws, while serving to enhance the wage-earning ability of adults at the bottom of the educational ladder, also served to keep the young out of the labor market until midadolescence. The paradox has become that while societies have taken adults out of the home to a greater extent than at any other time in history, they have left the young on their own with fewer and fewer roles reserved for them to realize economic usefulness and to become other than creatures of leisure.

Economic Forces Affecting Parents

Both economics and technology have brought forces to bear on parents as primary wage earners in the family. These forces have created enormous strains. In general, the adult parent can no longer rely on an institutional parent such as a company with which to live out his or her entire working life.

Adults can expect to change their employment many times and may have to change their occupational identity and training several times within their working lives. This has led to pressures on adults that at times make the days of economic stagnation with employment security look attractive. As corporate entities that govern the commercial life of modern society have come to exist in an increasingly competitive milieu, the economic life of the adult has become more uncertain than ever. Corporate buyouts, deaths of corporations and their products, cycles of inflation and stagflation, and unstable currency levels in the global economy threaten the family's confidence and ability to survive economically. These changes often occur outside and beyond the control of the individual adult parent. The pressures on the family generated by the modern economic system have yet to be appreciated. One wonders whether we are generating two types of families, those that must remain stagnant because of their lack of education and those that can move occupationally and geographically. The reality is that the families of the lower and underclasses may retain ties with extended family members, while the more economically successful families trade their economic and educational adaptability for loss of family ties.

Social and personal consequences of these frequent moves, up to once every five years for the typical mobile family, are staggering. Children in "successful" families face the daunting and potentially harmful prospect of repetitively losing their friends and peer-based supports. Schools must be changed frequently. Parents lose friends and social support settings, and relationships with families and parents are disrupted. All relationships may come to be experienced as temporary and subject to inevitable premature loss.

Establishment of the Paired Relationship and Marriage

One of the foremost tasks of the family is to perpetuate and preserve the art of human relationships. Part of this task is training of the offspring. All else springs out of the function of the family to provide the matrix for emotionally charged and meaningful human relationships.

In the traditional view, the family serves to provide the status of marriage for a new couple that seeks to establish its own social unit. This new marital unit is viewed with care by society. It is expected to take some period of time to establish itself and to cement the emotional relationship with formalized mechanisms of temporary retreat, such as the honeymoon. Relationships with outsiders are attenuated for a time or restricted to other "young marrieds" until the new family is sure enough of itself to endure increasing degrees and forms of separation as dictated by occupations and so on.

The couple is faced with developmental tasks arising from its new station. The individuals are expected to separate emotionally and physically to a greater or lesser degree from their families of origin and to begin to depend more on themselves. For the couple's relationship to sustain itself, trust formation is an all-important task. Without this basic ingredient, the couple faces the chore of remaining loyal to each other with little reason other than those of circumstance and tradition. In the past, these reasons may have sustained couples now in their elderly years, but with the ease of obtaining divorces and the slowly increasing equity possible in division of property, this is no longer the case. The partners in the new family must present themselves as reasonable substitutes for each other's parents, friends, and siblings. Mutual dependence becomes the norm that facilitates the development of trust.

In trusting each other, the couple performs a number of tasks important to the pair, including affirmation of each other's values, interests, likes, dislikes, and so on and providing for each other a safe haven and confidant. This goes hand in hand with another essential function of the young couple: the establishment of an interpersonal genre of what psychiatry has long called "reality testing." The growth of individual reality testing permits the personality to distinguish between external reality and internally driven reality, or "fantasy." The interpersonal reality testing is the vision of the world outside the couple. Couples begin to forge a commonly held catechism of priorities of relationships that face them in the outside world of commerce, competition, and relationships. Whether accurate or not, this marital reality testing helps form the common emotional ideology of the marriage.

Many couples come to wish for offspring in order to perpetuate their family line, to extend their care-giving needs to additional members, and to complement their own relationship. When the wife becomes pregnant, momentous changes ensue. The wife's energy may decrease, and the husband may assume an increased work load in the home in preparation for the arrival of the infant. The wife often goes through periods of emotional introspection and neediness, which the more mature husband can supportively accept and process with his wife. Again, the power of the dyad sets the stage for how the triangular relationship will be handled. The husband may become jealous of the presence of the third party, the unborn child, and become distant from his wife or react with dependent behaviors that stress the marriage. In the extreme, the husband, unable to face the responsibilities of partner to the expectant wife, may manifest irresponsible behavior such as substance abuse or extramarital affairs in reaction to the needs presented by his wife.

Separation-Individuation of the Adolescent from the Family

The family provides for the separation-individuation of the new marital unit from their parents. This function is best done in a spirit of compromise and middle-of-the-road course charting. Young adults who cannot establish themselves independently of their parents often do not do well later. Those who have to forgo the support of extended families because of enforced moves away from the available support of parents also experience additional stress.

As noted earlier, a basic task of the parental unit in the family is providing nutritional, economic, educational, and other types of support for the development of the dependent adolescent member. The parent faces the paradox of knowing that almost everything done to further the development of the adolescent serves to hasten the day when the child takes leave of the parent. Just as the adolescent faces developmental hurdles—the "tasks of childhood" or the "tasks of adolescence"—so, too, the parent faces time- and role-based developmental functions that make up the hierarchical chain of tasks contained in parenting. Many of these tasks of parenting are themselves responsive to the developmental phases of the adolescent. The usual tasks of parenting, difficult for even the most ably emotionally grounded and mature parent, prepare the adolescent for the task of eventual separation.

A brief review of the psychodevelopmental theory of the process called "separation-individuation" may be useful. This theory began in the early days of psychoanalytical practice when the followers of Freud began to realize that the bonds between the parent and the preschool child had enormously important long-term consequences for personality development. With the blitz bombing of London during World War II, child psychoanalysts began to study the effect of separation from parents on subsequent personality development in children who were transported to the countryside of England. In general, they found that with such separation, the usual developmental parameters were disrupted, and reactive symptoms predictably appeared, some nonspecific and some specific to the meaning of separation. Since then, the causal effects of separation leading to the developmentally framed symptoms seen in school phobia and avoidance have become a focus in child psychiatry. Metaphors that conceptualize the ingredients in the early study of separation-centered conflicts focused on aberrations in the interactions between parent and child. Terms such as *overprotectiveness* were used in attempts to characterize some of the processes that undermined the successful outcome of separation-individuation. This was a difficult subject to study and was not widely appreciated outside psychoanalytical circles for several decades. Nonpsychodynamically trained health care professionals had only a dim understanding of the developmental processes involved. This superficial view of separation-individuation was shown in the metaphor of symptoms as "phases" that would be "grown out of." Symptoms of emotional and interpersonal conflicts in the preschool and elementary-aged child founded on separation issues, such as dependency, night terrors, separation from parental beds, school avoidance, social phobias, and excessive shyness, were not seen as indications for detailed psychiatric intervention in the young child. Instead, these potentially disruptive symptom constellations were naively viewed as time-limited "phases." This approach relied excessively on the normal press of developmental impetus in most children to at least ameliorate and modify such symptoms. The lack of professional awareness and recognition of important personality growth issues involved in the process of separation-individuation impeded a long-term appreciation of the consequent effects that cause personality-based conflicts in adults and even in adolescents. These future residues of a faulty developmental process in children were seen only by therapists who treated adults left with the results of developmental interference and by psychoanalysts and psychiatrists who treated the more severely disturbed character neurotics, borderline psychotics, and psychogenically psychotic adults and adolescents. Practitioners geared toward timely interventions stressing problem solving, such as school-based counselors and behavioral pediatricians, could not address such entrenched psychopathology and saw psychological issues through the metaphors of the transient phases of biological and cognitive development.

Reconstruction of childhood emotional experiences as a means of helping severely disturbed adults has long been a venerated, though highly criticized, tenet of psychiatric practice. This retrospective psychological practice has led to theories that have paved the way for incisive observational studies of child development and have sharpened and advanced our understanding of processes taking place in the preschool and childhood years. This view of the continuum development of the personality as originating in the preschooler's resolutions of the painful dilemma of separation-individuation has taken years to formulate and can best be appreciated through training that affords long-term and intensive psychotherapeutic clinical work with patients of all ages. This is necessary when the consequences of an early process such as separation-individuation are apparent only some two decades later. Only then can the importance of early developmentally based personality deficits be appreciated in adolescents and adults who fail the more complex tasks of emotional and interpersonal life.

The theory of the psychological process of separation-individuation is most closely associated with the work of Margaret Mahler. Mahler, a child psychoanalyst, found that there are age-specific phases in the process of moving away from the exclusive and dyadic orbit of the parent by the infant and young child. These seem to be rooted partly in neurocognitive mechanisms of the developing infant and toddler but have an innate psychodevelopmental timetable of their own. First, there is an early autistic bond of the infant with the parent caretaker in which the infant functions mostly as a dependent extension of the parent and there is little distinction between the self of the infant and that of the parent. Second, there is a phase during the middle to later months of the first year of life when there is a symbiosis between infant and parent but the infant is more self-aware. The child recognizes in a rudimentary way that the parent is separate from the self, but autonomous functioning on the part of the older infant and young toddler is piecemeal and partial. The dependent symbiotic functioning of the dyad is preferred and is appropriate to buffer and protect the inadequately developed psyche of the young toddler.

In the later part of the first year of life and through the second year, rudiments of modestly independent functioning of the child appear. These are the beginnings of movements toward emotional separation. They may be manifested by the appearance of the ability to make demands on the parent, to play separately for short periods, and to tolerate being alone for short intervals. Parents begin to separate from their young children and leave them for periods of time to the care of others, such as baby-sitters. This process is accelerated with the advent of walking. Physical locomotion promotes separation of the toddler from the parent and helps to propel the preschooler to much more autonomous and semi-independent functioning by age four or five. Acquisition of simple and then more complex language skills permits self-expression, and the ability to make verbal demands and to say no to the parent also speeds the work of separation-individuation. The success of this process permits the child to enter into early peer-based relationships in day-care centers, to substitute other adults for parents for the part of each day spent in child care, to sleep alone at night, and to enter programs such as day care, kindergarten, and formal school at ages four through six. Without successful completion of the tasks contained in these phases of development, separation-based constellations of aberrant emotional development begin to appear, including the familiar school-refusal phobias, night terrors, eating disorders of early childhood, childhood anxiety and depressive disorders, and the more malignant disorders that are forerunners of childhood psychogenic psychoses, such as hyperactive disorders and oppositional disturbances.

The importance of emotional separation or emancipation becomes more evident with each succeeding year, as the child is faced with ever more complex and socially stressful hurdles, such as making the transition into larger peer groups, sharing a teacher within larger classrooms, encountering strangers outside the home, facing the temptations of adolescence that require youngsters to make choices of right and wrong, and consolidating complex issues of self-image and confidence and competence. The youngster who has a shaky and deficient sense of self often cannot say no to wayward influences. Insecure preteens and teens will attempt to please and affiliate in a dependent manner left over from earlier stages of development where psychic autonomy was not sufficiently internalized and solidified in the practicing world of the family. This results in the herding together of uncertain teens as a temporizing means of defining self. These are the incompletely individuated teens who display the emergence of a number of unhealthy adjustments and account for the huge upsurge in behavioral and psychological casualties in the teenage population. These unhealthy adjustments include premature and infantile clinging to "best friends" with constant bickering and near-paranoid imagings of insults and slights. Tempestuous relationships mark these attempts at close and dyadic bonds. When the relationships are sexualized, the problems multiply, and sexuality substitutes for sharing. The gradual deepening of relationships through self-revelation and getting to know each other is replaced by impulsive and anonymous sexuality. Teens with strong dependencies resulting from incomplete separation processes can be seen walking together in schools and malls, literally acting out their inability to separate through the physical-behavioral metaphors of clinging to each other obsessively and using physical touching and premature sexual overtures. The rush of early adolescents toward lovelike bonding alternating with abrupt termination of such relationships when they get too close may be inappropriately perpetuated in the older adolescent and young adult. What is lost is the ability to sustain and deepen relationships to the mutual benefit of the growth of both personalities. There is the normative brittle safety mechanism of the junior high schooler that prevents relationships from going too far, too fast. This is inappropriately utilized by the personality-disordered late adolescent and adult who have not been able to achieve emotional emancipation and are unable to move toward the achievement of longer-term relationships. This produces the pathology of serial and self-defeating relationships in the adult who cannot sustain a marriage or long-term bond. Still more disturbed is the more primitively arrested individual who remains tied to the parent emotionally, the borderline personality, so common in the psychiatric populations of the last two decades. This person's truncated personality has the pattern of severely chaotic relationships, whether in marriages or affairs, with outbursts of paranoid jealousy, rage, and self-destructive behaviors.

Substance abuse, also a nearly ubiquitous problem of modern times, often has major etiological ingredients contributed by the residues of an incomplete emotional separation-individuation process. Another result of abnormal separation-individuation is the intolerance of painful internal affects in the impaired personality. Again, the combination of impulsivity and proclivity toward pleasure seeking in the adolescent sets the stage for the use of pleasure-producing substances to shore up a shaky personality. Use of hallucinogenics, alcohol, stimulants, and soporifics serves to induce states of antidepressant euphoria and to suppress states of loss, despair, normative depression, disappointment, and so on. The pleasure-producing substance serves as a substitute for the lost relationship and an ever-ready coping mechanism, resulting in substance abuse that is notoriously difficult to change without substantive internally directed personality change. Personalities thus impaired—and they are very common in the modern adolescent population—require thorough personality rehabilitation through intensive psychotherapy or total environmental life changes, such as religious conversions or immersion in all-encompassing communities such as cults, authoritarian religions, or military-like groups.

What is needed in the all-important process of individuation? Simply put, it is the "standard emotional issue" akin to the minimal equipment of the government issue of the field soldier—minimal provisions for approaching and effecting the job of individual emotional autonomy. This is provided by a relationship with a reasonably empathic and supportive parent who intu-itively supplies reliable emotional support and compliments the child's en-deavors, while simultaneously inviting the adolescent to achieve what he or she is able to accomplish at each stage and gently exhorting progress to the next stage. The supportive recipe is sensed by most well-equipped parents and is also illustrated by the styles of the disturbed parent who cannot support the child's move toward autonomous functioning.

An example of this problem is provided by a mother and young child seen for "separation problems" at a walk-in psychiatric clinic. The mother was referred originally to an orthopedist for unusual and severe degenerative changes in the femoral head without corticosteroid use or advanced age. The mother was found to be depressed and referred for psychiatric evaluation. A spot diagnosis could be made as soon as the mother presented herself. She walked in carrying her late-preschool child on one hip and declined to let the child walk on her own. The child, who was nearly six years old, functioned at the level of a two-year-old and refused to physically separate from the mother. Both evinced severe anxiety at the suggestion of being interviewed separately. Since the mother had never permitted or initiated much of a separation process between herself and her daughter, the daughter was school phobic, had never attended school, was incompletely toilet trained, and was com-pletely dependent on the mother for most daily activities. The mother was house- and child-bound, depressed and anxious, unable to face the inevitable separation from her child, who was under community edict to enter school. The physical changes in the heads of her femurs were caused by lugging her child around long after the child had become too heavy to be routinely carried.

Another contemporary example is that of a mother who sought evalua-tion for her daughter who in her early twenties was still unable to separate from the mother after her own second marriage and balked at going on her honeymoon. When they were interviewed by a psychiatrist, the mother spoke for the daughter until the psychiatrist intervened and structured the inter-view to permit expression by the identified patient. The appearance of the pair was most striking: The mother and daughter were almost identically attired, with the same shades of dyed blond hair, yellow clothing, and facial makeup. The daughter wished to "get on" with her life but experienced inexplicable separation anxiety at any life event that took her out of her parents' home. She had already lost one spouse, who had quit in disgust over the inability of his new wife to take leave of her mother, her inability to stop weeping, and her frequent phone calls to her mother to the exclusion of attention to her husband. The mother spoke at length in the initial interview of her daughter's many social accomplishments, speaking of them as if they were also her own. Delicate and carefully created work utilizing the daughter's secret wishes to accomplish other deeds, not envisioned by the mother, permitted gradual work with the daughter to the exclusion of the mother from the sessions. Gradually, the mother came to exhibit her own separation-anxiety reactions and to be socially phobic as her daughter was able to save the second marriage and "step out on her own."

Parenthood as a Developmental Phase

The tasks of early parenthood are related to important functions of the family. These phase-specific tasks complement and spur the maturation of the individual as a young adult. Personal wishes and selfishness undergo revision, and higher levels of impulse control are called upon. Young parents take pride in providing for their young at their own expense. Mutual responsibility develops at levels usually not seen previously in the life of the individual. Empathy for the tasks of the mate is stimulated, and mutual respect and supportiveness are mustered as common tasks demand the cooperation of the spouses. They become for each other a safe emotional haven from the outside competitive world, the confidant-consultant that they have perhaps not had to such a degree in their own families of origin. In a well-functioning marriage, each spouse becomes the replacement for the other's adolescent peers and the other's best friend.

The increased stress upon the marital relationship stimulates emotional fidelity, another of the essential functions of the family. Relationships of the preteen child are marked by rivalry about different developmental crises and needs. The world of the adolescent moves from crises of loyalty in same-sex friendships to the tumultuous world of affectionately and sexually charged relationships. Emotional bonding is still largely governed by selfish needs and wants. The family of the young adult serves to temper the internally driven impulsiveness of such relationships and to make them more reliable and sustained. When this function is not well accomplished, marital dissension, separation, and distance or divorce ensue.

An often neglected function of the young family is enabling the transition from the person dependent on his or her parent to the independent adult entering a mature and even-handed relationship with an adult spouse. If development of a person is conceived as a continuum, an orderly progression through successive stages of maturation, then the business of parenting becomes immensely important to the development of the child. In each critical stage of development, children reactivate their parents' own developmentally based conflicts, urges, and strivings. This can either bring about further psychopathological deterioration in the parent or initiate solution of conflict issues such as narcissistic wishes to be cared for, dependency, and so on.

Against this backdrop of the handling of the changes in the behavioral and emotional demands of the child, there is parental modulation that gives rise to a grand and unending conflict of closeness and dependency versus separation and autonomy, constituting the ongoing and lifelong unfinished business of the family. Some of this unfinished business involves not only the separation-individuation process but also the reconstruction of relationships between the parents and the grown offspring. Contained within this task are the need to understand the reality of the parents, the developmental exigencies of the parents, the development of empathy for the parents, and the acceptance of limitations of the parents in order to take responsibility for later origins of one's own behaviors.

The reactions of the parent to the adolescent become crucially important to the attainment of maturity by the teenager. E. James Anthony has written eloquently of the reactions of parents. He describes parental reactions as due largely to stereotypical images of adolescents fostered by society and the media, by idiosyncratic, personalized, and experiential characteristics of the parents themselves, and by archaic psychological transference reactions on the parts of the parents that are based on experiences from earlier emotional phases of their lives that exert unknown influences on their behaviors and attitudes toward their own adolescents and adolescents in general.

The aggressiveness of some adolescents contributes to the view of teenagers as victimizers who stalk helpless adult parents. This view of adolescence, born out of the parents' memory of their own aggressiveness, makes for contradictory reactions to the adolescent. Institutional overprotectiveness is seen in the legal restrictions placed on entry of adolescents into the workplace and in child labor laws. Legislatures and courts continually struggle over the issue of how to handle the juvenile offender, whether as a figure who deserves harsh punishment or as a dependent individual who needs protection and merciful and humane rehabilitation with partial forgiving or responsibility for antisocial behaviors.

The parent has no small ambivalence toward the adolescent as a sexual being and object. Intensely ambivalent reactions are seen, ranging from attempts at rigid prohibition and delay of sexual activity in the adolescent to the laissez-faire attitudes of both psychopathic and morally conservative parents who look the other way and ignore out-of-control sexual behavior of their adolescents. The internal reaction of the parent, based on a lack of resolution of his or her own adolescent sexuality, determines how the parent will help the adolescent govern sexual wishes and urges. When these issues in the parent are poorly handled or unacknowledged, intense sexual rivalry, sexual jealousy, and sexual overprotectiveness by the parent may result. The adolescent, who has enough difficulty handling sexuality, is then forced to assume the weight of the parent's unresolved sexual conflicts that are projected onto the teen. The teen can then only react, either with externalized acting out in the sexual arena or with internalized reaction formation of overly severe prohibition and inhibition.

On another axis of parental governing, the rejection or seduction of the adolescent by the parent determines how the incest taboo is respected within the family. If the parent fails to defuse the overtly sexual appeal of the offspring, then incest may occur, which traumatizes the teenager, making sexuality an area of intense suffering and conflict for years or for life.

The adolescent as an "object of envy" assumes importance in the adult who must strive to govern intensely personalized reactions. Parents who have had insufficient narcissistic developmental supplies given to them in their earlier years because of emotional neglect or abuse may find themselves envying the luxuries that they give to their adolescents. Reactions often take the form of complaining that the parent never had it so well as the adolescent, with mechanisms of inappropriate guilt induction and feelings of rage over the dependency fostered by the parent. The parent can unwittingly foster abnormal narcissism in the adolescent by identifying with the youth out of envy. In such cases, adolescents are exhorted to adhere to overly high expectations, and failure is not tolerated by the parent, who attempts to live unfulfilled fantasies displaced onto the adolescent.

Parents may also react to the adolescent as a lost object or as a replacement for a lost figure from earlier life. In the former scenario, the all-important process of separation-individuation is stymied as the mourning or depressive reaction of the dependent parent ties the adolescent to the parent. In this case, the adolescent feels compelled to take care of the parent or impelled to effect an abrupt and often tumultuous separation from the parent, often unable to tolerate contact with the parent for more than brief periods. In the latter case, in which the adolescent substitutes for a lost object of the parent, the ties may be more subtle and also stronger, with almost invariably the same effect.

Psychosocial Development of the Adolescent

During the entire process of maturation and separation-individuation, the adolescent has a personal set of tasks to be accomplished in the service of identity formation. During early adolescence, the intensity and exclusivity of earlier attachments to the parents begin to give way. At a time of increased urges and physiological readiness for erotic and aggressive action, closeness to family members can be quite threatening. While an expanded peer life and increased social activities facilitate this distancing, the need for an internalized autonomy from early objects is not easily resolved. Indicators of the severity of the struggle are behaviors such as insolence, disparagement of the parents, and a devaluation of past connections. This lessening of earlier attachments is a necessary developmental step if the identity and the idealized self-image of an adolescent are to take on their own uniqueness. When deficiencies exist in this area, they show up in the form of adolescents who appear to be copies of the parental models. They exhibit the typical developmental impairment of an individual who has not been able to expand beyond the earlier types of identification with parental figures. Part of the need for separation results from the requirement that sexual attachments occur outside the family. Without this process, the adolescent may initiate incestuous relationships within the family or may forgo sexual self-differentiation altogether.

Adolescence has been viewed by Peter Blos, Sr., as the second major period for individuation. The first such process was during infancy, when, by roughly twenty-four to thirty-six months, the goal of attaining object constancy was reached. Object constancy is the emotional surety about the other person, essentially the parent. If a stable sense of individual autonomy is to be achieved by adolescence, it requires an acceptance that emotional dependence on others is going to be present, that it is relative, and that it will vary in different contexts. The focus is on emotional, not physical separation. In contrast, the main task is an internal one, that of gaining emotional independence from the inordinate degree of control that internalized ties to the parents or "objects" continue to exert on the adolescent. If conflicts from earlier childhood over dependency, ambivalence, and control have not been resolved by adolescence, a variety of defenses and character traits emerge to handle the anxiety that arises over the need to individuate. These defenses may take the form of displacements, substitutions, or behavioral repetitions with others in the environment, or they may show up in the form of ego disturbances such as acting out, negativism, learning disabilities, exaggerated moodiness, or episodic acts of violence. Achieving individuation is a hallmark of both ego maturation and ego strength.

During middle adolescence, the person, if permitted by his or her development, native intellectual endowment, and social and familial educational stimulation and support, moves into the Piagetian stage of formal thought operations. These mental operations make possible many of the complex steps taken in the development of the mature adult personality. Formal thought operations are those that involve reasoning based on verbal propositions. Through this mode of more abstract thought, the adolescent can make hypothetical deductions and entertain ideas and concepts of relativity, ambiguity, and multiple causality. These operations facilitate the growing tools of self-observation, empathy for others, altruism, and abstract psychological insight. These faculties permit the controlled expression of emotions and greater titration of impulsivity in behavior, a necessary task if the adolescent is to achieve maturity. Adolescents who do not reach these levels of abstraction remain tied to the constraints of linear cause-and-effect thinking. Growth makes possible an outwardly directed, altruistic view of the world and lessens selfish impulsiveness.

Many more abstract emotional and psychological tasks await the adolescent during this middle stage. The push toward individual autonomy continues. The ability to control impulses, sublimate physically based urges, and relate to the social and personal productivity of the world of work begins to solidify. The ability to delay gratification through impulse control and sublimation plays no small part in the progression of the older teen who moves into the world of adults and the demands of the more impersonal world of work. Adolescents who remain tied to earlier and more dependent, self-centered attachments to parents view the adult authority figures in high school and the job site as ungiving and uncaring. They tend to provoke loss of jobs as they expect their bosses to care for them as dependent beings.

Egocentrism, while important as narcissistic fuel for separation and achievement, nonetheless must be toned down as the adolescent moves into the outside world beyond the immediate environment of family and peer group. Forerunners of stable capacity for intimacy and tolerance for the needs and wishes of others begin to appear in the later adolescent. Concomitantly, affective or emotional control continues its development. This capacity makes possible temper control and curbing of earlier rageful states more typical of the moody and irritable early teen. Adolescents unable to muster affective control come to use aggressive affect in bullying fashion to influence and govern relationships with others and to assuage their own anxieties borne out of incomplete self-esteem.

Self-esteem, a much overused term, nonetheless is all important for the middle to late adolescent. Many factors go into the development and stability of self-image and self-esteem in this stage of adolescence. Moral value development, with clarification of personal beliefs about religion, denotes the successful beginnings of curbing personal egocentrism and defensive narcissism. Body image, the pride, pleasure, and surety of one's physical image, is an all-important ingredient in the self-image of the adolescent. That this is well recognized in the outside world is shown by the hype and emphasis of merchandising feeding on and stimulating the insecure adolescent striving for consolidation of personal body image. Adolescents are expected to become accustomed and adjusted to the fact that their bodies have been out of their control and changed through the forces of biological growth and maturation into adult bodies.

Self-image is further evidenced by the ability of the adolescent to consolidate role identity with flexibility. Those adolescents who are not successful in this transitional skill on the way to adulthood come to be unfocused in their roles, unable to decide on their place in small or large groups, and unable to choose college majors or occupations. Others become frozen in place and rigidly define themselves out of personal instability. These are the teens who use their rebellion against parents and authority figures to construct identities solely out of their opposition to the standards and styles embodied in such figures.

Sexual definition is one of the most controversial tasks of late adolescence. It has been commonly held that an end stage of successful adolescent development is selection of a stable sexual role and self-image. This is spoken of as "gender identity." When this is not achieved, the adolescent is not able to achieve or sustain stable, enduring, and truly intimate personal sexual relationships, heterosexual or homosexual. Emotionally archaic dependent attachments in the late adolescent and early adult come to dominate their relationships, and patterns emerge of serial, repetitive, tumultuous pairings with little stability. These can be seen in the "macho male" who must have affairs with multiple women before and after marriage, revealing earlier dependent ties to parents in his quest for the perfect woman who will care for him. Likewise, the insecure gay adult may demonstrate prodigiously serial relationships with tendencies toward anonymity and lack of closeness. On the other side of the equation, some heterosexual and homosexual late adolescents and young adults establish patterns of defensively dependent closeness, tying them to hostile dependent relationships that last too long. Often they are unable to terminate these relationships even when it is best for them to do so.

The Black Family and the Adolescent

The impact of poverty and low socioeconomic status on the functioning family is unfortunately amply shown within the families of poor minorities. As Spurlock and Lawrence have written, being poor and still enmeshed in economic and racial deprivation and discrimination or regarded socially as a product of slavery adversely affects family structure. The pervasive effects on families in turn severely influence the development of adolescents, producing teens at risk, who develop antisocial syndromes as adults or who are socially and occupationally unsuccessful in disproportionately high numbers.

In spite of economic gains for the more educated black individuals and families, the numbers of black families that lived in poverty increased in the 1970s and early 1980s. For many black families, the effects of a fluctuating economy brought to a halt the economic progress of preceding years.

The adolescent in the black family faces an arduous set of developmental hurdles in addition to those posed by adolescence. By the time the black child reaches adolescence, alienation from society is often a pervasive influence. Adolescents in poverty, black as well as white, experience severe exacerbation of the usual adolescent process of disillusionment with their parents as they move toward separation and autonomy. This disappointment is made worse by the fantasized superiority of the adolescent to the parent and by the witnessing of economic stagnation or failure of the parent to make headway toward achieving the American dream. Poor adolescents experience estrangement from their parent or parents and may come to identify with antisocial and more successful adult figures, such as drug dealers.

For many years in contemporary American thought, there has been a vituperative debate regarding the strengths and weaknesses of the poverty-stricken minority family and its relationship to the spawning of antisocial outcomes in its young. Numerous authors have documented the strengths of the black family even under conditions of single parenthood, abandonment, and poverty. The survival metaphor of black children and teens has emerged as a means of conceptualizing the apparent resistance of some youth to social influences considered hostile to personality and occupational development. Black authors have become advocates for the black family by detailing the previously overlooked strengths of the black family, whether an intact nuclear family or one that is matriarchal in structure. From defense of the black family structure, some black authors have come full circle to reflect a more conservative trend toward seeing the resurgence of more traditional and cohesive family structures as beneficial.

Conclusion

The family is the original and most enduringly important formative influence in the life of the child and adolescent. The power of attachments and patterns of managing relationships and emotions internalized from within the family experience determine the shape of the personality of the young adult. Whether this newly grown young adult will function productively within the society of adults rests on years of complex and intertwined psychological, biological, and interpersonal processes that take place in the matrix of the family. The family is the most influential arbiter of the outcome of the individual. The family is, in turn, exquisitely sensitive to outside influences that affect its well-being, including poverty or affluence, illness of family members, presence or absence of parents, and interpersonal loss. The past three decades have seen an enormous increase in our understanding of ways in which the family inscribes its signature on the script of each individual family member. The family and its tasks, needs, and functions point the way toward wider societal support. The shape of society depends on the care with which the family as our ultimate social institution is nurtured by us all.

Suggested Readings

Adelson, J. "The Mystique of Adolescence." *Psychiatry*, 1964, *27*, 1–5.

Anthony, E. J. "The Reactions of Parents to Adolescents and to Their Behavior." In E. J. Anthony and T. Benedek (eds.), *Parenthood: Its Psychology and Psychopathology*. Boston: Little, Brown, 1970.

Billingsley, A. *Black Families in White America*. Englewood Cliffs, N.J.: Prentice-Hall, 1968.

Bloom, M. V. *Adolescent-Parental Separation*. New York: Gardner Press, 1980.

Blos, P. "The Second Individuation Process of Adolescence." In A. H. Esman (ed.), *The Psychology of Adolescence*. New York: International Universities Press, 1975.

Carlson, R. "Stability and Change in the Adolescent Self-Image." *Child Development*, 1965, *36*, 659–666.

Chunn, J. *The Survival of Black Children and Youth*. Washington, D.C.: Nuclassics and Science Publishing, 1974.

Chunn, J. *Portrait of Inequality: Black and White Children in America*. Washington, D.C.: Children's Defense Fund Press, 1980.

Hill, R. B. *The Strengths of Black Families*. New York: National Urban League Press, 1972.

Lidz, T. *The Family and Human Adaptation*. New York: International Universities Press, 1963.

McAdoo, H. P. (ed.). *Black Families*. Newbury Park, Calif.: Sage, 1981.

Mahler, M. S. *On Symbiosis and the Vicissitudes of Individuation*. New York: International Universities Press, 1968.

Malmquist, C. P. "Development from Thirteen to Sixteen Years." In J. D. Nospitz (ed.), *Basic Handbook of Child Psychiatry*. Vol. 1: *Development*. New York: Basic Books, 1979.

Spurlock, J., and Lawrence, L. E. "The Black Child." In J. D. Nospitz (ed.), *Basic Handbook of Child Psychiatry*. Vol. 1: *Development*. New York: Basic Books, 1979.

Staples, R. *The Black Family: Essays and Studies*. Belmont, Calif.: Wadsworth, 1971.

5

Effects of Poverty and Affluence

Paul L. Adams, M.D.

Many unemployed, demoralized, and unmotivated young people live in the United States today. Some of these young people need to be evaluated from the standpoint of mental disorder. In some cases that have been referred to me for evaluation during the past decade, while the young adult's parents have felt that the referred individual was depressed (sometimes they *were* suicidally depressed), they offered, oddly, to pay for an evaluation only, leaving any extended care for me to negotiate, on a sliding-fee basis, with their offspring. This is odd because the young offspring are so poor economically and because the parental abandonment of the youth to manage his or her own psychiatric bill often has been the parents' first dramatic act to "emancipate" their offspring; parents turn them over, in effect, to the adolescent psychiatrist. Such parents are especially fearful of financially coddling late adolescents; they appear delighted to hand them over to a psychiatrist.

Work with these demoralized, burned-out young people has led me to enlarge my psychiatric approach by adding the perspective that the young person is also an economic specimen, although usually not an economic success story. Increasingly, economic failure in young people may be seen as less indicative of personal psychopathology than of some institutional structures that go beyond the motives of individuals and values of families. The institutional approach does not supplant but rather complements customary psychiatric work whenever the latter scrutinizes family, school, and peers.

Advanced capitalism, it is generally theorized, has segmented economic institutions into three different domains: (1) a monopolistic sector of

118

huge corporations; (2) a state capitalism sector; and (3) a free-market competitive sector. As Marxists are fond of declaring, the economy has made
definite moves away from a strong and viable sector of free competition
while showing a vigorous growth in both monopolization and state capitalism. Thus, it is the first two sectors that have reached paramount importance economically; while a competitive free market has been extolled loudly,
it has been declining rapidly. Both monopolies and state capitalism are
strengthening rapidly. For the present, it is not only their dominance but also
their honeymoon, this truce between the state and the monopolies, that has
come into being. Competition has been squeezed out of many fields, even the
health field, as Curtis Bergstrand showed in a study of nursing homes in
Kentucky. What, then, does an economic structure of monopolies and government in coexistence mean for the unempowered young people of
America?

Several economic matters must be considered. First, young people are
consumers more than producers; economists view youth as a nonproducing
dependent group who receive income transfers from producers. As consumers, they are catered to when capitalists pitch their toys, clothes, books,
breakfast cereals, toothpastes, and games toward young people. Certain
adolescent and child fashions influence adults to mimic them, causing
adolescents to become pacemaking consumers. The clothing industry, for
example, may undergo drastic shifts in styling, but a continuous and recurrent theme is that all ages are urged to dress like adolescents. Blue jeans are an
example of how an older generation is persuaded to mimic adolescent dress
patterns. One new consumer age group is preadolescents, now called
"tweens" to indicate their ages between nine and thirteen, between childhood
and adolescence. In 1987, some 82 percent of a sample of the sixteen million
young people in that age range said that their primary wish was for money to
buy more of the fashionable clothes, cassettes, and records that have become
very dear to them. They have made shopping malls into their gathering
places. Youth are, indeed, a special market for consumer goods purveyed with
advertising "hype." However, youth are also potential producers. Many do not
consider them as producers simply because the economy is structured to
make youth demur from being productive.

Children and adolescents are not only dependent on adult producers
but also shut out from ownership and paid labor. In short, youth are pres-
sured toward becoming economic nonentities in our capitalistic system.
Their powerlessness and redundancy from the standpoint of economic
exchange make them a true underclass from an economic perspective. They
have nothing; they control nothing; they earn nothing; and they are superfluous. When the time would ordinarily have come for them to "get started in
the labor market," they find that full labor is not needed and full employment
is not a national policy.

Young people from affluent or working-class families who are ready to go to work find themselves encouraged, instead, to linger on in college beyond four years, prolonging the earning of baccalaureate degrees and doing graduate work. Having obtained a terminal degree in the humanities or social sciences, many no longer truly young people find that academic employment is not available to them, despite the fact that their whole preparation as graduate students was for a nonexistent academic post. Youth who drop out of high school and do not go to college fare even worse. If adolescence was an early capitalist invention in a previous era of increasing industrialization, the prolongation of adolescence today is a creature of postindustrial, advanced capitalism.

Youth, both as a phase in the life cycle of individuals and as a communally shared experience, embodies structurally induced incompetence and dependency. We must inquire how these young people reaffirm their incompetence in their life-styles but also ask what—in the structure of economic institutions—breeds and reinforces the incompetence of youth, giving youth psychosocial stressors and economic stressors that are institutionalized. This warrants a closer look into the economics of being young in America.

The Shrinking Demand for Youth as Competent Workers

Youth are in no real demand as producers. They are paid subminimum wages that cause them to be debilitated as a class; they are urged to add more years to the quasi-compulsory ten years of education; they find quickly that the "welfare" state is structured to offer them only casual, off-and-on employment and unemployment. Youth cannot even collect unemployment insurance, since they have not been previously employed.

The very location of productive industries is increasingly remote from high-youth populations; that is, remote from large urban areas. The number of formal and informal apprenticeships available to youth has decreased radically during the past two decades. For example, in June 1978, electrical and plumbing unions in New York City opened their apprenticeship programs to 550 youths. The weekend before the applications were distributed, more than a thousand youths camped out for two nights on sidewalks outside the union halls, hoping to be hired as apprentices to plumbers and electricians.

Self-employment and family-centered employment, traditionally attainable in agriculture and small business, have become a thing of the past for youth, as monopolization of capital has squeezed out the small entrepreneurs in both farming and commerce. Simultaneously, youth confront an escalating number of rules serving to exclude them from work seniority, such as work permits, "protective" maximum hours to work, driver's licenses, workers' compensation, complex safety regulations, and statutes requiring that youth cannot operate forklifts or be near or deal with other "dangerous" equipment or moving machinery.

The legal labor force of America has been subdivided by economists into a force that is composed of core workers, called the *primary labor market*, and a population of underdogs, called the *secondary labor market* and consisting of young people, illegal aliens, and similar factions. Among the secondary labor market's salient features are that the workers are poorly paid, their work is unskilled, and the enterprise is labor-intensive but not unionized. When the secondary labor market grows, living standards decline. The secondary labor market waits in the wings for youth, matching the adolescent's own desire to hibernate and procrastinate. Even in the primary labor market, there have been structural changes in recent years. In aerospace and "defense" industries, for example, it is not production workers who shape the industry; instead, it is the engineer, a nonproduction worker. And if youth have any talents at all, they are to work hard and productively, not to be engineers and idea people.

Youth as a class are shut out from legal employment at a rate five times that of adults. Teenage joblessness is twice that of the middle-aged in good times and bad. For black youth, the unemployment rate rises to as high as 50 of every 100 youths. Because youth are shut out of the primary labor market and find numerous obstacles to working even in the secondary labor market, jobs in the "hidden economy" are appealing. Both the primary and secondary labor forces deal in the "legitimate" economy, but the hidden economy has far more to offer young people. In the hidden economy (also called "illicit," "illegal," "pariah," and "underground" by some writers), no records are kept; there is little red tape—the mission of the enterprise may be altogether illicit or merely tax-evading.

The impoverishment of women and children and youth under eighteen years, sometimes called the "feminization and juvenilization of poverty," is an escalating phenomenon in the United States. More women are taking on the arduous job of producing the entire income to be transferred to the young in America. It has been estimated that, at the present rate of pauperization, by the year 2006 few people except women and children will be dirt poor in the United States. The economic demolition of women and the young does not bode well for our national future. Nevertheless, America remains as the sole holdout among all of the world's industrialized nations in *not* having a national policy to support families with children.

The Supply of Youth

Most of the circumstances already noted would be called "demand factors" by an economist. In brief, the economic demand story is that there is little demand for youth in the economic institutions of America. However, demand is not the entire story, since youth can be viewed also from the standpoint of available *labor market supply*. When the labor force is larger than the job market, glib explanations often are offered. If the labor market is glutted by oversupply, then oversupply is often advanced as a reason for gravely high unemployment in a particular sector of the work force. Can the chronically high unemployment be explained by an oversupply of youth resulting from the indirect or second-generation effects of the post–Korean War baby boom? Have youths merely multiplied faster than jobs in our economy? The answer to these questions is simply no.

Only in 1974 was there an appreciable increase—an oversupply—in people aged fifteen to twenty-five years. The increased supply of youth coincided with two things in 1974: an economic recession and a heavy migration by black youth into cities. By 1960, two-thirds of such youths had taken up residence in cities, swelling the ranks of the unemployed. By 1974, some effects of a baby boom were evident, but by 1984, that was no longer a sizable factor in youth unemployment. During economic recessions, heavy unemployment among youth often occurs; truly, they are the last to be hired and the first to be fired. But the business cycle is not the main causal circumstance for youth unemployment.

Is youth unemployment due to the high turnover of youth? Is their economic incompetence compounded by their quit rate? Are youth frequent entrants, dropouts, and then reentrants into the work force? The answer again is no. Instead, unemployed youth are never hired in the first place for the most part; they are principally an *unwanted* supply. They are the school dropouts, the nonwhite, the inexperienced and unskilled. Also, they are students who unsuccessfully seek part-time work. Since many students do work, and most of the remainder wish to work, the Bureau of Labor Statistics considers youth who are students as among the jobless whenever they have no work. Other countries do not calculate their youth unemployment in that manner, and their inclusion in the United States may artificially elevate our figures on youth unemployment.

The most remarkable *supply* issue is the competition for jobs that youth encounter. Who is squeezing these lumpenproletarians out of their point of entry into both the primary and secondary labor markets? American youth have been moved aside by two principal competitors for jobs: adult married women who want to work and illegal aliens who have entered the U.S. work force. The aliens have probably had some deleterious effect on the economic chances of American youth, but it may be a different matter with women entering the work force. Economists concede only that married women did not account significantly for the high jobless rate of youth in any jobs except those requiring the driving of cars, trucks, and other vehicles. Employers and parents know that insurance for company vehicles increases significantly when a young male is listed as the driver of the vehicle.

Supply factors soon pale as determinants of youth joblessness when they are compared with demand factors. There is not an overabundance of youth in America. The supply of teenagers stopped growing late in the 1970s, and in 1983 the supply of all people in their early twenties began diminishing. However, the supply of black and Hispanic youth has risen steadily during the 1980s. The fifteen- to twenty-five-year-old age group today is almost 20 percent black.

Many forecast that youth will continue to be confined to entry into the underdog secondary labor market or into the underground economy. Despite that reality, it is anticipated that most governmentally subsidized youth training programs will be geared only to the *primary* labor market and will overlook the secondary market. And, naturally, the underground economy will be neither countenanced nor eliminated.

The economist Martin Trow gave considerable attention to the mechanisms by which youth might enter the secondary market, or even the illegal market, in a way that would augment their economic life chances—specifically, the chances to move from secondary to primary status in the labor market. Briefly put, Trow found that movement into the primary labor market was facilitated by two things: (1) on-the-job training that prepared youth for primary labor market jobs (good examples being informal apprenticeships and nonunion construction jobs; poor examples being crime, marginal manufacturing, and casual labor) and (2) on-the-job links to primary labor market jobs (good examples being apprenticeships that expose one to primary labor market openings; bad examples being fast-food chains). There are some unskilled jobs from which youth can move upward economically with greater ease than from other jobs. Many jobs in the secondary labor market are dead-end jobs, quite literally getting youth nowhere, and often these are the only jobs available.

Trow acknowledged that youth, not a unified bloc, should be subdivided on economic grounds into four groups: (1) advantaged youth, (2) alienated or dispirited youth, (3) disadvantaged youth, and (4) deprived youth. It goes without saying that no public support programs are required for either advantaged or alienated youth. Probably, too, no additional special programs are required for many of the merely disadvantaged youth. Disadvantaged (but not deprived) youth demonstrate what a social support network can do economically in communities all across America: These youth have used their families and friends to make economically fruitful contacts. They often squeeze out the deprived from federally funded programs, and they are often co-opted and show a declined militancy. They and their families have spawned a complex apparatus of ethnic patronage across America; black or Hispanic or whatever their ethnicity, they have been able to land the Cooperative Educational Training Administration jobs and the Youth Education and Training Program jobs and to cash in on job opportunities in a way that deprived youth are unable to do. The truly deprived lack the "pull" (*palanca*, for Hispanics) that the disadvantaged know very well.

Disadvantaged and truly deprived youth often choose the option of becoming soldiers. When youth were conscripted into military service during the Vietnam War era, disproportionate numbers were drawn from working-class or lower status; with a voluntary armed force, the situation stays the same. Middle-class people have been neither drafted nor volunteered in sizable numbers; the poor and working-class youths are our warriors. Young blacks and Hispanics appear in numbers at lower military echelons far beyond their proportion in the general population. Still, not even the intensified war economy of the 1980s has benefited the economic fate of poor minority youth. Of all youth, the economy demands them least.

Doctrines That Blame Youth for Economic Dependency

Our age is one of blaming victims. We wonder what the victim of rape did to encourage her attacker(s), what the sexually molested child did to welcome the abuse, what the elderly lady did to invite the mugger to assault her, what it is about the poor that invests them in an unending cycle of poverty and shiftlessness, what it is about youth that makes them unduly dependent.

Psychiatry contributes its share of victim blaming. Psychiatrists who do not keep their conceptual frameworks open to multiple etiologies beyond simply that of the individually based psyche may utilize their guild's well-established cognitive patterns to ignore socioeconomic influences on behavior. They may think more of the lusty motives of wicked children than of the beam in the eye of wicked adult seducers and con artists. Witness our terminology: oedipus complex of children, the wife-beater's wife, the Cinderella complex of sexually abused girls, and the culture of poverty. This victim blaming is apparent, too, in doctrines that blame youth for their economic dependency. We look to youth themselves for a motivation that could account for their being so deprived of economic life chances. We are ever fond of asking what youthful motives, skills, and personal traits are associated with young people's becoming productive workers, as if the key were mental. Terms such as "youth culture," "cultural unemployment," or "culture of poverty" have wide currency and are preferred to institutional explanations that point to the very structure of our economy.

A doctrine that has considerable popularity among psychiatrists is that the increased hustling and illegal participation by youth in an illegal work force can be attributed to their lack of firm values and the rules of their "main chance" attitude. Youth are said to go into the pariah economy solely by free choice and not because of society-generated imperatives or necessities. We are inclined to impute motivations to youth that have no basis in social relations but are abstracted out of their social context. Youth are said to seek transitory jobs that do not tie them down to structured hours, regular work, and reliable obligations and responsibilities. They prefer, it is said, jobs that give them time to hustle, to study, and to travel—all with their age mates in the youth counterculture. We tend to regard alienation and disaffection within young people as the chicken and unemployment or unemployability as the egg. In truth, participation by youth in the subterranean economy is large—involving 10 percent of GNP and eight million workers—because most youth would rather go to work illegally than stay unemployed or stuck in the secondary labor market.

In a related doctrine, the increased delinquency and drug abuse among school dropouts and unemployed youth, although a reality, are seized on to "prove" that staying in school as long as possible adds to a youth's virtue, not just to his or her "bourgeoisification." Similarly, it is not the schools but youths themselves who are said to hold the key to the growing time gap between school and first job. The majority of youth, prepared as if for the primary market, ultimately enter the *secondary* labor market. The schools are academic-elitist, giving a "Mandarin" education but too little education in literacy and numeracy and too little practical training or counseling. Yet the mystique invested in education persists and functions as a self-fulfilling prophecy. Youths who do not go those two extra years do experience a disadvantage on their entry into the work force.

Robert and Helen M. Lynd discerned the relation of jobs and schools in 1937 when they wrote words that still ring true today: "Middletown's industries may be absorbing less and less of the population under twenty, leaving a helpless group too old for school and too young to get jobs. Under the circumstances, the prolonging of schooling through high school and into college may represent not only a desire for more education but a slowly growing necessity to choose between school and idleness" (p. 49).

While other advanced capitalist nations send only 15 to 20 percent of their eighteen- to twenty-four-year-olds to college, in the United Sates 50 percent of such youth are in college. Traditionally, Europeans have recoiled in fear from the rebellious potential of an unemployed intelligentsia, but Americans either have no such fears or do not believe that American colleges and universities can produce an intelligentsia.

Another of our cherished doctrines highlights the transition of youth from school to work while ignoring the transition from secondary labor market to primary. That shift in focus leads to our neglect of the true issue. For youth, the greatest difficulty is experienced in shifting to decent, stable jobs and leaving the dirty work of their first jobs behind. The social fact for most people is that the shift into the primary labor market now occurs five to ten years after they leave high school. That is a long delay, especially for youth with working-class or lower-class backgrounds. The horror, particularly for deprived youth, is that they stay put in poorly paid, transitory, uncertain, nonunionized, and dead-end jobs. For increasingly large numbers of youth who do not have a solid network of patronage and support to lean on, the reputed casualness of the adolescent–young adult moratorium in the secondary labor market has taken on a dreaded and compulsory permanency.

Some who are fairly advantaged will enter the secondary labor market only temporarily during their adolescent moratorium and then will leave the meaningless work behind. Some who are really advantaged will proceed directly into the primary labor market, while yet others, because of disaffiliation and counterculture participation or because of deprivation that is secular and enduring, will get stuck in the dirty work of either the secondary or the underground labor market or drift back and forth between secondary labor and chronic unemployment. Paul Osterman has noted, "The key characteristic of the U.S. labor market is the differential, in treatment and behavior, between youth and adults" (p. 151).

The world over, it is the adults who block youth's entry into the labor market. The adults shut out the youth, letting them in only when someone is needed to do the dirty work that adults reject doing. To be young in America is to be economically disadvantaged.

Cultural Contradictions Compounded

The general public's attitudes about adolescents' work in the United States show the operation of two conflicting imperatives. One is *to protect them* against child labor so that they might remain free of adult responsibility. The other is *to pressure them* to be more like adult workers.

Being more like adults means both to abide by the work ethic (even if done compulsively) and to be cynical and disaffected. Until age eighteen, the young male (and, less frequently, the young female) is exempted from the moral requirement to work and earn, but after eighteen, or earlier if the youth has dropped out of school, there is an urgent moral imperative to go to work for wages. Oddly, the pressure for sixteen- to nineteen-year-olds to go to work poses another dilemma, for that age group constitutes 25 percent of the unemployed in this country. They feel impelled to do what is socially structured as an impossibility for many.

Vocational training courses often are irrelevant to both the young people and their prospective employers. On-the-job experience might be thought to be just what is needed for adolescents—that is, some practical experience in working, in producing, and in acting responsibly. But high school students with jobs are often *more cynical* about work—that is, more like adults—than are nonworking students. And getting a job does not necessarily teach a young worker job-related skills such as punctuality, dependability, responsibility, or taking initiative. Most of the available jobs are in alienated work, at the bottom of the secondary labor market or patently illegal. Hence, working youth show higher rates of alcohol use, tobacco use, and sexual promiscuity than their nonworking age mates. Available work may initiate the young into manhood or womanhood but not into being dependable. In the 1980s, jobs have been debased markedly for adults, too—those jobs that have remained available are largely in the services sector.

What of More Affluent Youth?

Because of the escalating constriction of the American economy, most of today's middle-class youths are fated, in their adult lives, to live like the present working class. The middle class, while often regarded as a soft underbelly in our stratification system, has also been seen as a stabilizing element that transmits—even imposes—its sometimes straitlaced ways onto other classes and sets the moral tone for American social life. During my lifetime, the middle class has shown a decided propensity toward easy manipulation by governments, both in the world's democracies and in fascist regimes. The result has been a dramatic decline in morale and moral leadership. Today, in America, the middle-class stabilizer is radically destabilized. Middle-class dreams of a brighter world are being shattered, and the middle class's former optimism seems silly because it is compromised by our current economic and political dispensation.

Most middle-class youth will not grow up to live in privately owned homes; economists forecast that only 15 percent of those now under thirty years old will ever become homeowners. Nor will they find other survival essentials to be purchased as readily as by their parents. Even food and clothing will have to be budgeted and managed in a more stingy spirit than previously. In leisure and entertainment, the crimp will show conspicuously. International travel will be replaced in large measure by the necessity to "see America." Homegrown vacations using automobiles to travel to more proximate locations, camping and backpacking to the point of overflowing parks and public facilities, will be the standard way to vacation for the middle-aged middle class in the future.

The precariously constricted job market, with seldom a hope of respite for young people, will destabilize them still more. Job losses and structural unemployment will be the norm for young adults from today's middle class, and that norm will be compounded by youth unemployment based on age discrimination, the further demise of the smokestack industries in the United States, and the glut of doctors and lawyers in the United States that promises to decrease the attraction of these two traditionally chosen vocations for middle-class people. The onrush of women and children into poverty, so greatly augmented by recent administrations' economic policies, may continue for another decade or more, if a system of family subsidy is not enacted into American law. More and more children will grow up in want.

The wastage of the war economy, now made permanent in a highly structured reign of nuclear deterrence, adds to the demoralization of today's young people. The nation's productivity and taxes have been poured into the "defense" budget for past, present, and future wars instead of being deployed to more constructive channels. In the future, middle-class youths may be expected to take up military service that now is much more the preserve of working-class and underclass youth. If the economy constricts, the middle class will revert to more and more of the ways of the lower-than-middle classes.

The Really Rich Adolescent

A tiny minority, the really wealthy youth of America are unlikely to consult psychiatrists, vocational counselors, social workers, psychologists, and others in the human service professions. Their very wealth makes it hard for them to ask for competent professional help, and their unusual backgrounds and life-styles make it difficult for them to receive help even when they (or their family members) request psychiatric aid and comfort. They are accustomed only to solving problems on their own terms. Devoid of employment and of vocational plans, they often come across to those who are not rich as lacking in goals and unable to accomplish the tasks of adolescence. They defend their behavior by asking, "Why strive and strain if I don't have to?" In the terms enunciated by Erik Erikson, an adolescent's required accomplishments are sense of selfhood, vocational preparation and engagement, emancipation from parents, and sexual activity and commitments. How do the rich accomplish these tasks?

Reared principally by servants, these youth have learned by the time they achieved sexual maturity that class distinctions (and at times racial or other ethnic considerations) compel them to pull back from their earliest "love objects" and to take up instead an uneasy camaraderie with members of their own class. This knowledge produces an emotional discontinuity between their affectional attachments of earlier childhood and their "serious" obligations toward a future of identifying with extremely rich families and acquaintances. Ultimately, if rather late, they may be claimed by their family ties. Their infancy was spent in the company of nannies, their early childhood in the company of nursemaids and governesses, their school years in local private schools followed by boarding schools. Only in their later, developmentally formative years is the family eager to undertake a rather loose emotional affiliation with them. This is, however, not a close emotionally based attachment but a tight, clannish class bond occurring only when they have moved forward into late adolescence. Meaningful life in the original family has come too late for many highly wealthy youths. They feel lonely, unbonded, alienated, and unable to buy what they long for most of all.

But they try to buy happiness and can appear to do so while their extended youthful moratorium is drawn out interminably. It seems to end only when some agonizing self-assessment at middle age makes them dread their feeling empty, devoid of intimacy, unfulfilled, adrift. These youth may develop syndromes of narcissism, empty depression, cult membership, and other woes. This is not to say that the "poor little rich boys or girls" surpass the youth of the underclass or working class — or even the affluent middle class — in human suffering. It is still a truth in America that poverty does not necessarily make us happy (or miserable) and that all rich people do not feel miserable (or happy).

Differing Economic Pathways Related to Other Forms of Stratification

It is not only economic or class position that has a telling influence on youth in America; added to and interrelated with economic level are race, ethnicity, and gender. Let us consider how adolescence is stamped by growing up poor and white/black/Hispanic, or female, or of growing to adolescence in a mother-only family. In the commentary that follows, our attention turns back to youth in the working class, at the very bottom of the working class, or solidly in the underclass. These are the majority, vastly outnumbering the middle- and upper-class youth whom we have just been considering.

Racism and Classism

Class divisions are apparent by the time a young person reaches adolescence, even in such intimate matters as sexual behavior patterns, familism, respect for education, food aversions and preferences, and many more zones of personal life-style. When racism has been both attitudinally and institutionally structured in form during one's upbringing, stark differences will crystallize and consolidate by adolescence.

While the middle-class white adolescent has an advantaged position for attaining the accomplishments of Erikson's normal adolescence (sense of ego identity or selfhood, vocational preparation and engagement at least in learning, emancipation from parents, and being sexually active with some feelings of commitment), the working-class adolescent is relatively disadvantaged, and the adolescent of the underclass is deprived. The deprivation and disadvantage of the lower economic classes are compounded for black and Hispanic adolescents and, in many ways, recompounded for females in all those groups.

The social psychiatrist has a particular interest in deprived youth. Their situation economically and socially is a tangle of pathologies and a litany of disasters. Deprived youth are intimately involved in urban crime and in drug and alcohol addiction and abuse. They are prone to physical illness, chronic mental illness, and dependence on welfare and frequent psychiatric or correctional institutionalization. The deprived youth of America are a costly group because of the need for police to monitor and apprehend them, courts to "serve" their legal-judicial needs, and psychiatrists to "minister to their needs" in mental hospitals. Their spiritual losses in the realm of reduced quality of life constitute enormous drains and catastrophes in the lives of millions of deprived young Americans who are both poor and members of minorities. Some of their spiritual demoralization is readily apparent in the ways they face their adolescence.

Emancipation from Parental Authority

The emancipation of minority youth from their more authoritarian parents is often thwarted because their youthful strivings are interpreted as disloyalty (in Spanish, *faltas de respeto* — "lack of respect"). Consequently, quite benign youthful moves toward separation from parents are met with brutality and a persistence of parental intransigence. Often this leads to an incorrigible rupture between the two generations within the family, because the parents disallow negotiation or third-party mediation. Occasionally, a black teenager can call an aunt or uncle for aid, and a Hispanic working-class youth may avail herself or himself of a shrewd and tactful *madrina* or *padrino* (a godparent). As family enculturation advances, however, those resources usually disappear, especially for Hispanic youth.

Parents of minority adolescents often cannot abide any challenge or correction; they will not tolerate a rebellion within their own home and at their own hearth, not even if the clamoring subservients adopt loving and nonviolent tactics and hope ardently for no permanent breach. How well this kind of family experience prepares minority youth for democratic participation is a matter for conjecture and certainly of future consequence for the citizenship needs of the nation.

Vocational Preparation

Compared to middle-class whites, black and Hispanic youth are less frequently hired, are subjected to institutionalized antiyouth and antiminority practices in the marketplace, and are less enspirited about what formal education can do for one's chances in life. As a result, these youth are victimized by self-fulfilling prophecies that they will swell the ranks of dropouts and delinquents rather than become solid members of working or middle classes. Although some blacks and Hispanics have penetrated into affluence in the 1970s and 1980s, most of the working class has undergone economic deterioration, so that skilled minority workers, as an example, are worse off at the end of the 1980s than they were, relatively, in the 1950s, before civil rights legislation was enacted.

Do these changes imply that civil rights have not benefited minorities? Not really, because racism has actually lessened a bit since 1950, but it has merged with institutional disorganization and dysfunctional changes in the unregulated American economy to worsen the lot of ethnic minorities in the lower classes. Civil rights enactments have helped the minorities to forestall even greater suffering between then and now. If there had not been a civil rights struggle, the economic conditions of minorities, including minority youth, undoubtedly would have experienced an even greater erosion.

When the unemployment rate nationally was 7.6 percent in 1985, the unemployment rate for Puerto Ricans was 14.3 percent and for Mexican Americans 11.9 percent. Black unemployment in that period was higher still; added to that of other minorities, it gave a rate of 12.8 percent for minority women and 13.4 percent for minority men and averaged 35 to 36 percent for minority group members who were under nineteen years of age. Consigned to being second-rate and restricted to dead-end and dirty work, the bulk of today's ethnic-minority youth promises to swell the ranks of the underclass in America. Ethnic-minority women and their children promise especially to augment the numbers of America's dirt poor, since they suffer additively from classism, sexism, childism, and racism in this country. Often bearing children in their early teens, minority women account disproportionately for teenage pregnancies and deliveries. A sobering warning is that more than half of the black babies born each year in the United States are conceived out of wedlock, with an even higher proportion of babies being born out of wedlock to black teenagers.

Even Hispanics, with their undocumented but undisputed claim to a stability generated by family ties, have "illegitimacy rates" higher than those of whites. They also have more female-headed households (mother-only families) than the non-Hispanic population of the United States. Compared with the general population, Hispanics have more than five times the percentage of people with fewer than five years of formal education. In 1984, Hispanics had an unemployment rate more than twice that of the entire U.S. population and almost two and a half times the percentage of Anglos who lived below the poverty level. Those figures do not augur well for strong-but-poor Hispanic families in the United States.

Sense of Selfhood

Reaching adolescence laden with complexes and complications from earlier life stages is not salutary. Some of the woes, often blandly called "risk factors," of minority adolescents are parental absence during infancy (minority parents work out of the home with less adequate child-care provisions); subjection to stricter "discipline" and "toeing the line" during the walking and talking period of infancy (minority poor children, although motorically precocious and fending more for themselves, are made to be more obedient to parental will during the anal phase); having one's initiative curbed during the oedipal phase (minority children are often plagued by guilt about sexual desire and activities); encountering repeated episodes of feeling incompetent and inadequate during elementary school (minority school children are relegated disproportionately to special education programs in public schools and are considered to be slow learners and to have more behavior problems); and experiencing more loneliness and pseudomutuality than honest sociability and collaborative love during preadolescence. In a way, all of the precursors of adolescence show more losses than gains when one grows up poor. If one is also a member of an ethnic minority, the losses are augmented.

Classism and Sexism

Family life in the working class has not been a salutary or even benign experience for females. Today, more working-class women are repudiating marriage and the family or delaying them for a prolonged period while working in the primary and secondary job markets. Female children growing up in families with both parents working outside the home—now the statistical norm for Americans—experience an even greater need for auxiliary or surrogate parenting (child care, from the adults' perspective) during their upbringing. When they have matured out of adolescence, these girls face the necessity of getting jobs, now a common fact of life for them. They no longer are coerced into being solely homemakers but are expected to become "supermoms," with home management as an added burden to working for wages full time outside. The new pattern of overburdening women with two jobs exists in both capitalistic democracies and the "socialist" countries of Eastern Europe. While girls now have welcome alternatives other than motherhood's mandate imposed on them, they are correspondingly not an advantaged group within either the family or the marketplace.

In the workplace, some ancient patriarchal values persist: refusal to pay women equally for comparable work, an unwillingness to promote women equitably for competent performance on the job, consignment of women to work that does not compete directly or strongly — in good times — with jobs that have been the traditional realm of males, hiring women last and firing them first, giving no provisions for care of children, and so forth. Females are gradually closing the wage differential between themselves and males, but much of the gain has occurred by degradation of the jobs of males, not by higher pay for women. Still, the wages of the female employee typically are about 65 percent of the male's wages for comparable work.

Often the woman has a husband who is an equal of her children in demanding services in her second job as housewife and homemaker. Little responsibility for child care or cleaning, dishwashing, food purchasing, or preparation of meals is shared by her spouse, even if he verbally espouses his support of equality, women's liberation, and fatherly participation in child care. A young girl growing up in that atmosphere catches on rather quickly. If the family lives like the middle class, the girl discerns that she is somebody or at least has a chance to be someone later, provided that her family's ideology is not to perceive the female as a second-class person. If her family lives like the working class, she may sense that her future role as a breadwinner is not valued highly, her deformities and illnesses are treated more lightly, she is less likely to get orthodontia or psychiatric care than are her male siblings, and considerable pressure is exerted to influence her outcome as mainly a sex object who will turn into a mother sooner or later. If her family is lower-class, she may have only a mother, or perhaps no identifiable parent. More than a million children in the United States live in institutions apart from any parental care givers. The lower-class girl receives an upbringing in adaptive paranoia: Men mistreat women, adult males sexually abuse girls, and men rape one in three to four females before they attain the age of eighteen years; the streets are unsafe most of all for females.

In all classes, there is discrete socialization of the young male and female, but in the middle class, this is less conspicuous. In lower classes, it begins in the cradle and proceeds with escalating intensity until young adulthood. There are shapings of sexuality by class position throughout the life cycle.

Between the ages of twelve and eighteen, reproductive capabilities mature, the genitals enlarge, and the pudendum darkens and goes through hairy puberty. Procreation, seen as threat or delight, becomes feasible for the young woman at all economic levels. At this age, the adolescent woman shows a keener interest than ever before in the mere mechanics of sexuality; this is the age at which health and hygiene teachers usually propound a mechanistic version of human sexuality. Moral matters also begin to be highlighted, and a conscientious stand is taken on whether to engage in sexuality at all, and, if so, with whom and with or without promiscuity. In this period, orogenital practices are shown both in lieu of coitus and masturbation and in addition to them, especially in middle- and working-class females.

The teenage years bring an avid quest by all economic levels for the florid peer folklore about relations between men and women, a folklore that influences many youth to begin in earnest to pair off (done in elementary school also, but only in preliminary fashion). Pairing is accompanied by a progression in intimacy and caring concern about interpersonal and genital adequacy.

Before she reaches eighteen, the young woman usually has pretty well channeled her sexual desire along economic class lines. Economic type casting continues until the mid-twenties and then becomes stereotyped, almost ossified, for her and her partners. Lower-class adolescents frequently continue a pattern of premarital coitus, but middle-class youth may exhibit great caution and delay the time of their "invention" or "discovery" of frequent and regular sexuality. Working-class youth appear to be intermediate between lower- and middle-class females in their adolescent sexual activity.

In interaction with lower-class males, lower-class females learn to view sexuality as a power strategy, a love substitute, a medium of exchange for material commodities, an entertaining and playful diversion, a source of prestige, and a badge of identity. The working-class woman gets very similar messages but enshrouds her sexuality in more taboos and restrictions than lower-class female youth and fewer than the middle class.

By age eighteen, between 25 and 90 percent of females have masturbated, around 80 percent have petted up to orgasm, and 45 percent have had coitus. Black young women have surpassed even lower-class white males in frequency of coitus by the age of eighteen years. The young black woman's sexuality shows a scripting and meaning that combine class, ethnic, age, and gender influences (classism, racism, childism, and sexism).

After her eighteenth year, the patternings of class, ethnos, and gender exert greater influence over a woman's sexuality. The age of eighteen is a watershed year in other ways—leaving one's status as a minor; "deciding" (under classism's strong guiding arm) whether to go into the army, into the secondary or underground labor market, or to college; and being able to vote. For many young women, it will not be an age that ushers in economic security and stability but will instead be confirmation of "a lesser life."

Teenage Parenting

In 1985, black teenagers of all classes attained a pregnancy rate of 163 per 1,000—compared to 83 per 1,000 for white teenagers—to yield an overall teen pregnancy rate of 95 per 1,000 in the United States—almost three times the teen pregnancy rate in Sweden. Some 59 percent of pregnant young black women in the United States gave birth to the babies that they carried (54 percent for white teenage females), but only 8 percent of them were married when the babies were born (35 percent for white teenagers). Black teenagers showed a 41 percent abortion rate and whites 47 percent. Those who have abortions appear to receive contraception information that reduces future pregnancies, but those who give birth to children usually have multiple childbirth episodes before they reach thirty years of age. Since 1976, Congress has imposed escalating restrictions on public funding of abortions and family planning services for poor women.

Two generations are handicapped when a teenage mother delivers a living baby. Fewer than half of teen mothers complete high school; almost three-fourths of welfare mothers had their first baby when they were teenagers. From an obstetrical standpoint, they have more difficult and hazardous deliveries, and their offspring have lower birth weights at term, higher infant morbidity and mortality, and a higher incidence of neurological problems. The children are at risk for parenting distortions such as abuse and neglect, and ultimately they suffer from educational deprivation and lowered employment opportunities.

Teenage fathers show a bleak picture too, in contrast to men who wait until they are over twenty years old to be fathers. Their incomes are lower, their education is shorter because they drop out of school to try to get nonexistent jobs, and they go on to have more children than nonteen fathers. Few social supports are available for either teenage fathers or mothers, regardless of their marital status or race.

The Distinctive Economics of Being a Young Female

Since the mid 1970s in the United States, poverty has been "feminized and juvenilized," because females and children have disproportionately filled the ranks of the poor. Before that period, young women often were not expected to work outside the home, or, if they did, it was only as a temporary "secondary" worker, since it was the man of the family who was expected to be the primary breadwinner. But by the year 1980, two-thirds of American adults below the official poverty level were female, more than half of poor families with children were headed by women, and more than half of the mothers of young children worked outside the home.

Women traditionally occupied only about 20 of the 420 occupations listed by the U.S. Department of Labor; in those "women's occupations," they could earn only 50 to 60 percent of what men earned. Other women were the main competitors for these jobs, squeezing out male youth who desired to enter the labor force, and as a majority of women came to work outside the home, those jobs became further degraded in real-dollar terms. As I commented earlier, the degradation of working-class men's jobs continued throughout the 1980s: Typographers have been replaced by word-processor operators, machinists by unskilled operators, and department-store buyers by clerks who monitor the store's computerized inventory. Work in hospitals, laundries, and fast-food stores has drawn unemployed oilfield workers, off-shore divers, and auto and steel workers back to work — but these jobs have obviously degraded their skills and pay and thrown them into competition with women and youth, while decreasing "unemployment statistics."

Married or not, American women are working, often two jobs. Employed or not, women are poor in America. At their present rate of pauperization, only women and children will fill the poverty class by the year 2000. The tragedy is worst of all for women who are heading households with children.

Adolescents in Mother-Only Families

It is estimated that in 1989, about fifteen million U.S. children (eighteen years and younger) lived in mother-only families, but it is not certain how many of those were adolescents. In "fatherless" families, mothers lean heavily on their teenage offspring for practical help and moral support. Were they not to receive aid and boosting from their teenage offspring, mothers in mother-only families would be lonelier than they are already, more depressed, task-inundated, and emotionally overloaded, and more insecure and stressed. The son of a single female parent is the object of special maternal apprehension and trembling when he is young, for the mother may believe, until the son is eleven years old or more, that she is inept at disciplining and handling a fatherless son.

The single mother's trepidation is understandable when we read the facile statements by politicians and psychiatrists that a son without a live-in father is in peril. The single mother fears that her young son will turn out to be maladjusted and that she will not be able to deflect him from that course or to guide him toward a productive life. But by the time her son gets to be eleven or twelve, the mother often becomes relatively sanguine, feeling that her son will indeed turn out well. We may wonder, of course, what this "trial period" of maternal doubt and wariness means to the son. Nevertheless, by adolescence the son's moral probation in the eyes of his mother may come to an end, and he may feel appreciated as someone grown up and worthwhile.

A sexually mature youth, male or female, in a mother-only family is more likely than any other teenager to be a valued member of the household, doing assigned chores more faithfully than children in fathered families and in general showing earlier signs of cooperation and dependability, less rebellion, and more work, independence, and autonomy. Mothers in mother-only families are not very likely to regiment, infantilize, and overprotect their adolescent offspring. Hence, the adolescent tasks of parental emancipation and separation and individuation into selfhood are not typically impeded in

the mother-only family; nor are adult sexuality and sober vocational direc-
tionality generally interfered with in such a family.

One of the most telling differentiations in mother-only families is the
particular family's reason for being fatherless. Self-esteem varies according to
reason for fatherlessness — whether it was a result of never marrying, divorc-
ing, deserting, dying, working in a remote location, imprisonment, or prolonged hospitalization. A father who died as a moral and diligent worker but
left something for his heirs is more easily beloved than an unknown father
who never was around after insemination.

The influence indelibly stamping the mother-only family as institutionally vulnerable for all of its members is its economic poverty, not its
fatherlessness per se. Homelessness, hunger, and being ill-clad are all present
to haunt the mother-only family that is fatherless by virtue of never marrying
or from divorce or desertion. When divorce occurs, as it does in half of all
American families, the family often becomes poor overnight, because 80
percent of children whose parents divorce are fated to live with their mother,
and her income is usually insufficient to keep them above the poverty level.
The mother-only family that resulted from the father's desertion, imprisonment, or absconding without marrying is plagued by both poverty and often
a sense of shame. Nobody can give honor and praise to an absent father so
much as the children of a widowed mother. Hence, the family has no great
shame, usually, when dad has died; moreover, they are best off financially of
all the fatherless children — provided that the father qualified for benefits to
survivors.

Sociopsychiatric theory and research have devoted a great deal of
attention to the mental disorders, sex-role identification quandaries and
distortions, learning and academic problems, and delinquency that have
been imputed to fatherless children. Factoring out the tangled pathologies
resulting from poverty, racism, sexism, and childism so that they stand
independent of and apart from pure father absence is very difficult, leading
to the conclusion that father absence may play a very minor role, overall, in
the psychosocial noxae that enmesh the child and adolescent in a mother-
only family.

Recommendations

There are at least three positive changes that are attainable for poor families.
First, a *family subsidy* should be required for income transfer and support of
the nation's infants and children, whose plight has worsened each year since
1979. Infant mortality and infectious diseases and vitamin deficiency disorders that earlier had been reduced and almost eliminated have all risen again
in the past half decade. All families with children under eighteen years of age
are a needy but vital group for America, and a subsidy should be available to
them, not solely to those on welfare now.

In addition to family subsidies, there are two other ways in which a chastened and less affluent nation can benefit its youth between now and the year 2000: expansion of the welfare economy, or *human service sector* of the economy, and strong moves toward *economic equalization* of income, goods, and services, not merely of "opportunity." Were we to become a nation with incomes guaranteed and maintained at a livable level for all, a nation in which human service is vaunted and not decried, things would change from dismal to halfway hopeful.

With our national ideology today of espousing the ethic of warfare rather than welfare, we have a nation in which more than half the population receives economic support from a "welfare" or "social security" program of one form or another. As that grows and achieves legitimacy, regularization, and institutionalization, America may become more frugal but more secure for all. Even the middle class benefits from welfare programs, which, although often dubbed failures, have actually saved and upgraded the lives of millions in this country. For many, a national health service of one sort or another would seem to be an imperative for the United States.

When warfare and not welfare becomes the watchword, as it has in the United States during the past half century, inequality in the economic sphere becomes standard. By 1984, the poorest two-fifths of American families earned 15.7 percent of the national income, the middle fifth received 17 percent, and the wealthiest two-fifths of families received 67.3 percent. The lowest three-fifths of families, all together earning 32.7 percent of income, received the lowest income percentage recorded since 1947, the year when data collection began. For the top two-fifths of families, the percentage of economic holdings was the highest ever recorded. That inequality indubitably takes its toll on the youth of America, in the bottom three-fifths.

Extension and consolidation of America's welfare system is the only national policy of the future that makes sense for adolescents. The Scandinavian democracies may be the best models to follow, for they have consigned nearly all of their national priorities to support and provision of human welfare programs while at the same time maintaining democratic political forms and preserving individual rights and liberties. Their outlays for "defense" are relatively small. It seems mandatory that welfare must take precedence over warfare if the U.S. population is to survive economically. Human ingenuity must find ways to support our young in economic institutions that are far more serviceable than those to which American youth now have access.

Suggested Readings

Adams, P. L., Milner, J. R., and Schrepf, N. A. *Fatherless Children*. New York: Wiley-Interscience, 1984.

Ehrenreich, B., and Piven, F. F. "Women and the Welfare State." In I. Howe (ed.), *Alternatives*. New York: Pantheon, 1984.

Gordon, M. S. *Youth Education and Unemployment Problems: An International*

Perspective. Berkeley, Calif.: Carnegie Council on Policy Studies in Higher Education, 1979.

Greenberger, E., and Steinberg, L. *When Teenagers Work*. New York: Basic Books, 1986.

Hewlett, S. A. *A Lesser Life: The Myth of Women's Liberation in America*. New York: Morrow, 1986.

Lynd, R. S., and Lynd, H. M. *Middletown in Transition: A Study in Cultural Conflicts*. New York: Harcourt Brace Jovanovich, 1937.

Osterman, P. *Getting Started: The Youth Labor Market*. Cambridge, Mass.: MIT Press, 1980.

Price, R. H., and Burke, A. C. "Youth Employment: Managing Tensions in Collaborative Research." In R. N. Rapoport (ed.), *Children, Youth and Families: The Action-Research Relationship*. Cambridge, Mass.: Harvard University Press, 1985.

Wixen, B. N. "Children of the Rich." In J. D. Nospitz and I. N. Berlin (eds.), *Basic Handbook of Child Psychiatry*. Vol. 1. New York: Basic Books, 1979.

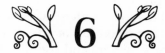

6

The Role of Education and Extracurricular Activities

William M. Kane, Ph.D.
Elias J. Duryea, Ph.D.

Health problems facing adolescents today can be categorized into two general areas. First are the unhealthy outcomes of which we are all painfully aware, such as suicide, pregnancy, injury and death caused by violence and automobile crashes, sexually transmitted diseases, and drug-related death and disability. These tragic outcomes are only the tip of the iceberg. Risky health behaviors, which may not yet be apparent as negative health outcomes, constitute the rest of the iceberg. These behaviors include tobacco and alcohol use and unprotected sexual activity, as well as risky health behaviors related to physical and psychological conditions such as obesity, eating disorders, and depression. Both risky behaviors and the consequences of those behaviors have a disproportionate impact on poor, disenfranchised, and lower socioeconomic groups, in which black, Hispanic, and Native American youth are overrepresented.

Professionals working in education and health fields as well as parents frequently encourage young people to remain in school and to take part in school health education classes, physical education and fitness programs, and school- and community-sponsored extracurricular activities. Many believe that education in general and health education, school physical education and fitness classes, and extracurricular activities in particular confer on adolescents a certain immunity from many social and health problems. These beliefs can be stated as hypotheses against which research evidence, pro and con, may be evaluated.

Hypothesis 1: Education contributes to prevention of adolescent health problems.

Subhypothesis a: Exposure to health education contributes to prevention of adolescent health problems.

Subhypothesis b: Participation in physical education and fitness-related activities contributes to prevention of adolescent health problems.

Hypothesis 2: Participation in school and community-based extracurricular activities contributes to prevention of adolescent health problems.

The remainder of this chapter explores the research related to the effects of health education, physical education, and extracurricular activities on the health of preadolescent and adolescent youth. Do education and extracurricular activities protect young people from health problems? What specific programs or activities make a difference? Programs and emerging trends that hold promise for the future are identified and discussed. The chapter concludes with recommendations for health and education professionals and parents regarding future action and research to prevent adolescent health problems.

Research Deficits

The relationship between the quality and quantity of exposure to health and physical education experience and subsequent development of risky or nonrisky health behavior in adolescents is, unfortunately, supported by little research. There is professional debate concerning the premise that more vigorous academic training in health education and physical education for young people results in lower rates of health problems later in life. While, for instance, the epidemiology of inner-city, poverty-level drug use is well documented, the confounding factor of heredity makes virtually impossible any conclusions about the absolute effect of educational exposure on later health status. In addition, mitigating variables such as teacher preparation and motivation, educational resources, family milieu and history, and community and environmental constraints make the picture even more confusing. Inner-city schoolteachers as well as their counterparts in affluent independent school settings all experience varying degrees of success in influencing student health, just as they do in influencing scholastic behavior.

Epidemiological Opportunities

Too few epidemiological studies have been conducted that delineate the dynamics that may determine what educational experiences and exposures would consistently predispose the adolescent away from health-debilitating actions and toward those that are health-enhancing. An array of epidemiological research designs is available to examine such questions. While the ability of such designs to provide definitive conclusions is limited, they can produce data with which subsequent investigations can be extended and refined. Educational researchers have not generally utilized these research approaches. The prospective cohort design is one such epidemiological methodology that investigators in education could implement. With this design, matched groups (cohorts), such as schools that have similar size, demographics, and resources but differing educational curricula, could be identified and followed over time and later assessed on a measure of interest (for example, proportion of students developing a certain health behavior, such as smoking). If one is able to make a compelling case that the schools are comparable except for educational curriculum and that they consistently differ on the measure of interest, then that difference could be cautiously attributed to the type of educational curriculum. The ability to replicate such outcomes in different regions of the country with different cohorts would support the proposition that the difference (for example, lower rate of smoking) is a result of the only differing variable (the type of educational experience). Such prospective design logic is well verified by the notable Framingham heart study as well as by many other epidemiological investigations.

The retrospective, or case-control, study is another possible epidemiological methodology that could be used to assess the effects of educational curriculum on later health status of adolescents. In contrast to the prospective cohort method, this process involves looking back in time at similarly configured groups that differed only on exposure to one variable (educational curriculum) and then examining them in the present time to measure the other factor of interest (proportion of students engaging in the risky health behavior of interest). Although inferences drawn from studies employing this design are attenuated by numerous sampling limitations, essential evidence can be produced. Moreover, the case-control method may be more efficient than the prospective cohort design, because with this method, data are collected and analyzed after events have already occurred. To date, neither cohort nor case-control design studies have been conducted on a national scale to examine the association between educational experience and later health problems in pediatric and adolescent populations. Without such investigations, the hypothesis concerning the relationship between educational exposure and later health problems in youth will remain unconfirmed.

Classic Studies of Stress, Coping, and Resilience in Children

Research focusing on the factors that enable young people to manage the stress of daily life is somewhat more abundant. In the attempt to understand what characteristics best help youth resist temptations and pressures to engage in risky health and social behaviors, it is important to look at several classic longitudinal studies that have examined coping skills and protective factors in children. With the increase in drug abuse, health-compromising sexual activity, alcoholism, homicide, and suicide, a new and burgeoning educational emphasis on coping skills has emerged.

In longitudinal research spanning more than two decades, Rutter investigated the attributes that foster greater coping behavior among adolescents. Rutter examined children from families where abuse, neglect, and punishment were consistently evident. His research identified factors that children use to overcome their environment and rearing history to become contributing, successful members of society. He labeled children who were able to overcome their deprived upbringing psychologically "resilient." These children did not become chronically involved with substance abuse, nor did they engage in delinquent or protodelinquent behavior during their early adult years. Nonresilient children, conversely, tended to engage in socially deviant acts such as stealing, abusing alcohol, taking illicit drugs, and engaging in risky sexual behaviors. A cluster of five psychosocial factors consistently emerged as predictors of a child's psychological resilience and ability to be successful and productive later in adult life. Secure relationships, adaptability, social problem solving, self-esteem, and self-efficacy were strongly associated with those deemed resilient.

With great consistency, Rutter's examination of resilient children's support networks reinforced generally accepted thought that if children are provided secure relationships that are stable, caring, and sharing during early adolescence, they will be less likely to fall prey to problem behaviors later. Although this factor by itself was less than maximally protective, it was inevitably present and potent when "resilient" children were evaluated. Children without secure relationships in their immediate milieu were at increased risk of entering into risky and health-debilitating behavior. Rutter found that resilient children were quick to report secure relationships as a major coping source, whereas nonresilient children could not report as great a level of such relationships.

Similar findings emerged when children's ability to adapt when circumstances or situations were abruptly changed was assessed. Resilient children somehow learned (possibly from resilient models) that even with a new and unexpected turn of events, one could survive and manage new demands. In seeing their significant referents (models) cope effectively with unplanned-for challenges, these children apparently learned how rewarding it was to adapt rather than give up and quit in despair.

Resilient individuals have been portrayed in Rutter's research as adept at social problem solving. They are skillful at generating a range of solutions when faced with a social dilemma. Children who learned, through observation, how adults around them deal successfully with social problems tended to perform similarly. Nonresilient children tended not to possess this ability to emulate adults and consequently had fewer skills to draw on when faced with pressures to take health-risky actions. Resilient children tended to have the ability not only to think of an array of ways to solve a social problem but also to assess the implications of various alternatives. Such an ability necessitates a more reflective style of thinking under pressure and frequently results in a better chance of beneficially resolving problems and conflicts.

A feeling of self-worth and esteem in children was also strongly associated with those children identified by Rutter as resilient. Nonresilient children tended to feel as though they were victims of fate and that they were not in control of their own destiny. Children who feel that they are worth something, that they matter and that they do indeed have some control over their lives, ultimately perform better under environmental stress. Children without this quality are more susceptible to a host of social and health-related problems. Once again, models were seen as critical precursors to a child's development of positive levels of self-esteem.

Health education research during the last decade has focused a great deal of effort on examining what Bandura and associates have called self-efficacy (a person's belief that he or she can do something and that this will result in the desired outcome). Rutter's work assessed this psychoemotional factor in children from traumatized backgrounds and determined that resilient kids possessed greater levels of this personality factor. Several model health education programs have recently been developed around this concept of helping young people develop self-efficacy through social skills and competence training. (A brief description of these kinds of programs is presented later in this chapter.)

In a series of investigations, Rutter and colleagues found that socially and emotionally deprived but resilient girls who had spent most of their lives in institutions and survived horrendous experiences reported a much higher level of favorable school experiences than did their nonresilient counterparts. The resilient girls in these studies reported a greater degree of success at school than nonresilient girls. It is striking that these "successes" were not generally academic, but were more often general or social. Succeeding at sports, achieving a position of responsibility, earning some recognition in music or art, having a faculty confidant, or even just being the "class clown" was protective (that is, seemed to correlate with ability to cope) for these girls. Whatever the success, it made the individual feel better, gave her some pleasure, and resulted in her acquiring some degree of resilience. Conversely, in a study comparing these girls to normal, noninstitutionalized girls, these protective factors appeared to add little additional resilience for the normal, noninstitutionalized girls. In other words, for a child raised in a happy, normal, stable family, these extra positive experiences did not contribute as much to the child's resilience.

Nonresilient girls from these institutions tended not to plan their marriages (non-planners), whereas resilient girls (planners) engaged in careful planning. Nonresilient girls often married to escape a bad situation, whereas resilient girls married men who were sharing, caring, and secure partners. Inevitably, girls who had some positive experiences at school were

much more likely to be planners. Good school experiences seemed to provide these girls with increased self-esteem, self-efficacy, and a sense of positive
accomplishment, thus giving them a feeling that they could also succeed at
others things—such as choosing a good partner.

In research spanning more than a decade, Block and colleagues followed children from ages four to fourteen and studied adolescent resilience
and vulnerability. Their research assessed factors that tended to be consistently associated with children who have been labeled "stress-resistant." Such
children were much like children studied by Rutter in that they were evaluated as able to overcome pressure and stress and still perform successfully.
Block found that some "stress-resistant" children had been mis-classified
because they actually used denial or lacked the intellectual capacity to
comprehend a condition that would for most people be stress-inducing.
Block reinterviewed subjects at ages four, five, seven, eleven, and fourteen to
examine developmentally how such children thought under stressful situations. Results repeatedly suggested that these children practiced both distancing ("that does not affect me") and minimalization ("it's really not that big
a deal" or "it's not very important"). Such psychological defense mechanisms
served to insulate these children from the environmental threats affecting
them. In real-world situations, such adaptive coping processes may become
detrimental rather than propitious because they lessen the child's exposure
to tangible real-life learning experiences. For children faced with the health
threats of contemporary society, insulation via denial and minimalization
does not help to provide the competence needed to deal with real-life
challenges.

Block developed a set of designations more precise in portraying truly
stress-resistant children. Block's "ego-resilient" child is a child who possesses
the ability to maintain integrated performance under conditions of frustration and stress. For example, consider a student who has only a little time left
to complete a test (stress) and has difficulty completing a problem (frustration). The ego-resilient child perseveres, trying different routes toward a
solution, while ignoring the impending pressure of time. The child without a
resilient ego submits to the pressure and frustration and ultimately ceases
performance—that is, gives up. Despite the difficulty of the problem, the ego-
resilient child is not threatened by possible failure and continues to try
different solutions. Such a child stands a better probability of negotiating
life's challenges and pressures than a child not so inclined.

Reducing Risks with Health Education

Research has provided health and education professionals with a general
sense of factors that tend to promote health-enhancing behavior in youth.
Educators at the primary-grade level must be cogently aware of these research
findings in developing pedagogical techniques that help promote such
attributes as resilience and ego strength in their students. The physical as well

as the psychoemotional threats our children face in the near future are immense. The cognitive, affective, and behavioral reserves that will be required to successfully negotiate these threats must in large part derive from the education they receive in the school setting. It is imperative that we evaluate the role of health education in the promotion of those characteristics and thus in the prevention of adolescent health problems.

Health education is a comparatively new discipline drawn from an eclectic foundation including education, psychology, sociology, medicine, and anthropology. The earliest research in health-related education focused primarily on providing students with cognitive knowledge. Critics were quick to point out that such increased information was of little relevance if it did not facilitate adoption of healthy behavior. Recent critics still echo this response whenever health education interventions demonstrate gains in knowledge but no overt behavioral changes.

As a new member of the larger family of education, health education has borrowed heavily from the broad base of educational science, theory, measurement, and practice-related research. The extension of this research base to specific health behavior issues (drug and alcohol abuse, nutrition, sexual activity, and fitness) has increased steadily during the last two to three decades. Current health education efforts utilize an array of pedagogical principles to stimulate healthy behavior in children. By integrating various cognitive, social, and behavior theories, researchers have been able to alter rates of health-compromising action in target subjects. Nowhere has this occurred on a larger scale than in pediatric and adolescent health promotion programs. Some noteworthy studies in this area are examined below.

Social Influences and Personal Skills Programs

Botvin's longitudinal research involving adolescents in New York City presents an excellent illustration of how health behavior can be favorably influenced by applying developmental and educational theory. Results from this exemplary research indicate that students can indeed be prevented from taking up cigarette smoking if the causative factors (high-risk situations, inability to resist peer pressure) in the development of the behavior are clearly delineated and addressed with appropriate intervention strategies. Botvin's Life Skills Program puts students into role-play simulations of situations that they will face in real-life settings. Students rehearse what they will say and do in the situation and examine the costs and benefits of various choices. In this fashion, students have some forewarning and practice in managing difficult situations that inevitably arise.

Botvin proposes that the development of risky adolescent health behavior, specifically substance abuse, is a function of two major antecedents. The first is the potent role of social influences, such as peer pressure, family modeling, and community media exposures. The young are largely unaware of how these influences operate to encourage experimentation with health-compromising behaviors. It is critical to note that high accessibility of health-risky products (tobacco, alcohol, drugs) is also a major antecedent to the adolescent's inclination to initiate risky health behaviors. While some propose a major prohibition in this area, it is probably more efficient in the long run to deter children from wanting chemicals than it would be to eradicate all potential access.

Inadequately developed personal and social skills constitute the second major factor that Botvin identifies as contributing to health-risky behavior among adolescents. The young are cognitively ill equipped to solve personal problems, make systematic and personally beneficial decisions, resist media appeals, or formulate and enact verbal counterarguments. Botvin's studies also indicate that students often lack the skills to know when and how to effectively assert oneself or how to initiate social interactions with the opposite sex. These deficits are seen as factors that predispose the young to substance abuse and health risks.

The Life Skills Program includes a multifaceted curriculum that addresses social influences and inadequate social skills and the causative factors within each. Students receive educational treatment that provides them with an awareness of the social influences predisposing them toward unhealthy behaviors. The program also provides behavioral training that helps students develop personal skills to actively resist the pressures that force them toward unhealthy acts. Results from Botvin's studies, as well as the results of other programs with similar orientations, indicate success in helping young people avoid unhealthy behavior. A reduction of between 50 and 87 percent in the number of new smokers has been shown in various research studies. These results far exceed results of past program efforts. Botvin's studies demonstrated a 50 to 67 percent reduction in the number of pretest nonsmokers who became regular smokers at a one-year follow-up with no reinforcement "booster." Pentz reported that her social skills intervention program produced a favorable effect on students' alcohol use and concurrently on academic performance. Her research found that the social skills development approach was an effective educational strategy for preventing teenage pregnancy. The application of social skills development to eating behaviors has also been tested with adolescents.

The School Health Education Evaluation

Many curricula designed to foster health enhancement among schoolchildren have been developed and implemented in the United States during the last decade. Without standardized measurement techniques or similar protocols (content, exposure time, implementation), precise evaluations of their effects have been difficult. Answers to the often-asked questions about school health education curricula — "Did the treatment make any difference?" "Did the time spent on this subject change or prevent health-risky behavior in those exposed?" — have remained inconclusive until recently.

The School Health Education Evaluation (SHEE), a three-year study, completed in 1985, that evaluated the effects of four different health education programs, has produced considerable evidence regarding the effectiveness of school-based health education interventions. The results of the study, involving more than 30,000 fourth- through seventh-graders from seventy-four school districts and more than 1,000 classrooms in twenty states, suggest that students exposed to comprehensive school health education exhibit significantly greater increases in health knowledge and positive changes in health practices and attitudes than do control groups not exposed. The results are best summarized in the comments of the project advisory panel: "The study shows, in general, that health education works; that it works better when there is more of it; and that it works best when it is implemented with broad-scale administrative and pedagogic support for teacher training, integrated material, and continuity across grades. It works best when there is attention to the building of foundations of basic health knowledge, rather than starting with categorical health problems later in the academic career of pupils."

There are now empirical data, rather than just anecdotal recollections and perceptions, that justify health education claims that comprehensive school health instruction produces favorable cognitive *and* behavioral effects. The schools implementing the four curricula were compared to schools not implementing a health curriculum, across the following four student test constructs: (1) overall knowledge, (2) attitude, (3) health practice(s), and (4) program-specific knowledge. Students receiving the health curricula scored higher than those not receiving them across each of these domains. Not surprisingly, evaluators found that it took many more hours to produce a favorable effect on children's attitudes than it took to show a positive impact on knowledge. In general, favorable changes in student behavior (for example, not taking up cigarettes) were achieved after thirty hours of these curricula, while a favorable impact on attitudes required fifty hours of curriculum time. When investigators examined various levels of program implementation for the four outcome areas, linear results consistently emerged: Regardless of the curriculum, the greater the degree to which the curriculum was implemented, the greater the difference between comparison and participating schools across outcome measures.

With most studies in behavioral science research, if a process is not followed in the way that it is designed to be followed (poor fidelity), the measurement of its influence is suspect. The potential results of numerous health behavior investigations have suffered from a deficit in program fidelity. The SHEE provides data for examining program fidelity. The success of the evaluation was divided into four distinct core elements: (1) teacher fidelity to the curriculum in concert with the duration of student exposure to the curriculum, (2) the extent to which exposure is accumulated year by year, (3) administrative support and commitment to school health education, and (4) adequately prepared and motivated teachers. Inevitably, given greater time and resources for both process and impact evaluations, school health education research will produce even more knowledge regarding the effects of adolescent risk-reduction programs.

Christenson and associates at the Center for Health Promotion and Education, part of the national Centers for Disease Control in Atlanta, have conservatively extrapolated that 146,000 seventh-grade students would delay the onset of smoking by having been exposed to the School Health Curriculum Project (SHECP). SHECP was one of the four curricula studied in the School Health Education Evaluation. Figure 6.1, taken from the SHEE report published in the *Journal of School Health*, portrays this extrapolation. The naturally low incidence of smoking among fourth-, fifth-, and sixth-grade students precludes any statistical difference between the SHECP and comparison classrooms. However, as students enter seventh grade and as smoking experimentation escalates, earlier exposure to a comprehensive school health program exhibits a potent prophylactic or delaying effect. Such an achievement has been the goal of health behavior programs in adolescent populations for many years. The ability of program interventions to utilize education to impede the development of health problems or health-compromising behaviors in children remains at the forefront of pediatric-based health promotion.

Researchers both within and outside health education have consistently emphasized the postponement of problem behaviors as an objective, because, it is reasoned, a certain proportion of those who postpone taking up a health-risky behavior will never take up the behavior. Intervention programs work both to postpone the acquisition of the risky behaviors and to help youth develop knowledge and skills that increase the likelihood that they will never experiment with those behaviors.

Current and Future Directions in School Health Education

The burgeoning area of adolescent-focused health behavior research provides significant cause for optimism. Further contributing to this optimism are recent changes in the preparation of school health educators, in school curricula, and in intervention projects within communities, resulting in increased support for school health education.

In the past, health education in the schools was often delivered by teachers with marginal or no preparation in the subject matter. Today, newly trained specialists in school health education are emerging. Their professional preparation includes course work in anatomy and physiology, as well as content competency in areas such as nutrition, drugs, alcohol, tobacco, infectious and chronic diseases, and human sexuality. The preparation of these teachers also includes course work in educational methods, materials, and philosophies; program planning and evaluation; and behavior change strategies.

The goals and content of school health education are also undergoing

Figure 6.1. Comprehensive School Health Education Makes a Difference: Estimates of Number of Children Who Smoke.

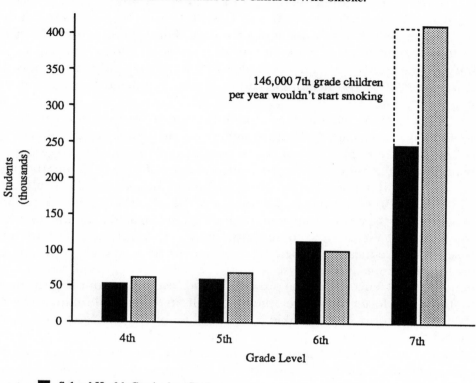

School Health Curriculum Project
Comparison Classrooms

Source: G. M. Christenson, R. S. Gold, M. Katz, and M. W. Kreuter, "Preface: School Health Education Evaluation." *Journal of School Health*, 1985, *55* (8), p. 296. Copyright 1985. American School Health Association, P.O. Box 708, Kent, OH 44240. Reprinted with permission.

dramatic changes. The goals, which once focused solely on the acquisition of knowledge about health and disease, have evolved to include the development of life skills such as decision making, resisting peer pressure, and self-reinforcement, as well as assistance to students in creating opportunities to practice healthy behavior. The content recognized as appropriate for school health education today includes prevention of drug, alcohol, and tobacco abuse; safety and injury prevention; adoption of health-promoting behaviors, including exercise, proper nutrition, and stress reduction; development of mental health and responsible sexual behavior; and the acquisition of skills and knowledge needed to appropriately utilize the health care system. Additionally, some innovative school programs work to help parents increase their health knowledge and thus ensure essential support to create opportunities at home and in the community to practice and to support healthy behaviors.

Increased community support has resulted in legislation and administrative decisions to strengthen school health education programs. Recent legislation has established an Office of Comprehensive School Health Education within the U.S. Department of Education. That office has been charged with the responsibility of working with state and local education agencies to improve the number and quality of health education programs in schools. A curriculum in school health education is now mandated by twenty-seven states.

The nation's schools offer a powerful vehicle for directing America's youth away from health-debilitating behaviors and toward health-enhancing behaviors. Careful planning of health education programs and targeting of behavioral interventions designed to meet the specific needs of the students are essential if schools are to have maximum impact on the health of adolescents. Other factors that will influence the success of health education programs are the preparation and motivation of the teacher and the support provided by the school and community. Characteristics of exemplary school-based health education programs designed to help young people make healthy decisions and establish healthy life-styles include exposure of students to the science of disease prevention and health promotion; assistance to students to foster their development of skills in reflective thinking, critical evaluation, and decision making; and facilitation of the development of students' ability to identify potential threats to their health and take action to resist those threats and minimize their impact. The end goal of health education is an individual armed with knowledge, skills, and the belief in his or her personal ability to act to prevent disease and promote health. The implementation of school-based health education programs with the characteristics described above is one action that communities can take to help youth grow up healthy.

Physical Fitness: Building the Foundation for Good Health

It is widely held that participation in physical education activities promotes healthy development. More than 97 percent of this country's elementary school children and more than 80 percent of its secondary school students have access to organized physical education. Students in elementary school take physical education an average of 3.1 times weekly, with 36.4 percent taking classes daily. At the high school level, students take physical education an average of 3.9 times weekly, with 36.3 percent taking classes daily.

Physical fitness has long been recognized as an important component of good health. *Mens sana in corpore sano*—"a healthy mind in a healthy body"—has been an accepted principle of good health for centuries. Plato recommended that individuals exercise both the body and the mind in order to maintain a healthy balance. The popular literature attributes a wide range of benefits to physical exercise, including improved cardiovascular and physiological functioning, reduction of stress, reduction of weight and fat, improved skeletal and muscle structure, and increased sense of self-worth. Indeed, research findings seem to support many of these popular beliefs. A brief review of the literature addressing these areas of physiological growth, cognitive enhancement, mental health, social development, and self-concept is presented below.

Physiological Growth

The book *Physical Activity and Well-Being*, published in 1986 by the American Alliance for Health, Physical Education, Recreation, and Dance (AAHPERD), provides an excellent review of research in the biological and behavioral sciences relating physical activities to the well-being of school-age children. In that publication, Malina concludes his review of the effects of exercise on growth and development by stating that physical activity is an important factor in the regulation of fat tissue in children and adolescents. Although weight loss is not common with regular activity, it generally results in an increase in lean tissue and a decrease in body fat. He also indicates that regular physical activity stimulates growth and integrity of bone and muscle tissue. Exercise enhances skeletal mineralization and density and produces wider and more robust bone growth. Regular high-resistance physical training results in hypertrophy of skeletal muscles. The beneficial changes in body composition and specific tissues are a function of the specificity, duration, and intensity of the exercise. Changes in response to short-term exercise programs are generally not permanent.

The importance of physical exercise early in life development supports the case for including such experiences in preschool and elementary school programs. Haubenstricker and Seefeldt concluded in the AAHPERD publication that the early acquisition and development of motor skills throughout infancy and early childhood provide a basis for the continued enjoyment of the benefits of movement and vigorous exercise.

Cognitive Enhancement

The benefits of exercise appear to extend beyond the physical domain to enhance cognitive development. Williams reports that, although limited in scope and design, research in motor development and cognitive growth indicates that development of basic and fine motor skills provides an important foundation for the development of more sophisticated perceptual and cognitive behaviors. Evidence suggests that at least a minimal set of neuromuscular skills is necessary for cognitive functioning. Sheppard found that in addition to gains in maximal oxygen uptake and increased muscle strength and performance, students who participated in additional physical education show improved language and math performance. These gains were posted despite a 13 to 14 percent reduction in classroom time. Similar findings were reported by Bailey.

Mental Health

Many have attempted to link physical exercise with improved mental health. There is some evidence that physically active individuals respond less intensely to stress and exhibit greater emotional stability and ability to cope with stress than inactive individuals. A review of eleven scholarly reviews on the psychological effects of exercise concluded that, although it is clear that physical activity is related to positive mental health, much remains to be learned regarding who can benefit from what types of exercise and under what conditions. The conclusions of a recent National Institute of Mental Health workshop on exercise indicate that physical fitness is positively associated with good mental health and wellness and that exercise is useful in reducing anxiety.

Social Development

Society has long expressed the belief that participation in physical activity and organized games and sports results in the development of "character" and acts as an important factor in social development. Many of the "health" problems of adolescents today are interwoven with their efforts to reach adulthood in "socially acceptable" ways. Drug and alcohol abuse, tobacco use, and indiscriminate sexual behavior, all with serious health consequences, might be described as misguided responses to the stresses of growing up. Parents, teachers, and many health professionals have often prescribed participation in organized physical activities as one means to help children avoid social ills. Sage, following an extensive review of the effects of exercise on social development, concluded that the personal-social effects of participation in physical activities are largely unknown. Sage's conclusions are supported by other reviewers, who agree that too little evidence exists to support claims that physical activities significantly contribute to overall personal-social development. Research focusing on possible relationships of organized physical activity (mostly sports) to personality and to social attitudes and values has been inconclusive. Research in the area of physical activity and self-concept has, however, suggested some interesting possibilities.

Self-Concept

Self-concept, believed to be a critical factor influencing behavioral choices related to health, can be seen as a result of experiences related to the development of cognitive, social, and motor skills. If one accepts this relationship, successful experiences in organized physical activities appear to have the potential to influence self-concept via both social and motor development. Indeed, a positive relationship between physical fitness and self-concept of elementary school–age children has been found by several researchers. Researchers have also produced similar findings among young adults. However, it is not always possible to determine the specific components of a physical fitness program that are responsible for the difference.

Participation in Sports

The literature tends to report positive effects of *fitness* on self-concept, but the effects of *organized sports* on self-concept remain unclear. Sage has reported that research on the relationship between participation in organized sports teams and self-concept does not show the same consistent pattern as does the relationship between physical fitness and self-concept. He states, "It appears that involvement in organized competitive sports produces a professionalization of attitude, meaning that greater emphasis is given to performance outcomes and the quest for victory and less to playing fairly. Indeed, persons who have extended experiences in organized sports display poorer sportsmanship attitudes than non-sports participants." While the slogan "sports builds character" is often used to support organized sports programs, this notion has rarely been subjected to empirical or longitudinal research. However, there is indication that structured games are effective in producing cooperative, socially interactive behavior.

Research indicates a consistent positive relationship between participation in interscholastic sports and academic achievement. Furthermore, at the high school level, it appears that sports participation does enhance educational aspirations, especially for youth from working-class families. Sports participants also tend to be less delinquent than those who do not participate in sports, with the greatest differences occurring among lower-social-class youth. Moreover, youth who regularly engage in conventional community and school activities may be less prone to take up problem behaviors such as marijuana and alcohol use.

The Progression of Physical Education Programs

Despite the growing body of knowledge regarding the effects of physical fitness and exercise on health and the long-time existence of physical education programs in America's schools, all is not well. Key findings from the National Children and Youth Fitness Study released in 1984 cited the following problems:

- Body fat of today's youth is significantly greater than in the 1960s.
- Only 50 percent of today's youth participate in appropriate physical activity.
- Only 50 percent of the students in twelfth grade participate in physical education classes.

- Physical education teachers devote most classroom time to competitive sports and other activities that have questionable health effects and that cannot readily be performed once one reaches adulthood.

Recognizing the importance of exercise for young people, the U.S. Department of Health and Human Services document *Promoting Health/ Preventing Disease: Objectives for the Nation* recommends that by 1990, 90 percent of ten- to seventeen-year-olds should participate in vigorous exercise and that 60 percent should be enrolled in daily physical education. That document, developed in the early 1980s, was an attempt to identify target health objectives to measure population health gains. One key assumption of these objectives is that school-based fitness programs embrace activities beyond competitive sports. The 1984 National Children and Youth Fitness Study found that the majority of school programs were not geared toward that end.

The typical student in the fifth through twelfth grades reports that more than 80 percent of his or her physical activity takes place outside of school physical education classes. Although some of this time is spent in school-related activities, the large majority of it is spent in activities sponsored by community organizations, including religious groups, parks and recreation programs, local teams, and private organizations. The variety and types of activities in which young people engage vary by gender. The top five activities for young females were (in descending order) swimming, bicycling, disco or popular dancing, roller-skating, and brisk walking. The top five activities for young males were bicycling, basketball, tackle football, baseball or softball, and swimming. The average young female spends 71 percent of her activity time on lifetime-oriented activities (that is, nonteam sports, such as golf or tennis, that can be performed for the rest of one's life), whereas the average young male spends only 56 percent of his activity time on these activities. Community-based exercise programs are more oriented toward lifetime activities (63 percent) than are school-based activities (48 percent).

The National Children and Youth Fitness Study found that year-round participation in appropriate physical activity and enrollment in and exposure to a wide variety of activities through physical education classes influence the fitness of school-age children. They further found that the greater the number of physical activities in which students participated and the greater the variety of community organizations through which they participated, the greater the level of fitness.

Youth can derive both physical and social benefits from carefully designed and implemented physical education and fitness programs based in the schools. Such programs should be implemented by schools wishing to increase young people's chances of growing up healthy.

The Phenomenon of After-School Hours

Adolescents appear to be far more susceptible to peer pressure to enter into risk-taking behavior during the unsupervised hours between 3 and 6 P.M.

than at any other time during the day. There is considerable research to support the hypothesis that much of this susceptibility is a result of the absence of supervision. For many adolescents, the time immediately after school and prior to the arrival of parents from work is unsupervised or "self-care" time. Studies to determine the number of children who spend this time unsupervised are contradictory and differ dramatically with age, geographical location, ethnic background, socioeconomic status, and family structure. A review of several studies indicates that the proportion of ten- to fifteen-year-olds (approximately twenty-two million) spending after-school hours unsupervised or in self-care ranges between 50 and 95 percent. Many of these youngsters spend this time with peers. The influence of peer pressure in stimulating adolescents' involvement in risk-taking and antisocial behavior has been well documented. For example, Steinberg found a significant correlation between parental permissiveness and adolescent susceptibility to peer pressure. He also found that susceptibility to peer pressure among unsupervised fifth- and sixth-grade girls varies as a function of where they spend their afternoons. Girls who spent their late afternoons at home were less susceptible to peer pressure than girls who spent their time at friends' houses. Girls who "hung out" (at the mall and other unsupervised sites) were more susceptible to peer pressure than were those who were either at friends' houses or at home. Some of the susceptibility among fifth- and sixth-grade boys was related to whether parents knew the whereabouts of the boys. Susceptibility to peer pressure to engage in deviant behavior was greater among boys whose parents did not know their whereabouts.

Authoritative parents appear to be able to protect young people from pressures of peers. Children may be more likely to adopt parental standards for behavior when they are raised in an authoritative fashion. In addition, the protective effect of authoritative parenting increases as adolescents move into after-school settings in which adults are not present. Reports suggest that the less supervision an adolescent receives during after-school hours, the more important it is for him or her to have been raised authoritatively.

Research conducted by Lipsitz at the University of North Carolina Center for Early Adolescence found that the goals of after-school programs differed widely from program to program. The goals of many programs included providing safe and supervised recreational activities and opportunities to acquire self-reliance and cognitive and vocational skills. Other programs focused on health education and service needs of adolescents, including the provision of information about sexuality, family living, child-rearing, and personal decision making. Health screening, referral, and, when feasible, even treatment were provided by various programs. Counseling aimed at preventing truancy, running away, and child abuse was provided for adolescents and families in some cases. Lipsitz concluded that "after-school programs do have the potential to be the delivery systems of preventive and remedial services that result from public policy initiatives." While the economic terrain of the United States may prohibit some parents from gaining more supervision time with their children, there is in all probability room for creative adults to begin to look at potential solutions. It is imperative that this previously ignored phenomenon be addressed. In blunt terms, if children are involved in an after-school program, such as sports, they are not accessible to those who might induce them to take part in health-risky behaviors.

What are the effects of extracurricular programs? Are these programs effective in preventing or delaying the onset of risky behaviors and the frequently resulting undesirable health outcomes? Unfortunately, these questions cannot be answered definitively. Lipsitz's review of the ERIC data base uncovered little useful data regarding the overall effects of extracurricular programs to serve youth. The majority of the evaluation data that do exist consist of attendance data and anecdotal testimonials. Researchers often cite lack of funding and data-collection problems as barriers to those types of program evaluation. Researchers report that the few studies available do suggest that community-based after-school programs can produce positive effects in skills acquisition, delinquency prevention, youth employment, and academic achievement. These findings may be summarized as follows:

- Several studies indicate that after-school programs increase young people's practical skills and knowledge.
- After-school programs provide increased contact with civic-minded adults who provide exemplary role models for community-oriented behavior, provide young people opportunities to practice formal leadership and community responsibility, and increase family involvement in the education of adolescents.
- Researchers have concluded that national voluntary organizations are capable of developing and implementing after-school programs that increase teenagers' parenting knowledge, attitudes, and skills.
- After-school programs and efforts involving the community in the prevention of juvenile delinquency can be successful in decreasing vandalism, truancy, suspension from school, school violence, recidivism referral, and justice-system encounters and in increasing leadership skills.

A summary of these propositions was forwarded by Lipsitz: "Searching for studies of program outcomes is frustrating. Hundreds of thousands of public dollars have been spent on categorical programs. At this point it is not possible to specify common features in apparently successful programs." She further concludes that, despite this dearth of valuative data, there is sufficient information to indicate that after-school programs can promote healthy development and reduce risk factors. In addition, "after school programs reduce risk to young people simply by keeping them off the streets."

The self-evident notion that adolescents can be in only one place at a time and the obvious observation that after-school programs keep youth off the streets should not be dismissed without further comment. Given that there are only twenty-four hours in a day, one could construct a paradigm that categorizes an adolescent's day into time periods each with its own varying level of potential risk. For instance, an average adolescent sleeps nine hours, spends seven hours in school, and spends at least one hour in transition between sleep and school. These seventeen hours are times during which direct parental or school supervision is available, thus presenting minimal opportunity for involvement in risky behavior. Moreover, another four hours of the young adolescent's time, between 6 and 10 P.M., represents a low-risk period if there is direct supervision by a parent, which is usually the case. How the adolescent spends his or her time between 3 and 6 P.M. becomes critical, since this is the only time when large numbers of adolescents are unsupervised and subject to peer and environmental pressure to engage in health-compromising behaviors. Because a significant number of early adolescents are unsupervised during this time, the availability of school- or community-based extracurricular activities is crucial. Time spent in supervised extracurricular school or community activities cannot be spent hanging out at the home of friends or at the mall, where susceptibility to peer pressure and social influences to engage in risky activities is potent. Supervised programs during this time interval thus provide possible structure and supervision twenty-four hours a day and could be viewed as important in impeding the development of adolescent health problems. In addition to the protective factor of keeping adolescents off the street, these programs, if carefully planned, present opportunities for the young to acquire socially useful knowledge and skills that may in turn foster more healthy behavior.

Despite the large number of young people who are responsible for their own care during after-school hours, not all "hang out" or involve themselves in other unsupervised activities. Many seek activities in the community in which they interact with adults. These extracurricular activities include sports and recreation, volunteer and salaried work, and clubs and other informal school, church, and community learning and social experiences. A recent study by the U.S. Public Health Service found that the average youth spends slightly less than thirteen hours a week in sports, active games, and exercise. Eighty percent of this time was in activities outside the school physical education class. Much of it was spent in community-based sports and recreation programs. However, this figure could be misleading unless one recognizes that most of these programs do not meet each afternoon, and many are only seasonal. Activity time peaked in the summer, fell off rapidly in the fall and winter months, and resumed in the spring. Because there is no national network of nonschool programs serving youth, and most programs are locally developed and operated, it is difficult to estimate the number of youth participating in extracurricular activities on a daily basis. Just as there are deficits in the epidemiological studies examining educational exposure and rates of health problems, there is a dire need for national studies comparing the rates of health problems of those involved in extracurricular programs with the rates of those not involved.

Carefully planned and implemented community-based extra-curricular activities can provide a safe environment for healthy develop-ment. Like the research on school-based physical education and health education, research on community-based extracurricular programs suggests that they have the potential to help young people develop specific life skills that increase the probability that they will choose healthy alternatives.

Summary

Schools represent the exemplary setting for the delivery of programs that can improve young people's chances of growing up healthy. However, the existing evidence indicates that many school-based health education and physical education programs are only beginning to reflect the best available scientific theories of learning, social development, and behavioral change. Unfortu-nately, many of these programs lack essential community, administrative, and financial support and regional diffusion mechanisms to be successful. Such programs are failing to achieve their full potential as positive influences on the health of adolescents. Likewise, community-based extracurricular pro-grams serving young people are not realizing their full potential because of the lack of research. Lack of trained personnel and inadequate guidance from federal, state, and local sectors also attenuate the full potential of these interventions. Such projects are piecemeal, offered in isolation and in loca-tions only sparsely dotted across the nation.

The needs of America's youth, specifically of those ten to fifteen years of age, are not being met. Early adolescence is a time of change, growth, and preparation for adulthood. During this time, young people need oppor-tunities to learn and to apply their knowledge and skills to daily tasks and challenges. Adolescents require guidance, adult role models, and oppor-tunities to practice social skills with peers as well as adults. They need physical health and emotional stability.

A review of the scientific literature reveals that, although we do know a great deal about those factors that help young people grow up healthy, we still have much to learn. But most of all, having reviewed the literature on the effects of education and extracurricular activities on the health of adoles-cents, one is struck by the absence of public policy based on research findings that address this population. Public policy aimed at meeting the health and health behavior needs of ten- to fifteen-year-olds is virtually nonexistent. Health professionals, parents, legislators, and community leaders need to move aggressively to influence boards of education to take action to close the gap between what we know can be done and what we are currently doing to improve the health of adolescents.

Recommendations

The lack of public awareness of the health status of adolescents is a major problem. Adolescents fall into the seam between public policies addressing the needs of children and policies focusing on employment issues for young adults. The following recommendations are intended to provide both energy and guidance to parents and to health and education professionals so that they all can become advocates for the health of adolescents.

Support for continued and expanded prevention research is essential so that we can establish a data base for program and policy development addressing the health and development needs of adolescents. Research needs include:

- Prevention research across ethnic groups with the expressed mandate of examining drug abuse, alcohol, sexual risk, and delinquency.
- Prospective investigations focusing on educational experiences and subsequent rates of risky health behavior and health problems of youth. Formal epidemiological methodologies such as the cohort study design should be integrated into research on education, with an emphasis on subsequent risk of developing health problems.
- Psychological research addressing how to produce more "resilient" children via health education treatments. Work in this area suggests the need to try to discover stronger and more efficient ways to help adolescents develop self-esteem, adaptability, social problem-solving skills, and supportive ties.
- Empirical research addressing the phenomenon of "high-risk time" after school. Research on the benefits of and mechanisms for providing adolescents greater after-school participation in organized activities is needed.
- Programmatic research addressing the kind and amount of physical education programs that favorably influence a child's academic performance, physical and mental wellness, and general sense of self-worth. The effect of these programs on the development of various adolescent health problems needs to be studied.
- Modifications of current data bases that include information on adolescents so that the data can be disaggregated by age, gender, socioeconomic status, and ethnicity.

The results of the School Health Education Evaluation, sponsored by the federal government, make a strong case for the beneficial influence of comprehensive curricula on adolescent health knowledge, attitudes, and behaviors. Dissemination of such information is currently haphazard and not well coordinated. Information dissemination needs include:

- A data base providing information regarding the need for and effects of programs serving adolescents.
- Establishment of a national clearinghouse and dissemination network on adolescent health. That network should be charged with working with states and local communities to ensure that all research findings are shared with groups at the federal, state, and local levels.

An investment in America's youth must be viewed as an investment in the future. An infrastructure that supports the healthy development of adolescents must be a cornerstone on which this investment is built. The following steps need to be taken in order to establish such a support system:

- Appointment of a presidential task force on the health of adolescents. That task force should be charged with advising the administration on a federal policy that increases young people's chances to grow up healthy.
- Establishment of a congressional commission charged with reviewing existing programs that address youth issues and making recommendations for future legislative and policy action to address the developmental needs of early adolescents.
- Formation of a national coalition involving organizations with agendas focusing on youth and with programs for early adolescents. Networking among these organizations is essential if an advocacy group supporting the needs and representing the potential of this age group is going to emerge.
- Establishment of a joint health and education task force by the secretary of the U.S. Department of Education and the secretary of the U.S. Department of Health and Human Services. The task force should be charged with making recommendations to guide programs that provide technical assistance and funding to state and local education agencies and community organizations.

America's youth are this country's most valuable resource. HIV infection and AIDS, drug and alcohol abuse, teen pregnancy, homicide, and suicide are potent threats to the healthy development of young people. This chapter has presented what is currently known about the role of education and extracurricular activities in preventing adolescent health problems. The recommendations for the establishment of a national infrastructure to help children grow up healthy are only the first step. The real action must take place at the local level. It is in our homes, schools, and communities that we can develop this nation's most valuable resource. Parents and community members must be proactive to ensure that local schools and communities take responsible action to invest in youth by establishing programs to promote adolescent health that are based on the current prevention and behavioral research.

Suggested Readings

Block, J. H. "The Role of Ego-Control and Ego Resiliency in the Organization of Behavior." In W. A. Collins (ed.), *The Minnesota Symposium on Child Psychology*. Vol. 13: *Development of Cognition, Affect and Social Relations*. Hillside, N.J.: Erlbaum, 1980.

Botvin, G. "Substance Abuse Prevention Research: Recent Developments and Future Directions." *Journal of School Health*, 1986, *56*, 369–374.

Lefstein, L. M., and others. *3:00 to 6:00 P.M.: Programs for Young Adolescents Center for Early Adolescence*. Chapel Hill, N.C.: University of North Carolina Press, 1983.

Lipsitz, J. S. *After School: Young Adolescents on Their Own*. Chapel Hill, N.C.: Center for Early Adolescence, University of North Carolina Press, 1986.

Office of Disease Prevention and Health Promotion. *Key Findings: National Children and Youth Fitness Study II*. Washington, D.C.: U.S. Department of Health and Human Services, 1984.

Paterson, G., and Stouthamer-Loeber, M. "The Correlation of Family Management Practices and Delinquency." *Child Development*, 1984, *55*, 1299–1307.

Pentz, M. A. "Prevention of Adolescent Substance Abuse Through Social Skill Development." In T. J. Glynn (ed.), *Preventing Adolescent Drug Abuse: Intervention Strategies*. NIDA Research Monograph no. 47. Washington, D.C.: National Institute on Drug Abuse, 1983.

"Results of the School Health Education Evaluation." *Journal of School Health*, 1985, *55*, 295–340.

Rutter, M., and Garmezy, N. *Stress Coping and Development in Children*. New York: McGraw-Hill, 1983.

Sage, G. H. "Social Development." In V. D. Seefeldt (ed.), *Physical Activity and Well-Being*. Reston, Va.: American Alliance for Health, Physical Education, Recreation, and Dance, 1986.

Seefeldt, V. D. (ed.). *Physical Activity and Well-Being*. Reston, Va.: American Alliance for Health, Physical Education, Recreation, and Dance, 1986.

7

Life-Style, Risk Taking, and Out-of-Control Behavior

Mary E. L. Vernon, M.D., M.P.H.

As noted in other chapters in this text, adolescence is generally considered a period of life characterized by constant change, rapid physical growth, emotional turmoil, and parental conflict. Adolescence in some instances has become synonymous with terminology such as "in crisis," "transitional," "risk-taking," "out-of-control," "eccentric," and "rebellion." Adolescence has allowed the young to experiment, seek independence, and prepare for adult life while still dependent on parents. With the earlier onset of menarche, a widening is observed in the gap between biological change and social maturity of adolescents. Adolescents want to be allowed to act grown up and indulge in adult privileges, but without the responsibilities and decisions that go along with adulthood, such as using contraception if sexually active or preparing for future job opportunities through higher education. In spite of these factors, the majority of adolescents survive and triumph over these tasks with successful adjustments. However, adolescence in the 1980s has become a more stressful and self-destructive period than it was just a decade ago. In fact, the adolescent population is the only age group in America with an increasing mortality rate over the past twenty-five years.

　　The last decade has revealed a most disturbing trend among America's forty million adolescents as we have observed confusion and pressures in this population that have resulted in a deeply troubled and vulnerable group of young people who are not becoming competent, self-sufficient, productive, and capable adults. In this chapter, certain life-styles and social issues are discussed that negatively influence adolescence and produce adolescents who are out of control and indulge in frequent risk-taking behaviors. Included is a review of the influences of the troubled family, divorce, single-parent households, changing moral values, television, and society on the lives of adolescents. Too many of our youth are growing up at risk for a number of negative life events in a society that lacks adequate skills and resources to identify and treat them. Some adolescents have given up on a vision of becoming a productive member of our society, as evidenced in the rising number of subcultures such as gangs. Identifying the youth at risk is a complex issue and a real challenge to those responsible for the care of these young people.

This chapter provides the reader with information that highlights vulnerable young people, defines the adolescent at risk, and encourages recognition of symptoms that may identify troubled, out-of-control adolescents. A partnership among health professionals and social workers, psychologists, and sociologists is needed. In addition, policy makers, businesses, federal and state governments, and the public and private sectors must work together to establish health care systems and innovative programs that effectively serve young people. Several model programs and networking efforts are presented that may provide insight into the prognosis of the problems and possible criteria for resolution.

Transition in Life-Styles

Fifty percent of all health care costs in this country are the result of life-style choices. The term *life-style* is used most frequently in connection with health problems such as smoking, sedentary life, and obesity and their contribution to cardiovascular diseases. Our life-styles are influenced by a number of factors, including family, cultural values and beliefs, societal influences, role models, and the media. The life-styles of adolescents today put them at risk for substance abuse, physical abuse, prostitution, violence, unwanted pregnancies, suicide, unintentional injuries, and antisocial delinquent behaviors. We do not know all the factors that cause adolescents to engage in such behaviors, but we do know that family types, socioeconomic backgrounds, racial groups, and social environments play an important role. Demographic, psychological, social, and behavioral variables interact to produce a syndrome of adolescent problem behaviors that may alert the health professional to intervene early in the life of vulnerable youth.

The American family has changed tremendously in the past fifteen years, and researchers are beginning to link risk factors for abnormal development and maladjusted adolescents with family backgrounds. Researchers are investigating the correlation of family types and adolescent problems, substance use, depression, and abuse. For example, research results document the fact that family dysfunction is a major factor in the process of a youth deciding to run away from home. The troubled family has become a frequent phenomenon in contemporary society at the same time as we have seen a marked increase in the number of troubled youth. The combination of families at risk and youth at risk leads to destruction of both. The family is not able to provide the support and structure needed to help the youth, and the youth lacks the buffer for normal progression through a turbulent adolescence. The family unit that we have traditionally known is in trouble.

The family unit in the past established a nurturing setting for adolescent growth, development, human relationships, identity, socialization, experimentation, and role modeling. The history of the family has been one of protection, support, and guidance that prepared us to deal with the stresses of growing up and provided coping skills for adaptation. Today, the typical American family is no longer parents and children with an extended family of grandparents, uncles, aunts, and cousins. New terms to describe the family include "single-parent households," "stepparent," "unwed mother," "broken homes," "suburban," and "homeless families." Along with these changes came different types of neighborhood dwellers that no longer concern themselves with correcting the behaviors of the neighbor's child. The term *community* has replaced *neighborhood*.

Many trends reflect the erosion of the family as it was known in the early 1900s.

- Today, less than 10 percent of the population lives in a two-parent family where the father is the sole financial support.
- The number of single-parent families has risen sharply.
- Within the past ten years, the number of working women with children under one year of age increased by 70 percent. By the end of 1985, 60 percent of women with children under the age of eighteen were in the work force. The "supermom" who has insurmountable demands and responsibilities of family and career is the woman of the times. What effect does this type of mother have on children and adolescents?
- Since 1983, 50 percent of marriages in the United States have ended in divorce. Each year, more than one million children deal with the consequences of a marital breakup; one in seven will be exposed to this situation more than once as a result of divorce of parents who have remarried.
- The stepfamily is becoming more common. Eighty percent of divorced men and 75 percent of divorced women remarry. Forty percent of remarriages end in divorce.
- The fastest-growing population of homeless people today is composed of families. In some cities, 50 percent of the homeless are members of families with children. It is estimated that one-third of homeless Americans are members of families with children and adolescents.

The impact of these massive demographic changes on the family lifestyle is reflected in the following observations. The single parent is the sole parent to offer children and adolescents education concerning social, emotional, and moral responsibilities and to provide financial support for the family. The number of individuals living in poverty among single-parent families increased by 27.1 percent from 1979 to 1986. Single mothers make up the majority of the labor force working at the minimum wage. In 1985, 67.8 percent of single mothers with school-age children were in the labor force.

Poverty has a devastating effect on families and especially on youth who are denied basic necessities, an adequate education, employment, and social support. Of all poor people in the United States, 35 percent live in families headed by a single mother. Teenage pregnancy is a major reason for the dramatic increase in single-parent families. How are rearing practices affected by an absent parent, and how are adolescents affected by poverty? Do they make unhealthy, destructive decisions because of lack of a role model, or are they forced into assuming adult responsibilities before they develop the skills of adulthood? Do limited choices force them to strike back at their parents or society? Do drug dealers, flashy cars, and freedom in the streets become more attractive to poor adolescents than working for a minimum wage for long hours, with little freedom to do the types of things that adolescents not in poverty are able to do?

Some parents have failed in their ability to supervise and control their youth. A survey in 1984 found 7.2 million children ages five to thirteen without supervision after school. They are known as "latchkey" children. Many are left without supervision for several hours a day. Researchers have found that most adolescent girls who become pregnant do so during the hours of 3 to 6 P.M. in their own homes. It is estimated that 76 percent of latchkey children are without adult supervision after school, 15 percent before school, and 9 percent in the evening.

Researchers have shown a correlation between watching television and maladaptive behavior. The media have become a major influence in the lives of youth. On television, adolescents view sexual relationships that are casually developed outside of marriage and are sometimes violent within a society that is alienated and without clear moral standards. They receive pressure from the media to be adultlike. The average eighteen-year-old today has watched approximately 22,000 hours of television and 350,000 commercials—more time than the total number of hours in schools. A modeling effect on vulnerable adolescents results in the desire to be sexy, use alcohol to become more sociable, or sell drugs to have power and control.

Adolescents who are socially isolated and depressed are known to be regular television viewers. A recent study showed evidence of an increase in suicide and crime after the viewing of related programs on prime-time television. Handguns appear in television shows an average of nine times per hour during prime time. Some adolescents imitate these actions in real life. For example, handguns are used in 50 percent of all suicides and murders in the United States. Suicide has become the second leading cause of death among youth today. Accidents involving guns are the fifth leading cause of death among children.

Homelessness of families endangers the health and well-being of adolescents. This chaotic environment of the family predisposes youth to emotional and/or behavioral problems. The problems observed most frequently among the children in homeless families are acting out, "wild" behavior, fighting, restlessness, moodiness, and frustration. These children have been found to have developmental lags, anxiety, depression, and learning difficulties. Homelessness disrupts the entire family structure and its dynamics through poverty, interruption of a child's education, lack of health care, inadequate nutrition, frequent moves, hostile environment, exposure to criminals and drug addicts, loss of disciplinary responsibilities to the shelter staff, separation of families, and eventually permanent family breakup. What type of individual would survive these negative influences in life? Can a healthy, functional, self-sufficient, caring adolescent be produced in this environment?

The literature clearly documents that troubled families lead to maladjusted adolescents. Consequences of dysfunctional families include substance abuse, adolescent pregnancy, depression, abuse and neglect, sexual promiscuity, and violence. National survey data show that about 50 percent of today's alcoholics had parents who were alcoholics; unwanted pregnancies occur more often in adolescents whose parents were also adolescent parents; suicide is more prevalent in families with a suicide history; of the thirty-two juveniles awaiting execution in 1986 for murder and other crimes, most were brought up in an abused background and never felt loved; runaway youth are often abused or neglected at home; child pornography and sexual abuse are linked; rebellious, antisocial, and delinquent adolescents are usually the product of antisocial, delinquent parents; more than 60 percent of identified delinquents had parents who were divorced or separated; children abused by their parents are likely to grow up and abuse their own children; and the primary reason that adolescents cite for running away from home is problems with a parent.

Adolescents are exposed to a number of different life-styles. One cannot always predict that if an adolescent is reared in a particular dysfunctional family life-style, the result will be a dysfunctional, maladjusted adolescent. There are many cases of adolescents who survived the worst possible family environments and became functional adults. The literature also clarifies certain life-styles that correlate with adolescent behavior problems, which allow service providers to identify at-risk family life-styles and provide intervention to protect vulnerable adolescents. The demographics of the nation indicate that the problems of our youth are getting worse. Therefore, health professionals and others should begin to work together to develop instruments and other materials that will help identify and serve troubled families and their vulnerable adolescents.

Vulnerability of Adolescents

Despite the magnitude of the problems affecting adolescents and the epidemic nature of most of them, very little is known about adolescents at risk and how to identify those at highest risk. Early identification of adolescents at risk would allow intervention and treatment before a crisis occurs.

There are a number of American youth who are considered vulnerable. Many of the problems occurring during adolescence begin in infancy and childhood, with a continuum through adolescence. Vulnerable adolescents are especially at risk for developing destructive behaviors. Unhealthy lifestyles, inadequate parenting, an unstable, unpredictable society, low self-esteem, negative peer influence, and stress in the environment produce susceptible young people.

Early adolescence is a time of particular vulnerability because of the combination of rapid physical, emotional, and social changes and a rapidly changing society that gives unclear values and mixed messages. Early adolescence is also the developmental stage of maximum conformity to peer norms. This tends to peak for girls at around twelve years of age and for boys at about fifteen years. Peer influence can act on a susceptible adolescent and encourage specific behaviors. Peer pressure is a major contributor to the development of risk-taking behaviors among early adolescents. This has been clearly documented by researchers observing peer pressure and the onset of sexual intercourse among adolescents.

Others have studied psychological risks and reported stress in the environment, high anxiety, and low self-esteem to be major influences for developing risky behaviors. These factors cause the adolescent to feel inadequate and to lose the ability to cope with them. This is followed by the need to seek relief, often through peer acceptance, running away, or use of drugs and alcohol in order to feel adequate. Adolescents often choose an action according to how it will make them feel rather than the consequences of the action. For example, alcohol may be used to seek immediate gratification and pleasure because it relieves anxiety and stress. Alcohol abuse by adolescents has been linked to violent crimes, suicide, auto accidents, and aggressive behavior.

Youth with low self-esteem often have few skills with which to cope with environmental stressors such as poverty, divorce, lack of community support, frequent family mobility, and unemployment. Low self-esteem may lead to self-destructive behavior. A strong concept of self appears to correlate with responsible decision making, effective coping abilities, social competence, cognitive abilities, and ability to communicate.

Minority adolescents must face racial prejudice in addition to the other risks. An adolescent from a minority ethnic group is more likely to live in poverty, lack positive role models, receive few educational opportunities, have an unstable family, and be reared in a single-female-headed household.

Promoting self-esteem among minority adolescents requires a different approach than work with majority-group adolescents. Lack of confidence, decreased achievement, and peer pressure make this population of adolescents most vulnerable and at greater risk for a number of problem behaviors. Several published reports from the Children's Defense Fund have revealed that, compared to white adolescents, black adolescents are twice as likely to see a parent die, have no parent employed, be unemployed, or be suspended from school; three times as likely to be poor, live with a parent who has separated, live in a female-headed family, be murdered between five and nine years of age, or die of child abuse; and four times as likely to live in foster care, be murdered as a teenager, or be incarcerated.

Blacks constitute approximately 12 percent of the U.S. population. Blacks are more likely than whites to be victims of rape, robbery, and assault. They make up 61 percent of the incarcerated juveniles and 54.9 percent of adolescents under eighteen who are arrested for violent crimes. Blacks and Hispanics are more likely than whites to be intravenous drug users and are at highest risk of AIDS. There is a need to obtain such data on other minority groups as well.

Recognizing Adolescents at Risk

Longitudinal studies have given us some clues about the identification of youth at risk. The indicators fall into three categories: (1) environmental characteristics, (2) social characteristics, and (3) academic performance.

Some groups of adolescents are reported to be more vulnerable to certain risk-taking behaviors because of environmental circumstances. For example, economically disadvantaged minority adolescents are known to be at higher risk than their peers across the country. It is their exposure to certain environmental factors that increases their chances of higher-than-average risk. Teasing out these environmental conditions may provide insight into the relative risks for these adolescents. Such conditions would include the single-parent household, unwed mothers, ethnic origin, economic status, and employment and education of the parents, as well as other conditions within a community. The following list, adapted from a Northwest Regional Educational Laboratory Program report by Gabriel and Anderson, summarizes the indicators of high-risk youth:

School
- Lack of basic skills
- Performance consistently below potential
- Poor grades or failure in subjects
- Record of nonpromotions
- Low standard test scores
- Irregular attendance and frequent tardiness
- Pattern of disruptive or aggressive behavior

- Poor study and work habits
- Lack of academic motivation
- Little or no participation in extracurricular activities
- Failure to read at grade level

Personal
- Alcohol or drug abuse
- Physical health problems
- Mental health problems
- Poor self-concept
- Marriage or pregnancy
- Poor social skills
- Friends who are not school-oriented
- Lack of realistic goals
- Lack of supervision
- Lack of ambition

Family
- Low educational level of parents
- Family pattern of dropping out
- Negative parental attitudes or low educational aspirations
- Broken home
- Frequent family moves
- Unstable home environment (severe conflicts between parents or be-tween parent and child, family violence, alcoholic parent)
- Parent unable to find employment
- Low economic status

Sociocultural
- Being disadvantaged
- Being a member of a minority group
- Being non-English-speaking
- Welfare support
- Low educational attainment of adults in family and community
- Lack of respect for authority

There is no known single characteristic that determines a youth's risk for running away, crime, violence, or homicide; however, there seems to be a relationship between these behaviors and clusters of environmental factors. A disproportionate number of youth exhibiting these behaviors are from economically disadvantaged communities. The lower the income of the family, the greater the chance of succumbing to these environmental stressors.

Social factors also appear to be most important for adolescents who engage in risky behaviors. Also noted is a sex difference in risk-taking propensity, which was greater for boys than for girls. These behaviors tend to occur as a result of peer models, the media, and dares by peers. Social factors are observed to have a correlation with substance abuse, delinquency, suicide, and violent crimes. Social pressures may lead the adolescent to self-destruction if no adaptation takes place.

School performance is another major category of indicators of at-risk youth. These risk characteristics are evident through low academic performance, school absenteeism, suspension, illiteracy, and learning disabilities. When low academic achievement is combined with poverty and peer pressure, the adolescent female is at very high risk for becoming an adolescent parent. School failure has been associated with adolescents who run away, commit delinquent acts, and use drugs. As a result, a large number of youth drop out of school altogether. However, the number-one reason stated by youth as the reason for dropping out of school is boredom.

The dropout problem is recognized as a crisis of national proportions. Not only are educators grappling with this problem; so are the U.S. government, social agencies, businesses, industries, communities, and taxpayers. The dropout rate in the United States is estimated to be 27 percent nationwide, with the rate exceeding 50 percent in some cities. According to a 1986 report by the Education Commission of the States, 700,000 secondary students drop out annually, and 300,000 are perpetual truants. The commission estimates that two million students currently enrolled in our schools are at risk of dropping out. We observe the problems that dropouts encounter— unemployment, low wages, unplanned pregnancies, inadequate education, inadequate health care, and poverty. The projected costs to society are enormous. The number-one reason for adolescent females dropping out of school is early childbearing. Females who drop out of school are more likely to be unemployed, to live in poverty, and to have a child out of wedlock. In the next decade, the jobs of the future will demand more highly skilled workers; many of today's uneducated youth will not be able to qualify.

Dropouts come from all types of backgrounds. Students who drop out of school do so for a variety of reasons, but truancy and frequent absenteeism seem to be two common warning signs. Some researchers have suggested that the warning signs of a potential dropout may appear as early as the third grade; difficulty with math and reading at this grade level seems to be related to subsequent truancy and dropping out. Unrecognized learning problems with poor school performance and concentration, parent-child conflict, inability to cope with stressful situations, and low socioeconomic backgrounds are all associated with dropping out. Those most likely to drop out of school do so as early as the ninth grade. School problems, including school failure, school phobia, underachievement, truancy, hearing disorders, and attention deficit disorder, account for 10 percent or more of adolescents who present to outpatient adolescent clinics. The symptoms of school problems may present as mental retardation, emotional difficulties, or even sensory impairments. Absence and truancy problems often are the result of social and emotional adjustment problems. The interview process of an adolescent by a health care provider should include questions regarding peer pressure, family conflicts, parental expectations, and abuse. Medical problems seem not to be a major factor in school absenteeism rates among adolescents. Extracurricular involvement by the student may afford some protection against the forces that encourage dropping out by contributing to improved school performance and resulting good grades. Participation in extracurricular activities does not guarantee improved performance as a student, but students who are active in extracurricular activities tend to get good grades and remain in school. When 30,000 high school sophomores and 28,000 seniors were surveyed in 1980, it was found that 79 percent of students with good grades were involved in one or more extracurricular activities.

There are subgroups of students that seem to be more vulnerable to dropping out of school. Among black youth, there is one dropout for every two students who graduate, and females are more likely to drop out than males. Early adolescent childbearing is the number-one reason why adolescent females drop out of school. Each day, 1,300 babies are born to adolescent mothers; 800 of these adolescent mothers have not completed high school, and 80 percent will never graduate.

The economic and social impacts of school dropout are overwhelming—costing the nation billions of dollars every year in lost productivity, lost taxes, and welfare expenditures. It is estimated that crime related to inadequate education costs $3 billion annually. Fifty-eight percent of the inmates in state correctional facilities in 1979 had not completed high school. Many of our youth will continue to remain illiterate and unwanted if we are unable to identify early those with the potential for dropping out of school.

Out-of-Control Behavior

Disturbances of adolescent behavior may manifest in symptoms often described as "out-of-control," "aggressive," "acting-out," or "antisocial." These terms may be used to describe adolescents who have lost the ability to maintain control over the impulsivity of mind and body. When control over impulsive and instinctive drives is lost, these factors may surface as acts of truancy, fighting in school, destruction of property, or hostile acts toward others, with the most aggressive directing pain on themselves and ultimately committing suicide.

The manifestation of these behaviors occurs across a spectrum. Some adolescents may express themselves through rebellion, anger, and misbehavior that can be considered normal for adolescents. However, other acts may encompass a wide range of risky behaviors, such as substance abuse, sexual promiscuity, depression, and running away. Because they lack adequate coping skills, these out-of-control adolescents succumb to the many pressures of just everyday living. As more and more demands are put on adolescents, they may feel threatened or uncomfortable with their environ-ment and behave impulsively, losing control of their behavior.

Out-of-control disruptive behavior is not well tolerated in the class-room. Most adolescents occasionally misbehave or lose control of their behavior in ways that are still acceptable to adults. However, when this behavior occurs in the classroom, in a library, or in public, it tends to create problems and often invokes punitive reactions from teachers, parents, and public authorities. Subsequently, the adolescent may be suspended from school, which can also lead to school failure, school dropout, and involve-ment with the court system.

Untrained adults working with adolescents may tend to respond to the surface behavior of the out-of-control adolescent without recognizing or investigating the underlying conflicts and causes. For example, the student who is late coming to class each morning and disrupts the class on arrival may be sent to the principal's office and ultimately suspended for a few days. Most schools do not investigate the home environment to determine why the student continues to be chronically late and disruptive. Many of these stu-dents are suffering from various environmental factors out of their control that have major implications as to why the adolescent is a habitual school offender. These influences may include alcoholic parents who may be loud and boisterous into the night, so that the adolescent oversleeps because he or she was not able to sleep during the night, or the simple fact that the family cannot afford an alarm clock, so that the adolescent sleeps late but still has to dress three other younger siblings because the single working mother left for work at 5 A.M. Most antisocial adolescent behaviors have an underlying social cause, and the adolescent cannot be helped by punitive measures directed to him or her alone, without an assessment that involves the adolescent's family and environment. Schools can provide in-service training for teachers and administrators concerning the maintenance of orderly classrooms. Does disorderly behavior occur because teachers just do not care about the prob-lems of adolescents, or is it that the problems are so pervasive that they feel that these youngsters have no future? Teachers and counselors sometimes give up on helping young people who are "troublemakers" and hope that they will drop out of school or become too old to attend. Teachers and counselors are often called on to deal with a multitude of behavior problems with little or no assistance from those who have been trained to deal with these adoles-cents, such as psychiatrists, psychologists, and social workers.

The first step toward helping the out-of-control adolescent is to recog-nize the underlying influences that make him or her susceptible to losing control. Symptoms such as frequent parent-child conflicts, truancy, under-achievement, shoplifting, fighting, sexual promiscuity, hostility toward oth-ers, destruction of personal property, or self-destructive behaviors may be the adolescent's plea for help. Therefore, it is important to assess the significance of such behaviors before they are totally out of control. There are clues that can be recognized in adolescents who are in the process of adopting out-of-control behavior. These clues are found through interactions of the adolescent with the family, peers, and classroom teachers. Often these adolescents are brought to the health professional or counselor after they have lost control. The three cases described below are examples of adolescents who exemplify the problems of out-of-control behavior, especially if the child is attending school.

The first case is a twelve-year-old girl referred by the school counselor because of frequent fighting in the classroom and on the school grounds. She has very poor social skills and often turns innocent interactions into situations of hostility and revenge. She is from a single-parent household, and her mother is pregnant. The adolescent states that she feels that her mother's pregnancy will force her to assume more responsibility around the household. She constantly complains of boredom in school and too many chores at home. She currently has more than fifty hours of after-school detention for frequent fighting in school. At each counseling session, she has bragged about the fight that she had been involved in the previous day and how she overpowered her opponent. She seems to make a conscious effort to participate in fights even though she is aware that she will be suspended for the remainder of the year if she continues to fight. She also states that she has a desire to be male and feels uncomfortable with the female role. It has become evident that she has a negative self-image, poor communication with her mother, poor school performance, and lack of close peer relationships.

The second case is a fourteen-year-old male who was adopted for the second time five years ago. At two years of age, he was dropped off at the day-care center by his biological mother, who never returned to pick him up. Following his first adoption, he was returned to the adoption agency by the parents because of frequent problem behaviors. The present adoptive mother knew of his prior problem behaviors but felt that these problems could be solved if he were placed in a loving home with people who cared about him. His history involves stealing, refusing to obey teachers as well as parents, taking unauthorized medication from the medicine cabinet, and fighting at school. He feels that his problems at school result from teachers asking him to do "stupid" things and that the teachers are responsible for his problems. His history also includes joining a gang at age nine and running away on several occasions in the recent past.

The final case is a thirteen-year-old obese sixth-grader who appears much bigger and older than her classmates. She was referred for counseling because of academic failures, constant disciplinary problems, and defiant behaviors, including fighting. She is from a single-parent household with a mother who is ill and two younger children, three years and one year old. This adolescent was the only child for ten years and admits difficulty in giving up this particular role in the family. She has been placed in the role of caring for her younger siblings and is often left to make decisions on her own. She has poor communication with her mother, as well as with her grandmother, whom she occasionally lives with. One month after she was referred to us, her mother abandoned her and moved to a shelter with the two younger children. The mother told the adolescent that she could manage on her own.

Some rebellion can be a normal expression of the adolescent's quest for independence and may manifest itself in problems in schools, frequent parental conflicts, wide mood swings, and erratic behavior. We may find it difficult to distinguish normal adolescent behavior from out-of-control behavior unless we know the background of the youth and the family. The three cases described above exemplify the underlying turmoil of adolescents, who often express themselves through acting-out behaviors.

Health Risk Appraisals

There are a number of health risk appraisals for adolescents that attempt to assess unhealthy behaviors and reinforce positive health practices. Health risk appraisals have the potential to motivate change in health behavior as well as assess risk factors that might negatively influence the adolescent's behavior. A number of commercial firms are now offering appraisal services with questionnaires. The Centers for Disease Control have developed a health assessment appraisal questionnaire that can be adopted for computer use.

With today's adolescents familiar with computer technology and the use of interactive computer games, there are several sources of computerized health risk appraisals for adolescents on the market. For example, "I'm a Health Nut," developed in St. Paul, Minnesota, is intended to effect a change in unhealthy behaviors and to reinforce positive health practices among adolescents through a computer printout of their health risks. Another interactive computer program, the Body Awareness Resource Network (BARN), was developed at the University of Wisconsin, Madison, Center for Health Systems Research and Analysis. These programs provide adolescents with confidential, nonjudgmental health information, behavioral change strategies, and sources of referral after completing their health risk assessment. Teen health computer programs from the University of Hawaii are used to obtain complete histories, evaluate responses, identify problem areas, and print a confidential health needs assessment focusing on high-risk areas among adolescents. The programs also provide individualized recommendations for the adolescent to share with the physician or other health care provider. A Teen-Link Health Risk Appraisal survey was adapted from the Centers for Disease Control health risk appraisal survey to obtain health risk data on inner-city minority adolescents ten to eighteen years of age at the Lincoln Community Health Center in Durham, North Carolina.

Early adolescence has been observed as the time when the more damaging behaviors are established. Researchers have found that many of the risk-taking behaviors are interconnected and believe that a common pattern of risk factors may exist to help the health provider predict which adolescents are potentially at risk for engaging in abnormal behaviors.

Intervention and Programmatic Strategies

A number of model programs have been designed to reach target groups of adolescents. These intervention strategies have focused on runaways, street youth, minorities, and school-age youth in an effort to reach those youth most at risk. There are five areas in which innovative approaches to adolescent care within today's context should be considered: (1) outreach to the community, (2) health promotive models, (3) school settings, (4) community based programs, and (5) networking and partnership with parents, health care providers, educators, businesses, and community agencies. There is no ideal approach to serving adolescents. However, a health promotion approach may prevent many of the unhealthy life-styles and risk-taking behaviors among today's youth.

Health Promotion

The W. K. Kellogg Foundation has devoted much of its philanthropic funds to supporting programs with a health promotion and disease prevention focus. Teen-Link, located in Durham, North Carolina, is an example of a comprehensive health promotion and disease prevention program with a multidisciplinary staff to meet the needs of youth. The key to the success of the program has been its outreach into the community, teen involvement, networking with other community agencies, school involvement, and comprehensive services. In addressing the problems of youth in the community, Teen-Link has sought to confront adolescents on their own turf, on their own terms, and in their own language. Teen-Link fuses compassion and sensitivity with professional discipline and social vision. These may be qualities more often associated with an individual than with a program—but that is precisely the point. If programs are to reach youth they must be culturally sensitive and allow the youth to take part in their development and implementation. The Teen-Link experience shows that addressing adolescent problems through a community-based program requires human bonding as much as medical and psychosocial skills. The program must be familiar and trusted as well as effective.

Teen-Link reveals a population of inner-city youth who lack adequate exposure to aid them in the internalization of principles of health maintenance. An alarming feature of this population is the extent to which adolescents are victimized by preventable behavior and health problems. Many of these problems are related and similar for all ethnic groups, although they may differ by sex and age. In addressing the interwoven health and social factors, Teen-Link initiated a series of activities designed specifically to engage the interest of youth. These efforts included special adolescent-oriented services in family planning, mental health counseling, an adolescent primary health care clinic, pregnancy testing and counseling, prenatal clinics, fun-oriented health promotion activities, school outreach, church-connected projects, and psychosocial support groups. It is through its partnership with local institutions, such as the city schools, the local churches, Duke University, North Carolina Central University, and the local health and social services departments, that the program has been able to relate to the deeply entrenched neighborhood network. Within this network, counselors and caretakers are accepted and trusted by neighbors who serve as advocates for at-risk adolescents as well as a means of service delivery. Teen-Link has revealed that many adolescents need a great deal of personal encouragement, patience, and hand holding to complete even the most basic beneficial activities.

School-Based Health Clinics

The role of the school in promoting adolescent health did not begin with the advent of school-based health clinics. In fact, schools have been recognized as important to the health care needs of students for at least the past thirty years. A number of innovative health programs have developed within schools, but school-based health clinics have become most widely known and controversial because they are primary health care centers located in the junior and senior high school settings. The prototype school-based clinic became operational in 1970 in St. Paul, Minnesota. Today there are more than 100 clinics across the United States that have been developed to meet the health needs of adolescents within a specific community.

In response to the 1981 national health statistics that revealed that young people between the ages of fifteen and twenty-four were the only age group with a rising mortality rate, the Robert Wood Johnson Foundation provided funds to twenty teaching hospitals to support community-based, comprehensive health services to high-risk young people living in communities with significant sociomedical problems, such as adolescent pregnancy, drug- and alcohol-related accidents, homicide, suicide, and depression. The goals and objectives of these programs are to improve the health of young people through (1) increasing services to high-risk youth, (2) training health providers to care for young people, (3) consolidating health services into one comprehensive care center, and (4) encouraging long-term financial support for programs to serve the target population.

As a result of the foundation's efforts, community-based organizations have collaborated with teaching hospitals as active partners in the planning and implementation of projects. These organizations include neighborhood health centers, public health departments, nonprofit community agencies, public schools, hospitals, health sciences centers, federal agencies, juvenile court systems, and Native American tribes. Through the projects, graduate students, medical and nursing students, psychologists, and social workers are trained in the problems of high-risk youth. The experience of the participating institutions suggests that high-risk adolescents need comprehensive health care services made available at one site. Community agencies and hospitals should collaborate to make these comprehensive services available to the high-risk youth in the community.

Other examples of programs within the community that provide services to high-risk youth include the Door, located in New York, the Larkin Center, in San Francisco, and the Bridge over Troubled Waters, in Boston.

Recommendations

Most of the medical and behavioral problems facing adolescents are reflections of problems existing throughout the larger society. Identifying, treating, and educating adolescents with these problems present an enormous challenge to those caring for this population of young people. Throughout this chapter, relevant issues affecting the future of adolescents have been discussed. Certain themes appear that suggest that we need a unified direction for identification, intervention, and treatment of at-risk youth. Without this unified approach, too many of America's youth will be compromised, and their problems will escalate.

These problems are complex but solvable. With all sectors of our society working toward a solution, the prognosis for future problems will be improved. Clearly, no one group can solve these critical issues, but each individual can make a strong contribution to solving them.

Collaboration is essential: The process of collaboration is evident in the nationwide call to action campaigns in support of America's youth developed through the initiatives of the U.S. Department of Health and Human Services, the U.S. Department of Labor, the U.S. Department of Education, the National Alliance of Business, and private foundations such as the W. T. Grant and Robert Wood Johnson foundations. Through their leadership, programs such as Youth 2000, Youth and America's Future, Workforce Readiness, and community-based health services for adolescents at risk have been established.

Everyone has a role to play, even though the approach and strategies will vary, among the private sector, businesses and industry, foundations, civic organizations, community groups, physicians, psychologists, counselors, social workers, sociologists, teachers, health professionals, and policy makers. Each has expertise to contribute to solving the problems facing adolescents. We must depart in some ways from the traditional approach; for example, we must change our attitudes to a greater emphasis on prevention and health promotion rather than focusing simply on treatment of diseases. For adolescents, by the time treatment is required, the resources for care are limited. Our goal for serving young people should be to foster healthy life-styles, economic self-sufficiency, and physical and emotional well-being rather than to treat sociomedical problems.

There are a number of individual and collaborative actions that professionals and advocates may undertake in an effort to address the problems affecting adolescents and to guide those at risk along the path of healthy and responsible life-styles.

Establishment of Partnerships

An essential requisite to real support in reaching youth is the development of partnerships among all sectors of our society. A variety of strategies for involvement can be implemented through collaborative efforts at the national, state, or local level among health professionals, businesses, families, schools, politicians, community agencies, government, and private foundations.

Advocacy

Many adolescents need a great deal of personal encouragement, patience, hand holding, and support. They are not given a place to express themselves, and the effects of this seem to spill over into their life-styles, where they take little responsibility for their own personal actions. They have not figured out what is good for them and what is bad for them. Young people should have a role and be involved in developing solutions to the problems facing them.

A Comprehensive Approach

A comprehensive plan needs to be established to deal with the multi-faceted issues affecting adolescents. The resolution of these issues must be approached holistically. A comprehensive interagency cooperation and a multiservice delivery system should be created. The Teen-Link experience shows the importance of providing activities that will attract adolescents to a program with a health model and provide them with an array of medical, social, educational, and vocational resources at one site. The experience of the Robert Wood Johnson Foundation illustrates the need to establish comprehensive community-based health services for high-risk adolescents and shows that these youth especially need consolidated one-stop services. Comprehensive assessments of adolescents must include a component of health promotion and disease prevention. Use of a case manager referral system provides an optimum approach for the prevention of diseases.

Culturally Sensitive Programs

Clearly, there is a need for the development of culturally sensitive targeted programs that provide care to minority youth. The type of educational materials and the staff and location of the program must be taken under consideration. If the program serves different ethnic groups, the individual needs of each group should be dealt with. Particular attention should be given to the problems unique to economically disadvantaged and minority youth. Health care providers need to understand the socioeconomic and cultural backgrounds of the population of young people they serve. For example, poor and minority youth are at higher risk than economically advantaged youth for a number of sociomedical problems that should be recognized by care givers.

Data Collection and Information Dissemination

Local and regional data bases need to be developed to analyze and understand the nature, incidence, and rate of occurrence of adolescent problems. It will be helpful for programs to create useful profiles of youth at risk for certain health problems and provide clues for projections of success and future funding resources. Foundations are important resources for providing seed money to initiate programs addressing adolescent health issues and for experimenting with new approaches to health service delivery to adolescents.

Today's youth are tomorrow's leaders, parents, workers, politicians, and educators. They represent our investment in the future. The problems of youth require real practical solutions. The extent of our success depends on our ability to work together in a unified effort to develop innovative strategies that will produce a healthy population of young people.

Suggested Readings

Dewart, J. *The State of Black America 1988*. New York: National Urban League, 1988.

Edelman, M. W. *Families in Peril: An Agenda for Social Change*. Cambridge, Mass.: Harvard University Press, 1987.

Fielding, J. E. (ed.). *Problems in Comprehensive Ambulatory Health Care for High-Risk Adolescents*. Washington, D.C.: Job Corps, Manpower Administration, U.S. Department of Labor, 1973.

Gabriel, R. M., and Anderson, P. S. *Identifying At-Risk Youth in the Northwest States: A Regional Database*. Portland, Oreg.: Northwest Regional Educational Laboratory, 1987.

Green, M. "Reaching Out to the Children of Divorce." *Contemporary Pediatrics*, 1988, *5*, 22–42.

Hawkins, R. P., and others. "Reaching Hard-to-Reach Populations: Interactive Computer Programs as Public Information Campaigns for Adolescents." *Journal of Communications*, 1987, *37*, 8–28.

Irwin, C. E., Jr., and Millstein, S. G. "Biopsychosocial Correlates of Risk-Taking Behaviors in Adolescence: Can the Physician Intervene?" *Journal of Adolescent Health Care*, 1986, *7* (supp.), 82S–96S.

Jessor, R., and Jessor, S. L. *Problem Behavior in Psychological Development: A Longitudinal Study of Youth*. Orlando, Fla.: Academic Press, 1977.

Kotulak, R. "Growing Up at Risk." *Chicago Tribune*, Dec. 1986, Jan. 1987, p. 68.

Lear, J. G., Foster, H. W., and Wylie, W. G. "Development of Community-Based Health Services for Adolescents at Risk for Sociomedical Problems." *Journal of Medical Education*, 1985, *60*, 777–785.

Lewis, C. E., and Lewis, M. A. "Peer Pressure and Risk-Taking Behaviors in Children." *American Journal of Public Health*, 1984, *74*, 580–584.

Robinson, T. N., and others. "Perspectives on Adolescent Substance Use: A Defined Population Study." *Journal of the American Medical Association*, 1987, *258*, 2072–2076.

Saucier, J. F., and Ambert, A. M. "Parental Marital Status and Adolescents' Health-Risk Behavior." *Adolescence*, 1983, *18*, 403–411.

Schetky, D. H. "Children and Handguns: A Public Health Concern." *American Journal of Diseases of Children*, 1985, *139*, 229–231.

Singer, D. G. "Alcohol, Television, and Teenagers." *Pediatrics*, 1985, *76* (supp.), 668–674.

Slovic, P. "Assessment of Risk Taking Behavior." *Psychological Bulletin*, 1964, *61*, 220–233.

Slovic, P. "Risk-Taking in Children: Age and Sex Differences." *Child Development*, 1966, *37*, 169–176.

Songer, D. "Does Violent Television Produce Aggressive Children?" *Pediatric Annals*, 1985, *14* (12), 804–813.

Strasburger, V. C. "Television and Adolescents." *Pediatric Annals*, 1985, *14* (12), 814–820.

Tonkin, R. S. "Adolescent Risk-Taking Behavior." *Journal of Adolescent Health Care*, 1987, *8*, 213–220.

Weitzman, M., and others. "High-Risk Youth and Health: The Case of Excessive School Absence." *Pediatrics*, 1986, *78*, 313–322.

Part Three

Adolescent Health Issues

PART EDITORS
Lawrence S. Neinstein, M.D.
Robert W. Blum, M.D., M.P.H., Ph.D.

Introduction

William R. Hendee, Ph.D.

Discussion and concern about the many problems and aberrant behaviors of today's youth are pervasive in our society, as well as in most other developed cultures. But for generations, even centuries, discussion and concern of adults have focused on the difficulties of dealing with wayward young people. While this dilemma is not simply a product of our time and culture, it may have some relatively new features. The temptations available to youth may be different in some respects today, and they may also be more numerous. Their impact on the physical and emotional health of adolescents and on their likelihood of a productive and rewarding life as adults may be more threatening and more potentially disastrous than in the past. When combined with the changing social and environmental climate in which young people are reared, these factors create a special vulnerability for today's youth. Adults who work as teachers, parents, friends, and counselors of young people can help them deal effectively with this vulnerability. First, however, they must understand it. The seven chapters in this part are designed to provide this understanding.

No aspect of today's youth culture is more widely discussed and worried about than the use of illicit drugs. By and large, drug abuse is a relatively new phenomenon in young people. Previous generations were concerned principally with alcohol and tobacco (certainly not benign substances), whereas today's youth include these items within a panoply of destructive and potentially addictive substances that by and large were unheard of two generations ago, at least within the adolescent population. This expansion of the illicit drug spectrum is discussed in Chapter Eight by Richard G. Mac-Kenzie, who suggests, as have so many others, that societal control of substance abuse must focus on the demand side as well as the supply side of the drug use problem. MacKenzie's recommendations for stemming the use of mood- and mind-altering substances by young people are sensible and specific and provide a reasonable starting point for societal programs designed to address the drug abuse problem.

Sexually transmitted diseases are occurring in epidemic proportions among sexually active young people in our society. Many adolescents do not regularly utilize health care services, and these diseases can go untreated for a considerable period, causing permanent harm to those infected as well as contamination of others. With HIV infection and disease, the risks of sexually transmitted diseases are now life threatening. These issues are discussed by Mary-Ann B. Shafer and Anna-Barbara Moscicki in Chapter Nine, which also includes a review of the pathogenesis and the clinical presentation and treatment of the more common sexually transmitted diseases.

Teen pregnancy, abortion, and childbearing are major societal problems that stress family relationships and deprive many young people of a productive and rewarding future. These problems are extremely costly to society, both economically and emotionally. As Janet B. Hardy emphasizes in Chapter Ten, the "most urgent task we face as a society" is to persuade adolescents to delay the onset of sexual intercourse until they have attained an appropriate level of maturity and developed a stable and supportive monogamous relationship. How this is to be done in a society that encourages the exploitation of sexuality and proposes sexual activity without consequences in advertising and the public media is a major question to be addressed.

In most discussions of adolescence and adolescent health, young people are portrayed as physically healthy individuals who may have emotional needs that lead them into trouble. These discussions ignore the many young people who suffer from chronic diseases and disabilities that present special difficulties during the transition through adolescence. The special problems and needs of these young people and their families are discussed by Gayle Geber and Nancy A. Okinow in Chapter Eleven.

Injuries are a major contributor to the morbidity of youth. In adolescence, physical, emotional, and intellectual growth occurs rapidly and frequently out of synchrony. During this period, adolescents are expected to master major challenges such as driving an automobile, responding to the temptations of addictive substances, and dealing with sexual desires and social expectations, including pressures from within their peer culture. These challenges make young people especially vulnerable to "accidents" and injuries. The role of intervenors in helping youth understand and accomplish these tasks without exposure to unnecessary hazards is explored in Chapter Twelve by Carol W. Runyan and Elizabeth A. Gerken, who emphasize the need for more research to gain a better understanding of the effects of injuries on the health and well-being of young people in our society.

Adolescence is the period when the individual begins to separate from the family and to gain a perception of self that is independent of family and friends. For most adolescents, this transition works fairly well, even though it does account for much of the tumult and turmoil of the adolescent years. But for some it does not work, and so they are unable to gain a reasonable image of self and the relation of self to others. Often these young people end up lonely and dispassionate and not infrequently hostile to society and prone to violent behavior. Occasionally, they become reclusive and remain very dependent on family or close acquaintances. Although these poorly adjusted young people are a minority of adolescents, they still constitute an impressive number of individuals. More often than not, they do not seek professional counseling, in part because influences, such as the family, that contribute to the maladaptation usually do not encourage the affected person to seek help. Infrequently, the signs of maladaptation are visible to people who interact with the affected adolescent, provided they know how to recognize them. As Daniel Offer, Eric Ostrov, and Kenneth I. Howard emphasize in Chapter Thirteen, intervention by these people may be essential to the adolescent's survival.

The neglect and abuse of young people are not a manifestation solely of the stress and strain of modern society. These problems have been present, although perhaps less well recognized as problems, since the beginning of modern civilization, and probably before it. Their growing acknowledgment in our society is a tribute to the increased value that we place on humanity, including those members who have not reached adulthood. Yet we still do not understand very much about the societal and familial influences that lead to neglect and abuse of our young people. These issues are explored in Chapter Fourteen by Joanne Oreskovich and Robert W. ten Bensel.

Young people are the future of a society. Maturation of young people into adulthood requires the successful hurdling of a variety of obstacles. If not negotiated successfully, many of these obstacles lead to destruction and death, or at least to deflection of the individual from a productive and rewarding life. Adults can help in many ways as young people attempt to maneuver through obstacles on their way to adulthood. First, however, adults must recognize these obstacles and the threat they pose to youth. This part is intended to help provide that understanding.

8

Substance Abuse

Richard G. MacKenzie, M.D.

Drug use and adolescence have become almost synonymous. For those who experienced their adolescence prior to the 1960s, the present epidemic of drug use among today's youth challenges comprehension. Tobacco and alcohol were the primary chemical health hazards to the teenager of thirty years ago. Tobacco "stunted growth," produced bronchitis, and was unacceptable as a teenage behavior. Adults smoked; teenagers did not. Freedom to drink alcohol was a privilege granted by social custom and legislative mandate. Much of what has become commonplace jargon today was foreign to teenagers thirty years ago. Words such as *Thai stick*, *sinsemilla*, *smack*, *crack*, *angel dust*, and *ludes* would have perplexed all within earshot of utterance. Little reaction would have been stirred, as these words had no meaning, by either hearsay or experience.

As we approach the close of the twentieth century, adolescence has taken on a new meaning. Negotiating a relationship with illicit drug use has become a significant new task of the teenage years and one that transcends socioeconomic status, geographical location, or family values. Recreational drug use is ubiquitous both in reality and by threat. The full impact of drugs as a health hazard is yet to be felt. The drug-sex connection, which in the past has been expressed by increased prevalence of sexually transmitted diseases and teenage pregnancy, now takes on the risk of lethality through acquisition of HIV infection. For most adolescents who do not use drugs intravenously, the threat is indirect. The risk originates from the sexual behaviors and freedoms that are facilitated by the breaking down of the barrier of personal value and conduct during the drug experience or use of the drug-sex trade-off to satisfy a chemical dependency need. Understanding drug use as a risk behavior with potentially serious and complex consequences, both direct and indirect, has now become fundamental to professionals working with or providing health care services for adolescents.

Recent longitudinal studies have shown that not all teenagers have the same risk profile for future serious complications from drug use. The majority of young people will not become habitual or regular users in their adult years. The risk for these experimental, transient, occasional users lies more in the setting and behaviors associated with the drug use than the intrinsic pharmacological properties of the drugs. Examples of those health hazards that indirectly arise out of the drug experience include drinking and driving, increased number of serially monogamous sexual encounters, drug-related pregnancy and fetal complications, and learning dysfunctions. In those individuals who develop a life-style with a commitment to continued use, these indirect consequences are compounded by the predictable complications of chemical dependency.

This chapter reviews not only some of the epidemiology of drug use but also etiological contributants, developmental issues, pharmacological characteristics of the more commonly abused drugs, intervention and prevention strategies, and recommendations for community action by professionals working with adolescents in medical, educational, juvenile justice, and social settings.

Demographics

Although the abuse of drugs has no respect for age, sex, socioeconomic status, cultural origins, or geographical location, there is greater use among young people than among adults. This predilection is not due to serendipity but is directly related to the rapid biopsychosocial growth and development that occur during adolescence. With this increase in velocity of change, the pressures for adaptation to perceived or declared norms are great. Teenagers search, experiment, and choose a variety of adaptations, social markers, mood modifiers, and facilitators to achieve any particular developmental task. The developmental task becomes the driving force. Behavior manifests as an attempt to modulate the discomfort of change and become more in harmony. The specific adaptational behaviors may vary depending on developmental pressures, previous experience, and purpose. Evidence of biopsychosocial maturation or arrest becomes expressed through situational behaviors.

Studies of drug use prevalence are best seen as a measure of situational behaviors arising from maturational forces, influenced by myriad factors. The annual survey of high school seniors carried out by the Institute for Social Research at the University of Michigan since 1975 provides a reflection of drug use in a national probability sample of 16,000 high school seniors. It also reflects the integration of drug use into the important developmental tasks occurring during the high school experience. Unfortunately, it provides no information on the 15 to 20 percent of young people who drop out of school. Despite this limitation, the study does provide an excellent cross-sectional view, with opportunity to compare, over a number of years, not only use prevalence but also attitudinal changes. Significant findings from the 1989 study include the following:

- Illicit drug use is a statistically normative behavior among American youth, with 51 percent of high school seniors reporting having used drugs sometime during their lives. An increasing proportion of students are discontinuing their use.
- Reported daily use of marijuana fell to an all-time low of 2.9 percent (peak use was in 1978, at 10.7 percent). Approximately 78 percent of the students surveyed in 1987 felt that smoking marijuana regularly put them at risk of physically or otherwise harming themselves. Only 35 percent felt similarly in 1978.
- In 1989, 10.3 percent of seniors reported having tried cocaine, with 4.7 percent reporting use of "crack." Both of these figures represent a downward trend. Changed attitudes toward crack use were also evident, with 75 percent believing that occasional use is dangerous (versus 70 percent in 1987). Students admitted to widespread availability of crack, and 47 percent said that it would be fairly easy for them to get, compared to 41 percent in 1987. Generally, there was a more negative attitude toward use and a decreased reported use, despite wider availability. Similar trends were also evident among previously surveyed high school graduates.
- Although approximately one-fifth of seniors (18.9 percent) still reported cigarette smoking daily, this represented a decline in use since a peak in 1978 (28.8 percent).
- Of those surveyed, 4.2 percent reported daily use of alcohol, 60 percent use in the past month, and 90 percent having tried the drug.

Etiological Considerations

No single etiological hypothesis explains all drug abuse. Perhaps what can be best identified is a vulnerability syndrome. The different degrees of expression of the syndrome are not dependent on one factor alone but result from a variety of interacting forces. The most important consideration is the vulnerable individual who, as a result of the interplay of genetic, familial, and early environmental influences, is more at risk. This multimodal paradigm is not dissimilar to that for coronary artery disease. The presence of atherosclerotic fatty streaks during childhood is ubiquitous, yet varies in degree of severity. These streaks initiate the process of biological vulnerability to future coronary artery disease. The mere presence of the streak is not predictive of disease. Other risk factors, such as diet, increased levels of cholesterol, elevated blood pressure, cigarette smoking, obesity, and poor physical fitness, must interact with this biological vulnerability. Many of these influences, which are derivatives of life-style, have their basis in habits developed during childhood and adolescence.

Research in the past decade has provided evidence that makes the theory of a progressive, multifactorial etiology for alcohol and drug abuse increasingly convincing. Although much of this knowledge has been gathered from the study of children of alcoholic parents, similar influences play a role in chemical dependency in general. This understanding of the evolution of drug dependency permits a more deductive approach to diagnosis and thus management planning. Clinical interventions become more directed in those individuals in which a more specific dynamic etiological diagnosis can be made.

There are four broad areas of influence that contribute to the syndrome of drug abuse: genetic, familial, environmental, and developmental. As with the example of coronary artery disease used above, boundaries between the influences of various factors are often blurred. It is the ongoing dynamic interaction in a changing psychosocial environment that leads to the substance abuse disorder. Consequently, the clinical manifestations of the syndrome appear within a spectrum of symptomatic expressions of the disorder. One end of this spectrum is represented by the mildest form of the disorder—the one-time user or "taster," who, through curiosity or peer pressure and without underlying vulnerability, experimented and discarded the idea of this option as important to his or her life experience. At the other end of the spectrum is the individual whose genetic and family profile is such that commitment to a drug life-style becomes manifest. Substance use and abuse find an important role in this individual's life, not only as a new or thrill-seeking experience but also to normalize and make tolerable daily interactions. Chemical dependency as a disorder rapidly encapsulates the individual in a life-style in which drug-seeking behavior and drug taking occupy a central role. This abuse may lead to paradependency activities ranging from petty theft from family members to armed robbery, burglary, assault, and so on. Between the two extremes of this spectrum are found the substance abuse behaviors of the majority of adolescents, among whom drug abuse is usually occasional and without pattern.

Abuse patterns at either end of the spectrum are quite evident and pose no difficulty in diagnosis. The gray middle zone, in which periods of use may be intense but episodic, creates a dilemma in diagnosis. Many drug treatment experts advocate that any drug use represents a chronic progressive disease without a cure. Effective intervention must consist of complete abstinence, peer support, family intervention, and environmental manipulation.

Although there continues to be disagreement regarding the exact nature of drug abuse as a clinical problem, most agree that early diagnosis through identification of a risk profile is optimal. This risk profile is based on known etiological contributants or antecedents to the disorder.

Genetic Influences

Most of the evidence for a genetic influence on the development of chemical dependency has come from the study of alcoholism. This research has elicited a vulnerability syndrome that has a biological basis but is not drug specific. This syndrome has been variably referred to as addictive-compulsive personality or antisocial personality. In their studies on substance abuse in adolescents, Jessor and Jessor have referred to this marker as the "deviance syndrome," or proneness to problem behaviors. The concept of the vulnerability syndrome implies that the specific drug choice, be it alcohol or other licit or illicit drug, is dependent on other factors, such as sociocultural influences, availability, peer norms, and so on.

Evidence for the biological-genetic influence derives from studies on siblings and half-siblings of alcoholics, on twins, and on adopted children either one or both of whose biological parents were alcoholic. Sibling studies noted that the offspring of an alcoholic parent were more likely to manifest subsequent alcohol abuse than their half-siblings who had been born to two non-chemically dependent parents. Twin studies provided further evidence by demonstrating a greater risk for chemical dependency in monozygotic than in dizygotic twins of alcoholic parents. The vulnerability was more significant in the males. Studies of adoptees were carried out to attempt to separate heredity from environment. A two- to ninefold greater risk for alcoholism was found in children whose biological parents were alcoholics but were raised by nonalcoholic adoptive parents. Conversely, studies have shown that children of parents who are nonalcoholics and who were raised in families in which the parents were alcoholic demonstrated no increase in the likelihood of alcohol abuse.

These three kinds of studies suggest that the family environment that incorporates chemical dependency into its value system must interact with a genetic predisposition or vulnerability that subsequently increases the propensity to similar behavior in the offspring. What has also become clear from studies on the nature-versus-nurture controversy is that not all children of substance-abusing parents have genetic vulnerability. Some parents themselves have developed their abuse patterns primarily because of environmental influences in their lives. They therefore would not have an increased propensity to genetically influence the vulnerability behaviors of their offspring. Conversely, some parents may be protected from expression of their own substance-abusing vulnerabilities by religious, social, or cultural pressures or personal preferences.

Familial Influences

Early infancy and childhood may amplify or modulate genetic or perinatal influences. It is the critical period of life during which the "primary scenario" gets imprinted. Within the environment of the family, attitudes and values are shaped and norms of relationships develop while trust and coping skills are acquired. Inadequacies and deficiencies of this early experience, compounded by genetic and perinatal vulnerabilities, may become the backdrop against which future adolescent drug use is enacted. The milieu of the family eventually gives way to that of the community, peer group, and greater social environment. Deficiencies of the "primary scenario" become further exaggerated, and significant dysfunction in the form of drug use may become manifest. Studies of families of serious youthful abusers demonstrate more emotional disturbances, inappropriate dysfunctional interaction patterns, and an increased incidence of other deviant behaviors. Raised in a dysfunctional family with often one or both parents chemically dependent, these young people grow up with poor models of behavior and socialization. Family and home-management skills are inadequate or absent. Healthy social interactions outside the family are lacking, and parental supervision is poor. Schooling is often neglected and basic needs such as food and clothing ignored. Family dysfunction is also characterized by an increase in conflict, a disorganized household with fewer rules and predictable schedules, fewer family rituals, frequent family moves, and increased day-to-day stress. Children and young people growing up in this type of environment often live their lives in chaos. A settled life is often considered boring. Self-esteem is low, frustration high, and anger easily manifest. Substance abuse temporarily relives their distress, but the chronic nature of their problems and the temporary relief provided by their substance abuse increase the risk for continued and patterned use.

Certain factors have been found protective for a child in a dysfunctional family and may ward off the negative family influences. Children with high intelligence, attentional competencies, even temperament, academic achievement, social responsiveness and dependency, and good coping skills are at less risk in later life for alcohol and drug abuse. Healthy school, community, and peer environments further augment this protective effect.

Environmental Influences

The family experience establishes the foundation for the adolescent's relationship to the greater community and social environment. Those families that have had a decreased articulation with the activities conventionally valued have an increased propensity to have children who are substance abusers. The children and adolescents from these families have fewer skills to negotiate the day-to-day interactions that promote a sense of competence and, thus, well-being. The school is often the single most important social environment for the adolescent. Those with serious chemical dependency problems are poorly integrated into the school environment, with decreased feelings of belonging and an increased rejection by school peers. Disaffection for schoolwork and related activities develops. Attendance at school declines, and tardiness increases. Educational performance subsequently suffers, which leads to placement in a special education or alternative school or, worse yet, school dropout. This alienation from the educational experience may appear early. Repeated episodes of rejection and failure occur over the subsequent years, with behavioral expression manifesting in the adolescent. Longitudinal studies have shown that young people who are susceptible to heavy chemical dependency have declared their differences through behavior and action prior to the actual onset of substance abuse.

Belonging to a drug-using peer group is one of the strongest predictors of drug use. Patterns of use established within that group will determine the commitment to use by any individual member. A peer group in which drug use is an occasional event will usually not attract young people who are committed to the drug life-style, or vice versa. Studies that have focused on the influence of neighborhood factors on drug use have found that characteristics such as high population density, high crime rates, secluded public areas, lack of a local neighborhood and community spirit, and a transient neighborhood population all promote increased delinquency in general and serious patterns of drug use specifically.

Adolescents who have the opportunity to grow up in an enriched, supportive, caring environment that offers options for their psychological and social development have less risk of developing serious abuse patterns. Adolescence as the period of rapid growth and development that prepares the individual for future social, educational, vocational, family, community, and personal achievements depends on congruent and nurturing childhood experience. The risk for developmental deviance is lessened by a healthy genetic influence and childhood experience. A social environment during the teenage years that provides a variety of healthy options for task accomplishment minimizes the risk for deviance, drug use, or chemical dependency.

Developmental Influences

Adolescence is a critical time for developing stress-alleviating behaviors to deal with the rapid changes that occur during this transitional period. Traditional views of adolescence suggest a number of essential tasks, such as independence, individuation, peer group acceptance, sexuality, intimacy, and emancipation. The forces that drive the individual to address the tasks evolve from a need for a sense of competence, empowerment, and control and a general sense of well-being. Adolescence may then be viewed as a period of incubation with a purpose: The outcome is to be a mature, responsible individual who may integrate him- or herself into the larger social system with clear options for life-style choices. Within this developmental phase, a variety of behaviors are learned and tried out, each serving a purpose or a role for the individual. Drug use becomes an option to facilitate the transitional events that require adaptational responses on almost a daily basis. As Jessor suggests, drug use becomes functional and purposeful rather than perverse. Drugs become the solution for resolution of the discomfort of the transition, rather than the problem in and of itself.

In support of this developmental view of drug use is the fact that most adolescents will greatly lessen or abandon their drug use with maturation into adulthood. The need for a reaction against conventional society is greatly diluted with the onset of the adult experience. Most grow up to lead normal lives, similar to their peers who have never used drugs. However, there are significant risks during the drug-using years that do not confront their non-drug-using peers. These risks are multiple, ranging from decreased academic performance to vehicular accidents. The risk for long-term dependency, although real in certain individuals, is overshadowed by the immediate risks to health from unintentional injuries.

Drugs of Abuse and Their Effects

The interaction of the variety of factors that determine whether any particular teenager is going to use drugs may be described by a Venn diagram. This concept, borrowed from epidemiology, suggests that there are three basic components that characterize a problem. The shape of the problem is the product of the contribution of each of these components (see Figure 8.1). The family and peer group constitute a very important part of the teenager's environment and, as would be expected, contribute greatly to it. The characteristics of the drug itself play a variable role in initiation and continuation of the drug habit.

Examined as a group, drugs of abuse have several common properties. They tend to promote an increased sense of well-being and sometimes a false sense of security. This effect may be produced indirectly by the creation of an altered state in which the individual avoids uncomfortable or dysphoric feelings. Common to the pharmacological properties of these drugs is the desired effect on the central nervous system (CNS). The desired physical and psychological actions may be complicated by adverse effects, such as a toxic reaction, a temporary loss of self-control, impairment of function, or chemical dependency. The drug phencyclidine (PCP) is a good example. The acute CNS effects are dose-dependent, with larger doses producing greater adverse effects. Also, the dose required to produce some of the desired effects is very close to the toxic dose. This drug then is notorious for its ability to produce dysphoric drug experiences. Other drugs, such as marijuana and alcohol, have predictable physical and psychological complications with prolonged and chronic use.

Used acutely, any drug has the potential to produce an idiopathic or inherent toxic effect. Over long periods of time, inherent effects of the drug are complicated and compounded by the blunting of the relationship between internal and external reality, stunting psychological development and impairing cognitive function. Drug-related morbidity is further compounded by the real risks to physical health posed by both acute and chronic

Figure 8.1. Factors Determining Drug Use.

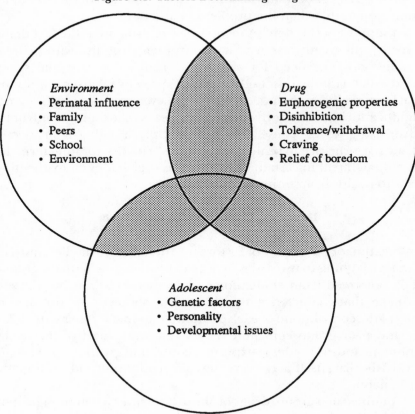

use. Most of the immediate consequences to physical health result from violence or associated trauma—the primary causes of morbidity and mortality in adolescents. Chronically, the drug itself may have inherent properties that with long-term use produce physical damage to various organs of the body. Well-known examples of the latter are cirrhosis of the liver associated with ethanol use and chronic bronchitis and emphysema, lung carcinoma, and coronary artery disease associated with tobacco use.

An understanding of the pharmacological issues of licit and illicit drugs helps to explain part of the problem of drug use and chemical dependency. Focus on this issue alone may deflect attention from the other two lobes of the Venn diagram. Unfortunately, the diagnostic nomenclature promotes the concept of the drug as the central issue, detracting from the importance of the others. Recently, the view that drug use is only one of many possible problem behaviors that contribute to a risk profile in young people has promoted the integrated approach to diagnosis. In this modified view, the issues of the entire adolescent experience are centralized, with decentralization of the risk behavior and recognition of the propensity for the clustering of problem behaviors within any one individual.

A knowledge of the pharmacological properties of the various drugs used by young people guides the principles of medical intervention during the acute phase but not necessarily during the drug-rehabilitation program. The latter incorporates multiple characteristics, most of which are independent of the pharmacological action of the drugs used. The following brief review of pharmacological issues in chemical dependency should serve as a topical overview.

The effect and risk of any drug for a particular individual are dependent on a number of factors, many of which are influenced more by the user than by the drug itself. Use of drugs whose primary effect is a modified psychological experience is extremely prone to external influences. The effect is influenced by the dose of the drug, the method of administration (orally, intranasally, intravenously, by inhalation, and so on), the setting in which the drug is taken, the user's expectations regarding the effects of the drug, the personality and psychological state of the user, the purity of the compound used, and the frequency with which the drug is taken. The teenager who smokes marijuana while driving a motor vehicle will have a very different risk profile from that of the one who does so in the quiet of his or her bedroom. The clinical pharmacological state produced in a naive, inexperienced cocaine user will differ greatly from that produced in a chronic user of crack.

Marijuana

Historically, marijuana is an ancient drug. It has had a wide range of uses, from relaxation to powerful psychic stimulation in order to facilitate spiritual ritual and experience. Around the world, this product of the hemp plant has a variety of names: hashish, charas, bhang, ganja, dagga, and so on. An estimated twenty million Americans, notably not all of them teenagers, smoke marijuana daily.

Pharmacology. Although the leaf and resin of the *Cannabis sativa* plant contain a number of psychoactive ingredients, the most active ingredient influencing behavior is delta 9-tetrahydrocannabinol (THC). Concentration of this psychoactive substance ranges from 0.5 to 9 percent depending on the source of the drug and the cultivated plant variety. Most marijuana is ingested through inhalation, with less than 50 percent of the active ingredient being absorbed. Inhalation produces effects in minutes, with peak plasma concentration occurring in ten to thirty minutes. The duration of the effect is variable, but it usually lasts from two to three hours. If the substance (marijuana, hashish, and so on) is ingested orally, usually in combination with chocolate (brownies being a favorite), onset of action is more gradual. Gastric acidity and detoxification by the liver diminish the concentration of the psychoactive metabolites by two-thirds. With oral ingestion, onset of action is delayed up to thirty to sixty minutes, and the effects last for three to five hours. This method of administration produces a much more variable psychoactive response. Despite the drawbacks, this method is often preferred, particularly when delayed onset of action is desired or the risk of discovery through smoking is great.

THC and its metabolites, particularly the carboxyacid analogues, are excreted via the urine (35 percent) and feces (65 percent). THC is a lipophilic agent and therefore accumulates in the fatty tissues of the body and thus can also cross the placenta. Following ingestion, the accumulated drug may be slowly released from the adipose tissue, and, depending on the experience of the user and the quality of the drug, it may be detected in the urine for a period of from three to thirty days. Tolerance does develop with continued use of the drug. After a chronic high-dose use pattern, a withdrawal syndrome manifests. Unlike the high of alcohol intoxication, that of marijuana may be overcome with intent.

Physiological Effects and Risks. Acutely, marijuana increases the pulse rate and, variably, the blood pressure. Both of these effects are augmented by cocaine. These effects may create a risk for young people with congenital cardiac abnormality, cardiac conduction defects, or labile increases in blood pressure.

Inhalation produces stinging and burning sensations in the posterior oropharynx and an irritative cough. A swollen and inflamed uvula has been reported in hashish smokers. Acutely, bronchodilatation occurs, but with continued use, there is bronchoconstriction. With long-term use, mild airway obstruction has been reported, along with inflammatory and preneoplastic changes. The bronchoconstrictor properties may aggravate attacks in asthmatics and may reveal a predisposition for asthma. Inhalation may further aggravate any preexisting bronchopulmonary disease, in addition to being a possible precursor to lung cancer.

THC decreases sweating and increases body temperature through a central effect. It may produce some impairment of vigilance, coordination, and reaction time and a multiple stimuli attention deficit. There is a preoccupation with drug-induced imagery and distraction from complex motor tasks. Hand steadiness is decreased, with increased body sway and decreased accuracy of fine motion. Learning and oral communication are impaired.

Alcohol

The pattern of alcohol use varies from person to person. During adolescence, its use is encouraged to the point of intoxication — often the first potent mood-altering experience for the young user. This experience will often lead to the use of other mood-altering substances — an outcome known as "the gateway effect." Alcohol, as a socially sanctioned intoxicant, is the most serious drug problem of youth.

Pharmacology. Because of their differing content of ethanol, alcoholic beverages will have varying effects on the consumer. The effect also depends on the absorptive state of the digestive tract, as alcohol is absorbed in both the stomach and the small intestine. Food with high fat content retards the absorption of ethanol. Maximum blood concentration is attained over thirty to ninety minutes. The rate-limiting factor for alcohol metabolism is the liver enzyme alcohol dehydrogenase. The rate of metabolism usually correlates with body size and the degree of metabolic tolerance that an individual has developed. Regular drinkers have increased amounts of alcohol de-hydrogenase and are therefore more tolerant to alcohol ingestion. CNS adaptation also contributes to this "tolerant" state. Ninety-eight percent of alcohol is oxidized in the liver, which has the capability of breaking down about an ounce of alcohol per hour, or ten to twelve ounces of beer per hour.

Physiological Effects and Risks. Alcohol is a direct irritant of the gastric mucosa, through both its inherent nature and its ability to increase hydro-chloric acid secretion through increased gastrin production. Ethanol also produces increased secretion of pancreatic enzymes. Ethanol increases the deposition of fats in the liver. Low doses increase high-density lipoproteins; moderate to high doses may increase low-density and very-low-density lipoproteins. Alcohol ingestion in adolescents poses the risk of superficial gastritis, irritative pylorospasm, and peptic ulcer disease secondary to irrita-tion and increased acid load. Chronic use may manifest as fatty liver with mild elevation of the liver transaminases. Acute alcoholic hepatitis and pancreatitis are rare complications of adolescent alcohol use.

The primary desired effect of alcohol is its effect on the CNS. It is essentially a depressant, affecting first the more highly integrated centers. Manifest expression of this effect may be disinhibition and what appears to be excitatory behavior. In moderate doses, ethanol affects cerebellar func-tion, producing slurred speech, ataxia, and horizontal nastagmus. Higher doses lead to lethargy, stupor, and coma. No good correlation exists between blood alcohol level and behavioral effects in adolescents. Most states use 100 milligrams per deciliter to define intoxication while driving. This value is probably too high for the naive adolescent drinker.

Risks to the CNS with alcohol use include the well-known drunken state, with decreased mental activity and impaired judgment. A comatose state may ensue from continued drinking. Paradoxical excitation from disin-hibition may produce erratic and uncontrollable behavior. Certain indi-viduals will experience a state of pathological intoxication upon drinking small amounts of alcohol. This is probably related to a genetic metabolic intolerance to alcohol. These individuals quickly learn not to drink. Certain individuals experience blackouts or temporary amnesia during periods of heavy drinking. The classic alcohol withdrawal syndrome is uncommon in adolescents, but in those who are beginning to develop a state of dependency, a modified abstinence syndrome is apparent. Drug-seeking behavior ap-pears, with irritability and irrationality being central to its expression.

The fetal alcohol syndrome is a complication of alcohol consumption during pregnancy. No amount of alcohol has been documented as safe to drink during pregnancy. Ethanol crosses the placental barrier and affects the developing fetus, producing an abnormal appearance of the face (micro-cephaly, short palpebral fissures, hypoplastic maxilla and philtrum, short, turned-up nose), mental retardation, cardiac abnormalities, congenital mal-formations of the genitourinary system, and skeletal deformities. Babies that are affected by the fetal alcohol syndrome are usually born small for gesta-tional age. This is important in that 17 percent of all pregnancies occur in adolescents, and the association between alcohol ingestion and fetal out-come is often ignored or denied by the teen mother.

Tobacco

The initiation of cigarette smoking has long been a rite of passage during adolescence and a significant source of revenue for the tobacco industry. The majority of new smokers are recruited from today's adolescents and young adults. Most cigarette smokers are habitual users. Rarely do smokers develop a pattern of episodic, irregular use.

Pharmacology. The burning of tobacco releases approximately 4,000 compounds in both its gaseous and its particulate phases. The variable composition of the smoke inhaled by the smoker governs the phar-macological effect. Nicotine produces the desired CNS effect through inter-action with specific receptors. Skeletal muscle relaxation accompanies an alerting effect and a decrease in anxiety and irritability. Appetite and craving for sweets are reduced, and thus overall caloric consumption is diminished. Pain threshold is increased, and thus so is pain tolerance, mediated through the release of endogenous opiates. Following inhalation, the nicotine sus-pended on minute particles of tar is quickly absorbed and reaches the brain within seven or eight seconds. Significant levels of nicotine are maintained in the bloodstream for thirty to sixty minutes following inhalation. Use of tobacco leads to the development of a dependence syndrome characterized by both tolerance and withdrawal. Relapse rates are high after attempts at permanent cessation of smoking. All tobacco products contain nicotine.

More than 90 percent of smokers initiate their habit during adoles-cence. Smoking during early adolescence has been reported to be predictive of other health risk behaviors, such as reckless driving, irresponsible sexual behavior, and alcohol and other drug use. Smoking has been identified as the greatest cause of preventable mortality in the United States today.

Physiological Effects and Risks. The constituents of tobacco in both smoke and smokeless forms expose the oral cavity to potent carcinogens, producing oral cancers and leukoplakia. Inhalation of tobacco smoke ex-poses the sensitive epithelium of the respiratory tract to carcinogens and ciliotoxins and interferes with proteolytic enzymes and immune mecha-nisms within the tracheobronchial tree. These effects lead to carcinoma of

the lung, larynx, and oral cavity, chronic obstructive lung disease characterized by chronic bronchitis and emphysema, periodontal problems, and
pulmonary infections.

Inhalation of tobacco smoke delivers not only nicotine and carbon
monoxide but also a variety of other physiologically toxic substances to the
bloodstream. Smoking of tobacco may increase cardiac rate and blood
pressure, free fatty acids in the plasma, low-density lipoproteins, and the
coagulability of blood. Risk for coronary artery disease, cerebral vascular
disease, and peripheral vascular disease is increased through nicotine's role
in increasing atherosclerosis.

Absorbed carcinogens from smoking increase the risk for cancer of
the esophagus, bladder, and pancreas. Smoking also increases the incidence
of spontaneous abortion, significantly reduces the birth weight of children
born to smoking mothers, and increases the incidence of sudden infant
death syndrome (SIDS) and other causes of perinatal mortality.

Tobacco, in both its smoke and its smokeless forms, produces considerable morbidity in the consumer. Recent studies demonstrate a significant
morbidity in passive smokers; that is, those who are in the environment
contiguous to the active smoker. Infants of parents who smoke are trapped
and have many complications from passive smoking. They have almost twice
as great a risk of SIDS as do other infants and are three times more likely to be
admitted to a hospital for pneumonia. Problems such as sinusitis, eczema or
hives, and skin infections are also more common. Hospitalizations of these
infants are prolonged as well.

Cocaine

The reference to cocaine as a recreational drug is an understatement.
It is so powerful in its effects that even sophisticated users have trouble
maintaining control over their habits. Cocaine can have a tragic impact on
the present and future lives of teenagers, who are still establishing boundaries of behavior and self-discipline.

Pharmacology. Cocaine is a derivative of the leaf of the plant *Erythrox-
ylon coca*, which is native to Central and South America. The principal active
ingredient is cocaine itself, which is available as the hydrochloride, alkaloid
(free-base, rock, crack), or paste (bazooka). It is a strong CNS stimulant that
blocks the initiation and conduction of nerve impulses. It also blocks the re-
uptake of norepinephrine. Half-life in the plasma is approximately one hour,
whatever the method of administration. The euphoric effect on the individual is dependent on the method of use and sophistication of the user; it
may last for thirty to fifty minutes. Metabolized by the liver and plasma
esterases, it is excreted primarily in the urine as benzoylecognine, or un-
changed cocaine. Its low molecular weight and high water and lipid solubility
facilitate transfer across the placenta, producing significant obstetrical and

neonatal complications. Tolerance develops fairly rapidly, with a withdrawal syndrome manifest on discontinuance of the drug. The euphoriant effect (high) of the various preparations varies in intensity; it is followed by an equally intense hypersomnolence and depression.

Physiological Effects and Risks. Direct contact with the nasal mucosa produces intense vasoconstriction and associated inflammation. Rebound nasal congestion follows. Mucosal irritation (xerostoma) is evident. Continued use may lead to recurrent epistaxis, mucosal atrophy, and, rarely, a perforated nasal septum. Deeper inhalation may produce hemoptysis and black-streaked sputum. Hyperventilation and pulmonary edema have been reported.

Both pulse rate and blood pressure are increased with cocaine use. Arterial vasoconstriction, especially of the coronary arteries, may occur. Cardiovascular morbidity and mortality related to myocardial infarction (coronary artery spasm), strokes (hypertension), and cardiac arrhythmias increase. These complications are not dose dependent but idiosyncratic.

Cocaine significantly decreases appetite, and ingestion of it may be accompanied by nausea and vomiting. Bowel sounds become hyperactive. Continued use may produce weight loss and malnutrition. Cocaine use may be associated with the pathology of eating disorders, as it may be used to decrease appetite and thus prevent weight gain. Aspiration pneumonia associated with drug-induced vomiting and seizures has been reported.

Acutely, cocaine delays ejaculation and orgasm in the male and also produces a generalized increase in sensory awareness and sensuality. This accounts for the drug's reputation as an aphrodisiac. Chronic use leads to impotence. Its powerful short-acting stimulant properties produce euphoria, alertness, and energy. It may give rise to hyperactivity, anxiety, and insomnia. Personality changes may occur, with suspicious and paranoid thinking appearing. This may lead to violent acts against self and others. Tactile, visual (snow lights), olfactory, and auditory hallucinations may occur. Tremors are often apparent. Generalized tonic-clonic seizures and status epilepticus may occur, with subsequent cerebral anoxia and risk of aspiration pneumonia. Lethargy and hypersomnolence appear in chronic users when cocaine is not available.

Miscellaneous Drugs

A number of drugs and chemical substances are used occasionally or gain popularity in certain geographical areas. Significant morbidity is associated with the use of many of them. A brief review of some of the salient characteristics of several of these drugs follows.

Phencyclidine pharmacologically is an anesthetic that when abused has stimulant, depressant, and hallucinogenic properties. Effects are dose-dependent, and risk of toxic reactions is great. Low dosages (one to five

milligrams) are associated with euphoria and dysphoria but may be complicated by numbness, blank stare, nystagmus, and hyperacusis. Higher dosages
(five to fifteen milligrams) are associated with seizures, hypertension, hyper-
reflexia, and psychosis. Violent and aggressive behavior is common, which
compounds the morbidity and mortality associated with the drug.

Methylenedioxymethamphetamine (MDMA), known on the streets as
Adam, Ecstasy, or E-tab, produces increased sociability, introspection, and
sense of well-being lasting four to six hours. Confusion, depression, and
anxiety may occur for several weeks following this experience. Several deaths
of cardiac origin have been directly and indirectly related to the use of
MDMA.

Volatile substances are occasionally used by less sophisticated young
people to obtain a high characterized by decreased inhibition, euphoria,
light-headedness, and illusionary experiences. All volatiles are lipid soluble
and thus produce a rapid onset of action. Low cost and ease of availability
make these substances attractive alternatives to illicit drug use. Loss of
inhibition may lead to impulsive behavior, increasing the risk of trauma. The
user may become confused and disoriented, leading to continued inhalation, CNS anoxia, and seizures. Cardiorespiratory arrest may occur. Specific
volatile substances such as toluene, gasoline, halogenated hydrocarbons,
nitrous oxide, and nitrites have particular complications in addition to those
listed above.

Use of *lysergic acid diethylamide* (LSD) persists among young people,
particularly on school and college campuses. It is a potent psychoactive
substance that has a wide safety margin of dosage. LSD is not easily detected
in urine. It is rapidly absorbed through the gastrointestinal tract and its
effects are felt within minutes. Dramatic subjective experiences include
visual and auditory illusions, synesthesias, increased sensitivity of touch, and
time distortion. Additional risk occurs when the user under the influence
misinterprets illusion for reality. Acutely, the drug may cause paranoid
ideation, depression, confusion, and fragmentation. With long-term use,
LSD may produce flashbacks, psychosis, depressive reactions, and personality changes.

The Integrated View: A Case Study

Given the availability of drugs, the congruence between the adolescent
experience and drug use becomes apparent. The genetic, perinatal, and
family factors set the stage. The childhood experience (primary scenario)
provides the deficiencies or the adverse behavioral responses to the ordinary
stress of daily life. Social and emotional constrictive and restrictive forces
limit the child's view of possibilities and options for adjusting to challenge
and circumstance. The usual developmental transitions for healthy psychological and social growth leave the child with a feeling of disempowerment,
poor self-esteem, and ineffectiveness. The adolescent experience rekindles

and activates the deficiencies and strengths of the childhood experience; on this foundation is built a structure on which future life experience may be based. The transitions demanded by biological changes, societal views, adult expectations, and peer behaviors demand resolution and reconciliation. The young adolescent struggles to maintain an equilibrium between the private experiences of self and the expression of them through behavior. Congruence between these two states, the solipsistic and the behavioral, creates the sense of well-being that is, of course, the goal of human life experience. Discord, on the other hand, prompts the young person to seek resolution of the discomfort—that is, to explore the options. Inherent in this search is the risk that the option chosen as the solution may well represent a problem in and of itself. The problematic nature of the chosen option may not be immediately apparent to the teenager but apparent only to those who have a broader view of life circumstances. The nature of the "solution" may involve not only risks that are inapparent to the individual but also inherent reinforcers that compound the magnitude of the problem. Drug use as an option often falls into the latter category.

Fortunately, for the majority of young people, the need is developmental, the driving forces situational, and the drug choice miniminally reinforcing. Some studies suggest that young people who try alcohol illicitly during their teenage years are likely to have healthier social lives and be less lonely than those who do not. This does not, of course, diminish the serious risks to health that drug use poses during the critical periods of puberty and adolescence.

Perry and Jessor suggest that health or the sense of well-being central to prime performance and enjoyment may be divided into four domains, or spheres, that are interactive and in a state of equilibrium (Figure 8.2). During adolescence, the teenager often feels an isolated uneasiness in one of these areas. In an attempt to alleviate this transient discomfort, a behavior is adopted or decision made that will pose great risk in the other domains. For example, isolation and fear of rejection from friends (social) and personal feelings of inadequacy and being different (psychological) may influence the young person to adopt a peer behavior, such as smoking, that poses an inherent risk to physical health; the individual is willing to take the risk for the benefit of the immediate value. Other choices not only may pose risks in other domains of health but, used over long periods of time, may significantly compromise health in the domain of which the benefit of well-being is sought.

Evaluation of an individual for drug use becomes an important activity of professionals working with teenagers. It is important not only to identify those individuals who are using drugs but also to make the specific-dynamic etiological diagnosis. The following case example exemplifies many of the issues of identification and evaluation.

Figure 8.2. Domains of Adolescent Health.

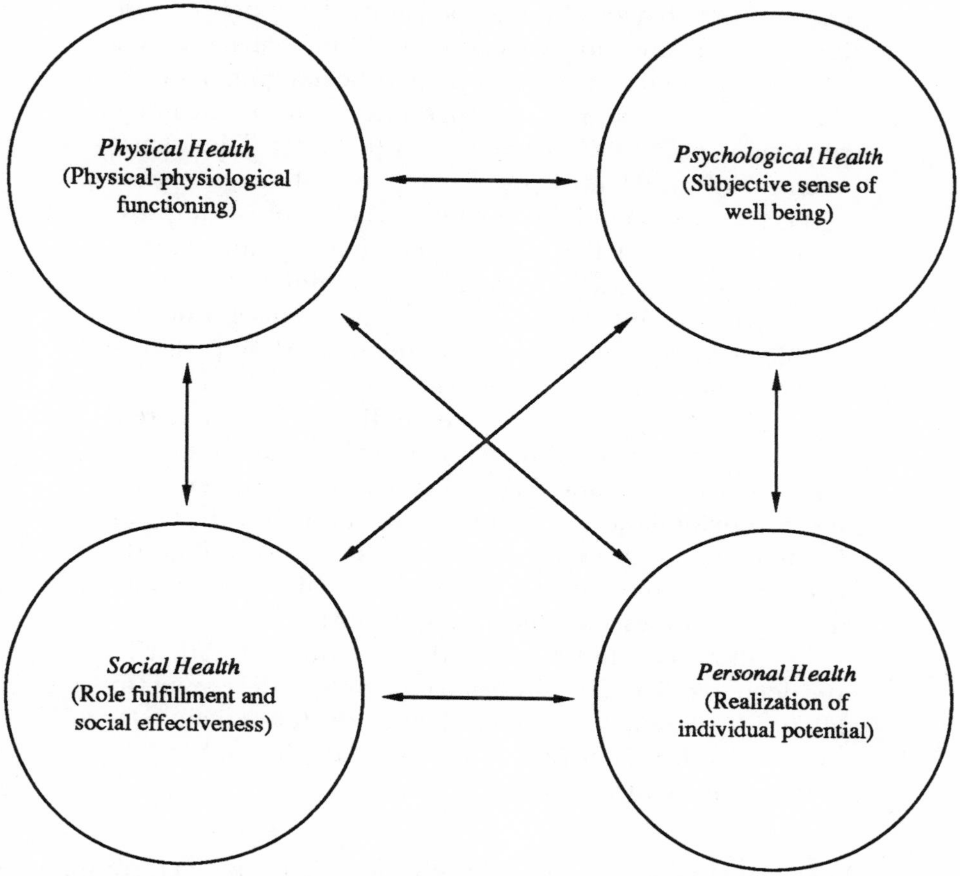

Source: Perry, C. L., and Jessor, R. "The Concept of Health Promotion and the Prevention of Adolescent Drug Abuse." *Health Education Quarterly*, 1985, *12* (2), 169–184.

Jill S.

Jill S. is a fifteen-year-old female student who was referred to the school counselor for frequent absences from class and failing grades. Review of Jill's cumulative school record showed that she had been an A, B, and C student through the sixth grade. In seventh grade, her academic performance began to decline, and her interest in the school environment began to wane. She no longer was anxious to participate in class projects or group activities. Teachers noted a general sullenness and isolation from her class peers. The school psychologist who evaluated her while she was in the seventh grade concluded that "Jill is a student of above-average intelligence, without evidence of a specific learning disorder. Her family has noted similar changes in behavior at home: becoming less interested in family events and not respecting nighttime curfews. The family expressed concern that Jill may be hanging out with the wrong crowd and using drugs, but a visit to the family physician could find no evidence of the latter. There have been no specific family problems, personal losses, or disagreements that could account for this behavior. My impression at this time is that Jill is experiencing an adjustment reaction to the anticipated change to middle school next year. I recommend alerting the academic counselor of Jill's problems to develop remedial academic work in conjunction with her homeroom teacher."

No improvement was noted in Jill's eighth-grade record in middle school; truancies became apparent, grades fell to a D average, and teachers generally noted her to be more rebellious and uncooperative, failing to hand in homework assignments, for example. The ninth-grade counselor recommended to Jill's parents that she be reevaluated by an adolescent medicine specialist.

Jill refused to be seen with her mother or father in the doctor's office. The physician encouraged the parents to allow Jill to establish a confidential doctor-patient relationship and, with their concurrence, had Jill sign her own consent for medical treatment.

Thus far, Jill has presented with a behavioral pattern that is compatible with a number of etiologies, including drug abuse, depression, attention deficit disorder, conduct disorder, personality disorder, and emotional response arising out of inapparent family problems. The possibility of an organic etiology, such as temporal lobe epilepsy, CNS lesion, or general chronic illness, must also be entertained. The physician's initial challenge was to establish rapport with Jill and utilize an interview style that would allow Jill to develop her anamnesis in a context of continuing trust.

Jill S.

The physician welcomed Jill to his office with a handshake and reiterated the contract of confidentiality, explaining, however, that if he received information indicating that Jill was going to do harm to herself or others, he would break the bond of confidentiality and recruit whatever help was indicated to benefit Jill. He also explained the state-mandated necessity to report certain conditions.

Medical history failed to reveal any particular physical complaints. Specifically, Jill denied headaches, visual complaints, syncopal episodes, dysthesias, loss of consciousness, or previous head trauma. Menarche was at eleven years, with initially irregular periods but now regular and with mild to moderate dysmenorrhea. Although Jill admitted to having a steady boyfriend for the past two years, she denied sexual activity. She also denied any gynecological symptoms. Past medical history was unremarkable, except for several middle-ear infections during childhood.

It was apparent to the physician that the underlying etiology of the presenting problem was not being elicited. Jill's affect was now more relaxed and confident. In order to maintain a balance of power in the interview, the physician had not been very aggressive initially. He now felt it necessary to reestablish the context to ask more probing questions that would further elicit problem behaviors most likely in an attractive fifteen-year-old. Following a reiteration of the confidential nature of their relationship, he elicited further information using the Childrens Hospital of Los Angeles "HEADSS" adolescent risk interview profile.

- *Home*: Lives at home with mother, father, brother, twelve, and sister, nine. Father is a university professor, mother a real estate agent. Jill was adopted at three years of age. No runaway behavior. Both mother and father spend most of their time with work.
- *Education*: Ninth grade, does not like school, not important to her future, no favorite subject, grade D's and F's, wants to be a model.
- *Activities*: Spends most of her time alone or with boyfriend (nineteen years old), who has an apartment. Likes to dance, has had occasional modeling jobs.
- *Affect*: Animated, with evidence of depression.
- *Drugs*: Smokes one-half package of cigarettes per day; has tried marijuana, both at parties and with boyfriend—likes the high; drinks wine coolers three to four times per week; has tried "crack"—boyfriend is a dealer. Doesn't like the drug scene and was told that biological mother was an alcoholic.
- *Diet*: Eats irregularly—not too often with family, always on a diet—finds that cocaine helps curb appetite, has used OTC appetite suppressants but not lately, has induced vomiting occasionally after "porking out."
- *Sex*: First boyfriend when twelve years old; was raped at thirteen while camping with parents (never told anyone), very uncomfortable with self sexually, sexually active with boyfriend—"helps me to lose weight," no contraception, never been pregnant, no past episodes of venereal disease.

- *Suicide*: Has had suicidal ideation, attempted once (overdose — ten acetyl-salicylic acid [ASA]) at thirteen years old. No family history of suicide.

The neutral stand of the physician helped to establish rapport and trust. The risk profile interview, deftly applied, elicited a profile of multiple problem behaviors, which created risk profiles in several domains of health. The symptom complex of poor school performance began to take on more "shape," and the specific dynamic diagnosis began to evolve. Alcoholism in the biological mother provided a genetic and perhaps a perinatal predisposition. Early family life may have amplified this. Adoption at three years of age, despite the apparent enrichment of the new family, was unable to completely negate this early life experience. Adaptive skills were developed during childhood but were challenged by the molestation and rape at age thirteen. Negative self-esteem was ameliorated by the boyfriend and drugs, while early developmental tasks of adolescence were satisfied (independence). The initial solution of drug use compromised Jill's social well-being and personal health (school) and manifested as a problem — though not to Jill.

Jill S.

Physical examination was remarkable for mild erosion of the enamel of the teeth, nail biting, mitral valve prolapse, and poor exercise tolerance revealed by office quick test. Pelvic examination was unremarkable, although chlamydia DFA was subsequently reported positive.

Following evaluation, a summary diagnosis was discussed with Jill. Positive aspects of her coping skills were emphasized and concern expressed about (1) substance abuse, (2) school problems, (3) unprotected intercourse, (4) eating disorder, and (5) poor exercise tolerance secondary to poor aerobic conditioning. Permission was obtained from Jill to schedule a family interview, again maintaining the bonds of confidentiality. A six-visit contract was also established to work on resolving some of the ongoing problems elucidated.

Evaluation clearly points out the need for an integrated management plan. Fortunately, Jill permitted a family interview, which allowed the physician to assess family dynamics, contributants, and resources. It also provided a forum that may allow Jill to share some of her problems. Options available to the physician at that time were ambulatory office-based care, inpatient short-term treatments, and residential care.

When *ambulatory office-based care* is considered, Jill's fragile developmental history with early childhood influences almost mandates a family-oriented approach. This may have to follow on an initial individual approach with Jill or be done concurrently. The benefits that Jill gets from her drug use are intertwined with her relationships, her sexuality, and her self-esteem. Ambulatory therapy limits environmental manipulation, introduction of reinforcers to positive problem solving, and exclusion of destructive and health-compromising behaviors. Developmental issues contribute significantly to her problem behaviors, and most options chosen for resolution have been unconventional. The skill of the physician and other members of the health team is paramount if continued office-based intervention is elected. An *intensive day-care program* may be a viable option if such a program is available.

Inpatient short-term treatment programs, ranging in length from thirty to forty-five days, provide for a period of intensive individual, group, and family intervention in a drug-free environment. Emphasis on sobriety and participation in a twelve-step program are central to most of these programs. The short-term inpatient program provides for environmental manipulation, adherence to intensive psychotherapeutic interventions, development of healthy life skills, and commitment to a healthy alternative to drug use — the twelve-step program. Unfortunately for many adolescents and their families, cost alone makes this option prohibitive.

Residential care programs are usually highly structured and require a commitment of six to nine months. They are ideally suited for young people who have multiple problems that may best respond to a diversity of intervention possibilities. The classic therapeutic community stresses open and frank communication, with admission of one's own inadequacies in personal life management but agreement to accept one's responsibility in the group. Several effective modified therapeutic communities have evolved around the live-in school experience, in which intensive adjunctive services are provided to deal with the multiple problem behaviors.

All therapeutic interventions, whether office-based, inpatient, or residential, require a program of continuing aftercare in the community. These aftercare programs must coordinate with the philosophies of the original care program and develop a well-identified system of community care that embraces all domains of health. Alcohol- and drug-free clubs and dances, knowledgeable and developmentally sensitive medical services, family meetings, twelve-step programs, and cooperative school personnel are a few of the essential components of this system. It is not unusual that initial control and alleviation of drug abuse patterns will give rise to problem behaviors in other areas. These must be anticipated and managed accordingly.

Projection and Recommendations

Early predictors of risk for drug and alcohol use have now been clarified. Many of the behavioral predictors appear in the family and school environment. Once a young person initiates a pattern of substance use, the influence of family and school greatly diminishes, while an increasingly deviant life-style evolves. Clearly, any effective attack on drug and alcohol abuse in our society involves many phalanges. All individuals working with young people — those from the health professions, law enforcement, education, recreation, and religious and political institutions — must work together from a common ground of understanding. Teenagers and young adults use drugs for a reason. Young people seek out solutions to the often difficult challenge of negotiating the teenage years. For some, the burden of genetic, perinatal, and family influences places them at great risk for the disease of chemical dependency. For others, without a multiple problem profile and with a strong family community and peer support system, drug use will be a transitional event — one that is employed to serve the developmental needs of adolescence and then discarded. Despite the transitional need, some will get caught up in the seductive euphoria produced by the drug itself and become entrapped in a dependent life-style.

The drug and alcohol use epidemic has been around for over a decade now. Is there any real hope for change in the future? Have we as a nation learned to live with this national crisis and accept the risks much as we have with other pollutants in our environment? Change is possible, but a concerted effort must be made to effect this change. The Monitoring the Future Study of the University of Michigan indicates that attitudes toward drug use are becoming more negative and prevalence of use is decreasing. Law enforcement has stepped up efforts to stem the supply of drugs entering the United States. Astoundingly, 85–90 percent of all illicit drugs produced in the world find their way onto the streets of U.S. cities and towns. Efforts will have to be extraordinary and massive to counter the ingenuity and greed of the world's drug brokers. The real impact will come from efforts to decrease the need for drugs and alcohol at the individual level. Efforts in this direction must include the following:

1. A system of care for adolescents and young adults who are already involved with drugs must be developed. Unfortunately, many young people who are in need of intervention and treatment and are willing to commit themselves are unable to do so for financial reasons. The expense of office-based, institutional, and residential care blocks access to quality care for young people emancipated by law but disarticulated from the work force.
2. Transitional options for young people must be broadened. The culture of the shopping mall society of youth must be enriched. With the encouragement of the media, young people have become spectators of life, rather than participants. Creative efforts to involve young people in social change, community programs, and personal development will only enhance all their domains of health and thus their personal sense of well-being.
3. Integrity, rather than personal wealth and greed, must once again be emphasized as an individual ethic. Young people look to mentors and

models in their aspirations and development. There are very few whose past or present does not send the message that "any means is justified by the end."

4.   The health professions and medicine in particular must get back to the individual person and not focus just on his or her disease. The inter-action of the host, agent, and environment truly determines the nature of the illness. The adolescent exemplifies the importance of the need for an integrated approach. Behavioral issues perpetuate the risk despite the removal of the agent. Negation of this integrated view will perpetuate the reservoir of illnesses that lay claim to young people in the twentieth century.

Suggested Readings

Bernardt, N. W., and others. "Comparison of Questionnaire and Laboratory Tests in the Detection of Excessive Drinking and Alcoholism." *Lancet*, Feb. 6, 1982, pp. 325–328.

Blum, R. H., and Associates. *Horatio Alger's Children: The Role of the Family in the Origin and Prevention of Drug Risk*. San Francisco: Jossey-Bass, 1972.

Bohman, M., Sigvardsson, S., and Cloninger, R. "Maternal Inheritance of Alcohol Abuse: Cross-Fostering Analysis of Adopted Women." *Archives of General Psychiatry*, 1981, *38*, 965–969.

Braucht, G. N., Brakarsh, D., Follingstad, D., and Berry, K. L. "Deviant Drug Use in Adolescence: A Review of Psychosocial Correlates." *Psychological Bulletin*, 1973, *79*, 92–106.

Cloninger, R., Bohman, M., and Sigvardsson, S. "Inheritance of Alcohol Abuse." *Archives of General Psychiatry*, 1981, *38*, 861–868.

Dowling, G. P., McDonough, E. T., and Bost, R. O. "'Eve and Ecstasy'—A Report of Five Deaths Associated with the Use of MDEA and MDMA." *Journal of the American Medical Association*, 1987, *257* (12), 1615–1617.

Garmezy, N., Masten, A. S., and Telegen, A. "The Study of Stress and Compe-tence in Children: A Building Block for Developmental Psychopathology." *Child Development*, 1984, *55*, 97–111.

Goodwin, D. W. "Alcoholism and Genetics: The Sins of the Fathers." *Archives of General Psychiatry*, 1985, *6*, 171–174.

Jessor, R., Chase, J. A., and Donovan, J. E. "Psychosocial Correlates of Mari-juana Use and Problem Drinking in a National Sample of Adolescents." *American Journal of Public Health*, 1980, *70*, 604–613.

Jessor, R., and Jessor, S. L. "A Social-Psychological Framework for Studying Drug Use." In D. J. Lettieri, M. Sayers, and H. W. Pearson (eds.), *Theories on Drug Abuse*. NIDA Research Monograph Series no. 30, DHHS Publication no. ADM 80-967. Washington, D.C.: U.S. Government Printing Office, 1980.

Johnston, L. D., O'Malley, P. P., and Bachman, J. G. *Use of Licit and Illicit Drugs by*

American's High School Students 1975–1987. Washington, D.C.: U.S. Government Printing Office, 1988.

Jones, M. C. "Personality Correlates and Antecedents of Drinking Patterns in Adult Males." *Journal of Consulting and Clinical Psychology*, 1968, *32*, 2–12.

Newcombe, M. D., and Bentler, P. M. *Consequences of Adolescent Drug Use: Impact on the Lives of Young Adults*. Newbury Park, Calif.: Sage, 1988.

❧ 9 ❧

Sexually Transmitted Diseases

Mary-Ann B. Shafer, M.D.
Anna-Barbara Moscicki, M.D.

Adolescents are engaging in sexual intercourse more frequently and are initiating this activity at younger ages than they were fifteen years ago. Fifty percent of adolescents have experienced their sexual debut by their sixteenth birthdays and more than 70 percent by their nineteenth birthdays. Sexual activity places the adolescent at risk for unplanned pregnancy and sexually transmitted diseases (STDs). As the sexual activity pattern has changed, there has also been a marked increase in the prevalence of STDs among adolescents. STDs are currently the most common infections among sexually active youth.

Adolescents and young adults under twenty-five years of age constitute more than 50 percent of the twenty million STD cases reported annually, and it is estimated that 25 percent will become infected with an STD before graduating from high school. STDs cause pelvic inflammatory disease (PID), which places young women at risk for subsequent development of ectopic pregnancy and infertility. With the advent of AIDS, it has become imperative for clinicians caring for adolescents to prevent, recognize, and treat STDs in

Note: The authors wish to thank the following members of the faculty of the University of California at San Francisco: Gail Boland, M.D., director of Sexually Transmitted Disease Clinics, Department of Public Health for the City and County of San Francisco; George F. Brooks, M.D., Department of Laboratory Medicine; and Julius Schachter, Department of Epidemiology. We would also like to thank Margot Duxler and Tracy Suitt Keogh for their careful preparation of the manuscript.

Figure 9.1. Reported Cases of Gonorrhea in United States by Age.

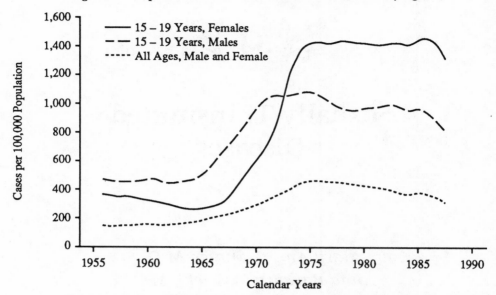

Source: Kevin O'Reilly, U.S. Department of Health and Human Services. *Sexually Transmitted Disease Statistics, 1985.* Washington, D.C.: Division of Sexually Transmitted Disease, Centers for Disease Control, U.S. Public Health Service, 1987.

our youthful population. This chapter reviews types of behavior placing the adolescent at risk for STD, common infections and clinical syndromes, and, finally, the approach to the sexually active adolescent boy and girl in office practice.

Prevalence of STDs in Adolescents

The rates of STDs are high among sexually adolescent females and males and decline dramatically with increasing age. While the exact causes of higher rates among adolescents remain unknown, they have remained at epidemic levels since the mid 1970s (Figures 9.1 and 9.2). Risk factors that may contribute to the prevalence of STDs among adolescents are discussed below. The prevalence rates of common STD organisms are outlined for females and for males. It must be remembered that gonorrheal rates reported by public health agencies such as the Centers for Disease Control are based on population by age and do not control for sexual debut. For example, approximately 50 percent of fifteen- to nineteen-year-olds have not become sexually active and therefore should not be included in the denominator when calculating the gonorrheal rate for adolescents. If one accounts for this sexual activity rate by increasing all reported gonorrheal cases by a factor of 2, it becomes obvious that the highest rate occurs among adolescent females.

Among sexually active adolescent girls reported in eleven studies,

Figure 9.2. Reported Cases of Primary and Secondary Syphilis in United States by Age.

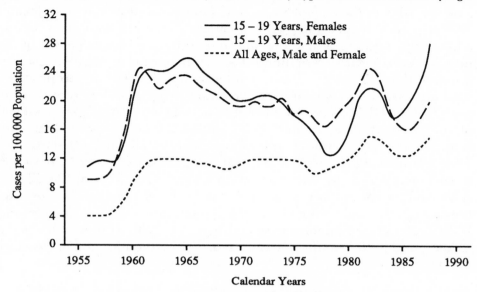

Source: Kevin O'Reilly, U.S. Department of Health and Human Services. *Sexually Transmitted Disease Statistics, 1985*. Washington, D.C.: Division of Sexually Transmitted Disease, Centers for Disease Control, U.S. Public Health Service, 1987.

Chlamydia trachomatis has been detected in 8–25 percent, *Neisseria gonorrhoeae* in 3–18 percent, *Trichomonas vaginalis* in 0–48 percent, herpes simplex virus (HSV) in 2 percent, and syphilis in 3 percent. Prevalence rates for common STD organisms among adolescent boys were not available until recently. In select populations where most of the subjects had symptoms of urethritis, *C. trachomatis* has been isolated from the urethra in approximately 30–35 percent of boys and *N. gonorrhoeae* in 12–20 percent. Among asymptomatic adolescent and young adult males screened with urethral cultures, *C. trachomatis* was found in 8–11 percent, and *N. gonorrhoeae* was isolated in 1–3 percent. Rates of human papillomavirus (HPV) infection have been difficult to obtain, since no culture method is available for detection, and HPV infection is not a reportable disease. With the use of the recent molecular genetics techniques, HPV DNA has been detected in 18 percent of San Francisco area sexually active adolescent females, and HPV has been identified in 33 percent of New York urban adolescent females. No studies have included asymptomatic males.

An indirect measure of the importance of the high prevalence rates of STDs, especially HPV, among adolescents is the increased rate of cervical intraepithelial neoplasia (CIN) among young women. The highest incidence of CIN occurs in women ages twenty to twenty-nine years old. Since HPV infection appears to be a developing event, progressive changes are probably occurring early in the adolescents' sexual life.

Adolescents currently represent less than 1 percent of all reported cases of AIDS in the United States. The number of cases is tenfold greater among people between the ages of twenty and twenty-four than among adolescents. Because of the long and unpredictable latency period of the disease (two to seven years or more), it is likely that in many cases young adults acquired the HIV infection during adolescence. Large-scale seropositivity data are available from military screening programs. The rate of sero-positivity for HIV has been reported to be 1.4 per 1,000 among screened military recruits. Rates among the 1.7 million U.S. active-duty military personnel were recently reported by the Centers for Disease Control to be 0.1 per 1,000 among seventeen- to nineteen-year-olds ($N = 322,506$) and 1.2 per 1,000 among twenty- to twenty-four-year-olds ($N = 568,920$) as of April 1988. These rates from active military personnel may be lower than the rate of sero-positivity in the civilian population for two reasons: homosexual males and IV drug abusers are underrepresented, as well as difficult to identify, in the military, and both hemophiliacs and seropositive recruits are denied entry into the military.

STD Risk Factors in Adolescents

After a review of these statistics, it becomes obvious that adolescents are at particular risk for acquisition of STD infections. A discussion of the risk factors associated with STD infections in adolescents can clarify the relationship between these high STD rates and youth.

High-Risk Behaviors

All age groups in the United States showed a decreasing trend in mortality rates between 1960 and 1980 except for the adolescent age group, which showed a rise in the mortality rate. Violent death rates among fifteen- to twenty-four-year-olds are epidemic (75 per 100,000 per year) and account for three-fourths of all deaths in this age group. High-risk behaviors such as substance abuse and early sexual debut have been found to be interrelated and may result in major health morbidities, including unplanned pregnancies and STDs. It has been shown that adolescents who use drugs (alcohol, cigarettes, marijuana, and other drugs) begin their sexual careers earlier and use contraception less effectively than their non-drug-abusing peers.

To better understand adolescent high-risk-taking behavior, Irwin and Millstein have developed an eloquent causal model and have adapted it to help explain the association between premature sexual behavior and substance use and the acquisition of STDs, including AIDS. Components of the model include the psychosocial, biological, and environmental factors that affect an adolescent's decision to engage in risk-taking behaviors. The link between drug use and sexual behavior is currently under investigation as a possible explanation for the recent marked increase in the gonorrheal rate among black adolescent males in several urban centers in the United States. This increase in infection may be associated with the onset of a crack cocaine epidemic among teenagers in the same urban areas. It is postulated that the use of crack cocaine leads to unsafe sexual practices, including multiple partners, nonuse of contraception, especially condoms, and prostitution to support cocaine use.

Gender and Age Factors

Infection rates for STDs have always differed by gender. Until recently, the male-to-female ratio for reported gonorrhea in the United States was greater than unity, but in 1973 this trend reversed, with a reported 1987 ratio of 0.62 (Figure 9.1). Several factors may be responsible for the recent change. First, it may be that, in the past, the male infection rate predominated because more men used public health facilities, and thus more were identified and reported. In contrast, young women traditionally have not frequented public STD clinics to the same extent. Second, there has been a recent decrease in gonorrhea cases among gay men compared to the adolescent female. Third, over the past two decades, young women have become sexually active at a younger age, and the rate of sexual activity for adolescent girls has risen to a rate more comparable to that for male adolescents. Fourth, adolescent females frequently have sexual intercourse with males who are two to four years or more older than themselves. The gonorrheal rate among twenty- to twenty-four-year-old males is higher than that among fifteen- to nineteen-year-old males (although it must be noted that this value does not account for differences in rates between heterosexual and homosexual males).

Changes in gonorrheal rates over time also differ by age. Between 1956 and 1975, when gonorrhea rates peaked, adolescents fifteen to nineteen years old experienced the greatest increase, with girls showing the largest change: 400 percent for girls and 240 percent for boys. More recently, between 1984 and 1987, adolescent males and females experienced the slowest decline (8 percent) in gonorrheal rates compared to all others of reproductive age. During the same three-year period, syphilis rates for fifteen- to nineteen-year-olds increased 11 percent for boys and 28 percent for girls. In addition to an increased rate of gonorrheal infection, adolescent females appear to be at greater risk for chlamydial infections and the associated morbidities of PID and ectopic pregnancy than are older cohorts. Even within the adolescent age group itself, age appears to be a factor. For example, we have shown that younger, sexually active adolescent females are significantly more likely to be infected with chlamydia than are older teenagers.

Several explanations for the age differences with infections such as chlamydia and gonococci have been postulated. It is possible that the adolescent, especially the young adolescent female, has not been immunologically challenged with STDs and therefore has a relatively "immature" urogenital immune system, with little or no local antibody prepared to respond to a repeat inoculation of an infectious agent. Histologically, the young adolescent has a larger area of "ectopy" on the exposed surface of the cervix than do older females. This "ectopy" represents columnar epithelial cells that are normally within the endocervical canal as squamous epithelial cells cover the cervical surface with increasing maturity. Chlamydia and specific phenotypes of gonococci appear to have a predilection for columnar epithelial cells. Others have postulated that the columnar epithelial cells are more accessible to culture and, therefore, that the isolation of the gonococci and chlamydia when present is more successful at younger ages. The role of behavior in placing the adolescent at risk for STD infection is unclear, since controlled studies by age and sexual behavioral history have not been done.

Ethnicity and STD Rates

Ethnicity is strongly linked to the presence of STDs and their sequelae. Epidemiological data show that black teenagers are at greatest risk for STDs. The average age-adjusted gonorrheal rate among black males aged fifteen to nineteen years is approximately fifteen times greater than that identified for their white counterparts. For black females aged fifteen to nineteen, the average age-adjusted rate for gonorrhea is ten times greater than that for their white counterparts. Black females have been shown to have higher rates of PID chlamydia, and secondary syphilis, as well as an increased relative risk of death attributable to PID and syphilis compared to white females. While black females have higher chlamydial infection rates than whites, we have found that the prevalence of chlamydial infection among Latina females (14 percent) appears to be intermediate between black females (23 percent) and whites (10 percent). Ethnicity is strongly associated with AIDS. Blacks and Latinos are overrepresented among diagnosed cases of AIDS, especially pediatric AIDS. Thus, minority youth appear to be at greatest risk for the acquisition of STDs and development of sequelae, including PID.

Contraceptives and STDs

Barrier methods, especially condoms, have been shown repeatedly in adult studies to prevent STDs, including gonococcal and chlamydial infections, and to have a role in preventing HIV infection as well. Yet contraceptive use appears inadequate, as evidenced by high pregnancy and STD rates among adolescents. Two-thirds of sexually active adolescent girls age fifteen to nineteen years use no contraceptives or ineffective contraceptives, and less than 17 percent reported using a barrier contraceptive method at last intercourse (15 percent condoms, 3 percent diaphragms). Contraceptive patterns among adolescent boys are less well defined, but available information indicates that the rate of condom use by boys is similar to that reported by girls. In a study of San Francisco youth attending three different clinics, only 13 percent of the boys reported using condoms consistently.

Among adolescents, the protective effect of barriers (mainly condoms) has not always been shown definitively. While some studies show a decreased infection rate for chlamydia among barrier users, others do not. Since it is logical to assume that condoms should afford some protection against STDs among users, these results may be best explained by the inconsistent use of barrier contraceptives by adolescents. Spermicides have also been shown to inhibit STD agents. A major component of many spermicides is non-oxynol-9, which acts as a surfactant to break down the infectious agent's cell walls. In in vitro studies, such spermicides have been shown to inhibit *N. gonorrhoeae, T. pallidum, T. vaginalis*, Candida, and herpes simplex virus I and II. More recently, nonoxynol-9 has been shown to kill HIV. While a combination of condoms or diaphragms and a spermicide seems to be the most effective protection that contraceptives can offer at this time, fewer than 10 percent of adolescents use spermicides, and fewer than a third use condoms.

The role of oral contraceptives in the establishment of an STD infection and subsequent development of PID is controversial. It has been well accepted that there is an increased incidence of candidal infections in oral contraceptive users. While many authors support the relationship between an increased risk for chlamydial cervicitis and oral contraceptive use, some do not. It has been postulated that the hormonal components of oral contraceptives may have different effects on different organisms. Progesterone inhibits the growth of *N. gonorrhoeae* while facilitating the growth of *C. trachomatis*. The estradiol component appears to enhance chlamydial growth, while its role in gonococcal growth is not clear. The role of oral contraceptives in the development of PID is discussed below.

Bacterial Infections

Sexually transmitted bacterial infections form the traditional core of venereology. Such infections have in common the advantages of convenient, definitive diagnostic laboratory tests and the availability of curative treatment regimens. The three most common infections are reviewed here: *Neisseria gonorrhoeae, Chlamydia trachomatis*, and *Treponema pallidum*.

Neisseria Gonorrhoeae

Neisseria gonorrhoeae is a gram-negative coccus. Typically, on stain of a clinical specimen, such as urethral exudate, the gonococci are seen as diplococci associated with or inside of polymorphonuclear cells.

Pathogenesis. Each gonococcus has the genetic ability to frequently change the expressed antigenic forms of surface-exposed structures that are important in the pathogenesis of infection. The following three examples illustrate how gonococci change their surface structures as if they had coats of many colors. First, pili are the hairlike appendages that extend from the gonococcal cell surface and function in the primary attachment of the gonococci to host epithelial cells. Each gonococcus has the genes for many antigenically different forms of pili and switches from one form to another with great frequency. It is these changeable antigenic forms that are seen by the human immune system. Second, another surface-exposed protein (protein II) has a secondary role in immune response. Gonococci also switch the antigenic forms of this protein with great frequency. Different protein IIs play distinct roles in the formation of certain colony types on agar and may have similar roles in the formation of microcolonies on the host's epithelial cell surfaces. A third example of a changing surface component is the gonococcal endotoxin. This lipooligosaccharide (LOS) causes damage to host epithelial cells, such as those of the fallopian tube. Gonococci have the genes for multiple antigenically different forms of LOS and frequently transform from one type to another.

By frequently altering these three surface-exposed components, the gonococcus can change its characteristics during the acute infectious process and thus evade the host immune system. Because each strain of gonococci may have surface-exposed components that differ from those of every other strain, the development of a useful gonococcal vaccine directed at surface components has become one of the most formidable challenges to current gonococcal research. In addition to its capacity for changing surface structures, the gonococci have other mechanisms to evade host defenses. For example, the gonococcus produces an enzyme, IgA1 protease, that has the capacity to split and thereby inactivate IgA1, a major mucosal secretory antibody.

Protected by its elaborate system of changing surface structures from primary host immune response, the gonococcus can establish an infectious process. After inoculation of the gonococci onto the mucosal surface, attachment is followed by microinvasion of the epithelial cells by the organism. An inflammatory reaction ensues. In the more complicated disease of pelvic inflammatory disease, gonococci must travel through the cervical opening, infect the endometrium, and ascend to the fallopian tube, where the destructive invasion of tubal epithelium occurs. Since gonococci are not motile, it has been postulated that they may be transported to the fallopian tube by sperm, retrograde menstrual flow, uterine contractions, and white cells.

Clinical Syndromes. The most common manifestation of gonococcal disease among men is urethritis. Since screening of asymptomatic men for STDs such as gonococcal infections has not yet become routine, most men with gonococcal urethritis come to the attention of the health care provider with symptoms or as a contact to a partner with a positive gonococcal infection. After inoculation with the organism during sexual activity, it is estimated that it takes from two to four days for symptoms of dysuria and/or discharge to appear. The discharge may be scant and mucoid but in most cases tends to be more purulent in nature. The efficiency of transmission of

Table 9.1. Syndrome: Urethritis.

Symptoms:	Frequency; burning; dysuria; discharge
Signs:	Discharge: spontaneous, with urethral stripping, or none; erythema; and edema at meatus
Laboratory:	Gram stain of discharge: $\geq$ 4PMNs/oil immersion field, $\pm$ gram-negative intracellular diplococci; first-catch urine (15–20 cc.) in males: urinary leukocyte esterase positive on unspun urine or $\geq$ 15 PMNs/h.p.f. on spun urine sediment
Etiology:	*N.gonorrhoeae*, *C.trachomatis*, *T.vaginalis*, *C.albicans*, HSV, HPV, other

the organism to a partner is probably gender-specific, with less efficient transmission from the female to the male: Female-to-male transmission rates have been shown to be about 25 percent after one sexual encounter, with this rate increasing with subsequent exposures; male-to-female transmission rates have been shown to be approximately 50 percent, but the studies have not controlled for number of sexual encounters. Untreated gonococcal urethritis in males usually resolves over one to two months and rarely is associated with complications such as acute epididymitis and urethral strictures.

Females experience urethral infection as well, but in conjunction with an established endocervical infection. Most gonococcal infections in women affect the lower genital tract, with a particular predilection for the columnar cells of the endocervix. The clinical syndromes associated with ascent of the infection into the upper genital tract include endometritis and acute salpingitis (PID), which may develop into tubo-ovarian abscesses. Additional syndromes that affect both men and women are pharyngitis, proctitis, and disseminated gonococcal disease (DGI). Most cases of proctitis are asymptomatic and are spread by anal contact in both sexes or by local spread from an infected endocervix in women. DGI represents a blood-borne infection commonly manifesting as skin lesions, tenosynovitis, and septic arthritis (culture-positive in approximately 50 percent of cases only) and is often associated with particular gonococci as the Arg- Hyx- Ura- auxotype.

The clinical symptoms and signs of common syndromes associated

Table 9.2. Syndrome: Vaginitis.

Symptoms:	Pruritus; dyspareunia; discharge
Signs:	Erythema; edema; tenderness; discharge
Laboratory:	Vaginal pH: $\leq$ 4.5 in *C.albicans* and $\geq$ 5.0 (bacterial vaginosis, *T.vaginalis*) Vaginal wet mounts: KOH $\rightarrow$ pseudohyphae (*C.albicans*); saline $\rightarrow$ clue cells (bacterial vaginosis), or motile trichomonads (*T.vaginalis*)
Etiology:	Anaerobes, *G.vaginalis*, *T.vaginalis*, *C.albicans*, other

Table 9.3. Syndrome: Endocervicitis.

Symptoms:	Vaginal discharge; dyspareunia; postcoital spotting
Signs:	Edema; erythema; friability; swab test (+) mucopurulent endocervical discharges
Laboratory:	Endocervical gram stain: ≥ 5 PMNs/h.p.f. and/or gram-negative intracellular diplococci
	Vaginal wet mount: saline → trichomonads
	Cultures or indirect diagnostic tests (EIA, fluorescent antibody): endocervical *N.gonorrhoeae* and *C.trachomatis*
	PAP smear: inflammation, other
Etiology:	*N.gonorrhoeae, C.trachomatis, T.vaginalis, C.albicans,* HSV, other

with gonococcal infection—urethritis, endocervicitis, endometritis, epididymitis, and proctitis—are outlined in Tables 9.1 through 9.6. Acute salpingitis (PID) is discussed in a later section.

Diagnosis. In uncomplicated cases of gonorrhea, presumptive diagnosis of infection in males is made by (1) identifying gram-negative intracellular diplococci on smear of urethral discharge, (2) isolating the organism from selective growth media from anogenital specimens, and (3) identifying gonococci with the use of an enzyme immunoassay (Gonozyme, Abbott Laboratories) from urethral specimens. In women, while positive gram-stain findings from endocervical specimens indicate probable gonococcal infection, and rapid diagnostic tests such as Gonozyme show promise, it is currently recommended that the endocervix be cultured for *N. gonorrhoeae* in most clinical settings for a definitive diagnosis.

Treatment. Treatment regimens are outlined in Table 9.7.

Chlamydia Trachomatis

Organisms belonging to the genus *Chlamydia* are ubiquitous pathogens of animals and humans. Two species are known, *C. psittaci*, which is a common pathogen of birds and domestic animals and causes zoonoses in humans, and *C. trachomatis*, a human pathogen. *C. trachomatis* inclusions were first identified in the conjunctival scrapings from orangutans inoculated with human trachoma at the beginning of the twentieth century. Soon after, these

Table 9.4. Syndrome: Endometritis.

Symptoms:	Lower abdominal pain; discharge; fever
Signs:	Cervicitis: swab test positive; uterine tenderness
Laboratory:	Endometrial sampling: spotty inflammatory changes on cytology and histology
Etiology:	*C.trachomatis, N.gonorrhoeae,* anaerobes, mycoplasmas, mixed infections

Table 9.5. Syndrome: Epididymitis.

Symptoms:	Painful scrotal swelling; dysuria; discharge
Signs:	Tender scrotal swelling (most unilateral): early course → posterior and focal; late course → involvement of teste
	Urethral discharge (+ /–)
Laboratory	Pyuria on first-catch or midstream urine
	Gram stain of urethral discharge: urethritis
	Urethral culture: *C.trachomatis*; *N.gonorrhoeae*
	Doppler or radionuclide scrotal scan: blood flow increased
Etiology:	Males <35 years old: *C.trachomatis* and *N.gonorrhoeae* most common; *T.pallidum*, *T.vaginalis*, coliforms, and pseudomonas rare isolates

inclusions were found in specimens from infants with inclusion blennorrhea and from genital specimens from their parents, leading to one of the first clinical descriptions of chlamydial-associated nongonococcal urethritis. Little advancement in the study of *C. trachomatis* occurred during the first half of the twentieth century, because it was impossible to grow it on artificial media as can be done with other microorganisms because of chlamydia's intracellular growth requirements. A laboratory breakthrough occurred in the early 1970s when a tissue culture technique was refined that allowed propagation of the organism in as little as two to three days.

Pathogenesis. The pathogenesis of *C. trachomatis* infections has not been clearly defined. Chlamydiae are obligate intracellular parasites that destroy the host cell at the end of their growth cycle. Disease is most likely a result of both the destruction of cells during the growth cycle and the body's immune response to the infection, producing inflammation.

Clinical Syndromes. Uncomplicated infections include asymptomatic and symptomatic urethritis in men and women. In men, 20 to 50 percent of men with gonococcal urethritis are also infected with chlamydia, and it is the agent responsible for 30 to 60 percent of nongonococcal urethritis. Among women who complain of dysuria and frequency without vaginitis, many will have cystitis (significant bacteriuria), and a few may be shown to have "acute

Table 9.6. Syndrome: Proctitis.

Symptoms:	Most asympomatic; mucus in stool; loose stools; cramping; anal itching; pain with defecation
Signs:	Anal inflammation; mucopurulent discharge (+ /– bloody)
	Anoscopy: mucopurulent discharge; erythema; friability; ulceration of mucosa
Laboratory:	Rectal culture: *N.gonorrhoeae*; *C.trachomatis*; HSV
	Endocervical culture: *N.gonorrhoeae*, *C.trachomatis*
	Syphilis screen: RPR/VDRL
Etiology:	*N.gonorrhoeae*, *C.trachomatis*, HSV, *T.pallidum*

Table 9.7.[a] Treatment Regimens: Gonococcal Infections.

I. Uncomplicated Urethral, Endocervical, or Rectal Gonococcal Infections
   A. Recommended Regimen[b]
      Ceftriaxone: 250 mg. IM one dose
         plus
      Doxycycline: 100 mg. PO bid × 7 days[c]
   B. Alternative Regimens
      1. When patient cannot take ceftriaxone
         Spectinomycin: 2 g. IM one dose (followed by doxycycline)
      2. Proven non-PPNG strain
         Amoxicillin: 3 g. PO with 1 g. probenecid one dose (followed by doxycycline regimen)
      3. In *pregnancy* or when patient cannot take tetracycline/doxycycline
         Erythromycin base or stearate: 500 mg. PO qid. × 7 days or
         Erythromycin ethylsuccinate: 800 mg. PO qid. × 7 days
II. Pharyngeal Gonococcal Infection Only
   A. Recommended Regimen
      Ceftriaxone: 250 mg. IM one dose
   B. Alternative Regimens
      1. When patient cannot take ceftriaxone
         Ciprofloxacin: 500 mg. PO once (repeat culture in 5–7 days since experience with this regimen is limited)
      2. In pregnancy, see *STD Treatment Guidelines*, Centers for Disease Control (CDC), 1989, Reference 35.
III. Disseminated Gonococcal Infection (DGI)
   Hospitalization is recommended for initial therapy and to evaluate for evidence of endocarditis or meningitis.
   A. Recommended Regimens
      1. Ceftriaxone: 1 g. IM or IV q 24 hours
                        or
      2. Ceftizoxime: 1 g. IV q 8 hours
                        or
      3. Cefotaxime: 1 g. IV q 8 hours
   B. Alternative Regimens
      1. Patients allergic to β-lactams
         Spectinomycin 2 g. IM q 12 hours
      2. If gonococci proven to be penicillin-sensitive, change to Ampicillin 1 g. q 6 hours (or equivalent)
   C. Recommended Treatment Course
      1. Compliant patients with an uncomplicated disease may be discharged 24–48 hours after all symptoms resolve and may complete the *total* of one week of antibiotic therapy with:
         a. Cefuroxime axetil 500 mg. bid or
         b. Amoxicillin 500 mg. with clavulanic acid or
         c. Ciprofoxacin 500 mg. bid *if not pregnant*
IV. Adult Gonococcal Opthalmia (nonsepticemic)
   A. Recommended Regimen
      1. Ceftriaxone 1 g. IM one dose
   B. Recommended Adjunct Management
      1. Irrigation of eyes, opthalmology consultation, and evaluation for concurrent chlamydial infection
V. Treatment of Other Syndromes, Follow-up, and Partner Management
      1. Evaluation and/or treatment for concurrent chlamydial infections should be done.
      2. Treatment regimens for other conditions including meningitis and endocarditis, as well as treatment of infants and children, is described elsewhere (*STD Treatment Guidelines*, CDC, 1989).
      3. Partners within the last 30 days should be contacted, evaluated for both gonococcal and chlamydial disease, and treated. Condoms should be used.

Table 9.7.[a] Treatment Regimens: Gonococcal Infections (Cont'd).

4. Follow-up of patients should occur 4–7 days after treatment and definitive diagnostic tests should be done when possible to assess success of cure. Encourage safe sexual practices, including condom use.
5. All patients with gonorrhea should be tested for syphilis.
6. Treatment for PID is outlined in Table 9.14.
VI. *Epididymitis* (*N.gonorrhoeae* or *C.trachomatis* most likely cause in heterosexual male < 35 years)
   A. Recommended Regimens
      1. Ceftriaxone 250 mg. IM one dose
            and
         Doxycycline 100 PO IM bid. × 10 days
            or
      2. Tetracycline 500 mg. PO qid × 10 days

   [a] Other alternative regimens in pregnancy are outlined in *STD Treatment Guidelines*, CDC, 1989.
   [b] Most patients with incubating syphilis (seronegative and no signs) may be cured by any regimen containing β-lactams (for example, ceftriaxone) or tetracycline.
   [c] Tetracycline alone is no longer considered adequate therapy for gonococcal infections but is added for treatment of coexisting chlamydial infection.

urethral syndrome" ("sterile" pyuria). This latter syndrome is also associated with gonococcal, staphylococcal, and coliform infections, while in some cases no etiology is apparent. In addition, chlamydia is associated with mucopurulent endocervicitis in women, as well as proctitis and conjunctivitis in both men and women. It has been well documented that 60 to 70 percent of infants born to mothers with chlamydia in their genital tracts at delivery will themselves be infected with chlamydia, including conjunctivitis (30 percent) and/or pneumonia (20 percent). Like *N. gonorrhoeae*, chlamydia has been shown to cause biopsy-proven endometritis, including postpartum endometritis, and is a major etiological agent for PID, especially in the adolescent female.

Diagnosis. In uncomplicated cases of lower genital tract infection, *C. trachomatis* is considered to be the principal pathogen. In men, a diagnosis of nongonococcal urethritis (NGU) is considered in the presence of a negative gonorrheal culture and/or a gram-stained smear from the urethra showing four or more polymorphonuclear leucocytes (PMNs) per oil immersion field with no evidence of gram-negative intracellular diplococci. Men with NGU may also present with the typical symptoms of urethritis, including discharge and dysuria, or may be identified only by a positive history of contact with a chlamydia-positive partner. Asymptomatic males are presumed to be infected with chlamydia if they have any of the NGU criteria and lack only the typical urethral symptoms.

Approximately 50 percent or more of chlamydial lower genital infections among women are asymptomatic. An uncomplicated chlamydial endocervicitis is presumed with or without symptoms of a lower genital tract infection if the following clinical signs are present on pelvic examination:

(1) mucopurulent endocervical discharge on a white swab (swab test positive) and/or (2) ten or more PMNs per high-power field on gram-stained specimen from the endocervix that is not vaginal contaminant and/or (3) endocervical friability (bleeding from endocervical tissue after contact with one swab). Since *N. gonorrhoeae* infection as well as such STD organisms as *Candida albicans* and *Trichomonas vaginalis* can also produce cervicitis, it is recommended to screen for alternative causes at the time of the pelvic examination and to perform a definitive diagnostic test for endocervical chlamydia when available. When a diagnosis of endometritis or PID is made, chlamydia and the gonococcus must be presumed as leading causes of PID in the adolescent female. Again, an attempt to perform definitive diagnostic tests to determine etiology should be performed on the patient and her partner(s) when possible.

The laboratory "gold standard" for the clinical diagnosis of chlamydial infection remains the inoculation of material from a clinical specimen and identification of chlamydial inclusions on cell culture lines when stained by Giemsa or iodine or with a fluorescent antibody technique. Because of the expense, the length of time for incubation (three to seven days), and the lack of availability in many clinical settings, there has been a great deal of energy devoted to the development and refinement of the rapid diagnostic techniques. The two main tests in use currently are a direct immunofluorescent antibody test, MicroTrak (Syva, Palo Alto, California), and an enzyme immunoassay, Chlamydiazyme (Abbott Laboratories, North Chicago, Illinois). Recent studies show that the performance profiles (specificity, sensitivity, predictive values negative and positive) of the two rapid tests are similar. The sensitivity and specificity for MicroTrak ranged from 70 to 100 percent and from 85 to 100 percent, respectively. The Chlamydiazyme profile was similar. The lower sensitivity values of 70 percent reflect the performance for both the MicroTrak and the Chlamydiazyme tests in male urethral specimens. When they were studied, it was reported that the performance of the tests is independent of the presence or absence of clinical signs of infection. In low-prevalence populations of women, the sensitivity of rapid chlamydial tests may be as low as 70 percent as well. From these data, it appears that the rapid diagnostic tests can be used in specimens from the endocervix but that these rapid diagnostic tests require more evaluation before they are used as definitive diagnostic tools in men and in low-chlamydial-prevalence populations of women. Clinical syndromes produced by *C. trachomatis* parallel those caused by *N. gonorrhoeae* and are reviewed in Tables 9.1 through 9.6 and 9.13.

Treatment. Treatment regimens are outlined in Table 9.8.

Treponema Pallidum

Treponema pallidum is a member of the order of Spirochaetales. The small size of *T. pallidum* renders it below the resolution of light microscopy,

Table 9.8. Treatment Regimens: *Chlamydia Trachomatis*.

Uncomplicated Urethral, Endocervical, or Rectal Infection
A. Recommended Regimens
   1. Doxycycline 100 mg. PO b.i.d. × 7 days
              or
   2. Tetracycline 500 mg. PO q.i.d. × 7 days (may have decreased compliance because of q.i.d.protocol)
B. Alternative Regimens
   1. Erythromycin base or stearate: 500 mg. PO q.i.d. × 7 days
              or
      Erythromycin ethylsuccinate: 800 mg. PO q.i.d. × 7 days
   2. Additional alternative when erythromycin not tolerated
      Sulfisoxazole: 500 mg. PO q.i.d. × 10 days
   3. In *pregnancy*
      Erythromycin base or erythromycin ethylsuccinate in doses stated in B-1 above
C. Partner Management
    If sexual contact within 30 days of onset of symptoms, partners should be tested and treated or treated when testing is not available.
D. Treatment regimens for acute epididymitis are found in Table 9.5.
E. Treatment regimens for PID are described in Table 9.14.

Source: Adapted from 0445, *STD Treatment Guidelines, 1989.*

and therefore dark-field microscopy is required for identification of the organism in a specimen from a moist lesion. As with chlamydia, the study of *T. pallidum* prior to the 1970s was greatly restricted by the lack of an in vitro technique for growth. Syphilis is becoming of interest to clinicians caring for the adolescent, as the prevalence of primary and secondary syphilis doubled among fifteen- to nineteen-year-old females between 1975 and 1987 (see Figure 9.2).

Pathogenesis. From human and animal studies of the natural history of the disease, it appears that the organism gains entry through the epithelial layer of tissue through small abrasions in the skin during sexual activity. It has been estimated that transmission of the organism occurs in about one-third of people who have sexual intercourse with an infected partner. A local immune response occurs at the site of entry, resulting in the formation of a chancre. Shortly after entry, it is spread hematogenously and replicates at peripheral sites, resulting in the characteristic lesions of secondary disease.

Clinical Syndromes. Primary Syphilis. Approximately three weeks after inoculation (range of ten to ninety days), an ulceration at the site of infection develops that is painless and has a raised, firm border. The ulcer evolves from a macule to a papule, which then erodes to form the ulcerative chancre. The chancre may become painful if a secondary bacterial infection develops. This chancre is frequently missed, because the site of inoculation may be the vagina, cervix, or rectum. Local adenopathy is common at this stage. Chancres frequently occur in the glans penis, the coronal sulcus, and the shaft in the male and the vulva, labia, and cervix in the female. Some authors estimate that these classical lesions in genital sites occur in only half of the cases. Atypical presentations include multiple chancres in genital and extra-genital sites. Extragenital sites include the perianal area, mouth, tongue, tonsils, lips, breasts, axilla, and fingers, among others. Untreated primary chancres usually resolve spontaneously in two to eight weeks. The differential diagnoses of ulcers resembling chancres include herpes simplex virus, staphylococcus, streptococcus, and trauma. Rare causes of ulcers include LGV, chancroid, and Donovanosis. To establish a correct diagnosis, these etiologies must be considered along with syphilis.

Clinical Syndromes. Secondary Syphilis. The hallmark of this stage of syphilis is the generalized skin rash on the face, trunk, genitalia, and extremities, especially involving the palms and soles, which often appears six weeks after the onset of the primary chancre if untreated. Other skin manifestations include mucous patches of the mouth and tongue, condyloma lata, and patchy alopecia, or "moth-eaten" hair loss. Common systemic signs of disease include generalized lymphadenopathy, fever, arthralgias, and myalgias. More rarely, other organ systems show disease, including the liver (hepatitis), kidney (nephrotic syndrome), and CNS (aseptic meningitis). Primary and secondary syphilis are considered highly infectious stages.

Clinical Syndromes. Early Latent or Late Latent Syphilis. These stages are not discussed in depth here, since they occur rarely in adolescents. Early latent syphilis is characterized by (1) duration of less than one year, (2) asymptomatic presentation, (3) occurrence in the presence or absence of a history of primary and/or secondary syphilis, (4) current positive Venereal Disease Research Laboratory (VDRL) or Rapid Plasma Reagin (RPR) test or a significant rise in serology titer, and (5) a positive confirmation with a direct treponeme test such as the fluorescent treponeme antibody absorption test (FTA-ABS). Late latent syphilis is characterized by a duration of greater than a year, is asymptomatic, and has a positive serology with VDRL or RPR and FTA-ABS as well. Tertiary syphilis, or neurosyphilis, occurs years to decades after acquisition and is therefore out of the sphere of this discussion. It is characterized by the presence of central and focal neurological signs and cardiovascular disease, such as aortic aneurysm and gummas.

Diagnosis. The definitive diagnosis of primary syphilis is made through observation by an experienced dark-field microscopist of viable treponema obtained from a fresh specimen of a chancre. However, when this technique is unavailable, the client should be evaluated as described below for secondary disease. The diagnosis of secondary syphilis is usually determined by the presence of the typical clinical signs (especially of the skin) and a positive nontreponemal serology for syphilis or a fourfold titer rise in the serology between serial tests. All positive nontreponeme tests must be confirmed with treponeme tests such as the FTA-ABS and MHA-TP (microhemagglutation test — *Treponema pallidum*), which are more specific. If a diagnosis of primary syphilis is considered with a lesion consistent with a chancre, and the screening nontreponeme test is negative, it may be necessary to repeat the nontreponeme test every two weeks until a definitive diagnosis is made and/or to perform serial dark-field examinations.

Serum nontreponeme tests commonly employed include the VDRL and the RPR. Both test for the presence of "reagin," which is a complex of antibodies that join with cardiolipin antigen to produce a positive test. These nontreponeme tests are in wide use because they are inexpensive and easy to perform. Nontreponeme tests have a sensitivity (percentage of clients with the disease who have a positive test) of 50 to 70 percent during primary syphilis, which rises to 100 percent in secondary syphilis. The nontreponeme tests can be quantified and titers of the same test can be followed to evaluate response to treatment (RPR and VDRL titers are not interchangeable and therefore not directly comparable). False-positive nontreponeme tests can occur in the presence of a febrile illness, after immunization, and with immune diseases and can be evaluated with a direct treponeme test. Within two years of appropriate treatment, most nontreponeme tests resolve after both primary (97 percent) and secondary (76 percent) stages of the disease.

We do not routinely screen all sexually active adolescents for syphilis in our teen clinics. Screening adolescents for syphilis is recommended if the index of suspicion for syphilis is sufficient. Criteria suggested include: (1) a diagnosis of one or more STDs, (2) a history of contact with any STD, including syphilis, (3) the presence of clinical symptoms and signs consistent with syphilis, (4) sexual behavior that places the client at high risk for acquisition of STDs, including syphilis (prostitutes, people with multiple partners, and homosexuals, among others), and (5) a client's being a member of a population that has been shown to be at particularly high risk epidemiologically for syphilis.

Treatment. For primary and secondary syphilis, the treatment consists of one of the following regimens: (1) benzathine penicillin G 2.4 million units IM at one dose or, for the penicillin-allergic client, (2) tetracycline 500 milligrams PO qid for fifteen days. In pregnant women, erythromycin is no longer considered adequate therapy because of its high failure rate. The pregnant penicillin-allergic woman who elects to continue her pregnancy must be hospitalized, desensitized to penicillin, and then treated with penicillin under expert care. All pregnant women with syphilis must be closely followed after treatment with a monthly RPR or VDRL. Infants born to such infected women should be evaluated and should have a treatment plan devised in consultation with a medical expert such as a pediatrician and/or an officer in the local public health department. The treatment for latent and tertiary syphilis is beyond the scope of this text; it is discussed in local public health clinic guidelines and recommendations from the Centers for Disease Control (CDC).

Protozoan and Fungal Infections

While protozoan and fungal infections are ubiquitous and known to cause sexually transmitted infections in man, their importance has increased among STDs, paralleling the rise of HIV infections and their associated immunodeficiency diseases. *Candida albicans* and *Trichomonas vaginalis* will be discussed here. A complete discussion of related infections among homosexual men is beyond the scope of this chapter.

Candida Albicans

The acceptance of *Candida albicans* as a genitourinary pathogen has varied since 1849, when Wilkinson first described the association in women between the presence of yeast in the genital tract and a profuse vaginal discharge. By the turn of the century, *C. albicans* was considered "normal flora" in women. But in 1931, *C. albicans* as a pathogen was "rediscovered." *C. albicans* has a worldwide distribution and is isolated from the mucosal tissues of warm-blooded animals, including humans. There are about 500 species of yeast, many have been isolated from humans, and approximately 90 percent of human isolates are pathogenic. Fifty percent of human yeast infections are genital. Among pathogenic species in humans, *C. albicans* is by far the most common (72 percent), with *C. glabrata* (torulopsis) infecting 10 percent and a variety of other species responsible for the remaining 18 percent of infections. Except for *C. albicans* and *C. glabrata*, pathogenic candidas originate from nonhuman sources. From a number of studies, it is estimated that *C. albicans* is isolated from body sites in the following frequencies: skin, 0.1 to 2 percent; oral cavity, 6 to 62 percent; feces, 15 to 70 percent; and vagina, 2 to 40 percent. *C. albicans* has also been isolated from inanimate objects, fomites, and hospital air, among other sites. Two serotypes of *C. albicans* have been described, A and B, which differ in their global geographical distribution and may differ in degree of pathogenicity in humans.

Until recently, it has been difficult to define the epidemiology of *C. albicans* infections because of the lack of an appropriate method to differentiate strains. Three methods for separation have been developed: the "resistogram," which measures differences in resistance to a panel of six preselected chemicals; biochemical characteristics, which differentiate strains by their reaction to exposure to specific biochemical tests; and killer toxin factors, which differentiate by their pattern of killing specific genera of yeasts. Using the "resistogram" technique, Warnock and co-workers have isolated the same strain of *C. albicans* from the lower genital tract of women with candidal vulvovaginitis and the intestines and genitals of their male consorts. In addition to this work, others have described evidence from studies in both men and women that supports the sexual transmissibility of *C. albicans*. Although sexual transmissibility of *C. albicans* occurs, its importance to the overall infection rate among sexually active women is unclear. We found no significant differences in the isolation rate of *C. albicans* between virginal and sexually active adolescent girls. Other researchers have found similar isolation rates for yeasts in clients of an STD clinic and those attending a non-STD-clinic site.

Pathogenesis. The exact mechanism of the pathogenesis of candida has not been delineated. An association between the presence of symptomatic disease and the pseudohyphae form of candida has been shown. Unlike the case with bacterial vaginosis, the presence or degree of vaginal symptoms does not appear to be related to the number of organisms present. The pathogenicity of the organism seems to depend on the degree of candidal adherence to epithelial cells and host factors, especially immune status. *C. albicans*, for example, has been shown to be more adherent than less pathogenic types of yeast. Many newborns are colonized with candida from their mothers' genital tracts during the birth process. Nonpregnant adults have developed delayed hypersensitivity reactions to candidal antigens, and testing for this hypersensitivity reaction is a common screening device for immune status. Immunocompromised patients, including AIDS patients, are known to be vulnerable to disseminated and mucocutaneous candidiasis. Other host factors appear to play a role in the development of candidal infections. Pregnancy, oral contraceptive use, and diabetes mellitus appear to increase the risk for candidal infections. It has been postulated that the increased glycogen stores found in these conditions in some way enhance the growth of yeast or have a negative impact on cellular immunity.

Clinical Syndromes. Vulvovaginitis is the most common syndrome of candidiasis in women. The classical presentation includes complaints of a discharge without odor, external dysuria, and intense pruritus. On examination, the vulva may appear normal, may have mild erythema, or may be markedly swollen with evidence of excoriations. On vaginal inspection, an abnormal discharge characterized by increased amount and a creamy or curdlike appearance with no odor may or may not be present. Plaques of adherent discharge on the vaginal walls may be noted, and marked erythema and edema can be seen on both the vaginal mucosa and the exocervix. In males, an inflammation of the glans penis, balanitis, is associated with infection with *C. albicans*. Inflammation of the prepuce has also been described. Dysuria may be the presenting complaint.

Diagnosis. In women, the presumptive diagnosis is made in the presence of the classical symptoms of candidal vaginitis and confirmed with the identification of candidal forms (pseudohyphae and/or blastospores) by microscopic examination. Specimens are obtained from the lateral vaginal walls and from the vulva (as indicated) with a swab or plastic spatula and placed on a glass slide. The specimen is then examined by either the gram stain or the wet-mount technique, which includes the addition and mixing of a few drops of 10 percent KOH or saline with the slide specimen. Specimens obtained from infected male sites are processed in the same manner. The gram and wet-mount techniques are capable of confirming the diagnosis of *C. albicans* infections in only 40 percent of cases. Definitive diagnosis is made by direct culture technique using Stuart's, Sabouraud, or Nickerson media. Culture may be helpful in cases of wet-mount or gram-stain-negative vaginitis where other etiologies have been eliminated as the cause and in cases of treatment failures where clear definition of the organism is warranted. Papanicolaou smears and serology have not proved helpful in the diagnosis of acute infections.

Treatment. The imidazole derivatives have been shown to have cure rates of more than 90 percent with the use of two 100 mg. vaginal tablets for three or six nights. Unanswered questions regarding candidal infections include the following: Should asymptomatic carriers be treated? Why do some individuals live in apparent harmony with yeast while others have recurrent symptoms? What are the host and environmental factors that encourage the transformation of yeast infection from a symbiotic relationship to a pathogenic one? These questions need to be addressed in order to develop effective preventive strategies with yeast.

Trichomonas Vaginalis

Trichomonads are flagellated protozoans with three species linked to disease in humans: *Trichomonas tenax* (mouth), *Pentatrichomonas hominis* (intestine), and *Trichomonas vaginalis* (genital organs of men and women). Because of their geographical specificity, these species are rarely if ever isolated from other anatomic areas. *T. vaginalis* has been shown to be sexually transmitted, is rare or absent in female virgins, and occurs in from none to 25 percent or more of the women tested. *T. vaginalis* has been noted in 4 percent of men attending an STD clinic and in 5 to 15 percent of men with NGU.

Pathogenesis. The pathogenesis of this disease in humans is not completely understood. *T. vaginalis* is known to attach to epithelial cells. The response to infection varies from little or no reaction (carrier state) to a marked acute inflammatory response characterized by the presence of numerous PMNs. It is known that half of the asymptomatic carriers of *T. vaginalis* will become symptomatic within six months. The mechanisms that cause the development of clinically recognizable disease, determine the degree of inflammatory reaction, and encourage the change from the carrier state to the symptomatic disease state are unknown but are most likely dependent on both host and environmental factors. Development of disease appears to be related to the menstrual period, to pubertal development, to pH, to the environmental microbiological flora, and to gender. For example, most men who are consorts of infected women are asymptomatic, and their disease is self-limited. Among prepubertal girls, the *T. vaginalis* is found in the urine and not typically in the immature vaginal mucosa. *T. vaginalis* does not appear to cause acute salpingitis, as only one case of *T. vaginalis* isolation from an inflamed fallopian tube has been reported. While serum antibodies to *T. vaginalis* can be measured, the presence of such antibodies does not seem related to the presence of an acute infection. While the organism requires the human as host, it apparently can live for short periods of time outside the host, as it has been isolated from contaminated tap water, toilet bowls, and toilet water.

Clinical Syndromes. Since the target tissues for *T. vaginalis* infection in humans are so specific, the syndromes associated with the organism are very limited; they include vaginitis and cervicitis in women and urethritis in both men and women. In women, genitourinary symptoms include vaginal discharge, dyspareunia pruritus, lower abdominal pain, and symptoms of urethritis including dysuria and frequency. On examination, the vulva is often erythematous, and vaginal discharge may be present externally. On speculum examination, the walls appear granular in more than half the cases. While a discharge is common, the "classical" frothy yellow-green discharge occurs in only 12 percent and has been described in other vaginitis as well. The "strawberry cervix" (punctate hemorrhages on the exocervix), which is pathognomonic for *T. vaginalis* cervicitis, occurs in only 2 percent of the infections. In men, the infection is usually self-limited, and most men are asymptomatic or present with the symptoms and signs of NGU. Infrequently, epididymitis or proctitis may develop.

Diagnosis. The clinical diagnosis is presumed in the presence of vulvovaginal symptoms, a vaginal pH of $\geq$ 5.0, and the organisms identified on wet mount, Pap cytology, or direct culture. The ability to detect the organism is dependent on the number of organisms present in the inoculum for both wet mount and culture and the ability to maintain the specimen at body temperature and examine the wet mount immediately to preserve the motility of the organism. Even under the most controlled research clinical settings, the wet mount and Pap smear detect only about 60 percent of infections, with the Pap smear having the added disadvantage of a 31 percent false-positive rate. Culture techniques such as Diamond's media detect from 82 to 95 percent of infections. In a study comparing the wet mount, Pap smear, direct culture, and direct monoclonal antibody technique, the rapid immunofluorescent diagnostic technique was comparable to the two- to seven-day culture method and superior to both the wet mount and cytology techniques.

Treatment. The treatment for uncomplicated genital infections in both men and nonpregnant women is 2.0 gm. PO metronidazole. Both multiple-day and one-day regimens have a cure rate of 90 percent, but the one-dose regimen, because of better compliance, is the treatment of choice for the adolescent. In the young woman who is pregnant or where pregnancy is possible (last menstrual period not documented, rapid pregnancy test unavailable, history of unprotected intercourse), it is recommended to use the low-cure-rate regimen of clotrimazole, 100 mg. tablets or one applicator of vaginal cream at bedtime for seven nights.

Viral Infections

Viral infections share common properties as STDs. They are probably the most common STDs (especially human papillomavirus), they are long-term infections, no curative medications are available for treatment, and they are linked to the development of carcinomas in the reproductive tract—especially the cervix in the female. Herpes simplex virus and human papillomavirus will be discussed here. A complete discussion of the human immunodeficiency virus is beyond the scope of this chapter.

Herpes Simplex Virus

Herpes simplex virus (HSV) is a linear double-stranded DNA virus with an approximate molecular weight of 100×10^6 known to encode more than seventy gene products. The viral genome is enclosed in an icosahedral capsid with 162 capsomeres, and its outer layer is a lipid-containing envelope derived from a modified host cell membrane. This outer envelope is acquired from the host as the DNA-containing capsid "buds" through the host cell nuclear membrane. The virus modifies the membrane by embedding glycoproteins later used for host cell attachment. Two types of HSV have been described on the basis of differences in DNA content with approximately 50 percent DNA homology conserved between the two types. Despite this difference, both HSV 1 and HSV 2 cause a similar spectrum of clinical disease in genital HSV infection.

Pathogenesis. The virus appears to enter the human host through either mucosal surfaces or abraded squamous epithelium. After attachment to host cells within the epidermis and dermis, fusion occurs between the host cell membrane and viral envelopes, resulting in intracellular release of viral DNA. The viral DNA advances into the host nucleus, where expression of viral genes occurs in a regulated fashion, resulting in 50,000 to 200,000 virions per cell. The replicated viral genomes and the newly synthesized structural proteins are assembled into "nucleocapsids." Envelopment (formation of outer membrane) occurs as the nucleocapsids "bud" through the inner nuclear membrane into the perinuclear space. These infectious virions are then transported through the endoplasmic reticulum and the Golgi apparatus to the cell surface, where they are released to then infect sensor and autonomic nerve endings.

The virus is thought to migrate by several mechanisms: centripetal spread within the nerve axion from the distal site of infection to the nerve cell body; centrifugal spread from sensory nerve bodies along the axon to multiple surface sites, resulting in the multiple clinical lesions that may occur during a primary or recurrent infection; and contiguous spread to neighboring nerve cells. After resolution of primary disease, latency occurs. The mechanism involved in latency is unknown, but it involves HSV infection without detectable replication of the virus. The control of this dormant state and the reactivation mechanism are not well understood. Reactivation involves viral replication and migration, resulting in appearance of clinical disease.

The host's immune response to HSV infection affects the severity of disease and both latency and frequency of recurrences. Both humoral and

Table 9.9. Clinical Course of Primary HSV.

Event (Days)[a]	Days from Onset of First Symptom[a]	Duration
Incubation	–6	7
Systemic symptoms	0	4 to 7
Lesions		
Vesicle	0	6
Open ulcer	6	6
Crusted ulcer	12	8
Total	—	20
Viral shedding	0	12

[a] Mean days: 0 = day of first symptom; negative refers to number of days prior to onset of first symptom; positive refers to number of days after the onset of first symptom.

cell-mediated immunity appear important, although their specific roles need to be defined. Prior HSV 1 may offer some protection against HSV 2 acquisition, and most appear to attenuate clinical symptoms.

Clinical Syndromes. In primary genital herpes, both HSV 1 and HSV 2 are associated with genital infections, with HSV 2 linked to 85 percent of primary genital disease. Many individuals with serological evidence of a past HSV 1 or 2 infection have no history of clinical symptoms associated with a primary infection. Thus, some HSV infections may not be clinically apparent. The clinical course for primary genital infection is outlined in Table 9.9. The incubation period for primary herpes ranges from one to twenty-six days (mean six days). Forty percent of men and 70 percent of women with primary HSV infection will experience systemic symptoms, including fever, headache, malaise, and myalgias, for four to seven days. Localized symptoms include pain or itching, dysuria, vaginal and urethral discharge, and tender inguinal adenopathy. Within one to two days, the painful primary lesions appear anywhere within the anogenital tract and anal region where contact has occurred. Primary sites for infection are the vulva, vagina, and penis. More than 90 percent of women with primary HSV infection will have viral shedding from the cervix in the presence of vulvar and vaginal lesions. HSV cervicitis may present as visible ulcers or mucopurulent cervicitis or may be clinically undetectable. Women appear to have a longer duration and more severe symptoms than men. HSV proctitis has been increasingly recognized in those who practice anal intercourse. (Symptoms of proctitis are outlined in Table 9.6.)

Lesions and symptoms of primary infection usually resolve within twenty to twenty-six days of onset. Tender adenopathy appears in the second week of clinical disease and is the last symptom to resolve. Viral shedding from lesions can be detected for about twelve days, which parallels the mean time for the appearance of crusting lesions. However, virus can be detected in some up to the time of complete healing or re-epithelialization of ulcers. A history of prior HSV 1 infection appears to ameliorate symptoms in primary

HSV 2 genital infection. Complications of primary HSV infection include aseptic meningitis, autonomic nerve dysfunction (constipation, urinary retention, and sacral anesthesia), transverse myelitis, pharyngitis, development of extragenital lesions, vaginal superinfection, and in some cases disseminated HSV infection. Dissemination, which is often fatal, occurs predominantly in immunocompromised hosts.

Eighty percent of those with primary genital HSV 2 infection will have clinical recurrences within the first twelve months, compared to 55 percent of those with primary HSV 1 genital infection. Frequency of genital recurrences each year differs by viral type: HSV 2 recurs 2.6 times where HSV 1 recurs 1 time. Forty to 50 percent of patients with recurrent lesions will have prodromal constitutional symptoms, and the mean duration of viral shedding from lesions is four days, with complete re-epithelialization in about ten days. Only 12 percent of women with recurrent HSV will have cervical shedding. While complications are rare in recurrent disease, transmission to partner and infant is possible. Although viral shedding from asymptomatic patients has been documented, symptomatic clients shed virions in numbers from 100 to 1,000 times greater and, therefore, may more efficiently transmit infection than their asymptomatic counterparts.

Diagnosis. The diagnosis of genital HSV infection is often based on presentation of clinical symptoms and signs, not on a definitive diagnostic test. Because of the potential psychological and biological impact, documentation of HSV infection by diagnostic tests should be made when possible. Standard tests employ identification of HSV cytopathic changes in commercially available cell culture systems that can provide a method for typing the virus as well. These changes are detectable in as little as twenty-four hours when immunofluorescent antibody is combined with the cell culture technique. Under current study are newer monoclonal antibody and DNA hybridization methods that may prove to be sensitive and rapid in viral detection. Current tests are not capable of detecting the presence of virus late in the disease course. While serology is not helpful in determining acute infection, it may be useful to identify past infection.

Treatment. Oral acyclovir has been shown to help both alleviate and shorten the duration of symptoms from primary HSV infection. The current schedule is outlined in Table 9.10. Oral acyclovir may have some benefits for recurrent episodes. Currently, routine use of acyclovir for recurrent episodes is not recommended. Suppression of recurrent HSV infections has been successful using long-term (six months) oral acyclovir. However, the recurrence rate returns to the pretherapy rate after discontinuation of acyclovir. Although long-term daily administration of oral acyclovir appears to be safe, further information is needed on its toxicity, its effect on the emergence of resistant strains, and its effect in blocking transmission of infection to a partner. Thus, long-term therapy should be considered in selective compliant patients with disabling frequent recurrences.

Table 9.10. Treatment Regimens: HSV.

Primary:
Oral acyclovir 200 mg. 5 times a day for 10 days.
Recurrent HSV:
Currently, oral acyclovir is not recommended for all episodes. Some may benefit if recurrences are especially painful or frequent.
Suppression of recurrences:
Daily oral acylovir 200 mg. 3 times a day for 6 months. Recurrences after discontinuation usually occur.

Human Papillomavirus

Human papillomavirus (HPV), a member of the Papovavirus family, is a closed, circular double-stranded DNA virus. The viral genome is enclosed in an icosahedral capsule, composed of several protein capsomeres. A distinguishing feature is the lack of a lipid-containing envelope seen in many other viruses, such as herpes simplex. Because of the variety of papillomavirus occurring in a wide species of vertebrate animals, it is possible to study HPV in an animal model to assist in understanding human disease.

The common clinical presentation of HPV is in the form of genital warts or external condyloma acuminatum. While warts were described as early as A.D. 500, it was not until 1907 that the viral etiology of skin warts was established. In 1930, the Shope (cottontail rabbit) papillomavirus was the first oncogenic DNA virus to be isolated and characterized, leading to the association between HPV and human cancers. For years, the lack of an in vitro culture technique has hampered HPV research. However, with the advent of recent DNA techniques, it has been possible to link HPV, genital warts, and genital cancer. These new molecular genetic techniques have also permitted the subclassification of HPV into more than sixty types on the basis of differences in degree of DNA homology. Common skin warts are associated with types 2 and 4, whereas benign genital condyloma are usually associated with HPV types 6 and 11. In contrast, anogenital neoplasias are commonly associated with types 16, 18, 31, 33, and 35.

Pathogenesis. The exact mechanisms of HPV infection are not well understood. HPV appears to require direct access to basal epithelial cells. For the establishment of infection, active cell division is required. In vivo human sites where basal cells not only are physically accessible to viral inoculation but also are actively dividing include the active squamous metaplasia of the transformation zone of the female cervix and areas of genital wound healing of columnar tissue. Such wounds may be related to other STD infections, such as *C. trachomatis* or HSV. Present epidemiological and microbiological evidence has associated HPV with anogenital cancers. The natural progression to cancer, however, is even less understood than infection. It may be that cells infected with virus lie relatively dormant until active viral replication is activated by some unrecognized stimulus. In addition, it has been postulated that cofactors are necessary for the progression to neoplasia. Cofactors that may have a role in the neoplastic process include HSV, *C. trachomatis*, other sexually transmitted agents, hormonal influences, and immunological responses to infection or injury.

Clinical Syndromes. HPV is a sexually transmitted organism capable of causing multicentric disease within the anogenital area. In women, this includes the vulva, vagina, cervix, perineum, and anus. In men, genital warts are usually localized to the penis, including the prepuce, frenulum, corona, glans, and shaft. The anus and the scrotum may be involved as well. Common genital warts, condyloma acuminatum, seen on the skin surfaces present as a polypoid mass with a fissured and irregular surface. These warts are often multiple and polymorphic and will commonly coalesce into large masses. Condyloma acuminatum on mucosal surfaces appear as fingerlike projections with central dilated capillary loops.

Recently, a new clinical-histological type of flat condyloma, "condyloma planum," has been described. In contrast to the condyloma acuminatum, these lesions are invisible to the naked eye and are noted only at colposcopy. These flat condyloma may occur anywhere and at multiple sites within the anogenital tract. These lesions are often difficult to distinguish colposcopically from higher-grade neoplasias.

Diagnosis. The diagnosis of condyloma acuminatum frequently is based on gross visual clinical inspection of the anogenital area. Because of the subclinical nature of the flat condyloma (invisibility to the unaided eye), other methods for diagnosis of such lesions are required. In some, cytology has been the most common method to identify women with disease. Detection of the "koilocyte" on Pap smear examination has been associated with the presence of HPV. However, the presence of the "koilocyte" does not confirm HPV-related disease. The next step in the diagnosis of HPV is the colposcopic examination. With the aid of acetic acid and magnification, flat condylomas appear as discrete flat or slightly raised white epithelia with or without granular surfaces. Specific colposcopic appearances of HPV lesions include vessel patterns described as coarse punctuation or mosaic patterns. Other colposcopic patterns of HPV include the spiked condyloma, florid condyloma acuminatum, cerebriform condyloma, and condylomatous cervicitis or micropapillary formations. It must be emphasized that the flat condylomatous lesions cannot always be distinguished from neoplasias even on colposcopy, and this technique should be used to direct biopsy, not to confirm the diagnosis of HPV infection. The diagnosis usually is confirmed by the histopathological changes consistent with HPV infection. Many researchers firmly believe that HPV infection is a continuum of a neoplastic process and that its condylomatous lesions are simply very-low-grade neoplasias.

In men with HPV infection, similar colposcopic findings have been

Table 9.11. Treatment Regimens: HPV.

---

1. *Condyloma acuminatum*
   A. *Antimitotics*
      Podophyllin[a,b] 25% resin
   B. *Ablative*
      Trichloroacetic acid (TCA) 80%[a,c]
      Liquid N_2[a,c]
      Cryotherapy
      Laser
   C. *Antimetabolites*
      5-fluorouracil (5-FU)[d]
      Interferon
2. *Flat condyloma*[e]
   A. Cyrotherapy: Best for localized lesions on the cervix
   B. Laser: Best for multicentric disease and large areas of involvement
   C. TCA: Good for small localized lesions on penis, vulva, or vagina
   D. 5-fluorouracil (5-FU):[d] Appears excellent for extensive vaginal, vulvar, and penile disease

---

[a] Therapy is based on weekly application for up to four to six weeks. If no improvement, alternative therapy, such as laser, may be required.
[b] Should not be used on mucosal surfaces or in pregnancy.
[c] May be used in conjunction with podophyllin.
[d] Not FDA approved.
[e] Regimens efficacious by type of lesion.

found that are similar to those described in women. With acetic acid and magnification, flat lesions can be detected in men as well, especially in those men who are known contacts to women with either genital condyloma or genital neoplasia. Again, diagnosis always should be confirmed by the use of rigorous histological criteria. Currently, there is no tissue culture method available for detection of HPV infection. While HPV DNA detection tests currently remain experimental, they may prove useful in the future as a cancer screening test by detecting the oncogenic potential of specific HPV types in the anogenital area.

Treatment. Table 9.11 outlines the treatment for condyloma acuminatum and flat condyloma. Treatment of these flat condyloma is similar to that recommended for neoplasia. Cervical condylomas are frequently treated with ablative methods, such as cryotherapy or laser. Extensive multicentric disease is best treated with laser therapy. New therapies for widespread multicentric disease, especially vaginal disease, include intravaginal 5-fluorouracil (5-FU). Small doses of topical 5-FU have also been used to treat external disease including condyloma accuminatum and flat condylomas of the penis and vulva. As with any STD, treatment must include close examination of partners and treatment of visible lesions and follow-up. These examinations must include both acetic acid application and magnification in men and women.

Human immunodeficiency virus (HIV) is the newest viral STD to threaten youth. An in-depth description of its clinical syndrome of AIDS is

Table 9.12. Syndrome: Bacterial Vaginosis.

Symptoms:	Discharge; dysuria
Signs:	Homogeneous white adherent discharge;[a]
	Amine test: fishy odor with 10% KOH added[a]
Laboratory:	Vaginal pH $\geq$ 4.5[a]
	Clue cells on saline wet mount (>20% of epithelial cells)[a]
	Gram stain: gram variable coccobacilli without
	lactobacilli present
Etiology:	*G.vaginalis*; anaerobes; other?

[a] Diagnosis of bacterial vaginosis: three of the four items noted.

beyond the scope of this text. For primary care clinicians, the focus regarding HIV infection is prevention; this is addressed in the section on assessment of the adolescent for STDs later in this chapter.

Syndromes

The constellation of symptoms and signs that are characteristically associated with a particular pathological clinical entity and caused by one or more sexually transmissible organisms defines a sexually transmitted disease syndrome. Common syndromes are vaginitis, endocervicitis, endometritis, and acute salpingitis (pelvic inflammatory disease) and bacterial vaginosis in women; epididymitis in men; and urethritis and proctitis in both. The syndromes are presented in outline form in Tables 9.1 through 9.6, 9.12, and 9.13. These tables should be integrated with the previous descriptions of each STD microorganism and with the medical assessment protocol described below for a full appreciation of the comprehensive approach to the diagnosis, treatment, and prevention of STDs in the adolescent male and female. Bacterial vaginosis and pelvic inflammatory disease are discussed specifically below. While the syndrome of AIDS is important, the clinical presentation and course are beyond the purview of this chapter. The approach to the prevention of STDs and AIDS is outlined in the following section.

Bacterial Vaginosis

Evidence for the existence of a vaginal syndrome in the absence of candidal or trichomonal infections was first presented by Gardner and Dukes in 1955. These authors described the association between vaginal findings and the presence of a small gram-negative organism that they termed *Hemophilus vaginalis*. The confusion as to the nature of the syndrome is best reflected in the variety of terms used to describe it over the years, including *H. vaginalis vaginitis*, *nonspecific vaginosis*, and, most recently, *bacterial vaginosis*. Bacterial vaginosis was chosen because it appears that other

Table 9.13. Clinical Criteria: Diagnosis of Acute Pelvic Inflammatory Disease (PID).

All three of the following should be present:
1. Lower abdominal tenderness
2. Cervical motion tenderness
3. Adnexal tenderness (unilateral or bilateral)
   Plus:
One of the following should be present:
1. Temperature ≥ 38°C
2. White blood cell count ≥ 10,500/mm.3
3. Purulent material obtained by culdocentesis
4. An inflammatory mass present on bimanual pelvic examination and/or sonography
5. Erythrocyte sedimentation rate > 15 mm./hr.
6. Evidence of the presence of *N.gonorrhoeae* and/or *C.trachomatis* in endocervix:
   a. Gram stain reveals gram-negative intracellular diplococci
   b. Monoclonal antibody for *C.trachomatis* positive
7. Presence of ≥ 5 PMNs/oil immersion field on gram stain of endocervical discharge

Source: Sweet, R. L. "Pelvic Inflammatory Disease and Infertility in Women." *Infectious Disease Clinics of North America*, 1987, *1*, 199–215.

bacteria in addition to *G. vaginalis* may be responsible for the clinical presentation ("bacterial") and that epithelial inflammation does not appear to play a prominent role in the disease process ("vaginosis," not vaginitis). Controversy has been linked with this "syndrome" ever since it was first described, including questioning of its very existence, the role of *G. vaginalis*, anaerobes, and other bacteria, its pathogenesis, and the clinical criteria for its pathogenesis and diagnosis.

The importance of bacterial vaginosis as a sexually transmitted syndrome is not clear. Bacteria related to the syndrome, including *G. vaginalis* and anaerobes, have been isolated from non-sexually active adolescent girls and from sexually active girls with and without signs of the syndrome. Among sexually active girls, it has been shown that a greater quantity of *G. vaginalis* is isolated from the vaginal specimens of girls diagnosed with bacterial vaginosis than of girls with no signs of the syndrome. It therefore may be not only the type but also the quantity of organism present that determines the development of bacterial vaginosis. Although bacterial vaginosis has been linked to PID, definitive data supporting this hypothesis are lacking. Current clinical criteria for diagnosis of bacterial vaginosis are outlined in Table 9.12. The treatment currently recommended by the CDC is metronidazole 500 mg. by mouth twice daily for seven days.

Pelvic Inflammatory Disease (PID)

Pelvic inflammatory disease (PID) poses the most important reproductive health problem for women, especially sexually active adolescent girls. The term *PID* as used here refers to a sexually transmitted infection involving the uterus, ovaries, and peritoneal tissues as well as the fallopian tubes. An estimated one million cases of acute PID are diagnosed annually, with more than 250,000 women hospitalized for treatment and 150,000 women requiring surgical intervention for complications. As a direct result of PID, women may experience one or more serious threats to their fertility: one-fifth of all women who have had PID will develop long-term sequelae, including ectopic pregnancy and involuntary infertility. Tubal factor infertility has been implicated in as many as one-third of cases of involuntary female infertility.

Risk Factors. The syndrome of PID has been associated with a number of risk factors that may predispose women for the development of disease. First, younger age appears to be important. Sexually active adolescent females are diagnosed with PID 3 times more frequently than their twenty-five to twenty-nine-year-old counterparts. Suggestions have been made to help explain the apparent PID-age association. For example, adolescent girls have more cervical ectopy (both *N. gonorrhoeae* and *C. trachomatis* preferentially infect such tissue), may not possess local immunity to the infecting agent (at primary infection), may use barrier methods less effectively (unproved), or may engage in sexual behaviors that place them at greater risk for STDs (unproved) than older women.

A second risk factor is the acquisition of a sexually transmitted infection, since STDs have been closely linked to PID. STDs have been isolated from the fallopian tubes of women with laparoscopically verified PID: *N. gonorrhoeae* (30 to 50 percent); *C. trachomatis* (25 to 40 percent); mixed infections with anaerobes and facultative microbial agents (25 to 50 percent); and possibly genital mycoplasmas. A third factor related to the development of PID is a history of previous gonococcal PID, predisposing young women to recurrent episodes of infection. It is likely that other organisms, such as *C. trachomatis*, follow a similar pattern of recurrent infection. A fourth factor includes sexual behaviors, such as increased numbers of sexual partners, that have been linked to the development of PID.

IUDs are a fifth factor linked to PID; their use has been associated with a two to four times greater risk for PID. As a foreign body, the IUD may establish a local endometritis that may lead to upper-tract disease. In contrast, although its role in PID is controversial, most authors have shown that the oral contraceptive affords some protection from PID, especially gonococcal and possibly nongonococcal, nonchlamydial PID. It appears that oral contraceptive users have fewer endocervical gonococcal infections, and when gonococcal PID is established, the oral contraceptive ameliorates its severity. The role of oral contraceptives with *C. trachomatis* infections remains confusing, since many authors have reported an increase in the endocervical infection rate among pill users while others have not. However, recently, a Swedish group has reported a decrease among pill users in the risk for chlamydial-associated PID as well.

Pathogenesis. The pathogenesis of PID involves the ascending canalicular spread of the causative sexually transmitted agent(s). The STD agent is first inoculated into the vaginocervical compartment during sexual intercourse and spreads contiguously through the mechanical and immunological barriers of the endocervix, along the endometrial surface to the tubal mucosa and onto peritoneal surfaces through the leakage of organisms from the tubal fimbria. Since etiological agents such as gonococcus and chlamydia have no known inherent motility, several possible explanations for their movement have been postulated: transport by attachment to sperm; movement with reflux of menstrual blood; transport with uterine contractions; and mobility through attachment to the surface or ingestion and transport by migrating inflammatory cells at the endocervix. In addition, it has been shown that the IUD string facilitates access of bacteria from the vagina and/or cervix to the normally sterile uterine cavity.

Diagnosis and Treatment. Acute PID presents with a wide spectrum of clinical symptoms and signs, including lower abdominal pain, vaginal and endocervical discharge, cervical motion tenderness, and uterine and adnexal tenderness. Using these manifestations as clinical criteria for diagnosis of PID has been shown to be accurate in only approximately 60 percent of cases, even under well-controlled clinical situations verified by direct laparoscopy. The differential diagnosis to be considered in a young woman presenting with acute lower abdominal pain in addition to PID includes acute appendicitis, acute cystitis, acute cholecystitis, acute pyelonephritis, ectopic pregnancy, endometriosis, hemorrhagic ovarian cyst, intrauterine pregnancy, mesenteric lymphadenitis, ovarian cyst with or without torsion, ovarian tumor, septic abortion, severe constipation, and trauma.

While we recognize that laparoscopy is the only definitive diagnostic tool for PID, it is probably impractical and unnecessary to employ it in most cases because of its surgical risk, unavailability in many settings, and expense. The clinician must then rely on his or her clinical ability to elicit an accurate sexual history in as confidential and empathetic manner as possible and on the application of a standardized set of clinical criteria to assist in the diagnosis of PID. A set of criteria currently used in many settings is outlined in Table 9.13. These criteria are only to assist the clinician in making a decision about the most likely diagnosis in order to formulate a reasonable management plan.

Laboratory tests to be included in the diagnostic workup are outlined in Tables 9.3 and 9.13. Endocervical cultures or rapid diagnostic tests for *C. trachomatis* and *N. gonorrhoeae* and other STD screening tests should be performed when possible. A pregnancy test is essential in order to assist in the differential diagnosis and in the determination of the appropriate treatment regimen. Principles to remember in the clinical approach to PID include (1) using the standardized clinical criteria to guide, not dictate, the diagnosis, (2) erring on the side of "overdiagnosis" of PID when doubt exists in order to begin therapy early and prevent sequelae, (3) treating aggressively with broad-spectrum antibiotics and beginning the course immediately upon diagnosis, and, finally, (4) following up with clinical evaluations (within twenty-four to forty-eight hours) in order to confirm the clinical diagnosis

Table 9.14. Treatment Regimens: Acute PID.

A. Recommended Inpatient Regimens
    Cefoxitin: 2.0 g. IV q 6 hrs
                            or
    Cefotetan[a]: 2.0 gm IV q 12 hours
                            plus
    Doxycycline: 100 mg. IV q 12 hours
    1. Use IV for minimum of 48 hours after patient improves.
    2. After discharge, continue doxycycline 100 mg. PO b.i.d. to complete 10- to 14-day
        course.
                            or
        Clindamycin: 900 mg. IV q 8 hours
                            plus
        Gentamicin: 2.0 mg./kg. IV or IM in one loading dose, followed by a maintenance dose
        of 1.5 mg./kg. IV q 8 hours in patients with normal renal function
    1. Use IV for minimum of 48 hours after patient improves.
    2. After discharge, doxycycline 100 mg. PO b.i.d. for a total of 10 to 14 days
                            or
    3. Continue clindamycin 450 mg. PO q.i.d. to complete a 10- to 14-day course as an
        alternative.
B. Recommended Outpatient Regimens
    Cefoxitin: 2 g. IM
                            plus
    Probenecid: 1 g. PO
                            or
    Ceftriaxone: 250 mg. IM or equivalent cephalosporin
                            plus
    Doxycycline: 100 mg. PO b.i.d. × 10 to 14 days
                            or
    Tetracycline: 500 mg. PO q.i.d. × 10 to 14 days
C. Recommended Alternatives for Patients Who Do Not Tolerate Doxycycline
    Erythromycin: 500 mg. PO q.i.d. × 10 to 14 days (based on limited clinical data)
D. Management of Sex Partners
    As in any STD, partners should be evaluated for STD and treated empirically for
    N.gonorrhoeae and *C.trachomatis* infection.

---

[a] Other cephalosporins such as ceftizoxime, cefotaxime, and ceftriaxone provide adequate gonococcal coverage; other facultative gram-negative aerobic and anaerobic coverage may also be used in appropriate doses.

Source: Adapted from U.S. Department of Health and Human Services. *STD Treatment Guidelines, 1989*. Atlanta, Ga.: Division of Sexually Transmitted Diseases, Centers for Disease Control, U.S. Public Health Service, 1989.

and reevaluate the treatment regimen. Management of the sexual partner is an important step in preventing STD infection and PID.

Treatment. The overall goals for treatment of PID are aimed at fertility preservation and prevention of ectopic pregnancy as well as other long-term sequelae. The treatment regimens currently recommended address the polymicrobial nature of PID; they are outlined in Table 9.14.

Assessment of the Adolescent for STDs

STDs pose a major threat to the future health and fertility of our youth, with AIDS adding a new dimension to the threat. Primary care clinicians therefore must become skilled in the recognition, treatment, and prevention of

STDs among young males and females. To meet this challenge, clinicians should be guided by several principles that may affect clinical practice, including the epidemic proportions of youth infected, the unique approach to adolescents as patients, the frequency of asymptomatic infection, the sensitive nature of sexuality and sexual behaviors placing adolescents at risk for STDs, and the importance of prevention in the master plan for STD management in adolescents.

Principle	*Impact*
Epidemic of teen STDs	STD management is integrated into practice.
Adolescent as patient	Cognitive and pubertal changes are addressed in management plan.
Asymptomatic STDs	Clinicians initiate STD history, exam, and screening tests.
Sensitive nature of STDs	Clinicians develop rapport and trust and ensure confidentiality.
Prevention of STDs	Clinicians incorporate health prevention in all visits and initiate discussion before sexual debut.

History

Obtaining an accurate sexual and medical history from an adolescent can be an uncomfortable experience for both the clinician and the adolescent. The clinician must establish rapport and trust with the adolescent. Ideally, this is accomplished as a part of routine well care before the adolescent considers initiating sexual activity. At the first signs of puberty, the primary care clinician can schedule a "transition interview and physical examination" for the annual physical assessment. The clinician can present the anticipated cognitive, emotional, physical, and environmental changes that will occur over the adolescent years to both parents and the young adolescent. Part of the visit can be used to discuss the need for the development of trust and confidentiality between the clinician and the adolescent. Parents can be informed that issues regarding sexuality and reproductive health, including STDs, are a normal part of preventive medicine for adolescents and will be appropriately discussed as a part of future visits. Encouraging parents to have their adolescent make and attend their own clinical appointments will provide a model for the parents of how to assist their adolescents in taking charge of health care.

While confidential management of STDs is provided by all states through their respective public health departments, it is imperative for primary care clinicians to integrate STD assessment into most adolescent health visits because of the ubiquitous nature of STDs and the unique developmental status of the adolescent. For the clinician to determine the presence of sexual activity, it is obviously crucial to ensure confidentiality and to use terminology that is appropriate to the adolescent's development. The topics to be addressed in an adolescent STD history are the following:

Subject	Focus
Puberty	Onset, menarche, last menstrual period
Sexual activity	Presence, frequency, type (vaginal, oral, anal)
Partners	Sex, number (last month, past year, lifetime)
Contraception	Type (debut, last intercourse, problems)
Pregnancy	Number of pregnancies or impregnations, abortions (type, number)
Drug use	Type, frequency, route
School and job	General risk for STDs
Support	Family's and friends' knowledge of sexual activity
History of STD	Type, frequency, treatment, problems
Symptoms	Self, partner(s)

Examination

The physical evaluation of the sexually active adolescent begins with a complete medical examination, since there is a wide range of presentations of STD infections, from few or no symptoms or signs to severe systemic disease requiring hospitalization. The clinician must prepare the youth by explaining the planned procedures and should use diagrams and models where appropriate. However, it is not always advantageous to overwhelm the anxious and/or ill adolescent with zealous presentation of educational material, including long explanations and direct demonstrations of reproductive anatomy. The young, inexperienced adolescent frequently wishes only to survive his or her first reproductive exam, while the older, more experienced youth may enjoy the detailed descriptions of anatomy and function and direct demonstration of reproductive organs.

It is recommended that the first pelvic examination be performed as part of a normal physical assessment at an appropriate time after menarche

Table 9.15. Common STD Symptoms and Signs in Males and Females.

Systemic	Fever, fatigue
Skin	
General	Rash +/− pruritus: papular/vesicular, ulcers, generalized/ genital erythema
Conjunctival	Purulent discharge
Joint	Erythema, swelling
Gastrointestinal	
Liver	RUQ pain +/− jaundice
Anal	Trauma, pruritus, pain, purulent/bloody discharge
Urethral	Frequency, burning, dysuria, discharge
Genitourinary	
Urethral	Frequency, burning, dysuria, discharge
Epididymo-testicular	Erythema, edema, pain
Vaginal	Abnormal discharge, erythema, edema, odor
Endocervical	Mucopurulent discharge, erythema, edema, friability
Uterine	Abnormal pain, cramping, abnormal bleeding (amount, periodicity)

and before sexual debut when possible. This approach will eliminate an unnecessary barrier of fear of the unknown in the future that could lead an adolescent female to delay seeking help for STD symptoms because of fear of the pelvic examination. During a routine annual exam or sports physical, the adolescent male can be taught both about normality and about symptoms of urethritis and other STDs so that he will be alerted to cues to seek appropriate medical care for possible STD infection.

Essential components of the STD-focused physical assessment are based on common symptoms and signs presented in Table 9.15. Indications for a pelvic examination in the sexually active adolescent female include unexplained abnormal vaginal bleeding, especially when prolonged, when intermenstrual, or when accompanied by unusual dysmenorrhea; pregnancy; unexplained frequency, burning, or dysuria; sexual activity; vaginal discharge; a history of lower abdominal pain; and a history of contact with a partner with a possible or verified STD. It may also be performed as a part of a routine physical examination or by request of the adolescent after menarche.

Laboratory Assessment

Laboratory assessment is reviewed in detail in the discussion of specific infections and syndromes above. However, since it has been established that many STDs are asymptomatic in adolescents, it becomes necessary to initiate screening for STDs as a normal part of a complete physical evaluation of a sexually active adolescent (Table 9.16). Screening for syphilis with an RPR or VDRL is recommended in the adolescent who has a current or past diagnosis of any STD. Screening for pyuria in the first-catch urine in boys indicates probable urethritis with chlamydia and/or gonococcus. Using

Table 9.16. Laboratory Screening for STDs Among Sexually Active Asymptomatic Adolescents During Health Maintenance Visits.

Gender	Test	STD	Syndrome
Females	Vaginal KOH wet mount	C.albicans	vulvovaginitis
	Vaginal NaCl wet mount	G.vaginalis (anaerobes)	bacterial vaginosis
		T.vaginalis	vaginitis
	Vaginal pH ≥ 5.0	G.vaginalis/ (anaerobes)	bacterial vaginosis
		T.vaginalis	vaginitis
Males	First-catch urinalysis (pyuria, esterase)	C.trachomatis,	urethritis
	Urethral culture	N.gonorrhoeae	
Both	VDRL, RPR if any past/current STD(s)	T.pallidum	syphilis

culture or rapid diagnostic tests to detect chlamydia and gonococci among asymptomatic girls is commonplace. Its cost effectiveness among boys is currently under investigation. In girls, Pap smear screening for signs of possible STD and dysplasia should be routinely performed annually. Using saline and KOH wet mounts in conjunction with phenaphthazine paper (pH paper) to detect asymptomatic *T. vaginalis*, *C. albicans*, and possible bacterial vaginosis should be a part of a routine pelvic examination.

Evaluation of the Sexual Partner

The sexual partners of adolescents diagnosed with STDs must be identified, examined, screened for STDs by culture and/or rapid diagnostic techniques, and appropriately treated or referred for management. When possible, the partner should be managed in the same clinical setting as the identified adolescent patient. If the adolescent consents and circumstances permit, nonjudgmental counseling with the sexual partner present may be an effective technique to maximize treatment compliance and prevent recurrent disease. Sexual abstinence or use of condoms by the male partner during the treatment course should be encouraged. Follow-up with a test-of-cure examination of both partners is important, and encouragement of continued use of condoms in the future is essential.

Evaluation of the Adolescent at High Risk for STDs and AIDS

The sexual practices of youth who identify themselves as homosexual may place such youth at high risk for specific STDs. Homosexual males appear to be at greater risk of acquiring pharyngeal gonorrhea, hepatitis B, syphilis, and some gastrointestinal parasites. The hepatitis B vaccine should be given to all HBsAg-negative homosexual or bisexual males. Risk of acquisition of HIV infection is high in this population, and appropriate prevention techniques should be specifically discussed.

It must be noted that many adolescent males engaging in anal-oral sexual practices with same-sex partners may not identify themselves as homosexual. It is also becoming apparent that heterosexual couples are engaging in oral and anal sexual practices at significant rates, which places them at risk for specific STD-infection-related syndromes, including STD pharyngitis and proctitis. It then becomes more important to emphasize the type and frequency of sexual activity and intravenous drug use that places the youth at risk for specific STDs, especially hepatitis B and HIV infection, than to elicit the youth's perception of his or her sexual identity during adolescence.

Screening youth at risk for HIV infection is controversial. Discussion of the positive and negative aspects of HIV screening for youth at risk should be undertaken by an experienced clinician in a supportive environment. The decision to test should be made freely by the youth after careful consideration of all alternatives and preferably with the knowledge and support of a responsible adult relative, counselor, or adult friend. However, routinely screening youth for HIV infection is not currently recommended.

It must be emphasized that the main role of the primary care clinician is the identification of youth at risk for acquisition of HIV and the prevention of that acquisition. Because of the fatal consequences of HIV infection, clinicians are obligated to counsel and assist youth to engage in behaviors that minimize HIV risk, including support of abstinence and delaying sexual debut during adolescence, encouraging monogamous relationships, educating the youth and partner about proper condom use, and assisting the youth to decrease or eliminate drug use. While intravenous drugs obviously place the youth at risk for HIV infection, drug use in general that results in impaired judgment and unsafe sexual practices (including anonymous sexual activity) may prove to be the greatest risk factor for HIV infection among adolescents in the near future.

Resources for the Primary Care Clinician

Information and recommendations regarding STD management, including prevalence, types, diagnosis, treatment and prevention, change rapidly in any one community and nationally. Textbooks discussing the clinical practice of STD management are available. The Centers for Disease Control in Atlanta, Georgia, periodically publish current recommendations for the diagnosis and treatment, as do the professional clinical medical journals. Staff members of community public health departments and STD clinics are excellent resources for the practicing clinician who wishes consultation, referral, and contact tracing services regarding STD management.

Suggested Readings

Adger, H., Shafer, M. A., Sweet, R. T., and Schachter, J. "Screening for *Chlamydia trachomatis* and *Neisseria gonorrheae* in Adolescent Males: Value of the First Catch Urinalysis." *Lancet*, 1984, *1*, 944–945.

Ajello, L. "Progress in the Diagnosis and Therapy of the Local Mycoses." *Acta Dermatologica Venereum* (Sweden), 1986, *121* (supp.), 13–18.

Alexander-Rodriguez, T., and Vermund, S. H. "Gonorrhea and Syphilis in Incarcerated Urban Adolescents: Prevalence and Physical Signs." *Pediatrics*, 1987, *80*, 561–564.

Bingham, J. S. "Vulvo-Vaginal Candidosis: An Overview." *Acta Dermatologica Venereum* (Sweden), 1986, *121* (supp.), 39–46.

Brunham, R. C., and others. "Mucopurulent Cervicitis — the Ignored Counterpart in Women of Urethritis in Men." *New England Journal of Medicine*, 1984, *311*, 1–6.

Campion, M. J. "Clinical Manifestations and Natural History of Genital Human Papillomavirus Infection." *Obstetric and Gynecologic Clinics of North America*, 1987, *14*, 363–388.

Chambers, C. V., and others. "Microflora of the Urethra in Adolescent Males: Relationships to Sexual Activity and Nongonococcal Urethritis." *Journal of Pediatrics*, 1987, *110*, 314–321.

Corey, L., and Spear, P. G. "Infections with Herpes Simplex Viruses, Part I." *New England Journal of Medicine*, 1986, *314*, 686–691.

Fiumara, N. J. "Treatment of Primary and Secondary Syphilis: Serologic Response." *Journal of the American Medical Association*, 1980, *243*, 2500–2502.

Holmes, K. K., Mardh, P.-A., Sparling, P. F., and Wiesner, P. J. (eds.). *Sexually Transmitted Disease*. New York: McGraw-Hill, 1984.

Irwin, C. E., Jr., and Millstein, S. G. "Biopsychosocial Correlates of Risk-Taking Behaviors During Adolescence: Can the Physician Intervene?" *Journal of Adolescent Health Care*, 1986, 7, 82S–96S.

Jacobson, L., and Westrom, L. "Objectivized Diagnoses of Acute Pelvic Inflammatory Disease." *American Journal of Obstetrics and Gynecology*, 1969, *105*, 1088–1096.

Krieger, J. N., and others. "Diagnosis of Trichomoniasis: Comparison of Conventional Wet Mount Examination with Cytologic Slides, Cultures and Monoclonal Antibody Staining of Direct Specimens." *Journal of the American Medical Association*, 1988, *259*, 1223–1227.

Schachter, J. "Are Chlamydia Infections the Most Prevalent Venereal Disease?" *Journal of the American Medical Association*, 1975, *231*, 1252–1255.

Schachter, J. "Chlamydia Infections." *New England Journal of Medicine*, 1978, *298*, 428–435, 490–495, 540–549.

Shafer, M. A. "Educational Approaches: AIDS and the Adolescent." In R. F. Schinazi and A. Nahmas (eds.), *AIDS in Children, Adolescents and Heterosexual Adults: An Interdisciplinary Approach to Prevention*. New York: Elsevier North Holland, 1988.

Shafer, M. A., Irwin, C. E., and Sweet, R. C. "Acute Salpingitis in the Adolescent Female." *Journal of Pediatrics*, 1982, *100*, 339–350.

Shafer, M. A., and others. "*Chlamydia trachomatis*: Important Relationships to Race, Contraceptive Use, Lower Genital Tract Infection and Papanicolaou Smears." *Journal of Pediatrics*, 1984, *104*, 141–146.

Shafer, M. A., and others. "The Microbiology of the Lower Genital Tract of Post-Menarchal Adolescent Females: Differences by Sexual Activity, Contraception, and Presence of Nonspecific Vaginitis." *Journal of Pediatrics*, 1985, *107*, 974–981.

Shafer, M. A., and others. "Prevalence of Urethral *Chlamydia trachomatis* and *Neisseria gonorrhoeae* Among Asymptomatic Sexually Active Adolescent Males." *Journal of Infectious Disease*, 1987, *156*, 223–224.

Sweet, R. L. "Pelvic Inflammatory Disease and Infertility in Women." *Infectious Disease Clinics of North America*, 1987, *1*, 199–215.

U.S. Department of Health and Human Services. *Sexually Transmitted Disease Statistics, 1985*. Washington, D.C.: Division of Sexually Transmitted Disease, Centers for Disease Control, U.S. Public Health Service, 1987.

U.S. Department of Health and Human Services. *STD Treatment Guidelines, 1989*. Atlanta, Ga.: Division of Sexually Transmitted Disease, Centers for Disease Control, U.S. Public Health Service, 1989.

Washington, A. E., and others. "Oral Contraceptives, *Chlamydia trachomatis* Infection and Pelvic Inflammatory Disease: A Word of Caution About Protection." *Journal of the American Medical Association*, 1985, *124*, 2246–2250.

Westrom, L. "Effect of Active Pelvic Inflammatory Disease on Fertility." *American Journal of Obstetrics and Gynecology*, 1975, *122*, 707–713.

Wolner-Hansen, P., Swensson, L., and Mardh, P. A. "Laparoscopic Findings and Contraceptive Use in Women with Signs and Symptoms Suggestive of Acute Salpingitis." *Obstetrics and Gynecology*, 1985, *66*, 233–239.

Zelnik, M., and Kantner, J. F. "Sexual Activity, Contraceptive Use and Pregnancy Among Metropolitan Teenagers 1971–1979." *Family Planning Perspectives*, 1980, *12*, 230–237.

❧ 10 ❧

Pregnancy and Its Outcome

Janet B. Hardy, M.D.

The premature onset of sexual activity and subsequent pregnancy, abortion, childbearing, and parenting and the acquisition of sexually transmitted disease are all parts of a chain of events that have become serious, vexing, and controversial issues in our society.

The United States has by far the highest rates of pregnancy, abortion, and childbearing among females fifteen through nineteen years old of all similarly developed countries. Among girls under fifteen years of age, the rates are four times those of any other westernized country. Yet, high as these national rates are, they mask the diversity that exists within the United States, by region and population subgroup. They understate the serious problems arising from the extremely high rates of teenage pregnancy, childbirth, and sexually transmitted diseases among the poor and socially disadvantaged in our inner cities and among Native Americans. Some population subgroups, such as those of Asian descent, particularly the Chinese and Japanese, have by comparison very low birthrates among teenagers.

During the past decade, issues concerned with various aspects of the teenage pregnancy problem have attracted a large amount of serious research. Many research findings have received massive public attention and have raised public concern, with but limited response by federal, state, and local governments. Lack of general understanding of some of the underlying factors and lack of consensus and controversy regarding ethical issues and the role of the family have seriously hindered the development of integrated and well-evaluated preventive efforts. As a result, the abortion rate among teenagers remains at record levels, and an intergenerational pattern of

250

unintended and mostly undesired childbearing is developing among the poor in our large cities, helping to create an underclass characterized by✓ female-headed, single-parent families, at high risk for unemployment, poverty, social disadvantage, and chronic welfare dependency. This subgroup is also at risk for other social problems, such as crime, drug abuse, alcoholism, mental health problems, and child abuse and neglect.

Valid solutions to the problems generated by early childbearing and the urgent need to prevent premature sexual activity and its consequences depend on a thorough understanding of the dimensions of the problem. What are the circumstances that surround unintended and premature conception and decision making with respect to pregnancy resolution? Who are the teenagers, male and female, who become involved in unintended and out-of-wedlock pregnancy? What are their legal rights and responsibilities, and what are those of their parents? Who has abortions, and who bears children? What are the correlates and consequences for the young parents, their children, and society? What can be done to minimize the impact of premature childbearing? Most importantly, what can be done to prevent the premature onset of sexual activity and its possible adverse consequences? The purpose of this chapter is to provide some answers to these questions.

Definitions

One of the factors that have hindered the development of consensus at federal, state, and local levels as to ways of resolving the problems stemming from adolescent sexual activity and its consequences is confusion over definitions. The terms *teenage pregnancy* and *adolescent pregnancy* are frequently used synonymously. The Bureau of the Census lumps all births to teenagers aged fifteen through nineteen in one group for most analyses, even though there are marked developmental differences between the youngest and oldest members of the group. Most policy makers consider the group to be homogeneous.

Adolescence

In a social sense, adolescence is defined as that period in the life cycle that extends from childhood to adulthood, when independent adult roles are assumed. During the past fifty years, as American society has changed from a largely agricultural and heavy-manufacturing base to dependence on advanced technology, the educational process has been greatly extended, and the time when independence and adult roles are assumed has advanced, sometimes well into the twenties.

In a biological sense, adolescence extends from the onset of puberty until physical growth is complete, at about eighteen years of age. Puberty may occur as early as age ten and as late as age fifteen with corresponding rates of change in body size, shape, and function. Furthermore, the development in the cognitive and socioemotional domains and in moral reasoning may not parallel rates of physical and sexual development, particularly for those in whom puberty occurs early. As a result, adolescence is an anxious and turbulent period for many young people.

Some of us consider those under eighteen years of age as adolescents and eighteen- to nineteen-year-olds as older teens; others use the term *school-age* to define younger teenagers. In any event, pregnant adolescents age seventeen years and younger appear at higher risk for adverse medical and social outcome than those eighteen to nineteen years old. Physically, the adolescents are generally less mature and still growing, most are still in school (or should be), and most are still immature in cognitive and socioemotional development. Many are still in the cognitive stage of concrete operations, which impedes planning for the future, projection of self into another's situation, and abstract thinking—all basic to effective contraception and good parenting. Their problems are frequently compounded by poverty and single parenthood, as most of those who bear children come from poor families and thus have lacked the ready access to the information and services needed to protect them from the adverse consequences of premature sexual activity. Increasingly larger proportions of adolescent mothers are not married; among blacks, all but a tiny proportion are unmarried.

Older Teenagers

By contrast with younger teenagers, eighteen- to nineteen-year-olds have generally completed their physical growth, their cognitive and socioemotional development is more advanced, and larger proportions have finished high school. While single parenthood is frequent, especially among blacks, somewhat larger proportions in this age group are married. Prenatal care usually begins earlier, and pregnancy risks are less than those of younger mothers. Social risks may, however, be considerably greater than those experienced by more advantaged, older mothers, who delay childbearing into their twenties. Pregnancy risks are considerably higher for all teenagers having a second- or higher-order birth. Thus, for optimal results, intervention to prevent premature sexual activity and pregnancy and to prevent and manage adverse consequences must take into account the developmental level of the young people involved.

Sources of Information

Sources of information for this chapter on teen pregnancy fall into two broad general categories: literature and Johns Hopkins research programs.

Literature Review

During the past fifteen years, there have been many hundreds of journal articles and a significant number of books devoted to discussion of the various aspects of teenage sexuality, pregnancy, abortion, childbearing, and parenting. Two general groups of sources are discussed here.

The first group of sources includes the indispensable national statistics contained in the *Monthly Statistical Reports* of the National Center for Health Statistics, particularly the *Advance Reports of Final Natality Statistics* for 1984 and 1985 and *Induced Terminations of Pregnancy: Reporting States, 1984*. The former reports include demographic descriptions of mothers and fathers (age, race, marital status, and education) and data on pregnancy care and infant outcome. The latter also includes demographic information in addition to that pertaining to abortion.

Also in this group of sources are four important books. The most recent of these books is a two-volume report, published in 1987, prepared by the Panel on Adolescent Sexuality, Pregnancy and Childbearing of the National Research Council in Washington, D.C. This report, entitled *Risking the Future: Adolescent Sexuality, Pregnancy and Childbearing*, provides a comprehensive and current review of teenage pregnancy, its antecedents, and the adverse consequences that may follow. The first volume, edited by C. D. Hayes, provides an overview and a series of recommendations for action. The second volume, edited by S. L. Hofferth and C. D. Hayes (1987), contains the working papers and statistical analyses that formed the basis for volume one. These reports together provide a historical perspective on changing trends in teenage sexuality, pregnancy, abortions, birth, and parenting.

The second book, edited by J. B. Lancaster and B. A. Hamburg and published in 1986, is entitled *School-Age Pregnancy and Parenthood: Biosocial Dimensions*. This is a scholarly volume that provides information about the biological, emotional, cognitive, and psychosexual aspects of development and their interrelationships with the physical aspects. Of particular interest are the chapters that provide historical and cross-cultural perspectives. A chapter by Arthur B. Elster and Michael E. Lamb provides a review of what is known about adolescent fathers. R. J. Gelleis reports on school-age parents and child abuse and L. V. Klerman on the economic impact of school-age childbearing. In the final chapter, C. M. Super makes the point that the developmental consequences are socially constructed. School-age motherhood, by itself, does not have a straightforward influence on the developing child. Other influences, biological and environmental, prenatal and postnatal, interact to determine the development of the child.

Also recent is *Adolescent Mothers in Later Life* (1987), by F. F. Furstenberg, Jr., J. Brooks-Gunn, and S. P. Morgan. The twenty-year follow-up of a group of adolescent mothers delivering their first children in the mid 1960s shows the remarkable diversity of outcomes and examines some of the factors related to good and unfavorable outcomes. Educational attainment and social supports, particularly within the family, that are available to the young mother appear to reduce their vulnerability and to be conducive to more favorable outcomes in later life.

The fourth volume, *Pregnancy in Adolescence: Needs, Problems and Management* (1982), contains an excellent chapter by B. W. Paul and P. Schaap that details the legal aspects of adolescent sexuality and pregnancy and their management and the rights of minors with respect to pregnancy care, including abortion.

The Johns Hopkins Experience

The second general set of sources is provided by several research and clinical research programs that have been carried out at Johns Hopkins University since the early 1970s. The surveys of sexual experience, contraceptive use, and pregnancy among a nationally representative sample of young, unmarried women (age fifteen through nineteen) in metropolitan areas in the United States carried out by J. E. Kantner and M. Zelnik during the 1970s made a major contribution. These surveys document the extent and increasing frequency of both sexual experience and contraceptive use by teenage women between 1971 and 1976, with some leveling off by 1979. The data base they established has been used by Kantner, Zelnik, and their colleagues to address a number of adolescent fertility issues, such as the timing of first intercourse, sex education in relation to teenage sexual activity, pregnancy and contraceptive use, and the risk of adolescent pregnancy following the first months of intercourse.

A twelve-year follow-up of urban women and their children enrolled in the Johns Hopkins Collaborative Perinatal Study demonstrated the disadvantage of primiparous adolescent mothers younger than eighteen and their children in terms of both immediate pregnancy outcome and risk of long-term adverse consequences, as compared with similar, older mothers and their children in the same population.

The results of these and other studies in the adolescent pregnancy and parenting clinics in the Johns Hopkins Hospital set the stage for the development of intervention to improve outcomes for young mothers and their children and subsequently, in collaboration with the departments of education and health of the city of Baltimore, to prevent pregnancy among inner-city junior and senior high school students. The results of this program have been evaluated by L. S. Zabin, J. B. Hardy, and their colleagues. In addition, in 1983 an additional research program, undertaken by J. B. Hardy and A. K. Duggan, involved the use of birth certificates to describe teenage pregnancy, abortion, and childbirth in Baltimore and to select a random sample of adolescent births for further intensive study. These and other Johns Hopkins studies are described in a book entitled *Adolescent Pregnancy in an Urban Environment: Issues, Programs, and Evaluation* by J. B. Hardy and L. S. Zabin, published in 1991 by Urban & Schwarzenberg.

The remainder of this chapter will provide a brief description of the national scope of the problem followed by a more detailed description of the urban adolescents who became pregnant, their pregnancy outcome, the fathers of their babies, and the children themselves. Our intervention efforts will be briefly described and brief recommendations for action at local, regional, and national levels made.

Demographics

A National Perspective

During the past twenty-five years, there have been marked changes in American society and in the status of women. The ability to control fertility by means of contraception and abortion and the liberalization of sexual attitudes and beliefs that underlie the so-called sexual revolution have reached down to affect the sexual behavior of teenagers, even young adolescents.

Sexual Activity Among Teenagers

Underlying the pregnancy rates are frequency of intercourse in the population, the age at which it is initiated, and contraceptive practices. Fewer than half of unmarried teenage females in the United States are sexually active (that is, have had sex at least once). However, the proportion of those who are sexually experienced increased markedly, from 28 percent in 1971 to 46 percent in 1979. There was a subsequent slight decline to 42 percent in 1982. There has been a substantial difference by race throughout the period, with larger proportions of black teenage females (more than 52 percent) sexually active than of whites (40 percent). However, rates of sexual experience have increased more rapidly among whites than among blacks, and the differential, just over 12 percent, is the lowest since such data have been available. By age twenty, most unmarried males and females—80 percent of males and 70 percent of females—have become sexually experienced. By age eighteen, 64 percent of boys and 44 percent of girls report having had intercourse at least once. The frequency of experience increases substantially with age. Black teenage women initiate intercourse at earlier ages than their white counterparts, and, at each age, the proportion of sexually experienced blacks is larger than that of whites. Within each race, boys, in general, become sexually active at earlier ages than girls. The experience of Hispanics appears to be more similar to that of whites than to that of blacks.

Teenagers from socially disadvantaged backgrounds, as measured by parental education and by the dropout rates in the schools they attend, are at higher risk for the early initiation of coitus, failure to use contraceptives, and pregnancy and sexually transmitted diseases than those from more favorable backgrounds. However, despite the increase in the proportion of sexually experienced unmarried teenagers in all levels of American society, intercourse among them is often sporadic and infrequent. This is a factor that must be considered in relation to contraceptive use. Both the rationale for

Table 10.1. Pregnancy Outcome Among American Teenage
Females Ages Fifteen Through Nineteen Years, 1984.

	Number	Percentage
Total pregnancies	1,004,859	100.0
Live births	469,682	46.7
Elective abortions	401,128	39.9
Spontaneous fetal death	139,049	13.8

Source: Data extracted from Hayes, C. D. (ed.). *Risking the Future: Adolescent Sexuality, Pregnancy and Childbearing*. Vol. 1. Washington, D.C.: National Academy Press, 1987, p. 54.

and the motivation to practice oral contraception may be affected by this behavior pattern.

Teenage Pregnancies, Abortions, and Births

More than one million teenagers and preteens become pregnant each year. The total number of pregnancies among teenage females fifteen through nineteen years of age increased from 839,663 in 1960 to 1,151,851 in 1980 and then gradually declined to an estimated 1,004,859 in 1984. Since 1960, births in this age group decreased markedly, by over 25 percent, from 644,708 to 469,682 in 1984 and 467,485 in 1985. The number of elective abortions, however, has steadily increased, from an estimated 150,000 in 1970 to 401,128 in 1984, with a corresponding increase in rate per 1,000 fifteen- to nineteen-year-olds from 6 to 44. Spontaneous fetal deaths (miscarriages and stillbirths) accounted for an additional 134,049 teenage pregnancy terminations (13.8 percent) in 1984. The proportion of pregnancies among teenagers (fifteen through nineteen) is shown by type of termination in Table 10.1. Of all pregnancies in this age group, fewer than half (46.7 percent) resulted in live births. In addition, there were 9,965 live births among girls under fifteen years of age. It should be noted that consideration of teenage births alone, without spontaneous and elective fetal loss, greatly understates the scope of the teenage pregnancy problem. The distributions of elective terminations of pregnancy among teenagers are shown by age and race in Table 10.2.

Maternal mortality in the United States has persisted at very low levels for the past ten years. The risks of mortality following legally induced abortion are very low for all women and lower than average for teenagers. In fact, the risks of mortality associated with a legally performed abortion are less than those associated with childbirth.

The striking decline in both number of births and the birthrate among teenage females and the lesser decline in the number of pregnancies reflect several opposing forces. Between 1975 and 1985, the number of teenagers in the population declined by 14 percent, and the use of contraceptives increased steadily from 1970 to 1976, after which it leveled off somewhat. Both

Table 10.2. Abortion Ratios by Race and Age of Young Women, 1984,
and Percentage Change, 1983–1984: U.S. Thirteen-State Area.

Age of Woman	Abortion Ratio		Percentage Change	
			1983–1984	
	White	Black	White	Black
Under 14 years	2,089	1,884	10.9	–10.7
14 years	1,846	1,291	17.2	5.6
15 years	1,239	914	15.4	–3.6
16 years	984	748	3.6	3.1
17 years	811	664	7.3	1.0
18 years	804	668	2.7	–0.3
19 years	599	611	3.0	–0.1

Source: National Center for Health Statistics. *Induced Terminations of Pregnancy: Reporting States, 1984.* Monthly Vital Statistics Report, vol. 36, no. 5 (supp.). Hyattsville, Md.: National Center for Health Statistics, 1987.

factors have tended to reduce the number of teenage pregnancies. In addition, since the legalization of abortion in 1973, the rate of elective termination of pregnancy in this age group has increased steadily, with a concomitant and marked reduction in both number and rate of live births.

Forces acting in the opposite direction have included an increasing frequency in the proportion of sexually active teenagers in the population and the initiation of sexual activity at ever younger ages. The net result of these opposing factors has been a pregnancy rate among fifteen- to nineteen-year-olds that increased from an estimated 88 per 1,000 in 1970 to a peak of 111 per 1,000 in 1980; the rate was level at 109 per 1,000 in 1984. While the number of births has decreased by more than 25 percent, the birthrate in this age group decreased less sharply, from 68 per 1,000 in 1970 to 53 per 1,000 in 1976. However, the rate has changed little since then, to 51 per 1,000 in 1984. As might be expected, the pregnancy rate among the sexually experienced is much higher than that among fifteen- to nineteen-year-olds in general. Among the sexually experienced, the pregnancy rate declined from 272 in 1972, to 245 in 1980, to 233 in 1984, only rather small declines. It was estimated that in 1986, 40 percent of white and 63 percent of black females reaching twenty years of age would have been pregnant at least once.

There are differences in rates of teenage pregnancy, abortion, and childbirth by state and, within a given state, by geographical area as well as by race. Local differences reflect socioeconomic factors as well as racially determined cultural patterns. These differences are important because of their relevance to strategies for pregnancy prevention. This point is discussed in greater detail in the following section.

Correlates of Live Births

Table 10.3 shows the distribution, by age of mother and race of child, among teenagers delivering a live baby in 1985. The bottom line in the table

Table 10.3. Live Births by Age of Mother and Race of Child, United States, 1985.

Age of Mother	All Races	White	Black	American Indian	Asian or Pacific Islander				
					Chinese	Japanese	Hawaiian	Filipino	Other
All ages	3,760,561	2,991,373	608,193	42,646	17,880	9,802	7,193	21,482	59,259
15–19 years	467,485	318,725	134,270	7,983	196	285	1,139	1,235	3,380
Under 15 years	10,220	4,101	5,860	149	2	3	3	18	77
15 years	25,002	13,276	11,001	425	5	11	58	54	157
16 years	53,474	33,052	18,913	871	14	23	109	117	345
17 years	89,313	59,714	26,895	1,564	30	51	185	213	610
18 years	129,563	89,950	35,399	2,332	59	94	337	368	951
19 years	170,133	122,733	42,062	2,791	88	106	450	483	1,317
Percentage under 20 years	12.7	10.8	21.4	19.1	1.1	2.9	2.0	5.8	5.8

Source: National Center for Health Statistics. *Advance Report of Final Natality Statistics, 1985. Monthly Vital Statistics Report,* vol. 36, no. 4 (supp.). Hyattsville, Md.: National Center for Health Statistics, 1987.

Table 10.4. Distribution of Births to Teenagers
by Mother's Age and Race of Child, United States, 1985.

	Under 15 Years	15–19 Years
White		
Total	4,101	318,725
First births	3,951	252,887
Second order and above	150	65,838
Percentage second order and above	3.7	20.7
Black		
Total	5,860	134,270
First births	5,646	95,619
Second order and above	214	38,651
Percentage second order and above	3.7	28.8

Source: National Center for Health Statistics. *Advance Report of Natality Statistics, 1985.* Monthly Vital Statistics Report, vol. 36, no. 4 (supp.). Hyattsville, Md.: National Center for Health Statistics, 1987.

shows the marked differences in the proportions of total births that were to teenagers of different racial origins. Black teenagers accounted for more than 21 percent of all black births and Native American teenagers for 19 percent. Only just over 1 percent of all births to Chinese and just under 3 percent of all births to Japanese women in the United States were to teens. It is interesting to speculate about the family and sociocultural factors that may account for these differences.

Age of Father. While 12.7 percent of all births in 1985 were to teenage mothers, only 3 percent of all U.S. fathers in 1985 were teenagers, reflecting the fact that the great majority of fathers were considerably older (on average, two to four years) than the mothers.

Parity. Information about prior pregnancy history for the nation as a whole is not readily available. However, there are data pertaining to prior births, and, particularly among older teenagers, substantial proportions of those who delivered in 1985 already had one or more live-born child. The proportions are shown by age of mother and race of child in Table 10.4.

Marital Status. Table 10.5 shows the changes that occurred between 1964 and 1980 in the proportions of teenagers married at the time of conception and at the time of delivery of their first child. While there were many fewer married in 1980 than in the mid 1960s among teens of both races, the decline among blacks was marked, from 42 percent in the 1960s to only 11 percent in 1980.

Education. Among teenage mothers in the United States, 61 percent of whites and 65 percent of blacks had twelve or more years of education at the time of delivery in 1985. The proportions completing twelve grades or more are shown by age of mother and race of child in Table 10.6. On average, educational attainment was quite low among teenagers becoming pregnant.

Prenatal Care and Low Birth Weight. Obstetrical outcome is associated with both the time of onset of prenatal care and the number of prenatal visits.

Table 10.5. Trends in the Distribution of First Births to Teenagers,
Fifteen Through Nineteen Years, by Marital Status and Race,
1964–1966 (Average) and 1980, United States.

	1964–1966 (Average)	1972	1980
Number of first births	340,000	294,000	305,000
White			
Percentage married at:			
Conception	50.0	52.0	30.5
Delivery	85.0	75.5	63.9
Black			
Percentage married at:			
Conception	15.1	12.1	4.8
Delivery	41.9	20.7	10.6

Source: National Center for Health Statistics. *Trends in Marital Status of Mothers at Conception and Birth of First Child.* Monthly Vital Statistics Report, vol. 36, no. 2 (supp.). Hyattsville, Md.: National Center for Health Statistics, 1987.

Table 10.7 shows the trimester of onset of prenatal care by age of mother and race of child. Black teenagers, on the average, registered for care later in pregnancy than whites, and the younger adolescents of both races initiated care later or had no care more frequently than older teenagers. Not surprisingly, as seen in Table 10.8, the frequency of low birth weight (below 2,500 grams, or 5.5 pounds) nationally was higher among the infants of the youngest teens and decreased progressively with increasing age. Black teenagers had higher frequencies of low birth weight than whites.

Costs of Teenage Childbearing and Child Rearing

Because a teenage mother is often unmarried and undereducated when her child is born and may not continue school afterward, she tends to

Table 10.6. Distribution of Teenage Mothers' Educational Attainment of
Twelve Years or More at Delivery, 1985, by Age and Race of Child.

	White			Black		
Age	Number with Education Stated	Number with 12 or More Years of Education	Percentage	Number with Education Stated	Number with 12 or More Years of Education	Percentage
17	43,507	6,440	14.8	23,039	3,921	17.0
18	66,569	29,863	44.9	30,363	15,084	49.6
19	91,122	55,698	61.1	35,535	23,100	65.0

Source: National Center for Health Statistics. *Advance Report on Final Natality Statistics, 1985.* Monthly Vital Statistics Report, vol. 36, no. 4 (supp.). Hyattsville, Md.: National Center for Health Statistics, 1987. Calculated from data in Table 22.

Table 10.7. Live Births by Time of Onset of Prenatal Care Among
Teenagers, by Age of Mother and Race of Child, United States, 1985.

Age in Years	Total Number	Number with Prenatal Care Stated	Trimester Care Initiated Percentage Distribution[a]			
			First	Second	Third	None
White						
Under 15	4,101	3,947	58	40	15	7
15	13,276	12,887	45	40	10	5
16	33,052	32,169	52	37	9	4
17	59,714	58,234	54	35	9	3
18	89,950	87,628	57	33	8	3
19	122,733	119,770	62	29	7	3
Black						
Under 15	5,860	5,656	34	46	14	6
15	11,001	10,603	40	43	12	5
16	18,913	18,227	43	42	11	5
17	26,895	25,966	46	40	10	5
18	35,399	34,220	48	38	10	4
19	42,062	40,653	51	35	9	4

[a] Rounded percentages may not add up to 100.
Source: Calculated from figures in Table 25, *Advance Report on Final Natality Statistics, 1985.* Monthly Vital Statistics Report, vol. 36, no. 4 (supp.). Hyattsville, Md.: National Center for Health Statistics, 1987.

face a bleak future marked by difficulty in obtaining an independent status with adequate employment to sustain herself and her child. This is particularly so if she soon becomes pregnant again and has another child. Even if she marries, this relationship is likely to be highly unstable.

It has been estimated that the public costs, in 1985, for Aid to Families with Dependent Children and Medicaid totaled $16.65 billion for families in which the mother had her first birth as a teenager.

Table 10.8. Frequency of Low Birth Weight (Below 2,500 Grams) Among Infants
Born to Teenagers, by Age of Mother and Race of Child, United States, 1985.

Age in Years	Race of Child			
	White		Black	
	Number	Percentage	Number	Percentage
Under 15	428	10.5	863	14.8
15	1,265	9.5	1,537	14.0
16	2,835	8.6	2,649	14.0
17	4,759	8.0	3,673	13.7
18	7,067	7.9	4,693	13.3
19	8,393	6.8	5,341	12.7

Source: National Center for Health Statistics. *Advance Report on Final Natality Statistics, 1985.* Monthly Vital Statistics Report, vol. 36, no. 4 (supp.). Hyattsville, Md.: National Center for Health Statistics, 1987.

An Urban Perspective

We now turn to a consideration of urban teenagers, their pregnancy and childbearing experiences, and the relationships of these outcomes to underlying personal and environmental factors. A general discussion of these issues as they pertain to all teenagers living in an urban setting is followed by a more detailed discussion of the problems of pregnant and parenting adolescents.

Urban Teenage Pregnancy, Abortion, and Childbirth

The studies conducted at Johns Hopkins University in Baltimore show that statistics for the nation as a whole markedly understate the dimensions of the teenage pregnancy problem in large cities, where substantial proportions of all births are to unmarried teenagers.

Among cities with a population in excess of 500,000, Baltimore is one of the poorest, with high rates of school dropout, unemployment among people fifteen through twenty-four years of age, single-parent families living below the poverty level, pregnancy among adolescents and older teenagers, sexually transmitted disease, including HIV infection, and alcohol and drug abuse. Blacks make up 55 percent of the total population. There are very few Hispanics. While poor whites make up a smaller proportion of all whites than is the case with blacks, they generally experience consequences of teenage pregnancy that are equally severe as and, in some respects, more severe than those experienced by blacks.

In 1983, there were 5,221 pregnancies among Baltimore teenagers; 2,969 terminated in a live birth, and 42 percent were aborted. Data from birth certificates recorded in 1983 show that 28 percent of all live births in Baltimore during that year involved at least one parent below twenty years of age. This is more than twice the proportion reflected in national statistics. In 12 percent of the live births in Baltimore, both parents were teenagers; in 14 percent, the mother was a teenager and the father was twenty years of age or older, and in 2 percent, the father was a teenager and the mother was older. The children born to parents who were both teenagers were at considerable disadvantage, both biologically and socially, compared with those both of whose parents were age twenty or older. The degree of disadvantage was, in general, inversely proportional to the age of the mother at delivery, for both whites and blacks.

Characteristics of Childbearing Teenagers. Thirty percent of white teenagers in the Baltimore studies were married at delivery whereas only 3 percent of blacks were. Eighteen percent of the white teenagers and 30 percent of the blacks had completed high school; only 1 and 3 percent, respectively, had education beyond the high school level. Both the proportion completing high school and the proportion married decreased with maternal age. Sixty-one percent of the whites and 74 percent of the blacks were sufficiently poor to be eligible for Medicaid assistance to cover all or part of the cost of their obstetrical care.

Prenatal and Obstetrical Care. Just over 64 percent of white urban teenage mothers having a first birth registered for care in the first trimester of pregnancy, and 5 percent had no care in the third trimester; these mothers made an average of 11.2 prenatal visits each. Among blacks, there was even less adequate prenatal care: Only 49 percent registered for care in the first trimester, 10 percent received no care in the third trimester, and the average number of prenatal visits was 9.4. Where the teenage mother had a second- or higher-order birth (20 percent of whites and 22 percent of blacks), slightly larger proportions were married — 40 percent of the whites and 5 percent of the blacks. But larger proportions required Medicaid assistance — 74 percent of the whites and 81 percent of the blacks. Also, there was, on the average, a greater delay in this age group in seeking prenatal care and larger proportions with no care at all: 7 percent and 12 percent, respectively. Fewer prenatal visits were made — an average of 10 for whites and 8 for blacks.

Complications of Pregnancy. Complications were reported most frequently among the youngest teenagers and more frequently among blacks (19 percent) than among whites (14 percent). Complications of labor and delivery were frequent — 38 percent among blacks, 32 percent among whites. Overall, 17 percent were delivered by cesarean section, with no significant difference by race or age of mothers.

Preterm Delivery. At less than thirty-seven weeks preterm delivery was twice as frequent among blacks as among whites — 24 percent versus 12 percent. Similarly, low birth weight (LBW) was more frequent among black infants, with 16 percent weighing less than 2,500 grams and 4 percent less than 1,500 grams, while among white infants, the respective proportions were 8 percent and 2 percent. Among first-order births, the overall distributions of LBW were essentially as listed above; among blacks, however, the youngest girls (those under fourteen) had the lowest frequency of LBW, 13 percent, while those age sixteen had the highest, with 19 percent. By contrast, it was the youngest girls, both black and white, having a second- or higher-order birth who had the highest frequencies of LBW. Among adolescents, multiparity is a significant risk factor.

Adolescent Childbirth and Parenting in Baltimore

The youngest mothers, those under eighteen years, have greater than average pregnancy and parenting risks. This group constituted nearly 46 percent of teenage and preteen deliveries in Baltimore in 1983, and their pregnancy rates have shown little decline. To provide insight into the underlying sociobiological factors, the discussion here reviews the characteristics of the young mothers, the fathers of their babies, and the babies themselves, as discerned from an intensive study of a citywide, random sample of 389 births to adolescent (seventeen years old or younger) residents of Baltimore in 1983. Data were collected by lengthy interviews during home visits at three and fifteen to eighteen months after delivery. Those from the first interview, supplemented by information from birth certificates, are used to describe the adolescent and her pregnancy, her family, the father of the baby, and his relationship with her and their child. Those from the second interview, just over one year later, update the information. Comparisons of data from birth certificates of those interviewed and those of nonrespondents indicated no bias, suggesting that the random sample was representative of births to all Baltimore adolescents in 1983. During this period, 46 percent of all adolescent pregnancies were terminated by abortion.

Age, Race, and Marital Status. Of the 389 adolescent mothers, 272 (70 percent) were black and 117 (30 percent) were white. The youngest was aged ten, and 6 percent were age thirteen or younger. Fifteen percent already had one or more living children. One percent of the blacks and 24 percent of the whites were married at the time of delivery.

Education. Among black adolescents, 85 percent reported being in school at the time of conception, whereas among whites, only 44 percent were in school. Of those who were in school, 28 percent of the blacks and 74 percent of the whites dropped out during pregnancy. Educational attainment was deficient for both groups; 5 percent of the black but none of the white girls had graduated from high school by the time of delivery. Three months later, 60 percent of the black adolescent mothers but only 10 percent of those who were white were attending school. By eighteen months after delivery, 47 percent of the black and 82 percent of the white mothers had dropped out of school without completing twelfth grade. The rest either had graduated or were still in school.

Religion. Sixty-four percent of the black and 45 percent of the white adolescents reported being Protestant, and 7 percent and 29 percent, respectively, were Catholic. However, only 44 percent and 36 percent, respectively, said that they belonged to a specific church or attended services on a regular basis. These proportions are quite similar to those reported for all junior and senior high school students in the Johns Hopkins Pregnancy Prevention Program.

Family Background and Marital Status After Delivery. Three months after delivery, most of the adolescents in the Baltimore sample were living in rather large and often single-parent families. Both parents were present in only one-quarter of the families. Among whites, 10 percent of the adolescent mothers were themselves the family head, but among blacks, the proportion was only 1 percent. Most families were poor: 59 percent of the blacks and 62 percent of the whites had earned income; 71 percent and 50 percent, respectively, received full or partial welfare support; 30 percent of the black and 20 percent of the white families reported an annual income of $15,000 or above, and 45 percent and 58 percent had annual incomes below $10,000.

Age at First Intercourse. The age at the initiation of intercourse among these mothers was very young. Some reported beginning before puberty; 42

percent of the blacks and 21 percent of the whites were thirteen or younger, and 86 percent of the blacks and 78 percent of the whites were under sixteen. These findings have major implications for intervention. To be effective, pregnancy prevention programs must begin early; the high school level is too late in urban communities.

Contraceptive Use. Unfortunately, the use of contraceptives lagged far behind the age at first intercourse in this population of young women. Even though only a very small proportion (9 percent) of the pregnancies were planned and most were unwanted, 55 percent of the black and 67 percent of the white couples had *never* used a method of contraception prior to conception; only 13 percent were using a generally effective method. A survey of several hundred mothers of seventh-graders in an inner-city junior high school revealed that they generally lacked sufficient information to control their own fertility, let alone be effective teachers for their children; only 12 percent knew the fertile period in the month, and only 25 percent believed oral contraceptives to be effective in preventing pregnancy. They expressed strong support for sex education in the schools: 94 percent were in favor of such programs.

Adolescent Pregnancy in the Environment. Adolescent pregnancy has become so prevalent in the inner city as to represent normative rather than deviant behavior. This impression was documented by the following data. Among these young mothers, 80 percent had mothers who were teenagers and 51 percent had mothers who were adolescents (under age eighteen) when their first child was born; 30 percent had sisters and more than three-fourths had other close relatives who were adolescent mothers; virtually all had either close friends or relatives who had given birth as adolescents.

Relationships Between Adolescent Pregnancy and Other Problem Behaviors. In the junior and senior high school populations included in the Johns Hopkins Pregnancy Prevention Program, youngsters engaging in one type of behavior generally considered deviant were at risk for engaging in another. Thus, constellations of behaviors such as cigarette smoking, alcohol use, and drug abuse tended to occur together and were positively associated with premature sexual activity and increased risk of pregnancy. Such constellations have important implications for intervention.

Relationships with Baby's Father. Few of these pregnancies resulted from "fly-by-night" affairs; more than half of the couples, 57 percent, had been acquainted for two years or longer and only 10 percent for less than six months. The possibility of pregnancy was not discussed prior to conception by 57 percent of the couples. In the 43 percent where such an eventuality was discussed, 54 percent of the fathers (52 percent of blacks and 61 percent of whites) were reported to have wanted a baby, as compared with only 12 percent of the black and 40 percent of the white mothers.

Pregnancy Resolution. Among these pregnant adolescents who eventually delivered their babies, 40 percent were initially uncertain and undecided about what to do about the pregnancy. Of these, only 43 percent discussed the matter with the father of the baby. However, 70 percent discussed their plight with family members and 33 percent with a professional, but 22 percent had no counsel from anyone. Where discussion took place, 88 percent discussed adoption and 86 percent abortion. However, none of these babies was placed for adoption. It must be remembered that approximately as many young women elected to terminate their pregnancies by abortion as those who bore a baby. Most of the families were not pleased about the pregnancies of their daughters. However, 88 percent were reported to be helpful to the adolescent mother during her pregnancy, with most remaining supportive after the baby was born.

Prenatal Care. A variety of prenatal care programs were used. Thirty percent of all pregnant adolescents and 41 percent of those fifteen years or younger enrolled in a comprehensive adolescent pregnancy program. Despite the fact that almost all pregnant adolescents would have been eligible for Supplemental Nutrition for Women, Infants, and Children (WIC) and food stamps, only 72 percent actually received WIC and 44 percent had food stamps. Almost all received nutritional advice from a professional (88 percent) or family source (73 percent) during pregnancy. Nonetheless, 11 percent encountered significant difficulty in obtaining sufficient food during pregnancy.

Complications of Pregnancy. The frequency of complications of pregnancy differed little by race. Anemia was frequent, occurring in 32 percent overall and in 53 percent of those having a second- or higher-order birth. Hypertension was noted in 19 percent but toxemia of pregnancy in only 3 percent. One of the significant costs of caring for pregnant adolescents is the need for antepartum hospital admission; 14 percent of black and 18 percent of white girls were admitted because of illness or pregnancy complications prior to the onset of labor.

Immediate Pregnancy Outcome. Cesarean section was used to effect delivery for 15 percent of the adolescents. Twenty-nine percent of black mothers and 12 percent of white mothers delivered prematurely (before thirty-seven weeks' gestation). Infant birth weight was below 2,500 grams (5.5 pounds) among 15 percent of blacks and 10 percent of whites. Fewer black infants (8 percent) than white (11 percent) were admitted to a neonatal intensive care unit. All infants in this study survived, but both the perinatal and infant death rates of children born to teenage mothers are generally higher than the rates of those born to older mothers. It seems likely that these higher rates, like those for low birth weight, reflect social disadvantage and the concomitant adverse effects on health and child care rather than the biological effects of low maternal age per se.

Depression. It is only recently that the occurrence of depression among children and adolescents has become a recognized clinical entity. Yet, to those caring for pregnant and parenting adolescents, it seems quite commonplace. In this random sample of urban adolescents, 54 percent reported being depressed, worried, or confused during pregnancy and/or the three months after delivery. These emotional problems were even more frequent (62 percent) among those young mothers having a second- or higher-order birth. Only 17 percent felt able to discuss this problem with the father of the baby. Overall, 28 percent received no help from anyone, either professionals or family members, and only 14 percent received professional help. This problem, with its potential for seriously adverse effects on parenting, has not received the attention that it merits.

Maternal Status Fifteen to Eighteen Months After Delivery. By fifteen to eighteen months after delivery, 2 percent of blacks and 24 percent of whites were married and living with their husbands, and, overall, an additional 6 percent were living with boyfriends. These were often not the same men as they had been living with one year earlier. The great majority (89 percent) of black adolescents had neither married nor lived with the baby's father. In contrast, conjugal living relationships were more frequent among whites, where 37 percent of mothers and fathers had lived together at some point; however, there were considerable instability and change in partners among them as well. Most of the young mothers who were not living with the fathers did not anticipate doing so in the future. It must be noted that 10 of the 389 children were placed in agency foster care because of the mothers' inability to care for them or because of abuse; 3 of the children were black, and the remainder were white.

Most of the adolescents and their babies were still living in female-headed households — 86 percent of the blacks and 73 percent of the whites. In a small percentage of the cases (6 percent of blacks and 17 percent of whites) the household was now headed by the teenager herself. The frequency of welfare support had changed little in the prior year, as had the distribution of annual income. The vast majority of these families were still very poor. During the period from conception to almost eighteen months after delivery, 90 percent of the young mothers and/or their children had received welfare and 95 percent had received Medicaid assistance for all or part of the time. Thus, urban adolescent childbearing is a major burden for society.

Continued Sexual Activity and Contraceptive Use. Seventy-seven percent of the adolescents reported being sexually active; of these, one-quarter reported intercourse less often than once each month. Almost 70 percent reported using contraceptives, and most reported using effective methods. However, 8 percent were using no method, and 16 percent had received no family planning services since delivery.

Repeat Pregnancies. During the first six months after delivery, 10 percent conceived again, and within twelve months, 22 percent were pregnant. Between delivery and the second interview, fifteen to eighteen months later, 46 percent of the young mothers had become pregnant or had had a "pregnancy scare." Among a number of white mothers, repeated conception appeared due to a combination of lack of money to buy oral contraceptives (prescribed at hospital discharge following delivery) or to pay for transportation to clinics where reproductive health services might have been obtained at little or no cost.

Mothers' and Children's Health. Health problems were frequent among these generally disadvantaged young mothers and their children. The white mothers and children were at significantly greater risk for health problems than the black. Eleven percent of all young mothers were attended by private physicians, 10 percent were enrolled in health maintenance organizations (HMOs) and 16 percent in comprehensive adolescent pregnancy and parenting clinics, and 11 percent had no source of care. These young women made an average of 6.5 ambulatory care visits during the fifteen- to eighteen-month period following delivery; 18 percent were admitted to a hospital. Of the hospital admissions, just over one-third were unrelated to pregnancy. Fifteen percent of the blacks and 24 percent of the whites reported that they had no type of insurance or assistance with health care costs. Overall, 9 percent of the mothers had been refused care because they could not pay. Only 3 percent had reported refusal by private physicians and comprehensive adolescent programs, 17 percent by HMOs and hospital emergency rooms. Public transportation was used by half of the girls to gain access to health services, but many appointments were missed because of the lack of transportation or money to pay for it.

The numerous health problems of the children should be even more worrisome from the societal viewpoint. Almost all mothers identified a regular source of health care for their children. The white children appeared to have had significantly more problems than the black. During the fifteen to eighteen months after delivery, they made an average of 3.1 visits to an emergency room and 5.3 illness-related visits to other sources of care, as compared with 2 of each among the blacks. Children of both races averaged 7.7 well-child visits, which is appropriate, but DPT immunizations were up to date for age for only three-quarters. White children sustained more injuries requiring emergency care (22 percent) than did black children (16 percent). Almost twice as many white (20 percent) as black (11 percent) children had chronic problems, and more than twice as many white (31 percent) as black (15 percent) were hospitalized during the eighteen-month period. Twenty-one percent of white children had no public or private health insurance, as compared with only 6 percent of the black children. Almost all children were receiving WIC — 94 percent of the blacks and 86 percent of the whites — even though almost one-third of the mothers reported encountering difficulty enrolling in the WIC program. Overall, 16 percent of the mothers also reported difficulty in obtaining sufficient food for themselves and/or their children since delivery. Breast feeding was attempted by only 12 percent of these young women.

Employment History and Child Care. In spite of less education, more of the white mothers (58 percent) had work experience than did the black mothers (31 percent). However, at the time of the second interview, only 17 percent of the white and 9 percent of the black mothers were working. Only 2 percent reported not wanting to work; these were among the older (sixteen and seventeen years at delivery) white girls. Three-quarters expressed the desire to go to work right away, but most were held back by child-care problems (only 4 percent had subsidized day care) and the scarcity of entry-level jobs for untrained teenagers. It should be noted that the minimum wage is not sufficient to cover child-care costs. Only 16 percent of those wanting to work had professional job-placement help.

Status of the Fathers of the Babies. In some respects, it seems inappropriate to describe teenage fathers separately at the end of a description of adolescent pregnancy. One of the major difficulties is that society tends to romanticize their essential but rather tangential role rather than face the facts as outlined below.

Overall, 16 percent of the fathers were living with the babies' mothers fifteen to eighteen months after the birth of their babies. Only 62 percent of these maintained their own household; the remaining couples lived with parents or other relatives. Of the 80 percent of fathers not living with the mother and baby, 60 percent lived with a parent, 6 percent lived with another woman, 4 percent were in the armed services, and 7 percent were in jail (another 1.3 percent had been in jail since the pregnancy began but had been released). Of the remainder, four were known to be dead, the whereabouts of thirty (7.7 percent) were unknown to the mother, and the rest had other living arrangements. According to the mothers' reports, 20 percent of the fathers overall had babies by other women. Among men age twenty or older, the proportions were greater: 29 percent for the whites and 36 percent for the blacks.

During the child's first three months, among fathers not living with mother and child, there was daily contact between father and child in 52 percent of the cases, weekly contact in 27 percent, and no contact in 7 percent. By months twelve through fifteen, the contact had significantly decreased; in 16 percent of the cases, there was none at all, and in only 24 percent was it every day. Half of the mothers believed that the fathers provided too little physical help in raising the child, and 61 percent believed that they provided too little financial support.

As indicated earlier, the fathers, particularly the white fathers, had severe educational deficiencies. Little additional education had been attained since the birth of the child. Fifty-three percent of white fathers were reported to have completed less than tenth grade; 36 percent of the white and 51 percent of the black fathers had finished high school, and 4 percent of the latter had higher education. Overall, 9 percent were still in school. Among white fathers, 75 percent were working, as compared with 47 percent among blacks. Twenty-three percent of the whites and 42 percent of the blacks were neither in school nor working, and 7 percent of the whites and 17 percent of the blacks were not looking for work. Of those fathers age twenty or older who were not working, 24 percent of the whites and 23 percent of the blacks were reported to have never worked.

Summary. With very few exceptions, the adolescent mothers in this random sample of urban births were poor and seriously disadvantaged in terms of education, employment, and material resources. They had not wanted to become pregnant, but, for the most part, they had neither the knowledge nor the means to prevent its occurrence. Furthermore, they were, in general, still in the adolescent stages of cognitive and socioemotional development, which make for difficulties in planning ahead. They were engaging in behavior that, while generally considered undesirable by their parents, was very prevalent in their schools and communities.

Most wanted to be good mothers and provide good care for their children but lacked the necessary emotional maturity, knowledge, and resources. Where adolescent childbearing had become intergenerational, they also lacked good role models. In addition, they faced the environmental context of poor housing, overcrowding, lack of outside space, and pervasiveness of alcoholism, drug abuse, and violence. In the inner city, the problems are compounded. Yet some inner-city adolescent mothers successfully overcome the challenges, become self-sustaining, and have healthy, well-developed children.

Longer-Range Outcome for Adolescent Mothers and Their Children

The short-term (eighteen-month) outlook for adolescent mothers and their children, as described above, appears bleak. What happens over the longer term? Data from our twelve-year follow-up of inner-city women delivering infants in the early 1960s and their children show that the outcomes for mothers and children were less favorable with adolescent mothers than with similar but older (twenty- to twenty-four-year-old) women in the same population. In fact, there were quite striking differences between the two groups along a number of parameters that affect the development of children.

First, the younger mothers were less often married at registration for prenatal care (17 percent) than were the older mothers (61 percent). After twelve years, 31 percent of the younger and 48 percent of the older women were married. Both groups experienced change, but the younger mothers had more unstable relationships, as indicated by the number of changes of partners they experienced; only 19 percent had none and 37 percent had three or more, as opposed to 39 percent and 4 percent, respectively, among the older mothers. Second, none of the young mothers had graduated from high school at the time of registration for prenatal care, while 64 percent of those age twenty to twenty-four had. After twelve years, 35 percent of the young mothers and 77 percent of the older mothers had completed high school. Third, the proportion of women in both groups eligible for public support declined with time, but when the children were twelve years old, 16 percent of the young mothers were supported entirely by welfare, and 40 percent received partial support from this source. Among the older mothers, less than half as many (7 percent) received full support and 21 percent partial support from public sources. Fourth, subsequent fertility was much greater among the younger than the older women. During the twelve-year period, the adolescents had an average of 3.25 additional children, as compared with 2.35 for the older women. Finally, the development of the children of the adolescent mothers during the twelve years was less favorable than that of those of older women. Their average intellectual performance, as measured by the Wechsler Intelligence Scale for children, was poorer. Their average full-scale IQ score at age seven was 89.7, compared with 93.8 ($p < .001$) for the children of older women. By age twelve, the children of younger mothers had failed and had to repeat a school grade more often, and their academic achievement test scores were significantly below those of the children of older mothers.

In their seventeen-year follow-up of adolescent mothers, F. F. Furstenberg, Jr., J. Brooks-Gunn, and S. P. Morgan noted significant poverty among the Baltimore mothers that they studied; 70 percent were welfare recipients at some point, and for 22 percent this was the case in three of the last five years of the follow-up. The adolescent mothers in their study also experienced greater fertility than the comparison group. The really impressive finding was the wide diversity of outcomes experienced by the adolescent mothers. There were no stereotypes in the group; some did very well, establishing self-sufficient, stable nuclear families, while others experienced chronic welfare dependency. While the definitive findings with respect to the children have not yet been published, the preliminary findings suggest that the children, on average, fared less well than their mothers. They experienced high frequencies of high school failure, juvenile delinquency among the young males, and pregnancy among the females.

Intervention with Pregnant Teenagers

While pregnancy and childbirth cut across all social levels, our studies of adolescents in Baltimore indicate strong relationships between poverty and high rates of pregnancy and childbirth. Abortion appears to be the recourse of more affluent adolescents, especially white adolescents, who become pregnant. Because an abortion usually requires an ability to pay for it, abortion is not an option readily available to poor white or black adolescents. As a result, many unintended and often unwanted pregnancies must continue through childbirth. The objective in those situations must be to ensure a healthy pregnancy and a healthy baby in order to provide the best possible chance for optimal adolescent and child development. The babies of urban adolescents are seldom placed for adoption.

Need for Services

A healthy pregnancy is not, by itself, enough. Provision must be made for meeting the multiple needs, including health, educational, and psychosocial, of the young family and helping the young mother to become self-sufficient. Intervention is essential both to improve pregnancy outcome and to improve the outlook for the young mother, child, and father.

Legal Rights and Responsibilities. In general, minors cannot give legal consent for their own health care. However, there are important exceptions to this rule, and every physician caring for adolescent patients must know what these are. As the legal requirements vary by state, the physician must be aware of both federal and state regulations. Among the types of care for which the adolescent may give legal consent are pregnancy diagnosis and care, abortion, contraceptive services (but not sterilization), the treatment of sexually transmitted infections, and the counseling and management of drug and alcohol abuse.

Adolescents who are unmarried and part of a family that provides financial and other support should be encouraged but not coerced to consult with their parents; however, sometimes it is not in their best interests to do so. Given a little help and a few suggestions about how to broach the subject with a parent, most all of those initially reluctant to discuss their pregnancy with a parent will do so.

Pregnancy Option Counseling. When a diagnosis of pregnancy is made, an adolescent should be informed of her options in a realistic way, so that she is helped to understand the problems with each. If she wishes to carry on with the pregnancy, she should be promptly referred for prenatal care. If she chooses not to have the baby, she should be counseled about abortion and her right to choose this option and promptly referred. In the event that the physician is subject to moral or institutional constraints with respect to abortion counseling, the adolescent should, if she wishes, be referred to someone else for abortion counseling. She should also be told about the option of adoption and referred for appropriate services if this is her choice. Parents cannot legally require that their daughter have an abortion, nor can the parents or the teen father prevent her from having an abortion.

Comprehensive Pregnancy Care. Intervention that meets the multiple and complex needs of the pregnant adolescent can improve pregnancy outcome for the adolescent and her baby. The adolescent pregnancy clinic established in 1974 at the Johns Hopkins Hospital, like several other comprehensive programs, has been highly effective in improving maternal health (Table 10.9) and fetal outcome (Tables 10.10 and 10.11), as shown by comparisons with similar adolescents delivering in the same obstetrical facilities but receiving care in other Johns Hopkins prenatal programs. The Adolescent Pregnancy Program has enrolled 300–325 adolescents under age eighteen years at registration each year. It has provided high-quality standard medical care, emphasizing prevention and treatment of adolescent problems such as anemia, sexually transmitted infections, and the nutritional requirements for maternal as well as fetal growth. In addition, comprehensive psychosocial support and health, childbirth, and parenting education have been provided.

A full-time social worker and an education specialist are part of the

Table 10.9. Effects of Prenatal Programs on Adolescent Pregnancy Outcomes.

	Johns Hopkins Adolescent Pregnancy Program (N = 744)			Other Prenatal Programs (N = 744)			P. Value (Significance Level)
	Mean	Standard Deviation	Percentage	Mean	Standard Deviation	Percentage	
Prenatal Characteristics							
Anemia (hematocrit < 30 mm.)			10.9 (81)			15.6 (116)	.002
Pre-eclampsia			3.5 (26)			5.9 (44)	.02
Weight gain, lbs.	28.9	12.8		23.5	15.1		.0001
Gonorrhoea			7.9 (59)			5.4 (40)	
Number of prenatal visits[a]	9.2	3.5		8.7	4.1		.006
Labor and Delivery Characteristics							
Gestation, weeks completed	38.5	3.0		38.4	3.5		ns
Gestation, ≤ 36 weeks			18.7 (139)			21.5 (160)	ns
Cesarean section			17.1 (127)			19.5 (144)	
at ≤ 4 months			0.5 (4)			1.7 (13)	ns
Premature rupture of membranes, > 12 hours			3.5 (26)			5.5 (44)	.03

Note: Patients over seventeen years at delivery have been excluded.

[a] Johns Hopkins Adolescent Pregnancy Program visits do not include initial visit for pregnancy diagnosis and counseling; controls include diagnostic visit.

Source: Reprinted with permission from The American College of Obstetricians and Gynecologists. Hardy, J. B., King, T. M., and Repke, J. "The Johns Hopkins Adolescent Pregnancy Program: An Evaluation." *Obstetrics and Gynecology,* 1987, *69,* 300–306.

health care team. The social worker screens each adolescent and, usually, her mother. Referral is made as needed for human services, medical assistance, and nutritional supplements such as WIC and food stamps. Helping to plan for the adolescent's continued education and mental health counseling are other important social work functions. The education specialist has responsibility for implementation of the program's educational curriculum. This curriculum includes a values-clarification discussion group emphasizing setting personal objectives and encouraging personal responsibility. Participation in an educational group is mandatory at each prenatal visit. Fathers are encouraged to attend and to participate in the preparation-for-childbirth sessions so that they may assist the mother during labor. The curriculum also includes a range of pregnancy nutritional, reproductive health, and infant-care issues.

Two full-time obstetrical nurses are an integral part of the program. They work in the clinic sessions and interview each adolescent as she leaves to

Table 10.10. Effects of Prenatal Care on Fetal and Neonatal Outcomes, 1979–1981.

	Johns Hopkins Adolescent Pregnancy Program (N = 744)			Other Prenatal Programs (N = 744)			P. Value (Significance Level)
	Mean	Standard Deviation	Percentage	Mean	Standard Deviation	Percentage	
Fetal Outcome							
Birth weight, gms.	3,083	576		3,038	685		
< 2,500 grams			9.9 (74)			16.4 (122)	.0006
< 1,500 grams			1.9 (14)			3.9 (29)	.02
Apgar, ≤ 6 at 5 minutes			4.0 (30)			6.7 (50)	.02
Stillbirth			1.3 (10)			1.0 (8)	
Neonatal death[a]			0.4 (3)			1.2 (9)	
Perinatal death[a]			1.7 (13)			2.2 (17)	
Hospital Days							
Infant	4.9	7.3		6.0	9.5		

[a] Small numbers preclude tests for significance; note threefold difference in neonatal deaths.

Source: Reprinted with permission from The American College of Obstetricians and Gynecologists. Hardy, J. B., King, T. M., and Repke, J. "The Johns Hopkins Adolescent Pregnancy Program: An Evaluation." *Obstetrics and Gynecology,* 1987, *69,* 300–306.

Table 10.11. Fetal Outcome by Maternal Age and Parity (N = 1,780).

		Perinatal Death		Birth Weight (in Grams)		
Age in Years	Number	Number	Percentage	Mean	Standard Deviation	Percentage Under 2,500 Grams
Primiparous						
Under 15	366	6	1.6	3066	572	11.5
16	439	3	0.7	3039	592	12.8
17	609	17	2.8	3043	611	12.5
18	199	4	2.0	3029	593	14.6
Total	1613	30	1.9	3045	595	12.6[a]
Multiparous						
Under 15	12	0	0	3176	587	8.3
16	37	4	10.8	2842	941	21.6
17	79	2	2.5	2996	697	17.7
18	39	0	0	3039	540	12.8
Total	167	6	3.6	2985	720	16.8[a]

[a] $p < .001$.

Source: Reprinted with permission from The American College of Obstetricians and Gynecologists. Hardy, J. B., King, T. M., and Repke, J. "The Johns Hopkins Adolescent Pregnancy Program: An Evaluation." *Obstetrics and Gynecology,* 1987, *69,* 300–306.

be sure that instructions are understood and questions answered. They assist the obstetrical director in reviewing each patient's record, planning for obstetrical care, and facilitating return of no-shows. About 80 percent of appointments are kept. The nurses are also available between clinic visits, either by telephone or in person in the clinic. In addition, they visit on the wards, providing postpartum instruction and contraceptives. Other staff include a clinic registrar and a licensed practical nurse, who provide additional support services. Each staff member is familiar with each patient. Individual case management is facilitated by means of weekly staff meetings. A postpartum visit is made four weeks after delivery to assess maternal health, provide family planning education and supplies, and arrange continuing health care for the young mother and infant.

Results of Pregnancy Intervention

As Tables 10.9 and 10.10 reveal, in the three-year period between 1979 and 1981, the Johns Hopkins Adolescent Pregnancy Program was effective in reducing the frequency of pregnancy complications, low birth weight, and low five-minute Apgar scores. In fact, the frequency of LBW was 9.9 percent in the special program, as compared with 16.4 percent for controls. There were concomitant decreases in neonatal and perinatal death rates. Table 10.11 shows the frequencies of perinatal death and mean and low birth weight by maternal age for primiparous and multiparous adolescents enrolled in the program. Two interesting observations stand out. The first is that the youngest mothers have the highest mean birth weight and the lowest frequency of LBW of any maternal age group. The second is the increased risks of low birth weight and perinatal death associated with multiparous pregnancy in adolescence. The youngest mothers had the highest average weight gain in pregnancy.

Comprehensive Care for Mother and Child

By the time the pregnancy program had been in operation for one to two years, both its beneficial effect on immediate pregnancy outcome and the shortcomings of a program that terminated with the postpartum visit were readily apparent. Young mothers returned with a subsequent pregnancy within a few months, and serious infant illness, even death, occurred in the early weeks and months after birth. Some of these pediatric events seemed directly related to poor child care and parenting. An intensive and comprehensive follow-up parenting program was initiated on a demonstration basis. Approximately 50 percent of the higher-risk mother-infant pairs were enrolled in this three-year program. The remainder of the young mothers and their infants were referred to other community resources, and several served as a comparison group.

The Teenage Clinic was designed to provide preventive and acute primary care for young mother and child, in a single site, by a small team of providers. This team included a pediatrician, two pediatric nurse practitioners, a full-time social worker, and a health and parenting education specialist, with nonprofessional supporting staff. The general concept was similar to that of the prenatal program. The schedule of preventive visits paralleled the standard for Early and Periodic Screening, Diagnosis, and Treatment (EPSDT) for well-child care. Family planning services were emphasized and supplies provided free of charge. Assistance in returning to school to complete education, in obtaining needed human services, and in finding jobs was provided to the young mothers by referral to appropriate agencies. Short-term counseling was available and referral made for obvious depression and other emotional problems. At the end of three years, the mothers and infants were referred elsewhere for continuing care.

This program component also was successful. Table 10.12 shows the frequency of completion of routine well-child care as compared with similar mother-child dyads cared for in another Johns Hopkins program (the Children and Youth Program). Table 10.13 shows the average number of clinic visits related to illness for children in the two groups, and Table 10.14 shows the average number of emergency room visits made by mothers and children in the two groups, by year after the index child's birth. All three sets of data attest to the effectiveness of the comprehensive program in improving the health of both mothers and children.

Intervention to Prevent Adolescent Pregnancy

Our experience with pregnant and parenting adolescents indicated that an intervention combining medical, educational, and social services specifically directed to meeting the complex needs of these young people was effective. However, most young mothers and their children would have been better off

Table 10.12. Completeness of Well-Child Care
in the First Two Years of Life, by Program.

	Percentage	
	Adolescent Pregnancy Program	Children and Youth Program
	(N = 97)	(N = 104)
Children having all required immunizations	89.4	74.0[a]
Children making all routine visits	60.8	31.7
Children missing 3 or 4 visits	5.2	21.2

[a] $p < .005$.

Source: Hardy, J. B., Flagle, C. D., and Duggan, A. K. Unpublished report on resource use by pregnant and parenting adolescents submitted to the Office of Adolescent Pregnancy Programs, Johns Hopkins University, June 1986.

Table 10.13. Average Number of Outpatient Illness-Related Visits Made by Children in the First Two Years of Life, by Program and Site of Visit.

	Number of Visits	
	Adolescent Pregnancy Program	Children and Youth Program
Visit Site	(N = 97)	(N = 104)
Adolescent Pregnancy or Children and Youth Program	5.4	12.4
Other clinic	0.9	0.3
All clinics	6.3	12.7

Source: Hardy, J. B., Flagle, C. D., and Duggan, A. K. Unpublished report on resource use by pregnant and parenting teenagers submitted to the Office of Adolescent Pregnancy Programs, Johns Hopkins University, June 1986.

had the pregnancy been delayed until the mother had attained greater maturity and completed high school.

On the basis of this experience, which indicated the need to reach students in their schools no later than seventh grade, a pregnancy prevention program was designed. The program included two large inner-city schools, a junior and a senior high school from which many of the pregnant adolescents came. The program was funded by a private foundation and was developed as a three-year research and service demonstration project in collaboration with the Baltimore departments of education and health. The department of education selected a junior and a senior high school, similar in their characteristics, for comparison and program evaluation purposes. These two schools provided the routine sex education available in the city but

Table 10.14. Mean Number of Emergency Department Visits Made by Mothers and Children, by Year and Program Affiliation.

	Adolescent Pregnancy Program			Children and Youth Program		
	Number Followed	Number of Visits		Number Followed	Number of Visits	
Year After Birth		Mean	Standard Deviation		Mean	Standard Deviation
Adolescent mothers						
First	260	.67	1.1	238	1.04	1.9 p < .02
Second	194	.73	1.1	182	1.42	2.8 p < .01
Third	65	.61	1.0	64	1.44	2.2 p < .01
Children						
First	264	3.1	3.3	227	2.6	2.9 N.S.
Second	192	1.6	2.3	179	2.2	3.3 p < .05
Third	67	1.2	1.5	54	1.3	1.5 N.S.

Source: Hardy, J. B., Flagle, C. D., and Duggan, A. K. Unpublished report on resource use by pregnant and parenting adolescents submitted to the Office of Adolescent Pregnancy Programs, Johns Hopkins University, June 1986.

no special prevention services. Parents were informed by mail of the program and were provided the opportunity to withhold the participation of their children.

The service program consisted of two components. The first was carried out in the school and included education and counseling. The other provided additional education and reproductive services for those who chose to be sexually active. This component was in a storefront clinic, close to the schools, operated under the egis of the Johns Hopkins University and Hospital. A nurse practitioner and social worker team in each school provided a bridge between the two components. These individuals provided both classroom instruction and individual or, more usually, small-group counseling in the school in the mornings and clinical services in the clinic after school hours. Educational and counseling visits could be done on a drop-in basis, but medical services required an appointment. Health services were provided by the nurse practitioners under the supervision of a gynecologist. In Maryland, minors may receive reproductive health care, including contraceptives, without parental permission. We did not require such permission; about 70 percent of those seeking medical services would have forgone the services had permission been required. However, we strongly urged that students inform their parents, and by the second or third visit, most had done so. When serious health problems were uncovered or pregnancy diagnosed (these conditions often initiated the first clinic visit), no problem was encountered in gaining the adolescent's permission to talk with parents. All services and contraceptives were provided free of charge, as most inner-city youngsters have little if any discretionary funds.

The educational program was designed to ensure wise sexual decision making by (1) encouraging personal goal setting and responsibility, (2) providing accurate information about puberty, sexual development, adolescent development, sexually transmitted infections, reproduction, and contraception, and (3) emphasizing the adverse consequences of premature pregnancy and childbearing and their relationship to living in poverty. A variety of pamphlets, books, games, film strips, and movies were available for use by the students.

The counseling and clinic services were widely used by students in both the junior and senior high schools. More than half of the junior high school males came to the clinic, motivated by anxiety about body size and sexual development and an avid desire for information. Just under half of the junior high school girls came, usually in small groups. A majority of the sexually active senior high school girls but only a small proportion (15 percent) of the sexually active boys attended. The males most often came because they suspected a sexually transmitted disease.

The program evaluation, which was based on data collected by voluntary anonymous questionnaires from 97 percent of students in the four schools, indicated the success of the program. During the two and a half school years in which the clinic was open, the rate of pregnancy was decreased by 31 percent in the program schools, as compared with a 57 percent increase among the students in the comparison schools. During these years, overall rates of adolescent pregnancy increased somewhat in Baltimore. The decrease observed appeared to result from two important changes in behavior that had occurred among students in the program schools. First, the sexually active adolescents improved their contraceptive practice, including the use of more effective methods and a greater proportion using any method. Second, the onset of intercourse was delayed; the average age at first intercourse advanced by seven months, from 15.7 to 16.2 years, between the beginning and end of the program. No changes in either contraceptive practice or average age at first intercourse were observed among students in the comparison schools.

In sum, this program designed to meet the needs of high-risk junior and senior high school students for information and services required to prevent pregnancy was highly effective, particularly among the youngest girls. The program resulted in a significant delay in the first sexual experience, contradicting the frequently heard statement that access to information and contraceptives merely encourages promiscuity. In addition, the program uncovered a major need and desire of these young people for information provided by someone with whom they could talk comfortably. These students were especially ignorant about puberty, with the result that they had suffered much needless anxiety. This program seems to have been most successful with the youngest adolescents, a group whose risks seem to have been overlooked by those concentrating on prevention programs for high school students. Our program stressed reproductive health because these services were those directly involved in preventing pregnancy, and they could be delivered without parental permission in a population where it has been difficult to motivate parents. However, a need for a greater breadth of health services was apparent, and it was our impression that students would have been more comfortable coming to a clinic that was not branded as a "sex clinic."

There seems to be merit to a system that provides sexuality education in the school and additional counseling and reproductive health (and other medical) services in a nearby but off-site location. An off-site medical clinic reassures parents who do not view the provision of contraceptives as appropriate for the school. It facilitates communication with students who hesitate to discuss sexual matters in the school setting. Furthermore, a health care–based service is open all year around and usually has provision for out-of-hours emergencies.

Summary and Recommendations

Pregnancy, abortion, and childbearing among unmarried adolescents and teenagers are costly problems for individuals, families, and society. The problems are generally most prevalent among those least able to deal ade-quately with them. It is axiomatic that the most effective way to reduce the abortion rate is to reduce the frequency of unplanned and unwanted pregnancy.

The most urgent task that we face as a society is to persuade adoles-cents to delay the onset of sexual intercourse until the time comes to establish a stable, monogamous relationship. The epidemic of AIDS lends a compel-ling urgency to this task. The "just say no" approach is not enough. Those who cannot be persuaded to wait must be encouraged to practice "safe sex," and it must be made easy for them to do so. A dramatic reduction in the teenage pregnancy rate would result. This task can be facilitated by the use of birth certificates and other records to identify and target areas for interven-tion, particularly high-risk communities and high-risk areas within those communities.

The interrelationships among problem behaviors such as premature pregnancy, alcohol and drug abuse, delinquency, and violence and their overall relationship to social disadvantage suggest that it is not efficient to have a unitary program to deal separately with each problem area. An integrated approach would be more efficient and less costly. It is most important that the needs of pregnant and parenting adolescents and their children not be overlooked. These needs include health care, social services, education, job training, and jobs. High-quality day care and preschool educa-tional programs are often required to make continued education and em-ployment possible for the mother. Grandmothers are often themselves in the workforce. The minimum wage is not sufficient to cover the cost of needed services. Furthermore, many jobs paying the minimum wage provide no health benefits and thus put young parents at risk of being refused medical care for themselves and their children. Finally, the fathers also need help to become self-sufficient members of society's mainstream. If and when adoles-cents can look forward to a decent, useful future, perhaps many of their problem behaviors will disappear.

Suggested Readings

Furstenberg, F. F., Jr., Brooks-Gunn, J., and Morgan, S. P. *Adolescent Mothers in Later Life*. Cambridge, England: Cambridge University Press, 1987.

Hardy, J. B., and Duggan, A. K. "Teenage Fathers and the Fathers of Infants of Urban, Teenage Mothers." *American Journal of Public Health*, 1988, *78*, 919–922.

Hardy, J. B., and Duggan, A. K. "Fathers of Children Born to Young Urban Mothers." Part II. *Family Planning Perspectives*, 1989, *21* (4), 159–163. "Rela-tionships with Mother and Child." Forthcoming.

Hardy, J. B., King, T. M., and Repke, J. "The Johns Hopkins Adolescent Pregnancy Program: An Evaluation." *Obstetrics and Gynecology*, 1987, *69*, 300–306.

Hardy, J. B., Welcher, D. W., Stanley, J., and Dallas, J. R. "The Long-Range Outcome of Adolescent Pregnancy." *Clinical Obstetrics and Gynecology*, 1978, *21*, 1215–1232.

Hardy, J. B., and Zabin, L. S. *Adolescent Pregnancy in an Urban Environment: Issues, Programs and Evaluation.* Baltimore, Md.: Urban & Schwarzenberg, 1991.

Hayes, C. D. (ed.). *Risking the Future: Adolescent Sexuality, Pregnancy and Childbearing.* Vol. 1. Washington, D.C.: National Academy Press, 1987.

Hofferth, S. L., and Hayes, C. D. (eds.). *Risking the Future: Adolescent Sexuality, Pregnancy and Childbearing, Working Papers and Statistical Appendixes.* Vol. 2. Washington, D.C.: National Academy Press, 1987.

Lancaster, J. B., and Hamburg, B. A. (eds.). *School-Age Pregnancy and Parenthood: Biosocial Dimensions.* New York: Aldine DeGruyter, 1986.

Paul, B. W., and Schaap, P. "Legal Rights and Responsibilities of Pregnant Teenagers and Their Children." In I. R. Stuart and C. F. Wells (eds.), *Pregnancy in Adolescence: Needs, Problems and Management.* New York: Van Nostrand Reinhold, 1981.

Zabin, L. S., Hardy, J. B., Smith, E. A., and Hirsch, M. B. "Substance Use and Its Relation to Sexual Activity Among Inner-City Adolescents." *Journal of Adolescent Health Care*, 1986, 7, 320–321.

Zabin, L. S., Kantner, J. F., and Zelnik, L. "The Risk of Adolescent Pregnancy in the First Months of Intercourse." *Family Planning Perspectives*, 1979, *11*, 215–237.

Zabin, L. S., and others. "Evaluation of a School and Clinic Based Primary Pregnancy Prevention Program for Urban Teenagers." *Family Planning Perspectives*, 1986, *18*, 119–126.

Zelnik, M., and Kantner, J. F. "Sexual Activity, Contraceptive Use and Pregnancy Among Metropolitan Area Teenagers: 1971–1979." *Family Planning Perspectives*, 1980, *12*, 230–237.

Zelnik, M., and Kim, Y. J. "Sex Education and Its Association with Sexual Activity, Pregnancy and Contraceptive Use." *Family Planning Perspectives*, 1982, *14*, 117–126.

Zelnik, M., and Shah, F. K. "First Intercourse Among Young Americans." *Family Planning Perspectives*, 1983, *15*, 64–70.

11

Chronic Illness
and Disability

Gayle Geber, M.P.H.
Nancy A. Okinow, M.S.W.

As children with chronic illnesses and disabilities move through adolescence and into adulthood, they and their families undergo numerous transitions that involve the educational, vocational, health, familial, and social services. These transitions have profound implications for the allocation of individual, family, and community resources. Adolescents with chronic illnesses and disabilities confront multiple obstacles, some of which are the consequences of normal developmental processes and others of which are the social sequelae of the chronic illness. These issues are a major public health concern because of the threatened loss of human potential as a result of the large number of youths in the United States with a chronic condition who may not be receiving optimal services.

This chapter discusses the prevalence of chronic illnesses and physical disabilities and their impact on the lives of adolescents, their families, and the communities in which they live, learn, develop, grow, and play. The presentation of the needs and psychosocial adjustment of these adolescents is placed in a developmental context that focuses on the multiple transitions of youth: transitions from child to adult, pediatric to adult health care, school to work, and home to community. Inasmuch as the larger social issues for chronically ill adolescents are emphatically ones that include the ensurance of civil rights, policy issues will be presented to guide future service delivery.

At the outset, it should clearly be noted that individual differences play a major role in the psychosocial course and outcomes of disabilities in adolescence. Although research has yet to definitely delineate all the factors

282

affecting resilience, it is certain that adolescents with disabilities are a hetero-geneous group. While they may be seen as "different" in some way as a result of the disability, neither the disability itself nor society's perception of it as being nonnormative imposes homogeneity on the adolescents. On the other hand, there do appear to be common themes to the experience of disability for adolescents and their families.

Demographics

According to the Developmental Disabilities Act of 1984 (Public Law 98-527, Section 102), a developmental disability is a severe, chronic disability that:

- Is attributable to a mental or physical impairment or a combination of mental and physical impairments
- Is manifested before the person reaches the age of twenty-two years
- Is likely to continue indefinitely
- Results in substantial functional limitations in three or more of the following areas of major life activity: self-care, receptive and expressive language, learning, mobility, self-direction, capacity for independent living, and economic self-sufficiency
- Reflects the person's need for a combination and sequence of special interdisciplinary or generic care, treatment, or other services that are of lifelong or extended duration and are individually planned and coordinated

This definition of developmental disabilities covers a wide range of con-genital and acquired conditions, including mental retardation, cerebral palsy, muscular dystrophy, severe vision and hearing impairments, and spi-nal cord injuries. Chronic illnesses, which do not always meet this definition of a developmental disability, are long-term disorders that can be progressive or fatal or that, on the other hand, may have no adverse affect on a normal life span. Often, chronic illnesses fluctuate between periods of remission and relapse or acute symptomatology.

The National Health Interview Survey indicates that more than two million children in the United States under the age of seventeen have a condi-tion that limits their participation in school or play and that the proportion of chronically ill children and adolescents with activity limitations has almost doubled from 1961 to 1981. In 1981, 3.8 percent of the population under seventeen years of age were estimated to have an activity-limiting condition. Children with chronic illnesses from single-parent families were more likely to be limited in activities for health reasons than children from two-parent families. Other data indicate that children from racial minorities are dispro-portionately represented among people with disabilities. Table 11.1 presents

Table 11.1. Average Annual Rates of Selected Chronic Conditions per 1,000 Children Under Eighteen Years, United States, 1983–1985.

Condition	Rate
Heart disease	21.4
Rheumatic fever (with or without heart disease)	1.1
Hypertension	2.3
Asthma	45.1
Blindness and other visual impairments	10.1
Deafness and other hearing impairments	20.6
Speech impairments	17.2
Mental retardation	9.9
Absence of extremities (excluding absence of fingers or toes only)	1.0
Paralysis of extremities, complete or partial	2.4
Deformities or orthopedic impairments	34.9
Cleft palate	0.9
Epilepsy	5.0
Arthritis	2.3
Diabetes	1.7
Anemias	9.6

Source: Collins, J. "Prevalence of Selected Chronic Conditions, United States, 1983–1985." *Advance Data*, 1988, *155* (May 24), 1–16.

data on the prevalence of selected chronic conditions for children and adolescents.

Although the number of children and adolescents with chronic illnesses increased between 1960 and 1981, it is unlikely that their numbers will significantly increase in the future, since 84 percent of those born with handicapping conditions currently survive through the teenage years (Table 11.2). Future increases in prevalence will likely be due to increases in the incidence of conditions of lesser severity. Although we are not faced with an ever-increasing number of youths with disabilities, the large number of teenagers living with these conditions and the community expectations regarding mainstreaming them pose special challenges for service providers.

Developmental Considerations

In approaching a study of adolescents with chronic illnesses or disabilities, one first discovers the diversity of this group of individuals. At times, this diversity is seen in behavioral adjustment problems, depressive symptoms, or intrapsychic conflicts; at other times, the diversity is seen in the complexity of normality that many adolescents with chronic illnesses experience. Diversity exists in the range of chronic illnesses that affect adolescents, as well as the severity of these conditions and the visibility of their symptoms. There is also appreciable variability in adolescents' psychosocial adaptation to the experience of disability. The examination of this diversity is complicated by the different theoretical frameworks used to study the lives of these adolescents.

Table 11.2. Estimated Proportion of Children Surviving to Age Twenty.

Illness	Percentage
Asthma (moderate and severe)	98
Diabetes mellitus	95
Cleft lip or palate	92
Hemophilia	90
Sickle cell anemia	90
Congenital heart disease	65
Cystic fibrosis	60
Spina bifida	50
Acute lymphocytic leukemia	40
Chronic renal failure	25
Muscular dystrophy	25

Source: Data extracted from Hobbs, N., Perrin, J. M., and Ireys, H. T. *Chronically Ill Children and Their Families: Problems, Prospects, and Proposals from the Vanderbilt Study.* San Francisco: Jossey-Bass, 1985. Original source Gortmaker, S., and Sappenfield, W. "Chronic Childhood Disorders: Prevalence and Impact." *Pediatric Clinics of North America,* 1984, *31,* 3–18. Reprinted with permission.

Further, many examinations lack theoretical frameworks altogether and simply catalogue adolescents' characteristics using noncomparable populations, methodologies, and instruments.

The normal developmental progression through the various stages of adolescence can be affected by chronic illnesses or disabilities; and the shifts in cognition during this stage of the life cycle can, in turn, affect an adolescent's perception of and reaction to the illness or disability. Perhaps one of the most noticeable effects of a chronic disability on normal development is either the precocious or the delayed onset of puberty associated with certain conditions, such as cystic fibrosis or spina bifida. At a time when conformity to peer standards of sexual development is paramount, any deviation from the norm can be painful. Cystic fibrosis has been found to be associated with a delay in the development of intimacy and sexuality related to delayed puberty. Girls with Turner's syndrome have been found to be less socially competent than girls with short stature. Research on boys with Klinefelter's syndrome has found that they had more problems with peers, less interest in girls, and a lower masculinity score on the Bem Sex Role Inventory than a control group; nonetheless, there were no significant differences between the two groups on a measure of masculine-feminine interests and activities.

Somewhat similar patterns for adolescents with virilizing congenital adrenal hyperplasia and pseudohermaphroditism are apparent. These adolescents have been found to have a normal sex-role identity but abnormal gender identities, suggesting that body image is more a function of self-perception than of environmental factors such as family influence. Further, adolescents with pseudohermaphroditism have reported a delay in dating and sexual relations when compared to other chronically ill adolescents.

Adolescents with short stature can experience rather favorable psycho-social adjustments. For example, adolescents with hypopituitarism compare favorably with healthy adolescents in terms of general adjustment, body image, sex-role development, and sex-related fantasies. Young adults treated with growth hormones have actually reported scores higher than the norms for self-satisfaction, personal worth, and sociality although lower than the norms for evaluation of physical self and self-criticism. They also reported problems with same-sex peer and heterosexual relationships. An age-related decline in psychosocial adjustment has been found for middle adolescents treated with a growth hormone, but a favorable adjustment was found for early and late adolescents. Nevertheless, lower than average employment and marriage rates have been found in young adults with growth hormone deficiency, which, apparently, were not related to their response to therapy.

With increasing age, youth with cystic fibrosis are more likely to express emotional conflicts through physical symptoms, be more anxious in social situations, and experience greater self-doubt, apparently a reaction to doubts about continued survival. On the other hand, five-year survivors of cancer from across the life span are more likely to experience developmental disruptions when in middle childhood or adolescence.

Adolescence is a time of dramatic physical, cognitive, ego, moral, and affective changes, many of which occur concurrently. These changes serve to focus the adolescent on her- or himself in what some have called the ego-centrism of adolescence. Given this intense self-scrutiny, adolescents are acutely sensitive to the evaluation of others. In addition, this intense self-focus often results in a misperception of many youth that adults intuitively know what is going on with them. Adolescents often picture an imaginary audience watching and judging their every action, as if constantly on stage. Along with this sense of preoccupation with self and an exaggerated notion of one's place in the world (either self-enhancing or self-deprecating), adoles-cents also frequently weave a "personal fable." This fable has as a component the belief that negative life events such as illness or disability will not affect oneself; and it is this fable that allows many youths to experiment behav-iorally with a sense of invulnerability not afforded to other generations.

Adolescents will selectively perceive, interpret, and sometimes deny their experience of illness or disability. Of young adults with a measurable disability, only some will consider themselves disabled. Additionally, for adolescents, the perception of being handicapped appears to be more of a transitory state than a stable trait. Reports of being handicapped are based on "hard" measures of illness or disability as well as subjective perceptions of the degree of disability and the adolescents' feelings about themselves. When adolescents report themselves to be handicapped over the course of their high school years, however, they are likely to experience problems with self-esteem, psychological well-being, and locus of control. Young adults may also actually perceive benefits from having a chronic illness or disability: greater appreciation of life, closeness to their families, involvement with others, maturity, and religious feelings. When a subjective reinterpretation of the experience of disability leads to successful coping, this process can be beneficial, but when the reinterpretation is based on a denial of reality, the outcome can be a disturbing noncompliance with necessary medical regimens.

The crucial issue for adolescents with chronic illnesses lies in the artificial social limitations placed on them by the nondisabled society around them. In fact, adolescents with cancer have been found to experience problems with exploring values, formulating goals, and making commitments, although there was no relationship between identity formation and severity of illness. These adolescents need to be integrated into every aspect of society to be able to take full advantage of the resources available to others. Ego and moral development can best proceed if social resources such as peer relationships, meaningful employment, and a challenging education are within the reach of chronically ill or disabled adolescents and reasonable accommodations are made for them to utilize these resources. Ego development requires the fullest possible exploration of the social world. Any adolescent's ego identity is grounded in interpersonal relations; but if discrimination against youth with disabilities and chronic illnesses prevents them from fully engaging socially on the same terms as their nondisabled peers, then the illness or disability will subsume all other aspects of the youth's identity, and the teenagers will come to define themselves primarily in terms of the disability or illness. Another component of the developmental process of adolescence is the assumption of personal responsibility for one's behavior. In relationship to health, this perceptual shift manifests itself in the increasing belief that the teenagers' health behaviors do influence their health status and outcome. Noncompliance with treatment regimens has been found to be related to the restriction of independence in daily life and an external locus of control.

Psychosocial Adjustment

Much research on chronically ill adolescents' psychosocial adjustment published in the 1980s is descriptive, with a cross-sectional design. When comparison groups are used in these studies, they generally consist of healthy controls selected to contrast with chronically ill adolescents from a single diagnostic category. Few studies have employed comparison groups of adolescents with different diagnoses along with healthy or acutely ill controls. By far, the chronic illnesses most frequently studied are cancer, cystic fibrosis, diabetes, and seizure disorders. The primary variables of research interest have included self-esteem, locus of control, independence, psychiatric symptomatology, peer relations, stress and coping, body image, family functioning, and cognitive maturity. Factors thought to influence psychosocial adjustment have focused on illness severity, age at outset, visibility of handicaps, gender, and socioeconomic status. Notably absent in most studies is the direct examination of the effects of race on psychosocial adjustment.

Many early reports predicting psychiatric disturbance for adolescents with chronic illnesses were anecdotal in nature. More recent empirical studies of mixed samples of chronically ill adolescents have found the earlier reports to be exaggerated. Typically, these latter studies find psychologically normal chronically ill adolescents. In one case, chronically ill adolescents actually had higher self-esteem than the comparison group. Admittedly, the sample size was small, yet the results challenge the conventional wisdom about chronic illness. Nevertheless, high self-esteem in chronically ill adolescents is often negatively related to depressive symptoms. Individuals with certain chronic illnesses tend to perceive less control over their health status than do other illness groups or healthy adolescents, but this externality is interpreted as being a realistic response to those particular illnesses. Nonetheless, when the chronic illness is associated with disability or impairment, certain areas of psychosocial adjustment are problematic: future planning, independence, underachievement, family life, and dating.

Many other recent studies compare a group of adolescents with one diagnosis either to a control group of healthy adolescents or to established norms. In general, these studies yield somewhat inconsistent results, in part, perhaps, as a result of differences in sample selection, sample size, age, and instruments used. The picture that emerges about adolescents with chronic illnesses or disabilities is one that describes a few areas of relatively poorer functioning (typically self-esteem) in a context of generally adequate adjustment. Often, as they grapple with the uncertainty of their lives, older adolescents with life-threatening illness may experience more emotional problems than younger adolescents.

Youth with cystic fibrosis, sickle cell anemia, and cancer have been found to perceive little control over their lives, but their coping styles are often quite adaptive. When their coping styles are maladaptive, however, their health status can be compromised. While the effects of stress on diabetic control in adolescents are not entirely clear, poor control has been found to be related to passive styles of wishful thinking and the avoidance of help seeking. When adolescents with cystic fibrosis or asthma have been compared to healthy adolescents on dimensions of control and independence, similarities between the groups are greater than the differences. Few differences are found for managing conflicts, living according to healthy rules, ideals, and opinions on politics, religion, and ethics. Adolescents with cystic fibrosis, in fact, have reported greater independence than healthy adolescents in terms of managing their own affairs. Again, the primary delays in the development of their independence were due to the realistic problems associated with coping with cystic fibrosis.

The types of stress with which adolescents with chronic illness or disabilities must cope differ widely. For some, it is the visibility of the impairment; for others, it is the uncertainty of life, although some investigations have found no relationship between adjustment and severity of illness. Others have found an inverse relationship between visibility of handicap and identity stability, social maturity, and self-esteem. It has also been found that visually impaired adolescents experience a greater number of fears and are more fearful of physically dangerous situations than their peers without visual impairments, while normally sighted adolescents have a greater fear of psychologically harmful situations.

Resiliency of self-esteem in coping with these stresses has been found to be associated with such factors as perception of self as disabled, involvement with household tasks, perception of self as being different from peers, having a network of friends, friends being nondisabled, and parental over-protectiveness. There is, then, an active interplay between adolescents with chronic illnesses or disabilities and the environment that speaks to the benefits of incorporating opportunities for success into the lives of all adolescents.

Social and Sexual Concerns

Sexuality issues for all adolescents are interwoven with issues such as self-esteem, peer relations, and attitudes toward sexuality. Adolescents with a chronic illness or disability have the additional task of integrating issues associated with the illness or disability into the process of their psychosexual development. In such an adolescent's coming to see herself or himself as a sexual being, though, the problem is not always the illness or disability or its medical management but, rather, both the individual's and society's attitudes toward the illness or disability.

Some illnesses or disabilities may complicate sexual expression, and it is reasonable to expect chronically ill or disabled adolescents to address these problems with no greater level of maturity than nondisabled teens. Sexual expression is further complicated for those adolescents and young adults who would compromise their health status by using certain medically contraindicated contraceptives or by becoming pregnant. Incontinence, coitus, orgasm, and masturbation can be problems for adolescents with sensory limitations, spasms, or decreased dexterity, and there can be problems in the management of menstruation for girls with mobility limitations. Although fertility is often unaffected by a chronic illness or disability, it can be a major developmental issue for those young adults who are unable to reproduce. In addition, many teens with chronic illness have misperceptions or a total lack of information regarding their fertility status. While genetic counseling is critical for many teens, it may be a source of embarrassment because of the associated need for comprehensive reproductive discussions.

Social handicaps caused by prejudicial attitudes regarding chronic illness or disability are especially troubling when they appear during adolescence, for such social limitations more often than not constrain the potential of youth. Incorporating opportunities for social interaction with both non-disabled and disabled peers into the lives of adolescents with chronic illness is crucial. Research has found that having nondisabled friends was related to lower self-consciousness, while those adolescents whose best friends were disabled had a more negative body image than those whose best friends were not disabled. Interestingly, having a friend of the opposite gender was related to lower anxiety levels, but dating or having a steady boy- or girlfriend was not related to self-image. Similarly, dating, sharing with friends, and being involved with school activities were characteristics associated with healthy adolescents, not those with a chronic illness.

The sexual consequences of chronic illness or disability can take many forms. Some illnesses, such as cystic fibrosis, are associated with delayed puberty. Adolescents who do not meet their peers' standards of acceptable physical maturity will be relatively unlikely to engage in dating or other social activities. Adolescents with cancer have experienced problems planning for career, marriage, and children, as a result, no doubt, of their realistic fears for the future caused by having cancer. Additionally, family-life education in schools and at home might not be meeting the needs of adolescents with certain disabilities, such as vision and hearing impairments, if methods and materials are not adapted to their needs.

Family

The health-related literature on families of adolescents with disabilities or chronic illnesses largely falls into two categories, one of which, often nonempirical, has a strong family advocacy perspective and typically emphasizes community-based, family-centered systems of care with well-organized case-management components. The second category consists of the empirical research on either the impact of the family on the adolescent's health status or parental stresses resulting from the demands of the illness or disability. Family interactions from a systems perspective are rarely studied. In other words, one body of literature views the family as direct, active participants in the adolescent's total care, while the other sees the family as more of a passive element in a social epidemiological model of dysfunctional development.

Over the past decade, a strong family-centered care approach for children and youth has emerged out of the family advocacy movement. At the very least, family-centered care involves the following components: parent-professional collaboration; comprehensive, flexible policies and programs that take parents' needs and strengths, as well as the developmental needs of their children, into consideration; and the mutual aid found in parent-to-parent support. Family-oriented care is not meant to diminish the role of the adolescent in his or her health care management. As the adolescent's role increases, the parent's role will change. Parents of adolescents often assume "guiding" roles while relinquishing the "directing" roles that had been appropriate for parenting younger children. This role transition can be a difficult one for parents of nondisabled adolescents and will tend to be more complicated for parents of adolescents with chronic illnesses whose care may require constant, life-sustaining monitoring and treatment.

Not only the parent's role needs to change as the child matures; so, too, does that of the child. Until the times of adolescence, the child's main loyalties lie within the family, but then peers increasingly become important, shifting relationships within the family. It is the family context, the family ecology, that is central in determining the ease with which the adolescent can shift these loyalties. A chronic illness or disability can complicate this normal developmental process by presenting additional tasks and roles that might challenge rules or norms in the family that govern the transition to adulthood. An example of this shift in family roles, structures, and relationships can be seen in insulin adjustment with diabetic adolescents, where it has been found that, as anticipated, parents become less involved with the insulin-adjustment process as their children grow older. On average, parental involvement stops when the adolescents are about fifteen years old. Unfortunately, adolescents do not always increase their involvement as their parents decrease theirs. Effective self-adjustment and metabolic control are positively correlated with adolescents' cognitive maturity, but such maturational shifts do not occur at the same time for all youths. Another example of changes in family functioning is found in families of young adults with recently acquired spinal cord injuries. These families experience problems with task organization, interpersonal relationships, family unity, communication, and power structures.

Research that considers family functioning as one factor in the chronically ill adolescents' adjustment often yields somewhat discrepant results. One longitudinal study of adolescents with seizure disorders found that a "disordered home" did not predict the level of independence achieved by the adolescents. A study of adolescents with diabetes found no significant relationship between adolescents' mood disturbances and family characteristics such as socioeconomic status, unemployment, large family size, single-parent family, or serious illness in any family member. These findings contrast with other studies of adolescents with cystic fibrosis and diabetes, which found several types of family functioning to relate to child distress and psychopathology, while permissive child-rearing practices and high educational and vocational expectations were found to be associated in a group of parents of high-achieving deaf students. Similarly, a study of adolescents with epilepsy indicated that a lack of harmony in family relations was related to the adolescents' noncompliance with their health care regimen.

Communication is crucial in families with chronically ill adolescents, although communication is not necessarily enhanced by the presence of a chronic illness, and its effects are not entirely clear. In some studies, communication patterns in families with diabetic adolescents have been found to be unrelated to the adolescents' self-concept and perceived responsibility for self-care and siblings' knowledge about diabetes. Other studies, although finding few family environmental differences between diabetic and acutely ill adolescents, nonetheless also found that greater family control was associated with greater symptomatology in acutely ill adolescents, whereas high levels of organization in families with diabetic adolescents were associated with less symptomatology. Within the diabetic adolescent group, family orientation toward independence, organization, and social recreational activities as correlated with the adolescent's perceived competence and diabetic control. Family characteristics such as overly strict or overprotective parents, however, are often associated with a number of long-term chronic illnesses, while more favorable characteristics, such as sharing and talking with parents and siblings, feeling close to parents, and doing things with the family, are associated with well adolescents.

With such diverse findings, it is difficult to draw many firm conclusions about the role and adjustment of the families of chronically ill adolescents. It is clear that families of chronically ill or disabled adolescents are a population at risk for adjustment problems as a result of the nature of the illness. Some theoretical models predict that a family's adaptation to a stressor such as a chronic illness or disability will depend on its resources, other urgent demands, perception of the significance of the illness, and coping styles over time. These factors account for a large share of the variation in family compliance with treatment for youth with cystic fibrosis, for example. In the same vein, mothers' subjective assessments of their children's illness severity were a more accurate indicator of maternal distress than were professional clinical ratings of the children's illness severity. Given this situation, the primary task for the family will be to attain an equilibrium of functioning that will accommodate both the changes brought about by the illness and the stability necessary for security and growth. Stability and change are related themes as families experience both developmental and situational transitions. With the co-occurrence of normative (adolescence) and situational (illness or disability) transitions, families are likely to experience a heightened sense of vulnerability as their usual patterns of functioning are challenged. Such challenges, though, need not inevitably predict dysfunction. If the appropriate resources—personal, family, community, and health services—are either helped to develop within or directed toward the affected families, a demand-capability imbalance can be avoided.

Knowing when to intervene or provide support or resources is a primary task for professionals. Family intervention services should be offered when the illness or disability is diagnosed, other family members are negatively affected by the illness or disability, family members' behaviors impede the adolescents' progress, the adolescent changes residence, a significant milestone is missed (for example, not graduating from high school on schedule), or the adolescent dies. The goal of intervention is to increase the family's resilience, either by decreasing stress and vulnerability or by increasing the availability of resources. As has been found in work with families of children with cancer, however, a decrease is not an adequate measure of the success of coping, because some stressors are so severe, and coping is so individualized, that an objective decrease in stress is not always a realistic goal.

Educational and Vocational Issues

Not all adolescents with special health care needs receive special education services in the public schools, nor do they all need them. Students eligible to receive special education services are those who have speech, hearing, or visual impairments, mental retardation, serious emotional disturbances, orthopedic impairments, multiple handicaps, learning disabilities, other health impairments, such as autism, or limited strength, vitality, or alertness as a result of an acute or chronic health problem that adversely affects educational performance. Also included are those students who have a specific learning disability as a result of any of these impairments and who need special education or related services. Nationally, for the school year 1986–87, nearly 1.7 million twelve- to seventeen-year-olds and 200,000 eighteen- to twenty-one-year-olds received special education services.

Students now graduating from high school have had the benefit of the educational protections of the 1975 Education for All Handicapped Children Act (Public Law 94-142), which mandates a free, appropriate education in the least restrictive environment. This education is to be facilitated by Individualized Education Plans (IEPs) written for each student with input from professionals, parents, and the students themselves. This law, as others, helped to establish as civil rights issues the special needs of individuals with disabilities. A 1981 government report on disparities in access to special education identified secondary school students and eighteen- to twenty-one-year-olds as an underserved group. In 1983, an amendment to the original law (Public Law 98-199) was passed to establish and fund services to assist in the transition of students from school to work and the community. Further, the vocational education of young adults was aided by the Carl Perkins Vocational Technical Education Act of 1984 (Public Law 98-524), which mandates the development or expansion of quality vocational educational programs with a 10 percent "set-aside" for individuals with disabilities. The Americans with Disabilities Act (ADA) passed in 1990 represents landmark legislation with respect to the civil rights of individuals with disabilities. The ADA provides Americans with disabilities the same rights as other Americans and will have a major impact on employment, accessibility, and transportation. These laws provide the rubric within which education takes place. If the goal of education in general is to help students achieve their potential and live successfully in the community, educating students with disabilities or

chronic illnesses can best be accomplished in a varied and flexible environment supported by individualized educational and vocational transition
planning.

Initially, "mainstreaming" meant offering separate classes in regular
education buildings. Only recently have some students with the more severe
disabilities been integrated into regular classrooms. Concurrent with this
trend has been the extension of related services (for example, intermittent
catheterization) to students with disabilities, affording them the opportunity
to remain in school. There has been a growing awareness that students who
have conditions, such as juvenile rheumatoid arthritis, that do not directly
limit their learning in the classroom may, nonetheless, need special planning
if their health conditions impinge on their awareness of or participation in
prevocational experiences.

On the basis of recent experience, the following have been identified as
key ingredients of special educational services: individualized planning,
functional curricula, long-term transition planning, interagency coordination, parent involvement, and the facilitation of peer relations. Other factors,
though, also influence students' success in school. School absence due to
chronic illness is one such factor. Children and adolescents with a wide range
of chronic illnesses miss more school than well students, but students with
psychosocial problems (for example, behavior, social, family relations,
school, and learning problems), as well as chronic illness, missed even more
school than those with a chronic illness but no psychosocial problems.
Poverty has been found to be associated with the mean number of days absent
for chronically ill youth, while race, sex, and level of maternal education are
not so related. Perhaps contrary to conventional wisdom, school absence
itself is not significantly related to school achievement; however, children with
some chronic illnesses (particularly those, such as epilepsy, that can affect
intellectual development) performed less well on standardized national
achievement tests than healthy peers. Chronically ill students who are of low
socioeconomic status are at special risk for school problems. It is troublesome to note that a significant number of teachers of chronically ill children
are not aware of the children's condition.

Youths with chronic conditions and their parents appear to experience
a number of problems at school. Some report problems coping not only with
restrictions on their school activities and unpleasant experiences with classmates but also with their teachers' lack of awareness of their problems and the
adjustments that they must make. The transition from a mainstreamed to a
segregated residential school is a difficult one for adolescents with hearing
impairments, for example, as they are thought to experience "culture shock"
in a new social atmosphere with a different intensity of communication.
Parents need to be strong advocates for their children in the educational
setting. In one study, nonmainstreamed hearing-impaired students were less
likely to be white, and mainstreamed students were more likely to be from
higher socioeconomic strata. It was found that parents of nonmainstreamed

students were not indifferent to their welfare in this discriminatory setting; rather, what they lacked were the sophistication, experience, time, and energy needed to successfully advocate their children's needs in the education system.

National studies have found that boys and black youths are somewhat more likely than girls and whites to be rated as having a disability that limits schoolwork or recreational activities. When teacher-identified limitations are compared to parental perceptions, it is clear that agreement regarding the need for special educational services is weak. Further, the lower the parents' education and family income, the less likely they are to perceive that their children either need or are receiving special education services. Race has not been found to correlate with either perception of need or awareness of service provision. According to teacher ratings, students with school or recreational limitations are thought to have greater difficulties with academic performance, social adjustment, and school behavior than students without these limitations. Disabled students themselves are more likely than non-limited students to say that they hate school, are only slightly or moderately interested in school, and are ashamed of making mistakes in school. While many educationally limited students' parents expect them to attend college, few of these students themselves expect to graduate from college, far fewer than their nonlimited peers.

According to the Federal Office of Special Education Programs data for the 1985–86 school year, every day more than 300 handicapped students ages sixteen through twenty-one drop out of school before graduation. The dropout rates are highest for students with learning disabilities (47.0 percent), mental retardation (23.0 percent), and emotional disturbances (21.0 percent). Much lower dropout rates are found for students with speech impairments (4.0 percent), hearing impairments (0.9 percent), multiple handicaps (0.8 percent), orthopedic impairments (0.7 percent), visual handicaps (0.3 percent), deaf-blindness (0.02 percent), and other health impairments (2.0 percent).

Perception of disability is an important factor in dropout rates. Students who consider themselves handicapped over the course of their high school years have higher dropout rates than students who consider themselves handicapped for a short period of time or who do not identify themselves as handicapped at all. Disability status, however, does not predict whether students pursue any type of postsecondary education within two years of high school graduation.

Results from an annual survey of two- and four-year public and private colleges and universities found that the percentage of freshmen reporting a disability rose from 2.6 percent in 1978 to 7.4 percent in 1985, although the percentage of enrolled students with disabilities is estimated to be 8.5 percent given full barrier-free participation. There are differences between disabled and nondisabled students, however. In 1985, students with disabilities were more likely to be older, have poorer grades, and be members of a racial minority group. Differences were also apparent in that students with disabilities had lower self-concept ratings and a higher degree of concern regarding finances. Nonetheless, the students with disabilities had higher educational aspirations in several areas than students without disabilities, and they showed a wide variety of career interests.

The impact of chronic illnesses is also seen in career decision making. When chronically ill adolescents were compared to well adolescents, those who were healthy tended to have career plans, while chronically ill adolescents made either indefinite plans for the future or no plans at all. This is a most unfortunate situation, given the significance of career to adults' self-esteem, quality of life, and ability to live independently. Schools are making major efforts in prevocational and vocational training for students with moderate and severe disabilities stressing functional, community-referenced curricula leading to competitive or supported employment. The vocational preparation needs of adolescents with chronic illnesses and less severe disabilities, however, must also be addressed. The loss of their full career contributions to society may be substantial.

Even given special educational and vocational services, youth with disabilities still are not fully employed. U.S. Department of Commerce data from 1988 indicate that 3.8 percent of the population sixteen through twenty-fours years of age have a "work disability" (4.1 percent for males, 3.6 percent for females). Work-disabled people are defined as those who have a physical or mental illness that affects the kind or amount of work that they can do or as those under sixty-five years of age who are covered by Medicare or are receiving Supplemental Security Income. The labor-force participation rates for March 1988 are 40.4 percent for males and 43.9 percent for females ages sixteen through twenty-four with work disabilities, whereas the comparable rates for young men and women without work disabilities are 69.5 percent and 62.4 percent, respectively. The percentages of sixteen- to twenty-four-year-old men and women with work disabilities working full-time year around in 1987 were, respectively, 10.2 percent and 8.7 percent. This compares with 26.6 percent of males and 20.8 percent of females without work disabilities. The presence of a work disability affects not only employment rates but also earnings. For all sixteen- to twenty-four-year-old workers in 1987, the mean earnings were $6,463 for males with a work disability and $7,851 for those without, while the comparable annual earnings for females were $4,910 for those with a work disability and $6,403 for those without. Caution should be taken in interpreting these data, however, because of the small numbers reported.

Policy Issues and Considerations

Most industrialized nations have carefully designed national policies to promote the well-being of their children with and without disabilities; however, that is not the case in the United States. Three factors evident in the past twenty years form a backdrop against which a policy can be considered. The first is the dramatic improvement in mortality rates for many chronic conditions, due, in large part, to advances in medical and surgical care. Survival rates for conditions such as spina bifida and leukemia have increased some 200 percent. Sixty percent of children with cystic fibrosis now survive into adolescence and beyond, with one-third living into their thirties. The National Health Interview Survey indicates an increase in prevalence from 1.1 percent to 2 percent of children in the United States with limitations in major activities of daily living. The cause of this increase is not entirely clear. In part, it may reflect earlier and more accurate reporting, more sophisticated assessment of children, differing survey techniques, and more awareness of disability on the part of the public and parents than previously. Irrespective of the cause, more children and adolescents live longer, more have some continuing disability, and more need changing services over a longer life span.

A second factor deserving consideration is the pervasive change in thinking about how to best provide services to individuals with developmental disabilities. Ideas such as "right to treatment," "least restrictive environment," "due process," and "civil rights" have served to inform policy and shift the provision of services from an institutional approach to one that is community-based. This community-based orientation stresses outcomes for individuals that promote their independence, productivity, and integration into the mainstream of community life.

An additional factor of importance was the passage, in 1975, of the Education for All Handicapped Children Act. This act provided that all handicapped children through the age of twenty-one have available to them a free and appropriate education that emphasizes special education and related services to meet their unique needs. The services were to be provided in the "least restrictive atmosphere" possible. The act made education possible for half a million previously unserved handicapped children and improved educational opportunities for several million others. In addition, the law and the educational opportunities that resulted from it created a new set of life expectations among a segment of society that had previously been socialized to expect little.

Policy through any one of several mechanisms (legislation, direct funding, provision of incentives, education) and at all levels (national, state, and local) can encourage or hinder the development of programs and services. Social policy is inevitably based more on ideology than on information. We know through research that adolescents with chronic illness and disability are more similar to than different from their nondisabled peers. Policy, then, must encourage community-based services designed to assist the adolescent to achieve maximum independence, economic self-sufficiency, and social participation, and to support families in this process.

The concept of family support is based on an awareness that the family remains the primary caretaker of the adolescent. It acknowledges that the

transition from childhood to adult life is complicated for youths with disabling conditions as well as their families. Such family support views the
family as a coequal partner in the therapeutic and rehabilitation process. For
such a partnership to exist, families must be given complete and realistic
information concerning their children's disability, thus allowing them to be
informed consumers and ensuring their involvement in the decision-making
process. Services provided in the community allow the family to be part of
the process, reducing the often overlooked costs of transportation and time
away from work. Recognition that having a chronically ill family member
creates additional stress necessitates the availability of support services such
as respite care, financial counseling, transportation, or equipment. The fact
that chronic illness increases the financial burden of most families necessitates the identification of new financing mechanisms to help them meet the
needs of their children.

Many of the needs and developmental tasks of teenagers with chronic
illness or disability are the same as those of their nondisabled peers. Policy
must be such that it encourages the inclusion of young people in the educational and social activities of school life by removing barriers (physical and
attitudinal) so as to provide opportunities for social maturation and development. The ability to participate in social activities with one's peers and
friends enhances the development of the necessary social skills required to
move away from one's family, work toward economic self-sufficiency, build
family relationships, and understand one's world outside the home and
school.

The adolescents, too, must be given information about their disability
and be actively involved in planning to meet their own health, educational,
employment, and social needs. Professionals of all disciplines need to create
an environment where the young person is comfortable bringing up sensitive
issues such as sexuality and reproduction. Acquisition of information and
knowledge is vital if adolescents are to assume responsibility for their own
health care needs, but knowledge alone is not sufficient. For the teenager,
there must be a shift away from parental supervision to the personal assumption of responsibility for one's illness, disability, and subsequent health
behavior. Planning for the adolescent's transition to adult life must begin
early and include the adolescent, the family, and the health, educational,
vocational, and social service providers in a collaborative team effort.

If the desired outcome is that young people have the opportunity to
work and live in their communities and develop friendships and positive
relationships, then what is needed to foster this outcome? Clearly, specialized
and technological services must be available, but communities must facilitate and nurture the adolescent's involvement in and use of the general
community resources available to other teens and young adults. Research has
shown us that teens with chronic illnesses and disabilities, as well as their
parents, utilize community resources less than do their nondisabled peers.

There is a sense of discomfort that causes such families to withdraw. Community educational activities to promote general public awareness and understanding of the adolescent with a disabling condition as an able individual rather than a handicapped person will positively support the family's and adolescent's development. For we must never forget that the most handicapping aspect of any chronic illness or disability is the social stigma that mainstream society imposes.

Conclusion and Recommendations

Adolescents with chronic illnesses or disabilities experience the same developmental transitions as their well, nondisabled peers, yet their illness or disability places them at risk for certain psychosocial problems in the transition to adulthood. The risk, however, is not solely in the medical complications of the illness or disability, although for some adolescents the health problems themselves are life-threatening. Rather, risk is related to the degree of fit between the adolescent and his or her environment: family, school, peers, health care services, work, and societal attitudes. The fit can lead to optimal integration and development, or it can result in isolation and low self-esteem.

What is needed is a new perspective for seeing adolescents, their illness or disability, factors contributing to problems in adjustment, interactions between parts of the service system, the treatment regimen, and, above, all, the adolescent's future. It is a perspective that would view the teenager in the context of his or her interactions with others, for social dysfunction often is the result of interaction with people rather than something within the adolescent. On the other hand, the favorable general adjustment typically characterizing chronically ill or disabled adolescents can also be attributed to functional interactions among the many factors affecting their lives.

If, indeed, the issues for adolescents with chronic illnesses and disability are complex and interactive, treatment and service planning must be strongly interdisciplinary, involving timely interagency and multisectoral collaboration to meet their many and diverse needs. Teaming and case coordination are essential to this process. Too often, adolescents must function in both a pediatric and an adult health care system, finding that neither alone nor both together will meet their needs for services. Vocational rehabilitation has not yet accumulated sufficient experience in working with young adults with chronic illnesses or disabilities to integrate their unique developmental needs into a planning model. Education has taken the lead in assisting special education students in making the transition from school to work, but very often students with illnesses not directly affecting the educational process do not receive transition planning. The development of an integrated service system, including streamlined financing mechanisms, is crucial to the long-term planning necessary to help youth to make the transition to careers and community living.

The overarching goal of all professionals is to facilitate autonomy, the capacity for engaging in meaningful relationships, and independent career functioning in adolescents with chronic illnesses or disabilities. Progress toward this goal will, in effect, help prevent the social morbidities of these youth. Frequently, attaining the goal of autonomy entails advocating for their needs as well as teaching them self-advocacy skills. Uniformly, this process involves the active involvement of the adolescents and, where appropriate, their families.

Systemwide planning for adolescents with disabilities will also emphasize access to community services that offer planning from a life-span developmental perspective; infants, children, adolescents, adults, and the elderly will all have their developmental needs and contributions addressed. Such services, consumer-oriented in approach and delivery, will operationalize an opportunity structure for adolescents so that they can take advantage of age-appropriate opportunities for community integration: recreation, mainstreamed education, competitive or supported employment, barrier-free housing and transportation, and community-based health care.

Suggested Readings

Anderson, E. M., and Clark L. *Disability in Adolescence*. New York: Methuen, 1982.

Blum, R. W. (ed.). *Chronic Illness and Disabilities in Childhood and Adolescence*. Orlando, Fla.: Grune & Stratton, 1984.

Blum, R. W., and Leonard, B. (eds.). "Youth with Disability: The Transition Years." *Journal of Adolescent Health Care*, 1985, *6* (2), 77–184.

Gavaghan, M. P., and Roach, J. E. "Ego Identity Development of Adolescents with Cancer." *Journal of Pediatric Psychology*, 1987, *12* (2), 203–213.

Gliedman, J., and Roth, W. *The Unexpected Minority: Handicapped Children in America*. New York: Harcourt Brace Jovanovich, 1980.

Hauser, S. T., and others. "The Contribution of Family Environment to Perceived Competence and Illness Adjustment in Diabetic and Acutely Ill Adolescents." *Family Relations*, 1985, *34* (1), 99–108.

Hobbs, N., Perrin, J. M., and Ireys, H. T. *Chronically Ill Children and Their Families: Problems, Prospects, and Proposals from the Vanderbilt Study*. San Francisco: Jossey-Bass, 1985.

Kellerman, J., and others. "Psychological Effects of Illness in Adolescence. I. Anxiety, Self-Esteem, and Perception of Control." *Journal of Pediatrics*, 1980, *97* (1), 126–131.

Office of Special Education Programs. *Tenth Annual Report to Congress on the Implementation of the Education of the Handicapped Act*. Washington, D.C.: Division of Innovation and Development, Office of Special Education Programs, 1988.

Orr, D. P., and others. "Psychosocial Implications of Chronic Illness in Adolescence." *Journal of Pediatrics*, 1984, *104* (1), 152–157.

Owings, J., and Stocking, C. *High School and Beyond: A National Longitudinal Study for the 1980's: Characteristics of High School Students Who Identify Themselves as Handicapped.* Washington, D.C.: Office of Educational Research and Improvement, U.S. Department of Education, 1985.

Resnick, M. S., and Hutton, L. "Resiliency Among Physically Disabled Adolescents." *Psychiatric Annals*, 1987, *17* (12), 796–800.

Smith, M. S. (ed.). *Chronic Disorders in Adolescence.* Boston: Wright, 1983.

Wallach, H. M., and others (eds.). *Handicapped Children and Youth: A Comprehensive Community and Clinical Approach.* New York: Human Sciences Press, 1987.

Wehman, P., Moon, M. S., and Everson, J. M. *Transition from School to Work: New Challenges for Youth with Severe Disabilities.* Baltimore, Md.: Brookes, 1989.

Weitzman, M., Walker, D. K., and Gortmaker, S. "Chronic Illness, Psychosocial Problems, and School Absences—Results of a Survey of One Country." *Clinical Pediatrics*, 1986, *25* (3), 137–141.

Zeltzer, L. K., and LeBaron, S. "Does Ethnicity Constitute a Risk Factor in the Psychological Distress of Adolescents with Cancer?" *Journal of Adolescent Health Care*, 1985, *6* (1), 8–11.

12

Injuries

Carol W. Runyan, M.P.H., Ph.D.
Elizabeth A. Gerken, M.S.P.H.

Today, traumatic injuries are the most serious health problem facing adolescents. In the United States, they result in more than 17,800 deaths and thousands more lifelong disabilities each year among those ages ten through nineteen. Because injuries affect youth disproportionately, more years of potential life are lost from injuries than from cancer and heart disease combined.

Attention to adolescent injury is relatively new, however. Before the turn of this century, adolescence was not even defined as a life stage. Injuries have gained recognition as a significant health concern only over the last two decades. The explanation for this failure of the health professions to address this critical issue may lie both in our concepts of accidents and injuries and in the unique qualities of adolescence as a life stage.

Many of the factors contributing to the excess risks for injuries among

Note: The University of North Carolina Injury Prevention Research Center provided support for the development of this chapter. The authors also acknowledge the conceptual, editorial, and technical contributions of Susan Gallagher, Melissa Kaluzny, David Klein, Jerrel Moore, Desmond Runyan, Laura Sadowski, Deborah Schoenfeld, and Irvin Wolf. The research reviewed in this chapter reflects the work of a considerable number of investigators. Because of space limitations, only a few selected references are listed. However, a complete bibliography is available from the authors.

adolescents are associated with their unique developmental characteristics. These include discrepancies among the physical, cognitive, emotional, and social development processes of youth and the relationship between the adolescents' developmental status and the physical and social environments in which they develop. For example, the hazards associated with mastering a complex social and physical task such as driving are magnified by the adolescent's challenge of adult authority (for example, failing to adhere to speed limits), desire for autonomy (for example, freedom from relying on parental transportation), experimentation with risky situations (for example, driving while intoxicated), and efforts to seek peer approval (for example, experimenting with drugs and alcohol) while enhancing self-esteem (for example, showing off the power of one's car).

However, there is much more to the story. While the characteristics of adolescent development contribute to the injury problem in important ways, their contributions can be understood only in the sociocultural milieu in which they operate. This includes the availability of alcohol and high-powered vehicles, media portrayals of fast driving, drinking, and the nonuse of seatbelts, and the lack of entertainment alternatives that do not require personal transportation. Because of the complex interactions of factors such as these with the adolescent's own development, the prevention of adolescent injuries requires a broad view of multifaceted approaches.

The past failure to adequately address injuries as a health concern is, in part, a function of the ambiguities that envelop our understanding of injury causation and injury prevention. Most early efforts focused on "accident" prevention. More recently, attention has been directed toward injury prevention, which includes the prevention not only of the events ("accidents") that lead to injuries but also of the injuries themselves.

The term *accident* carries connotations that probably have hindered progress in prevention. According to *Webster's* dictionary, an accident is an "unforeseen and unplanned event or circumstance . . . an unexpected happening." This definition implies that injuries are the result of unforeseen, unpredictable, and uncontrollable events. It supports the notion that accidents "just happen" and thereby may limit the scope of injury prevention by suggesting that injury-producing events are inevitable and must be tolerated and that injury prevention is futile. In contrast, *injury* is defined as sudden damage to the body resulting from exposure to a transfer of energy from thermal, chemical, mechanical, electrical, or radioactive sources or from the sudden absence of an essential agent; for example, oxygen in drowning or heat in the case of frostbite. Energy is the agent of injury in the same way that viruses or bacteria are the agents of infectious diseases. It is transmitted to the host by an inanimate "vehicle" (for example, a crashing car or scalding water) or a living "vector" (for example, a biting dog or a stinging bee). Both the disease and the injury processes result from the dynamic interactions among the human host, the agent, and both the physical and social environments.

The implication of this approach is that injuries can be prevented by directing efforts at any or all the elements of the host (for example, the adolescent's behavior), the agent or vehicle of energy transfer (for example, modifying the speed of the car), or the environment (for example, the design of highways or the availability of alcohol and driver's licenses). These interventions can be directed at preventing the initial event that might lead to injury and/or reducing the probability or severity of injuries if the event does occur.

Intentional injuries (homicide, suicide, other forms of assault) and unintentional ("accidental") injuries should be considered together within this conceptual framework. While there are obvious differences in the host's or the assailant's motives, the agent and environmental contributors are often the same. For example, a handgun in the bedside table functions as the injury agent in the unintentional shooting of a child, in a homicide resulting from a domestic argument, and in a teenage suicide, all of which can occur in the home environment. This suggests many very similar approaches to intervention. While the major focus of this chapter is unintentional injury, the problems of homicide and suicide are considered.

The science of injury epidemiology and the practice of injury prevention have begun to emerge. The application of the principles of both epidemiology and prevention to the adolescent injury problem forms the basis of this chapter. In addition, the chapter reviews some major deficits in the data available to provide understanding of the injury problem and suggests specific roles for health professionals in injury prevention.

Epidemiology of Adolescent Injury

Epidemiologists describe the occurrence of health problems at the population level by comparing both frequencies and rates of the problem. While frequencies are useful in understanding the overall size of the problem, rates adjust for differences in group size and permit comparisons among groups. Ideally, epidemiological measures take into account the element of exposure; for example, the hours of football played or mileage driven. This requires information that is often not available. Hence, the comparisons among frequencies and rates must be made with caution, considering the potentially different levels of exposure associated with a given activity. For example, the higher rate of football injuries in males than in females is undoubtedly a function of exposure time, not of some inherently greater sturdiness among females.

Two types of measures of frequency and rate are commonly used: incidence and prevalence. *Incidence* refers to new cases of illness or injury. In other words, each case is counted only during the time period in which it first occurs. *Prevalence*, in contrast, refers to the total number of cases in existence at any given time. When considering acute conditions, it is appropriate to measure incidence. However, chronic conditions are more accurately depicted with prevalence measures. Injuries are typically measured as incident cases, though when considering longer-term disabilities resulting from injuries it is useful to consider prevalence.

The statistic of years of potential life lost (YPLL) is a particularly useful one for making comparisons of problems within a population. This statistic is calculated by summing, across the population, the years between the time of death and a point representing life expectancy or retirement age. For example, if age seventy is defined as the age of life expectancy, years of potential life lost for someone dying at age sixteen would be fifty-four. In contrast, someone dying at age sixty-five would lose only five years of potential life. Summing the years of potential life lost for all people dying in a given year permits comparisons of the relative magnitude of different causes of death in a population.

Data on mortality are derived primarily from death certificates. At the federal level, every state's death records are compiled in a standard format by the National Center for Health Statistics. Included on the death certificate is information about demographics (age, sex, race, residence), as well as the "primary and contributing causes" of death. For injury deaths, causes are based on the International Classification of Diseases (ICD) external cause of injury codes, referred to as E codes. E codes are derived from the description of the injury-producing event. In many states, excellent data on injuries are also available from the medical examiner or coroner system, where more extensive descriptions of the injury event often can be obtained. In some states, this information is computerized, but in most states, the use of medical examiner data requires manual record review. Homicide data are also available, in the aggregate, from the U.S. Department of Justice, Bureau of Justice Statistics, where the reports from state crime control agencies are compiled.

Morbidity information is much less available and generally of poorer quality. The major sources of morbidity data include hospital discharge records, emergency room records, the records of emergency service personnel, private health care providers, or special studies. Because hospitals rely on diagnostic information for cost reimbursement, morbidity data are routinely coded according to diagnosis. In the ICD schema, these codes are N codes, referring to the "nature of illness or injury." The N code allows distinctions, for example, between a fractured femur, a lacerated liver, and a concussion. As mentioned above, another code (E code) is used to depict the external cause of the injury; for example, differentiating a fall down a flight of steps from a motor vehicle crash. Information about the circumstances of an injury that would permit coding of the appropriate external cause is not routinely included in sufficient detail in medical records. Undoubtedly, the extent of E code information included in hospital records is a function not only of the charting practices of clinicians but also of the coding practices of medical records personnel.

Information about injuries associated with consumer products can be obtained from the U.S. Consumer Product Safety Commission (CPSC), which operates the National Electronic Injury Surveillance System (NEISS).

This data-collection system operates in a representative sample of sixty-two hospitals nationwide. It includes routine, ongoing monitoring of all product-related injuries, with more in-depth study of specific products (for example, all-terrain vehicles). In addition to data on emergency room visits, deaths from consumer products are also monitored by the CPSC.

Two ongoing reporting systems catalogue injuries in organized athletics at the high school and college levels. One system, based at the University of North Carolina, monitors all catastrophic injuries, including those resulting in death, paraplegia, quadriplegia, and severe head injury. Another, the National High School Injury Registry, is managed by the National Athletic Trainers' Association and includes similar information on major high school sports.

Economic costs associated with a health problem are another way to gauge the magnitude and distribution of the problem. Usually, figures of dollar costs take into account both direct costs and indirect costs. Direct costs include medical care and rehabilitation expenses; indirect costs include measures of lost wages and productivity. Information about costs is gleaned primarily from health care billing or insurance records.

Mortality Trends

At the turn of this century, injuries were ranked well below the infectious diseases and heart disease as a cause of death. Over the past eighty years, the relative prominence of injuries as a source of mortality in the population overall has changed markedly. As of the mid 1980s, injuries were the fourth leading cause of death overall, following heart disease, cancers, and stroke. Among adolescents, the rate of death due to injuries has changed little. In fact, death rates from violence (homicide and suicide) have actually increased among adolescents in this century.

The injury death rates per 100,000 U.S. population across the age spectrum are depicted in Figure 12.1. As this figure shows, adolescents and the elderly have particularly high injury death rates: of 20 and 78 per 100,000 for youth ages ten to fourteen and fifteen to nineteen, respectively, and more than 80 per 100,000 for people older than age sixty-five. In considering the relative rate of injury death among the elderly as compared to youth, it is important to realize that the case fatality rates (that is, the proportion of all injuries that result in death) are higher among the elderly. That is, for every elderly person injured, the probability of death is higher than it is for a younger person with the same injuries. Consequently, total injury deaths among adolescents are actually reflective of many more injuries than are the total injury deaths among older persons.

Injuries are the leading cause of death among people between the ages of one and forty-four in this country. Among adolescents ages ten to fourteen and fifteen to nineteen, injuries account for 57 percent and 79 percent of all deaths, respectively. In contrast, for people between ages thirty-five and forty-four, injuries account for 30 percent of all deaths, dropping to 7 percent in

Figure 12.1. Injury Death Rates by Age, 1977–1979.

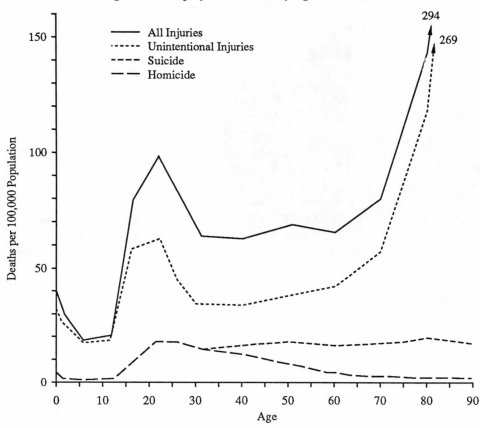

Source: Baker, S. P., O'Neill, B., and Karpf, R. *The Injury Fact Book.* Lexington, Mass.: Heath, 1984. Reprinted by permission of the Insurance Institute for Highway Safety.

the forty-five to sixty-four age group and 2 percent in the over-sixty-five age group. Figures 12.2 and 12.3 show the relative proportions of all deaths within adolescent age groups attributable to unintentional injury and intentional injury as compared to other causes.

Furthermore, injuries far exceed every other cause of death in terms of years of potential life lost (YPLL) before age sixty-five. In fact, in the U.S. population overall, injuries alone account for 40 percent of all YPLL, far exceeding the figures for cancer and heart disease. While cancer contributed, in one year's time, 1.7 million years of life lost, and heart disease and stroke combined contributed 2.1 million years, injuries accounted for 4.1 million years of potential life lost. This clearly shows the disproportionate injury mortality among youth.

Morbidity Trends

Deaths are just the tip of the iceberg. The numbers of nonfatal injuries are much larger. Data from the Massachusetts Statewide Childhood Injury

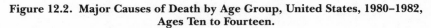

Figure 12.2. Major Causes of Death by Age Group, United States, 1980–1982, Ages Ten to Fourteen.

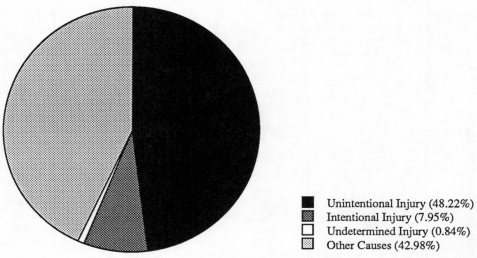

- Unintentional Injury (48.22%)
- Intentional Injury (7.95%)
- Undetermined Injury (0.84%)
- Other Causes (42.98%)

Source: National Center for Health Statistics. *Vital Statistics of the United States.* Hyattsville, Md.: National Center for Health Statistics, 1980, 1981, 1982.

Figure 12.3. Major Causes of Death by Age Group, United States, 1980–1982, Ages Fifteen to Nineteen.

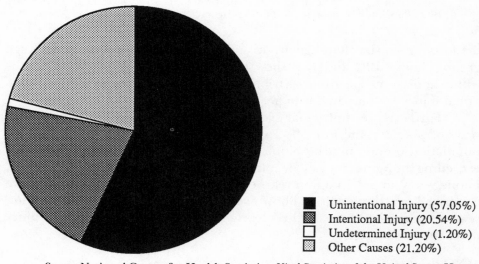

- Unintentional Injury (57.05%)
- Intentional Injury (20.54%)
- Undetermined Injury (1.20%)
- Other Causes (21.20%)

Source: National Center for Health Statistics. *Vital Statistics of the United States.* Hyattsville, Md.: National Center for Health Statistics, 1980, 1981, 1982.

Prevention Program (SCIPP) indicate that for every adolescent (ages thirteen through nineteen) injury death, there are 41 injury hospitalizations and 1,100 cases treated in emergency rooms. Good estimates of the additional number of injuries treated by private physicians, by clinics, by athletic trainers, and at home are not available.

Even data about injuries requiring hospital care are much less complete than is mortality information. There is no comprehensive and consistent nationwide system of hospital record keeping, although a number of states have routine discharge-data-collection systems as part of their hospital rate-setting commissions, and there is a National Hospital Discharge Survey that records information from a sample of hospitals nationwide. However, the inclusion of E code information varies considerably within this system.

Evidence from both North Carolina and Massachusetts indicates that adolescents suffer more hospitalizable injuries than members of other age groups under age twenty. In particular, in North Carolina, fifteen- to nineteen-year-olds alone accounted for 44 percent of all injury-related hospitalizations of people under age twenty in a one-year period (1980), or close to 10 percent of hospitalizations from all causes in the under-twenty population.

Information about long-term disability associated with injury is extremely sparse. Although not specific to adolescents, data from the 1977 National Health Interview Survey indicate that the prevalence of disabilities of at least three months' duration due to injuries was more than 1.7 million among people under age twenty-five. As many as 32,000 of these involved paralysis, and an additional 198,000 people experienced amputations of limbs, fingers, or toes.

Other studies suggest that the annual rate of head injury alone is 300 per 100,000 population of all ages, with the rates highest in the fifteen-to-nineteen age group, particularly among males. While an estimated 5 to 10 percent of victims die as a result of their injuries, most victims of head injury do survive. At least 10 percent of these have long-term neuropsychological sequelae. Until recently, milder cases of closed head trauma often have not been recognized and have been largely ignored as an injury problem. However, some recent studies have suggested that these milder injuries can have long-term behavioral and neurological ramifications.

Cost Trends

The total dollar costs associated with injuries are enormous. These figures include two components: direct costs associated with medical treatment and indirect costs, which are estimates of forgone earnings. As Figure 12.4 shows, adolescents are especially large contributors to the overall economic impact of injuries. The contribution by males in the fifteen-to-twenty-four age group are especially noteworthy. The direct costs are, in the aggregate, lower for adolescents than for the elderly, who frequently require more

Figure 12.4. Estimated Total Injury Costs by Age and Sex, United States, 1977 (Adjusted to 1982 Dollars).

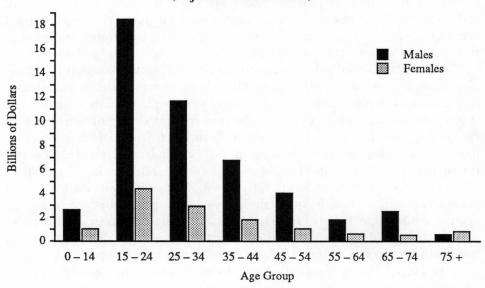

Source: Data extracted from Muñoz, F. "Economic Costs of Trauma, United States, 1982." *Journal of Trauma,* 1984, *24,* 237–244.

hospital care. However, the indirect costs associated with lost productivity are especially great during the adolescent years, particularly if the person suffers a permanent disability.

Etiology

The major causes of injury death among different adolescent age groups are shown in Figure 12.5. The height of each bar reflects the rate of injury death in that age group. Each segment of the bars represents deaths from particular causes. The largest share of deaths is associated with motor vehicles, followed by drowning.

Motor-Vehicle-Related Injuries. These can be subclassified according to whether they involve cars, motorcycles, bicycles, or pedestrians. Table 12.1 details the average annual number of deaths and death rates among adolescents for various types of motor-vehicle injury. Young drivers are especially vulnerable to fatal crashes at night. On a mileage basis, teenagers do 20 percent of their driving at night but suffer more than half of their crash fatalities during nighttime hours. Even taking into account the fact that males drive more than females, the nighttime fatality rates for teenage males exceed those for females by more than two to one. Not only do adolescent drivers suffer, but their passengers are also at increased risk. In fact, the majority of

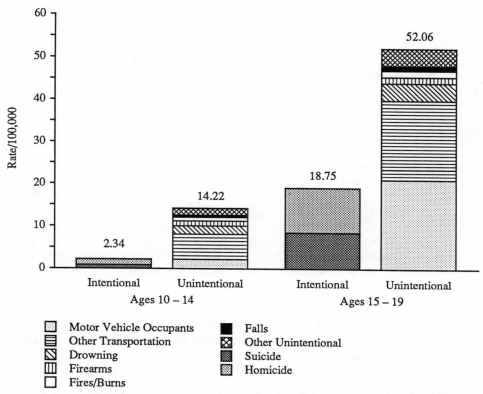

Figure 12.5. Major Causes of Injury Death by Age Group, United States, 1980–1982.

Legend: Motor Vehicle Occupants, Other Transportation, Drowning, Firearms, Fires/Burns, Falls, Other Unintentional, Suicide, Homicide

Note: The cause of injury is undetermined in approximately 1.5 percent of all injury deaths in each age group. These deaths are not represented on this graph.

Source: National Center for Health Statistics. *Vital Statistics of the United States.* Hyattsville, Md.: National Center for Health Statistics, 1980, 1981, 1982.

adolescents killed as passengers are passengers in cars driven by other adolescents. In addition, adolescents are disproportionately responsible for the deaths of other, nonadolescent drivers, passengers, and pedestrians.

Alcohol is an important contributor to the problem. The proportion of fatally injured adolescent drivers who have alcohol in their blood is lower than that of older drivers. However, the rate of alcohol-involved fatalities per miles driven is considerably larger among adolescents. In other words, while adolescents are less likely than older drivers to drive after drinking, those who do are subject to a higher risk of being in a crash than are their adult counterparts. In addition, the blood alcohol concentration in the fatally injured adolescent driver is less, on average, than it is in the fatally injured adult driver. This suggests that it takes less alcohol for the adolescent driver to be at risk for a serious or fatal motor-vehicle crash.

A number of studies have documented that adolescents are less likely to use seat belts than are other age groups. The evidence about the efficacy of seat belts is firm. The failure of adolescents to use seat belts consequently magnifies their risks of suffering serious or fatal injury in crashes.

Table 12.1. Motor-Vehicle-Related Average Annual Deaths
and Death Rates by Age Group, 1980–1982.

| | Ages 10–14 | | Ages 15–19 | |
	Deaths	Rate (per 100,000)	Deaths	Rate (per 100,000)
Motor vehicles	481	2.64	4545	22.12
Drivers	46	0.25	2469	12.01
Passengers	435	2.38	2076	10.10
Motorcycles	104	0.57	723	3.52
Pedestrians	367	2.01	723	3.52
Bicycles	223	1.22	150	0.73
Other and unspecified	203	1.11	1854	9.02
Average annual total	1377	7.55	7996	38.91
Average annual population	18,240,000		20,551,000	

Note: Sums of columns may not equal total because of rounding error in averaging.
Source: National Center for Health Statistics. *Vital Statistics of the United States.*
Hyattsville, Md.: National Center for Health Statistics, 1980, 1981, 1982.

Homicide. Homicide is also an important injury problem for adolescents, especially among minorities. In fact, homicide is the leading cause of death for black American males between ages fourteen and forty-four, with age-specific death rates as high as 99.8 per 100,000. Although homicide rates are highest between ages twenty and thirty-four, regardless of race, adolescents also are at significant risk. In 1983, the homicide death rates were 0.9 and 5.2 per 100,000 for whites in the ten-to-fourteen and fifteen-to-nineteen age groups, compared to 2.8 and 26.7 per 100,000 for blacks in the same age groups.

The homicide problem is primarily one of firearms, with 47 percent of ten- to fourteen-year-old victims and 64 percent of those in the fifteen-to-nineteen age group killed by guns. For adolescent homicides, the ratio of handgun involvement to that of other types of guns is more than five to one among the fifteen- to nineteen-year-olds. The vast majority of this violence is both intraracial and among acquaintances. Poverty is strongly associated with the incidence of homicide. In fact, in aggregate analyses when poverty is controlled, the excess risk among blacks virtually disappears.

Two studies have documented the ownership of firearms by youth. In a 1987 study by the Baltimore City Grand Jury, it was found that a full half of the male youth reported that they had carried a handgun to school, and 60 percent knew someone who had been threatened by a gun. In rural North Carolina, 75 percent of teenagers report that there are guns of some type in their homes, with 55 percent of males owning their own weapons.

As is true with other injury problems, alcohol plays a substantial role in homicide. One analysis has demonstrated that at least 40 percent of homicide victims between the ages of fifteen and twenty-four have measurable blood alcohol levels; 25 percent have blood alcohol concentrations of 0.1 milligram percent or more. Since alcohol content is not routinely assessed for decedents under age fifteen, the true extent of alcohol involvement is probably underestimated.

The impact of televised violence on children and youth has been studied extensively. Although it is impossible to implicate this as a direct causal factor for homicide, the evidence strongly supports the relationship between TV violence and aggressive attitudes and behaviors among youth. With children watching an average of two to four hours of television daily, when 80 percent of all programs contain violence, the potential impact of this factor on adolescent violence is considerable.

Suicide. Suicide among adolescents has gained increasing prominence during recent decades. It is the third leading cause of death for individuals between ages fifteen and twenty-four. As with many other types of injury, males are at greater risk than are females. However, the rates for whites and Native Americans are higher than those for blacks. The trend has shown dramatic increases, with the rates of suicide among adolescents ages fifteen to nineteen having increased from 2.7 to 8.5 per 100,000 population between 1950 and 1980. This rate translates to nearly 1,800 deaths among fifteen- to nineteen-year-olds in 1980. The trend is primarily due to the more than fourfold increase (from 3.7 to 15 per 100,000) for white males. The rate for white females increased over the same time period from 1.9 to 3.3 per 100,000, while the rates for minority males increased from 2.2 to 7.5 per 100,000. Black females experienced the least increase (1.5 to 1.8 per 100,000) during the period. Average annual deaths for 1980–1982 indicate that the overall trend was continuing (1,765 deaths per year; 8.6 deaths per 100,000).

During 1980–1982, approximately 170 young adolescents between the ages of ten and fourteen committed suicide, representing a rate of 0.9 per 100,000, increased from a rate of 0.5 in 1950. The sex and race differences are much less marked than for the older age group. For both age groups, it is likely that the figures are an underrepresentation of reality. Because of the stigma attached to suicide, some physicians are reluctant to record it as the cause of death. In addition, determining whether a given death is a suicide is sometimes difficult, particularly if there is no suicide note. The single-vehicle crash, for example, is a situation where determination of possible suicidal intent is often difficult.

As with homicide, firearms are the leading method of suicide chosen by males ages fifteen to nineteen, accounting for 65 percent of the cases, with hanging the choice in 22 percent. For fifteen- to nineteen-year-old females, firearms have supplanted poisoning as the method of choice since 1972. In 1980, 56 percent of adolescent female suicides were by handguns, 17 percent by poisoning, and 11 percent by hanging. A recent study in Sacramento County, California, indicated that this trend continues and that handguns account for as many as 70 percent of all firearm suicides among persons ages fifteen through twenty-four.

Adolescents are estimated to make about 500,000 suicide attempts each year. Across all ages, males are more likely to succeed in completing a suicide, though females attempt suicide four times as often. At least 80 percent of all people, regardless of age, who commit suicide have attempted it before, and 10 percent of those who attempt it will be successful in future efforts.

Identified risk factors associated with suicide among adolescents include mental illness, feelings of helplessness, family history of suicide, and substance abuse. Recent evidence also indicates that exposure to news stories or television movies about teen suicide may catalyze additional attempts, often with methods imitating those presented in the story. Other observable risk factors include talk of suicide or preoccupation with death; preparing for death by giving away personal belongings; symptoms of serious depression, such as expressed hopelessness or eating or sleep disturbances; and suicide attempt.

Blood alcohol level is not consistently recorded for victims under age fifteen in many locales. However, it has been demonstrated that as many as 25 percent of suicide victims between ages eighteen and twenty-four are legally intoxicated (blood alcohol levels at or above 0.10 milligram percent), with as many as 25 percent more with some alcohol present in the bloodstream. Furthermore, there appears to be a strong association between alcohol involvement and choice of suicide weapon. Suicide victims between ages fifteen and twenty-four who are intoxicated are more than seven times as likely to kill themselves with a firearm than are sober victims.

Drowning. Drowning is also a major injury problem for adolescents, accounting for more than 1,200 deaths in the ten-to-nineteen age group annually, with rates per 100,000 of 2.0 for ten- to fourteen-year-olds and 4.1 for those between ages fifteen and nineteen. The site of adolescent drowning is usually a lake, river, stream, pond, or canal, rather than an ocean or a swimming pool. While the vast majority of drownings occur during the summer months, recreation around cold water, including ice fishing or play on frozen ponds, lakes, and streams, is also a concern, as submersion in cold water poses the added danger of hypothermia and hinders rescue efforts.

Alcohol is involved in close to 40 percent of adolescent drownings. Alcohol not only influences the judgment of the person in a dangerous situation but also increases the likelihood of aspiration of water upon immersion. The extent to which knowing how to swim prevents adolescent drowning is not known. While it certainly cannot hurt, knowing how to swim undoubtedly is not sufficient to prevent drowning, especially if the potential victim or the potential rescuer is drunk.

Sports and Recreation Activities. These activities are leading sources of nonfatal adolescent injury according to data from Massachusetts, where they

**Table 12.2. Numbers and Rates of Injuries in Organized
School Sports, Springfield, Illinois, 1974–1975.**

Sport	Number of Injuries per Activity	Number of Participants	Rate per 100 Participants	Rate per 1,000 Participant Hours
Football	126	445	28.3	1.0
Basketball	29	283	10.2	0.3
Baseball	13	137	9.5	0.5
Wrestling	27	165	16.4	0.5
Gymnastics	2	15	13.3	0.4
Volleyball	4	105	3.8	0.1
Swimming	2	74	2.7	0.0
Track and field	23	289	7.9	5.7
Field hockey	2	65	3.1	0.1
Golf	—	—	—	—
Tennis	1	108	0.9	0.0
Cross-country	—	—	—	—
Badminton	—	—	—	—
All sports	229	1894	12.1	

Source: Zaricznyj, B., and others. "Sports Related Injuries in School-Aged Children."
American Journal of Sports Medicine, 1980, *8,* 318–324. Reprinted with permission.

account for one in fourteen hospitalized injuries among thirteen- to nineteen-year-olds. Injury rates vary considerably by type of sport or recreational activity, as shown in Table 12.2.

Football is one of the most hazardous interscholastic athletic activities, accounting for 28 injuries per 100 participants per year. Between 1973 and 1980, 260 high school and college football players died. Nationwide, the largest share of the injuries are to the knee or ankle, but a significant proportion are to the head and neck, where the severity of impairment is likely to be greater. Improvements in helmet design reduced the frequency of head trauma during the late 1960s and early 1970s but resulted in greater use of the head for blocking. In the early 1970s, this was associated with an increased incidence of neck injuries, including quadriplegia. However, the incidence of permanent quadriplegia declined from an average of 35 cases per year in 1971 to fewer than 10 per year as of 1986. This decrease has been attributed to the 1976 ruling by the National College Athletic Association (NCAA) and the National Federation of State High School Athletic Associations (NFSHSA) that eliminated spearing (using the head to block an opponent while tackling). This form of blocking poses particular risks for intracranial hemorrhage, craniocerebral death, quadriplegia, and other injuries to the cervical spine.

Other organized sports also contribute their share of injuries, with track and field, baseball, and basketball showing the highest rates among the predominantly male sports. In team sports with high female participation, gymnastics poses the greatest risks. Additionally, data from Massachusetts suggest significant risk for injury associated with roller skating among young adolescent girls. Interestingly, most sports injuries occur during practice rather than in actual competition. While this is certainly a function of the greater amount of time spent in training than in competing, it may also suggest problems with training practices.

Other recreational activities that contribute substantially to the adolescent injury problem are bicycling and the use of all-terrain vehicles. Bicycling injuries are greatest between ages five and fourteen, with approximately 70 percent of the 900 bicycling deaths and 550,000 injuries treated in emergency rooms occurring among riders under age fifteen. Among youth, the older the rider, the more likely the injury is to be the result of a collision with a motor vehicle. Crashes involving motor vehicles are more serious, with head injury as the major outcome. As many as 90 percent of all bicycling fatalities involve motor vehicles, and these are largely the result of head injuries. Among nonfatal cases, extremity injuries account for over half, with head injuries being associated with about a third. Across all age groups over age fourteen, as many as 65 percent of the victims of brain injury derived from bicycle crashes were intoxicated.

All-terrain vehicles (ATVs) have become a source of considerable injury and controversy since their introduction into the United States in the 1980s. Originally designed as tractors for use in the flat, wet rice paddies of Asia, these three- or four-wheel vehicles have been adopted for off-road recreational use, with some models capable of speeds as high as seventy miles per hour. Instability of these vehicles, particularly during turns, is a major problem. The injuries have been many, with 238 documented deaths to date and an estimated 85,900 emergency room cases in 1985 alone. For the three-wheel vehicles, 27 percent of the total cases are between ages twelve and fifteen, with an additional 35 percent in the sixteen-to-twenty-four age group. The twelve-to-fifteen age group accounted for 42 percent of the incidents involving four-wheel ATVs, while the sixteen-to-twenty-four age group accounted for 19 percent. Males are involved in close to 80 percent of the cases, most probably a function of increased exposure time.

Injuries from ATVs are primarily the consequence of either hitting an obstacle and/or tipping over. Among all age groups, head injuries are responsible for 70 percent of the deaths and are the major cause of hospitalization. Helmets are used by fewer than 20 percent of the victims, despite clear evidence of their potential to reduce the incidence and severity of head injury. Alcohol has been found to be involved in as many as 30 percent of the cases involving riders over age sixteen.

Occupationally Related Injuries. These injuries are not well documented specifically for adolescents. However, among workers of all ages, injuries account for 98 percent of all the cases of occupational injury and illness. With approximately eight million adolescents between ages sixteen and nineteen in the U.S. civilian labor force as of 1986, the opportunities for injury are considerable.

In the population at large, the occupations with the highest injury fatality rates are mining and quarrying, agriculture, and construction, followed by transportation and public utilities. Motor vehicles are responsible for the largest share of deaths across all industries, though injuries associated with other kinds of equipment and falls, as well as violence, are important sources of occupational mortality.

One study in Massachusetts using hospital-based injury surveillance data provides an indication of the risks for adolescents in the workplace. Among the study population, work-related injury accounted for 24 percent of all injuries to adolescents ages fourteen to nineteen for which the location of injury was known. Males were at four times the risk of females, and injuries were more frequent in the summer months, when more youth are employed and thereby exposed to unfamiliar equipment and environments.

Other investigators suggest that youth who work in retail establishments, especially convenience stores and gas stations, are at risk for shootings. Recent studies in both Texas and California demonstrate that on-the-job homicides accounted for a substantial proportion of all on-the-job deaths. Adolescents working in both gas stations and restaurants have been shown to be at increased risk of burn injury. In addition, it is estimated that 4,000 adolescents between the ages of ten and nineteen suffer nonfatal farm-related injuries each year, while an additional 186 are killed. Fatal farm injuries among teenagers occur at a rate of 16 per 100,000 farm residents, with the rate for males between fifteen and nineteen being more than 30 per 100,000 farm residents per year. The largest proportion of these fatal farm injuries are associated with machinery, but some result from drowning, suffocation, firearms, or trauma caused by an animal.

Risk Factors and Types of Intervention Methods

In order to develop interventions, it is important to understand the risk factors underlying injury problems. Risk factors are those characteristics of the host, the agent, or the environment that are associated with an increased likelihood of injury occurrence.

Risk Factors

As with many health problems, it is very difficult to pinpoint the exact contribution of any given factor, because very few operate independently. Risk factors in many cases are hard to quantify, and interactions among them can influence both injury occurrence and severity. Some factors that are associated with increased risk are considered below.

As has been indicated, injuries occur because of interactions among adolescents and the agents or environments with which they come in contact. Risk factors are associated with the demands of particular tasks and the individual's developmental characteristics, as well as peer, family, mass media, and other cultural influences on adolescent behavior and the injury process. While the specific contributions of some of these elements are not well researched with respect to injuries, their roles in other aspects of adolescent health probably can be generalized to the injury problem.

The availability of cars that are designed to travel at 120 miles per hour presents a considerable risk for youth. Similarly, the extent to which alcohol is marketed actively to adolescents represents a risk factor embedded in our culture. These are just two examples of the risk factors inherent in the products and environments that surround us. Efforts to control these kinds of risk factors differ from those directed purely at the adolescent's behavior.

Alcohol Use. Alcohol use is a major risk factor for all types of injury. Alcohol works in at least three ways in the injury process. First, it impairs the functioning of the user in terms of judgment, increasing the probability that the person will become involved in a potentially injury-producing activity or situation (for example, driving too fast, diving into shallow water, playing Russian roulette). Second, alcohol impairs the ability of the user to perform the tasks necessary to avoid injury (for example, negotiating a slippery curve, swimming to the shore without aspirating water, leaving a burning building). Third, alcohol serves to exacerbate the severity of whatever injuries are suffered.

Because adolescents typically are not experienced drinkers, small amounts of alcohol can have greater effects on them than on the more experienced drinker. This is evident in the case of motor-vehicle crashes.

Gender. Gender is a risk factor for injury in adolescence, as it is in all other age groups. Although there is some variation by cause, overall rates of injury death for ten- to nineteen-year-old males exceed those for females by as much as 9.9:1, as shown in Table 12.3. It is impossible to determine the extent to which this pattern is a function of differing exposures to situations where injuries may occur or to differing susceptibility based on some other factor. For example, it is known that males drive more than females, even in the teenage years, and they are certainly more likely to play football and may be more likely to acquire weapons or engage in activities that could result in drowning. Being male probably is not in itself what puts teenagers at risk; rather it appears that males are more likely to engage in more hazardous activities.

Race. Like gender, race is associated with injury patterns across the life span. For unintentional injuries as a whole, the rates for Native Americans exceed those for blacks and whites by a factor of almost 100 percent. Homicide occurs at considerably higher rates among black adolescents: 27 per 100,000 for blacks age fifteen to nineteen versus 5 per 100,000 for whites in the same age group in 1983. The rates of suicide are higher for both whites and Native Americans than for blacks. Asians are at the lowest risk for all types of injuries.

**Table 12.3. Male to Female Ratio of Unintentional
Injury Deaths by Cause and Age Group.**

| | Age Group | |
Cause	10–14	15–19
Motor vehicle occupant	1.4:1	2.4:1
Drowning	4.7:1	9.9:1
Firearms	6.8:1	8.7:1

Source: National Center for Health Statistics. *Vital Statistics of the United States.* Hyattsville, Md.: National Center for Health Statistics, 1980, 1981, 1982.

Social Class and Locale. In the aggregate, social class and rural versus urban locale have been shown to be associated with many types of injuries, but the specific relationships between these factors and injury in adolescence have not been well described. Certainly, the rural environment presents different types of exposure than does the urban; for example, the hazards associated with farm equipment versus inner-city violence. People who live in poverty, whether in the rural or urban environment, have greater risk for residential fires, homicide, unintentional shootings, drowning, and motor-vehicle-related deaths. It has been postulated that there are also social class differences with respect to the selection of specific types of recreational activities and their inherent risks. This is most likely a function both of the costliness of certain sports activities and of the sociocultural norms associated with choosing specific recreational activities.

Risk Taking and Experimenting. These are normal developmental components of adolescence, as are the processes of achieving autonomy and peer approval. There may be a tendency to want to devise some type of clinically based screening procedure to determine which adolescents are most likely to sustain injuries and thereby target interventions to them. This is impossible. Years ago, the term *accident proneness* was coined in an attempt to define personality attributes of individuals that predispose them to "accidental" injury. While there are clearly population groups, such as adolescent males, at increased risk of injury, it has not yet been possible to pinpoint specific characteristics of individuals that are associated with particularly high risk. Because the social development and behavioral characteristics associated with adolescent injury are universal, the practitioner should consider any adolescent to be at risk. This does not preclude developing individualized interventions suited to the developmental and environmental situations peculiar to any given patient.

Intervention Measures

Obviously, injury interventions need to be tailored to the particular problem at hand. Below, specific intervention measures are reviewed as they pertain to some of the major injury problems faced by adolescents.

Motor-Vehicle Injuries. Motor-vehicle injuries can be prevented by a variety of means. One clear intervention that has gained increasing acceptance over the past decade is the use of seat belts. However, because adolescents are more resistant than other age groups to using seat belts, special approaches to encourage adolescents to use seat belts are necessary. There has been at least one successful intervention to increase adolescents' voluntary use of seat belts. A cash-incentive program based in Chapel Hill, North Carolina, succeeded in increasing observed use among males from just under 20 percent to close to 39 percent and among females from 21 percent to 44 percent over a four-month period. The program involved soliciting donations from parents and private businesses paired with extensive publicity at the high school. Students' cars, identified by bumper stickers, were stopped randomly by study personnel as they entered the school parking lot; if the occupants were wearing their seat belts, they were rewarded with $5 in cash. For students not driving to school, their family cars were identified by bumper stickers. When the occupants were observed anywhere in the community to be wearing seat belts, they were rewarded with $5 the next day in school.

Passive-restraint devices such as airbags or automatic seat belts are becoming increasingly available as a result of federal regulation. These devices are each limited in ways different from standard shoulder-lap seat belts. Airbags, as they are currently constructed, are effective only in frontal collisions, which account for about 40 percent of serious or fatal car crashes involving adolescents. Their efficacy can be enhanced by the simultaneous use of manually operated seat belts. While the efficacy of automatic seat belts is somewhat more limited in side collisions than is the effectiveness of traditional lap and shoulder belts, the use of passive restraints could have a substantial impact on injury reduction, because, like airbags, they do not rely on active compliance with seat belt use each and every time the adolescent drives or rides in a car.

State laws requiring the use of seat belts have proved to be effective in increasing their overall usage. Current estimates suggest that in the thirty-two states with seat-belt laws (at the time of this writing), usage has increased, on average, from between 10 percent and 35 percent to an average of 48 percent after implementation of the laws. The usage patterns for adolescent drivers are less favorable. Adolescents are less likely to use belts voluntarily and also less likely to comply with seat-belt laws than are their adult counterparts.

Other measures that have been shown to be effective in reducing adolescent motor-vehicle injuries are nighttime driving curfews and changes in the drinking and/or driving age. It has been shown that states with nighttime curfews for sixteen-year-old drivers have reduced fatalities in this age group by as much as 69 percent. Since a full 50 percent of fatal crashes of sixteen- to nineteen-year-olds occur between 9 P.M. and 6 A.M., this measure has considerable potential for reducing injury. Drinking-age legislation has passed in all fifty states in recent years. In most states, these laws raised the legal age for alcohol consumption to twenty-one. The results from multistate studies clearly indicate that this is an intervention that is successful in reducing fatal nighttime crashes involving young drivers by at least 13 percent.

Similarly, it has been suggested that the age of driver licensure be increased so that the individual is more mature before taking on the complex task of driving. This approach does respond to the data that demonstrate a disproportionate involvement of young drivers in severe and fatal crashes. However, the approach does not account for the fact that it takes a long time to become a proficient driver, even at older ages. In response to this fact, a strategy that has been proposed by Patricia F. Waller, director of the University of Michigan Transportation Research Institute, is to develop a "graduated driver licensing system" whereby adolescents may actually start driving as early as age fourteen, but only under close parental supervision. Privileges of driving at night, without parents present, and with any alcohol use are phased in over the course of several years. Waller suggests that this could prolong the time in which adolescents are expected to master the task of driving and not force them to master learning to drive and learning to drink simultaneously. Rather, she contends, the two skills would be acquired more gradually, coupled with considerable supervised driving experience.

Driver education has long been endorsed as an intervention to reduce teenage morbidity and mortality due to motor-vehicle crashes. While completion of such a course has been reported to reduce crash involvement, this effect may be due more to the type of individual who enrolls in driver education courses than to the course itself. People who enroll in high school driver training tend to be better students and drive fewer miles, characteristics that are associated with lower levels of crash involvement. Controlling for these characteristics essentially eliminates the protective effects of driver education. In fact, it has been documented that the greater the availability of driver education, the greater the involvement of teenagers in motor-vehicle crashes. This may be the result of larger numbers of adolescents obtaining licenses. Thus, the driver education programs are of mixed value.

Homicide. Homicide prevention has not been well studied and is extremely difficult to study because of the multiple sociopolitical factors that are associated with it. It is also an area that has not received much attention in clinical practice, despite its public health importance. Considering the heavy involvement of firearms in homicides, gun control is one specific step that has been proposed. This measure obviously evokes considerable emotional and political sentiments. It is argued that guns do not kill, people kill, and that appropriate training in gun safety would be the best approach to preventing firearm fatalities. However, valid data in support of this position do not exist. The argument in favor of gun control is based on the correlation between the increased homicide rate and the proliferation in the sale of firearms, especially handguns, over the past sixty or seventy years. Carefully controlled studies of the effectiveness of gun control measures that have been implemented in specific locales, including Detroit, Washington, D.C., and other, smaller communities, have not been published to date, but they should provide useful evidence about the potential effectiveness of this counter-measure. Efforts to incorporate gun detection in some high schools have not been rigorously evaluated and, of course, would have potential impact only upon those assaults taking place on school grounds or possibly while students are going to or coming from school.

An innovative program developed by D. Prothrow-Stith has been targeted at increasing the skills of adolescents in dealing with conflict. The program's curriculum, which has been incorporated into a number of schools in the Boston area, is directed at improving the recognition among youth of hostile feelings and provides instruction and practice in alternative, nonviolent means of expressing anger. It is coupled with a mass media effort directed at dramatizing the adolescent violence problem and addressing the alternative means of conflict resolution. The full evaluation of this program is not yet complete, but the response to the program by the youth has been favorable. This program has relied on public service announcements and other advertising media. Other uses of television programming to foster prosocial behaviors have been suggested as being potentially effective in reducing aggressive and violent behavior among children and youth. In addition, reducing the amount of viewing of televised violence among children and youth may have promise. However, without regulations limiting what is aired, this approach to the problem may not be realized easily, given concerns about censorship.

Suicide. As with homicide, the prevention of suicide is exceedingly complex, and little information exists that demonstrates effective interventions. Given that close to 70 percent of adolescent and young adult suicides are handgun related, reducing the availability of these weapons would probably reduce suicides, although there is no firm evidence to demonstrate this from locales where gun control has been implemented. While it is argued that another method of suicide would replace firearms, it may be that an attempt by firearm is more likely to be successful than an attempt by some other means. This issue needs to be studied more carefully.

The striking contribution of alcohol to youth suicide suggests that reducing the availability of alcohol to teenagers may be an effective intervention. While one study in Massachusetts found no decrease in adolescent suicide after the drinking age was raised from eighteen to twenty, there may be greater promise for this intervention now that all states have implemented such laws and it is no longer possible to travel across state lines to obtain alcoholic beverages.

Other interventions directed at adolescent suicide, such as the provision of crisis centers, telephone hot lines, and secondary school suicide prevention programs, have had only limited success. However, evaluation of these interventions is very difficult. Crisis centers serve predominantly the population of suicide attempters. It is very difficult to determine whether they are working to deter these youth from suicide or whether the users of such services never would have completed the suicide regardless of the intervention. Similarly, hot lines are difficult to assess because the users are often not identified in such a way that it is possible to determine whether they either attempted or completed suicide. The effectiveness of school-based suicide prevention programs also is not easily studied. It has been suggested that the effects of these programs may be delayed until long after the program, when evaluation of impact is hard to document. Concern has been expressed that the programs may increase suicidal ideation and, subsequently, suicide attempts among the population exposed to them. While there is no firm evidence to substantiate this, the data demonstrating that greater media attention to suicide is associated with increased adolescent suicide suggest that the concern may be warranted.

Regardless of the effectiveness of these programs directed at youth, efforts to improve parents', health professionals', and teachers' awareness of the risk factors for suicide among adolescents are appropriate. It is also recommended that practitioners take a thorough psychosocial as well as family and medical history to help identify youth at risk for suicide and to provide appropriate preventive counseling.

Drowning. The prevention of adolescent drowning is very difficult. The major success story in drowning prevention is the use of adequate swimming pool fences. This measure has significantly reduced drownings of young children in Australia and Hawaii. However, most adolescent drownings occur in natural bodies of water so are not as amenable to this countermeasure. Reducing the use of alcohol among adolescents may be an effective means of preventing drownings. To date, there have not been any reports comparing drownings in states before and after the enactment of drinking-age laws.

It might seem that improvements in the overall swimming ability of the population would have a favorable impact on the drowning problem. However, there is no evidence of the numbers of drowning victims who knew how to swim or of the base-line rate of swimming competence in the population. For those adolescents who drown while boating or fishing, particularly those who have been drinking, the use of appropriate flotation equipment has the potential to reduce mortality. However, voluntary compliance with the use of life vests is unlikely to be high among youth, and enforcement of mandatory usage is exceedingly difficult.

Sports and Recreational Injuries. These types of injuries can be prevented through a variety of means. As noted above, changes in blocking and tackling rules implemented in 1976 and improvements in football helmet design have been helpful in reducing serious head and neck injuries among football players. Given that such a large share of sports injuries occur during practice, it is important to have well-qualified trainers and coaches who ensure that youth are properly conditioned and that there is appropriate

medical backup. While there is limited support for the benefits of preparticipation physicals in reducing sports injuries overall, identification of
incomplete rehabilitation of prior injuries appears to be important.

The use of bicycle helmets has the potential to reduce head injury
among cyclists. It has been found that helmets would be relatively ineffective
in most fatal crashes but have considerable potential for reducing the severity
of injury in nonfatal incidents. Several studies have indicated that hard-shell
bicycle helmets could reduce by as much as ten times the incidence of
significant injuries. Despite the demonstrated effectiveness, helmet use is low,
with estimates suggesting that as few as 10 percent of recreational cyclists use
helmets. As of 1986, the United States Cycling Federation made the use of
hard-shell helmets mandatory among all cyclists in sanctioned races. Local
school districts could require helmet use on school grounds and could
conceivably increase usage among students. The provision of bicycle paths,
appropriate maintenance of cycling equipment, and efforts such as incentive
programs to encourage voluntary helmet use all should be considered,
although their actual effectiveness has not been tested adequately.

There has been considerable furor over the use of all-terrain vehicles
during the past several years. As of March 1988, the Consumer Product Safety
Commission instituted a ban on the sale of three-wheel vehicles and ruled
that the sale of four-wheel vehicles must be more closely controlled. In
addition, there have been some local efforts to ban the sale of four-wheel
vehicles on the grounds that they, too, pose significant dangers, particularly
to youthful riders. Since a large proportion of the injuries to ATV users are
head injuries, the use of helmets is recommended. As with motorcycles and
bicycles, the required use of helmets is likely to result in more widespread
protection than is a strategy that relies on voluntary usage. However, there
have been no published evaluations of the effects of either the changes in laws
regarding sale of ATVs or the effectiveness of helmets in ATV crashes.

Occupational Injuries. The prevention of occupational injuries to youth
is, of course, dependent on the type of injury and setting in which they occur.
To a large extent, the occupationally related motor-vehicle and homicide
problems are amenable to many of the same prevention strategies as in
nonoccupational settings; for example, limiting the availability of firearms
and reducing driving hazards. In addition, robberies and shootings in retail
establishments might be addressed through modifications in the hours of
operation, isolation of the facility, access to police protection, access to cash,
or use of bullet-proof shields separating workers from clientele, either within
the shop or through drive-up windows. However, until more is known about
the injury risks faced by adolescents in the work force, few specific recommendations can be made about prevention.

Because agricultural injuries result from many different causes, interventions need to be varied. Some examples include the use of shields or
automatic shutoff devices on certain types of farm equipment to protect
against limbs getting caught in moving parts or rollover protection on

tractors and other riding equipment. Consideration of the appropriate role of youth in farm practices and the need for training to perform certain farming duties could also be more thoroughly addressed. In rural areas, health professionals can rely on the Agricultural Extension Service for considerable expertise on farm safety.

Approaches to Intervention

Because injuries result from the complex interactions of the agent (energy), the human host, and the physical and social environments, there are multiple approaches to prevention and multiple potential targets of change. One schema for conceptualizing the possibilities for prevention is the Haddon Matrix. This matrix combines the public health model of agent-host-environment interaction with the stages of primary, secondary, and tertiary prevention and serves as an extremely useful framework for conceptualizing possible intervention options. The agent-host-environment model serves to identify the elements of the injury process and the possible targets of intervention.

Just as interventions can be targeted at several elements, they also can be directed at several stages of the injury process: pre-event, event, or post-event. These parallel the public health concepts of primary, secondary, and tertiary prevention. Pre-event strategies are those that have their effect before the initiation of the injury-producing event. For example, reducing drinking among adolescents and reducing the availability of handguns are pre-event strategies in that they prevent the crash event or shooting event from occurring. Event strategies are those that are directed at reducing the effects of the event during its occurrence. Seat belts help protect occupants in crashes, just as bulletproof vests would protect in a shooting. Postevent strategies are directed at reducing the longer-term effects of the injury event after it has happened, such as through the provision of timely and appropriate first aid or medical services.

The Haddon Matrix combines these concepts of targets of intervention and phases of interventions. By considering interventions directed at each combination of target and phase, one can think of myriad possibilities. As an example, Figure 12.6 is a completed matrix showing some interventions pertinent to handgun homicide.

Choosing an Intervention

Generating ideas about prevention options is only half the task. Deciding which interventions to pursue and how to evaluate them is, in many ways, much more difficult. When one uses the Haddon Matrix to generate ideas about possible interventions, it becomes clear that there are many ways to intervene. They encompass efforts applied in clinical settings and in schools

Figure 12.6. Basic Haddon Matrix for Generating Countermeasures.

FACTORS

PHASES	Human	Energy Vector	Physical Environment	Social Environment
Pre-event	• Training people to recognize potential assault situations and respond in a self-protective manner	• Modifying guns so they cannot be easily concealed	• Providing a bullet-proof shield • Regular patrols by law enforcement • Surveillance systems, such as videocameras	• Making laws regarding gun ownership and access • Reducing TV violence
Event	• Providing people with bullet-proof vests • Training people in self-defense	• Modifying guns or bullets so they do not inflict serious injury when fired	• Regular patrols by area law enforcement to catch events in progress • Surveillance videocameras to monitor events and provide quick response	• Changing societal norms regarding resistance to assault
Post-event	• Training people in administering first aid for gunshot wounds	• Modifying guns so they must be reloaded after each shot	• Providing close, available medical emergency care • Providing rapidly responding, well-trained emergency personnel	• Ensuring access to emergency medical care for all categories of people, regardless of insurance coverage

as well as changes in various kinds of public policies. The types of interventions can be classified into four broad areas: education, regulation, legislation, and litigation. Health professionals have important roles to play in each.

Educational efforts might be directed at many different audiences, including the adolescents themselves, parents, teachers, manufacturers, and policy makers. For example, education could be directed at convincing adolescents to use their seat belts; parents could be taught how to discuss seat-belt use with their children; manufacturers could be educated about the public views regarding seat-belt design; and policy makers can be educated about the projected effectiveness of a law requiring seat-belt use.

It should be recognized, though, that educational approaches directed toward the individual at risk have traditionally been the least effective means of reducing injury. As with other issues in compliance, there are multiple reasons why a given set of recommendations may or may not be adhered to. These include (1) the complexity of following the recommendations (how difficult is it to make a safe turn on an ATV); (2) the frequency with which the task is required (the helmet must be remembered and used each and every time the ATV is ridden); and (3) the unpleasantness of the regimen (how hot and uncomfortable the helmet is).

In contrast to voluntary efforts that rely on education to promote compliance, regulatory measures typically are directed at changing the environment or consumer products. These regulations are frequently intended to provide passive protection by making changes that do not require individual action. For example, federal regulations require a wide array of safety features on cars (shatterproof windshields, collapsible steering wheels, and, more recently, passive restraints, such as air bags or automatic seat belts). Similarly, numerous aspects of highway design are the result of regulations concerning the physical environment.

While regulations are imposed by governmental agencies vested with regulatory authority by Congress or state legislatures, other measures are directly mandated by legislative action. Legislative measures are usually directed either at changing the environment or at requiring specific behaviors. Examples include the motorcycle helmet and seat-belt laws currently in effect in most states and local ordinances concerned with swimming pool fencing or the purchase of firearms.

Litigation also has been used successfully in some instances to bring about community-wide reductions in injury risk. These have primarily involved product liability claims directed at product manufacturers. Examples include efforts to hold handgun manufacturers accountable for the foreseeable harm associated with their products, lawsuits against toy manufacturers for the hazardous nature of some of their products, and suits against communities that fail to maintain playgrounds in safe condition. At times, the threat of litigation serves as an impetus for voluntary changes.

P. Z. Barry, a specialist in health policy at the University of North

Figure 12.7. The Barry Model for Sorting Countermeasures.

	Active	Passive
Voluntary	• Taking a driver safety training course • Extinguishing cigarettes before going to bed	• Purchasing air bags • Installing a smoke detector
Mandatory	• Seat belt and child safety seat laws • Regulations prohibiting smoking on airplanes	• Passive safety belt systems • Building codes that require smoke detectors in homes

Carolina, categorizes intervention options according to the extent to which they are active versus passive and voluntary versus mandatory. Figure 12.7 provides an example of a completed matrix. Active measures require action on the part of individuals in order to afford protection. In contrast, passive measures are those that involve product design or general environmental modifications. Mandatory measures are those that are required by legislative or regulatory authority, while voluntary measures rely on the cooperation of individuals, product manufacturers, or institutions. In general, mandated passive measures are the most effective. Those relying on voluntary active participation by the person at risk are least effective for all the reasons mentioned with regard to compliance. Measures directed at mandating behavior have some promise, although their effectiveness depends on the motivations of the at-risk population to comply with the law as well as the stringency of the enforcement system. Not surprisingly from a developmental perspective, the willingness of adolescents to comply with some required safety behaviors (for example, seat-belt use) has been demonstrated to be less than that of the adult population. Voluntary measures directed at passive improvements also are of moderate effectiveness. An example of such a measure is the parent's voluntary installation of passive seat belts in the car driven by the adolescent.

There are a number of factors that enter into the decision-making process for the individual clinician, the agency director, or the legislator. These factors have to do with balancing the trade-offs inherent in any kind of choice. Individual freedom is valued highly in our culture. Freedom is compromised by any mandatory measure, yet the gain in overall effectiveness of the measure may be deemed worth the loss in freedom. For example, limiting freedom to ride a motorcycle or bicycle without helmets may be judged appropriate when balanced against the resulting reduction in serious and fatal head injury. Similarly, there are concerns about equitable treatment of those being protected. One example is the concern raised about increasing the drinking age or having differential punishment for drunk driving among adolescents versus adults. While the treatment may be unequal, some would consider such a policy equitable as a means to compensate for the unusually high risk among youth; others would consider it discriminatory and unjustifiable. Certainly, the costs of interventions are an important consideration, but they must be weighed against the cost savings associated with the intervention's effectiveness in reducing death, injury, or long-term disability and all the inherent social and economic effects of those injuries. The balance of these issues will vary depending on the injury problem and intervention options that are available. In their roles as private citizens and community leaders, health professionals need to be aware of these issues and use their knowledge to help clarify the trade-offs in taking differing approaches to injury problems.

Needs for Improving Injury Data

Deciding what interventions to try and evaluating their effectiveness require good data. Data are needed to justify attention to the problem and the targeting of intervention resources to the appropriate population groups or in the appropriate settings. Evaluation is essential to determine whether interventions are working and to differentiate among the relative merits of the various approaches to reaching the desired goal.

Current data-collection systems need extensive improvement. Several specific areas of concern are (1) inclusion of cause-of-injury information (E codes) in medical record-keeping systems, (2) collection of data about injuries requiring treatment at all levels of care, and (3) greater information about exposure to injury-causing agents.

Evidence about the cause of injury is essential for determining appropriate interventions. While diagnostic information helps distinguish skull fractures from concussions or lacerations from contusions, it does not identify factors pertinent to the prevention of the injury. Rather, data about injury causation are essential to differentiate whether the skull fracture resulted from a fall from scaffolding, from a motorcycle crash, or from playing football. Each causal factor requires a different solution. In order to be useful, this information must be derived in the process of taking a medical history. It can be coded appropriately by medical record personnel only if full documentation is included in the patient's chart.

To monitor the injury problem adequately and to be able to define appropriate countermeasures require data collection about the full spectrum of injuries. The recent trend toward developing trauma registries has focused on collecting information about only the most severe cases. In fact, many trauma registries are developed with the expressed purpose of monitoring the quality of care in trauma centers. While this is undeniably an important issue, the data are insufficient to guide prevention planning and may, in many instances, be insufficient to address adequately the quality-of-care questions as well.

The inadequacies of trauma registries are several. There are selection problems associated with who is triaged to a trauma center. It may be, for example, that in some locales, burn cases go to the nearest hospital, while in other locales, they are taken directly to burn centers. If these facts are not considered, the survival patterns for patients in the two areas may be considerably different, yet the reasons may be misattributed to other characteristics of the care received. Trauma registries often define trauma in accordance with the definition put forth by the American College of Surgeons. This definition excludes major types of injury, such as drownings, poisonings, and electrocutions. Third, the emphasis within trauma registries has, to date, been on only those cases that are most severe; that is, cases admitted for treatment in tertiary-care facilities. By definition, injuries treated and released from emergency rooms are eliminated. However, this introduces a bias, not only because the majority of cases are missed but also because those may, in fact, represent a different pattern of injury than the cases requiring inpatient treatment. Just as it is clearly inappropriate to assume that patterns of death are similar to patterns of nonfatal injury, it is also inappropriate to assume that patterns of injuries treated in emergency rooms parallel those requiring admission to the hospital. For example, car-bicycle collisions are more likely to result in serious injury requiring hospitalization, while bicycle crashes not involving motor vehicles are generally less serious. Focusing only on hospitalized cases could potentially lead to conclusions about countermeasures aimed only at reducing car-bike crashes. In contrast, including the less serious cases could suggest other interventions that might have impact on a considerably larger pool of bicycle crashes.

Another injury-data issue is the measurement of exposure. This is a difficult task and typically requires data collection outside the health care delivery system. For example, in making adequate conclusions about the risk of motor-vehicle crashes involving adolescent drivers, it is important to document both the numbers of adolescent drivers and the extent to which they drive. This kind of exposure information serves as the denominator in calculating rates. It allows comparisons that take into account whether adolescents contribute disproportionately to motor-vehicle crashes or become involved in crashes at rates no different from those of their parents. Data from transportation or insurance authorities can be obtained to document the numbers of licensed drivers and, in some cases, estimate the numbers of miles driven by those drivers. However, this kind of exposure information is not available for most other types of injuries. For example, it is unknown how many people know how to swim or do swim; how much time or how many miles are logged on bicycles or all-terrain vehicles; or how ownership of handguns is distributed among the population.

Other data needs include information pertaining to long-term outcomes and the costs associated with injury. Documenting outcome requires a record-keeping system with the ability to track injured patients over time and through various systems of health care, educational, and rehabilitation services. To be able to document cost, there need to be options for linking data from the health and other service delivery systems with insurance records. Provision of the kinds of identifying information necessary to accomplish either linking or tracing is sometimes resisted because of fears of compromising confidentiality of either patients or health care providers. Both tracing and record linkage have been done in many settings without jeopardizing confidentiality. In any such deliberation, the gain in the ability to fully understand the injury problem and its consequences needs to be carefully weighed in the equation. The health professional must be involved in helping ensure that record-keeping systems are well designed and appropriately used.

The Roles of Health Professionals

Health professionals clearly have a role to play in all types of interventions: as counselors and educators of patients in the clinical setting, as educators of professionals and parents, as community leaders, and as policy advocates. They also can play a vital role in ensuring that clinical injury data are recorded carefully and completely. Specifically, practitioners can advocate for the consistent use of E codes in all clinical records and make concerted efforts to document clearly the external cause of injury events in their own case descriptions. Finally, there are important roles in conducting injury research and, of course, in providing care for the injured patient.

Clinicians can apply their influence and expertise in working with specialists in health behavior, health education, and social policy to effect changes in the whole complex of factors contributing to the adolescent injury problem. It is critical that the multiple, interacting dimensions of the problem be considered and that interventions be chosen with care. Efforts to change individual behavior probably will continue to have limited success unless they are based on sound tenets of health behavior and adolescent development. Furthermore, the approach must recognize the need for more broad-based modifications in the social and physical environments of the adolescent.

Working with decision makers and other community leaders is a vital activity for health professionals. Just as the enactment of the child restraint laws in all fifty states had its origins in the individual effort by one pediatrician in Tennessee, so can other injury initiatives be spearheaded locally by individual practitioners. This type of activity requires the development of coalitions with various health professionals, leaders in related fields, such as education, fire protection, and crime control, and a broad spectrum of parents, community leaders, and elected officials. While advocacy may not be as easy for those in private practice as for those working in other settings, the health care practitioner is well positioned to exert leadership even with modest investments of time. Likewise, it is important to remember that advocacy can take many forms, which include forming and leading community-interest groups; testifying before local, state, or national decision-making bodies; preparing papers and presentations to inform other practitioners about the nature and magnitude of the injury problem; participating in continuing education offerings about the topic; writing letters to elected officials about important injury issues within their authority; or serving as a resource person for community groups, the media, or technical and advisory bodies.

Over the next decade, the opportunities for research about injuries are bound to expand as the field matures and funding agencies become more aware of the magnitude of the problem and opportunities for intervention. Health professionals need to be involved in shaping the research agenda, helping to merge clinical and research expertise. Moreover, clinicians must become involved in improving the record-keeping systems that will permit themselves and others to study the injury problem, design appropriate interventions, and evaluate the effects of those interventions. Finally, health professionals should be willing to apply research findings in clinical settings and to facilitate the translation of research to policy through regular contact with decision makers.

Suggested Readings

Baker, S. P., O'Neill, B., and Karpf, R. *The Injury Fact Book*. Lexington, Mass.: Heath, 1984.

Berkelman, R. L., Callaway, J. L., Howard, L. B., and Sikes, R. K. "Fatal Injuries and Alcohol." *American Journal of Preventive Medicine*, 1985, *116*, 21–28.

Brent, D. A., Perper, J. A., and Allman, C. J. "Alcohol, Firearms, and Suicide Among Youth: Temporal Trends in Allegheny County, Pennsylvania, 1960–1983." *Journal of the American Medical Association*, 1987, *257*, 3369–3372.

Centers for Disease Control. *Homicide Surveillance: High Risk Racial and Ethnic Groups — Blacks and Hispanics, 1970–1983*. Atlanta, Ga.: Centers for Disease Control, 1986.

Centers for Disease Control. *Youth Suicide in the United States, 1970–1980*. Atlanta, Ga.: Centers for Disease Control, 1986.

Gallagher, S. S., Finison, K., Guyer, B., and Goodenough, S. "The Incidence of Injuries Among 87,000 Massachusetts Children and Adolescents: Results of the 1980–81 Statewide Childhood Injury Prevention Program Surveillance System." *American Journal of Public Health*, 1984, *74*, 1340–1347.

Haddon, W. "Options for the Prevention of Motor Vehicle Crash Injury." *Israeli Journal of Medical Science*, 1980, *16*, 45–65.

Klauber, M. R., Barrett-Conner, E., Marshall, L. F., and Bowers, S. "The Epidemiology of Head Injury." *American Journal of Epidemiology*, 1981, *113*, 500–509.

Kraus, J. F., and Conroy, C. "Mortality and Morbidity from Injuries in Sports and Recreation." *Annual Review of Public Health*, 1984, *5*, 163–192.

Kraus, J. F., Fife, D., and Conroy, C. "Incidence, Severity and Outcomes of Brain Injuries Involving Bicycles." *American Journal of Public Health*, 1987, *77*, 76–78.

National Academy of Sciences. *Injury in America*. Washington, D.C.: National Academy Press, 1985.

Newman, R. *Analysis of All Terrain Vehicles Related Injuries and Deaths*. Washington, D.C.: U.S. Consumer Product Safety Commission, 1987.

Prothrow-Stith, D., and Spivak, H. "The Violence Prevention Project: A Public Health Approach." *Science, Technology and Human Values*, 1987, *12*, 3–4.

Rivara, F. P. "Fatal and Nonfatal Farm Injuries to Children and Adolescents in the United States." *Pediatrics*, 1985, *76*, 567–573.

Rosenberg, M. L., Smith, J. C., Davidson, L. E., and Conn, J. M. "The Emergence of Youth Suicide: An Epidemiologic Analysis and Public Health Perspective." *Annual Review of Public Health*, 1987, *8*, 417–440.

Runyan, C., and Gerken, E. A. "Epidemiology and Prevention of Adolescent Injury." *Journal of the American Medical Association*, 1989, *262*, 2273–2279.

Runyan, C., Kotch, J. B., Margolis, L. H., and Buescher, P. A. "Childhood Injuries in North Carolina: A Statewide Analysis of Hospitalizations and Deaths." *American Journal of Public Health*, 1985, *75*, 1429–1432.

Waller, J. A. "Methodologic Issues in Hospital Based Injury Research." Paper presented at the 31st meeting of the American Association for Automotive Medicine, New Orleans, Sept. 28–30, 1987.

Williams, A. "Fatal Motor Vehicle Crashes Involving Teenagers." *Pediatrician*, 1985, *12*, 37–40.

Wintemute, G. J. "Firearms as a Cause of Death in the United States, 1920–1982." *Journal of Trauma*, 1987, *27*, 532–536.

Wintemute, G. J., Kraus, J. F., Teret, S. P., and Wright, M. "Drowning in Childhood and Adolescence: A Population Based Study." *American Journal of Public Health*, 1987, *77*, 530–832.

13

Disorders of Self-Image, Depression, and Suicide

Daniel Offer, M.D.
Eric Ostrov, J.D., Ph.D.
Kenneth I. Howard, Ph.D.

Much has been written in the clinical literature about disturbed adolescents who come for treatment. Recently, interest has shifted to disturbed adolescents in the community who are not receiving treatment. The goal of this chapter is to adduce evidence concerning adolescent self-image disorder, depression, and suicide among all adolescents so as to better inform prevention and intervention efforts.

Historical Perspective

Adolescents first became the subject of intensive study in the early 1900s, beginning with the work of G. Stanley Hall in 1904. Hall's thesis was that individual development recapitulates human evolutionary development. Hall viewed adolescence as similar to a prehistoric period when the human species began to break with the dictates of instinct and culture became preeminent. On the basis of this view, Hall characterized adolescence as filled with turmoil, rebellion, and *sturm und drang*.

Writers grounded in a different theoretical orientation have maintained and buttressed this view of tumultuous adolescence. Freud's position

Note: Preparation of this chapter was supported in part by a research grant awarded to Daniel Offer by the Chicago Community Trust, 1985–1988, and in part by research grant #RO1MH42901 awarded to Kenneth I. Howard by the National Institute of Mental Health.

was that individual development reflects the shaping, inhibition, or expression of human instincts. It is axiomatic in psychoanalysis that a prerequisite for normal development is resolution of oedipal instinctual strivings through the ages of about four through six. Psychoanalytical theory holds that this resolution is followed by a prolonged latency period during which instincts are for the most part successfully repressed, and less drive-dominated activities, such as mastering skill-requiring tasks, are pursued. In the Freudian tradition, adolescence has been described as an upsurge of instincts and disrupted interpersonal relationships. The ubiquity and stability of this characterization of adolescence have been bolstered by the experience of clinicians in their primary contact with disturbed adolescents who are patients or with adult patients who recall their tumultuous adolescence. Anna Freud probably represents the most extreme of psychoanalytical views. In 1958, she described adolescence as marked by an intensification of the struggle between ego and id. In her view, adolescent aggressive impulses are characteristically intensified to the point of unruliness and even criminal behavior. Anna Freud believed that being in equilibrium during adolescence is itself abnormal.

Later psychoanalytical authors sounded the same theme. Thus, in 1967, P. Blos, a major psychoanalytical theoretician in the area of adolescence, wrote that adolescence is the only developmental period during which ego and drive regression is an obligatory component of normal development. Recently, we showed that this view of teenagers as normatively in turmoil continues to hold sway among mental health professionals. Many of these professionals, our research shows, describe normal teenagers as being disturbed and as unhappy as hospitalized, psychiatrically ill teenagers describe themselves.

The likely consequence of clinicians' believing that turmoil and disrupted relationships are normative for adolescence is that they will not identify emotional disturbance or unhappiness during adolescence as a cause for concern unless it is so extreme that it is intolerable to either the adolescent or the adults with whom the adolescent has contact. Among clinicians who believe that adolescent turmoil or unhappiness is normative, only the most disturbing or undeniably disturbed adolescents may generate concern and inspire intervention.

Empirical studies of large groups of adolescents have revealed that the vast majority of adolescents are not in great turmoil. Most adolescents are not in a state of rebellion against other family members, and most have relatively smooth transitions to adulthood. Moreover, most report having adapted without undue conflict to the bodily changes and emerging sexuality that occur during puberty.

Ironically, then, early theories of adolescence, which emphasize the supposed inherent turmoil of this stage, may overestimate the extent of normative psychopathology among teenagers, while underestimating the amount of psychopathology among those who are truly disturbed. By describing only those adolescents who seek (or, more likely, are brought in to receive) intervention, some clinical studies tend to deflect attention from disturbed adolescents in the community, such as those who are depressed, shy, withdrawn, and even suicidal, who are not receiving help. Studies of the epidemiology of adolescent disturbance will help fill gaps in our knowledge, enabling us to more accurately identify the needs of disturbed adolescents and more efficiently direct mental health resources toward them.

Disorders of Self-Image

Clinically based theories of poor self-image among adolescents abound. These theories typically connect poor self-esteem during adolescence with negative childhood experiences that make the teenager less able to cope with the stresses and tasks associated with adolescence. These tasks include going through puberty, beginning to separate from parents, and forming a socially acceptable individual identity. Low self-esteem might be interpreted as an inferiority complex with origins in early experiences of failure or humiliation. Low self-esteem of teenagers might be viewed as a consequence of experiencing, on many occasions, feedback from others that one is not worthy or admirable. From a psychoanalytical, developmental point of view, as described by H. Kohut in 1971, low self-esteem in a teenager might have its roots in a lack of appropriate parental admiration or "mirroring" during his or her childhood. Kohut also has speculated that low self-esteem can conceal underlying grandiosity; the clue to this phenomenon is that overt low self-esteem stems from an adolescent's holding unreasonably high standards that subtly reflect an overinflated opinion of self.

Empirical studies of adolescent self-image provide a different perspective than do clinically derived theories on the consequences of low self-esteem in adolescence. The teenage years can be viewed as involving a series of tasks—including separation from parents, becoming autonomous, and forming one's own identity—that engender self-doubt. Research has shown that young adolescents are less self-confident than are older adolescents. Teenagers with low self-esteem are more likely to be lonely, bored, unhappy, and isolated than are teenagers with high self-esteem. Another clue to the role of low self-esteem during adolescence is provided by research that shows that over the course of several decades, there has been a strong correlation between the adolescent suicide rate and the proportion of adolescents in the total population of the United States (adolescent density). One explanation for this correlation is that disturbed adolescents become even more alienated, isolated, and unhappy when exposed to many peers—a large number of whom, presumably, they experience as more competent and happy than they are. Another explanation of this correlation is that an increased proportion of adolescents in the general population leads to a relative scarcity of resources for each adolescent. Adolescents with low self-esteem may be at a disadvantage in obtaining such resources, in the first place, and more sensitive to their not being available, in the second place. Thus, when resources become scarce, mortality in the low self-esteem group increases.

Epidemiological studies indicate that, of those tested at any one time, 10 to 30 percent of adolescents attest to being psychiatrically ill to a clinically significant degree. One study showed that about 20 percent of the boys and girls studied reported feeling depressed, with great difficulty sleeping and waking unnecessarily early in the morning.

In this country, there have been relatively few studies of the prevalence or types of emotional disturbance among adolescents. A 1974 study by T. S. Langner, J. C. Gersten, and J. D. Eisenberg in New York City showed that about 20 percent of the black and Hispanic children showed extreme impairment rates, whereas only about 10 percent of the white children did. And in a 1979 study of sophomores, juniors, and seniors attending a midwestern urban, lower-middle-class high school, A. Locksley and E. Douvan found that teenage boys experience a significantly higher frequency of aggression and feelings of resentment than do females; on the average, females report a significantly higher frequency of psychosomatic symptoms and feelings of tension. Unfortunately, these data did not include an estimate of the prevalence of psychiatric disorder among the adolescents studied.

Depression

Until recently, many mental health professionals believed that major depression could not be found among children; there is less question about whether it can be found among adolescents. One problem has been the tendency to assume that a wide range of behavior reflects underlying depression even if typical symptoms of depression such as tearfulness or lethargy are not present (the concept of "masked depression"). Given the theory, for instance, that acting-out behavior actually reflects or masks underlying depression, one could conclude that all delinquents actually are clinically depressed. Symptoms of adolescent depression appear to be similar to those found among adults. This phenomenon seems to have the same familial concomitants as does its adult counterpart and a parallel biological basis. Similarly, depression among adolescents appears to have the same cognitive and interpersonal roots as depression among adults. Cognitive concomitants of depression include negative thinking, pessimism, and hopelessness. Interpersonal roots of depression include identifying with a depressed significant other and "learned helplessness"; that is, a pervasive sense of incompetence that leads to expecting no reward for effort expended. Theoretically, depression may first be seen in adolescence, because it is at this stage that children can first make the consistently negative self-attributions that typify depression. At this stage, too, children become more able to reflect cognitively on the self, providing the preconditions for the pathologically low self-esteem often found in depression.

Studies of depressive symptoms among adolescents show that, compared with adults, adolescents have similar depression "persistence"; that is, they report feeling symptoms of depression most or all of the time during the preceding week at the same rate as adults. A study of seventh- and eighth-graders from one parochial school in suburban Philadelphia using the Beck Depression Inventory as a source of data concluded that about a third of the early adolescent sample exhibited moderate to severe depression, while only 2 percent exhibited severe depression. A seminal study of a representative sample of fourteen- to eighteen-year-old public high school students in New York State in 1971–72 found that adolescents from families with very low incomes were more depressed than those in any other group. Girls were more depressed than boys. One prevalence rate cited in this study was that 20 percent of the adolescents reported being very bothered about feeling sad or depressed in the past year.

Adolescent Suicide

Between 1956 and 1976, adolescent suicide increased dramatically in the United States. There was a 300 percent increase in adolescent male suicide and a 200 percent increase in adolescent female suicide. During the same time period, there was a decrease in suicide among people over sixty-five. It was the opinion of some epidemiologists that the rate of adolescent suicide would continue to soar. This has not, however, been the case. In a 1990 volume, P. C. Holinger and D. Offer summarize their work on adolescent suicide, which had originally predicted that the suicide rate among youth would slowly decline during the 1980s. As data from the *Vital Statistics of the United States* shows, suicide rate among youth (ages fifteen through twenty-four) between 1977 and 1983 did indeed decrease (see Table 13.1). Between 1984 and 1986, the suicide rate increased somewhat, but it was still below the 1977 level. There is no question that the suicide rate among youth has not continued to increase in the past ten years. Holinger and Offer developed a population model hypothesis to explain those changes. The model stressed that it was important to know the proportion of adolescents relative to the remainder of the population, since that would explain some of the changes in the suicide rate. They looked at the cohort theories of G. E. Murphy and R. D. Wetzel from a different perspective by showing that the post–World War II baby boom provided us with an unusually large adolescent population between 1960 and 1980, with resultant social and economic distress and, consequently, higher suicide rates in this group. Now that this group has moved on to young adulthood, the suicide rates for adolescents (and the crime rates from juvenile delinquency) have begun to fall.

Holinger and Offer's theory lends itself to a more flexible approach to suicide rates within a given cohort as it ages, rather than a more fixed view such as the one espoused by H. Hendin. Whereas Hendin's view predicts continued increases as the baby-boom cohort moves into old age, Holinger

Table 13.1. Suicide Rates Among the Young: 1977–1986 (Fifteen- to Twenty-Four-Year-Olds).

Year	Rate[a]
1977	13.6
1978	12.4
1979	12.3
1980	12.3
1981	12.3
1982	12.1
1983	11.7
1984	12.5
1985	12.0
1986	13.1

[a] Rates are calculated per 100,000 population.
Source: Holinger, P. C., and Offer, D. *Adolescent Suicide.* New York: Guilford Press, 1990. Data are originally from the Biomedical Division of the United States Department of Health Statistics.

and Offer's, by contrast, is consonant with the observed data (namely, decreasing rates in the elderly) by explaining that an increased proportion of elderly people in the population can bring about better legislation (for example, Medicare and Medicaid) and thereby sufficiently improve the quality of life for the elderly to cause decreased suicide rates.

Our data are related to M. H. Brenner's and R. A. Easterlin's work. Brenner demonstrated that indicators of economic instability and insecurity, such as unemployment, were associated over time with higher mortality rates, including suicide and homicide. His explanation for this association was that the lack of economic security is stressful — social and family structures break down, and habits that are harmful to health are adopted. Some data show that suicide, homicide, and accident rates are parallel over time and may all reflect self-destructive tendencies to some extent. Brenner's model suggests a reason for the parallel rates: economic cycles. Easterlin has related population increases and decreases in economic conditions among adolescents that correspond clearly to the decreases and increases, respectively, in the youthful population data.

Holinger and Offer's emphasis on "period effects" (events impinging on a cohort at any given point in time) rather than on "cohort effects" (effects described as though they were static over a given cohort's lifetime) provides a theoretical view that fits the data. Hence, we might expect to see further decline but definitely no increase in suicide rates among youth during the next decade.

From a clinical point of view, teenagers who commit suicide, the literature shows, consist primarily of socially isolated young white males. Feelings of abandonment, hopelessness, loneliness, and isolation are prominent among adolescents who attempt suicide. Progressive or continued isolation in early childhood is more indicative among youths of a serious prognosis for suicide than is an early history that indicates an ability to form interpersonal relationships. Depressive syndromes are common. One find-ing in the literature is that about a third of adolescents hospitalized with a history of attempted suicide did not subsequently receive any psychiatric care and did not tell about the attempt until much later. It is clear that many adolescent suicide attempts go unnoticed, or at least unreported. Suicidal adolescents have been described as "loners." As M. L. Peck described them in a 1982 article, in *Adolescent Psychiatry*,

> [The loner] frequently has a long history of spending much of his spare time alone. . . . These young boys tend to have very poor interpersonal relationships with peers and adults. They tend to feel isolated and lonely much of the time, with no one to confide in when they feel upset. When they do make friends, the relationship is often superficial. . . . When these youngsters are seen psychiatrically, the most common diagnoses are borderline state, schizoid personality, and depressive character. Unlike other kinds of adolescent suicides, these youngsters are less likely to communicate or signal their impending suicidal at-tempt. . . . Often, when faced with increased stresses such as dating, graduating, getting a job, going to college, or going away from home, he becomes overwhelmed with the hopelessness of that situation. He is unable to share these feelings with anyone, and may enter into a full-blown suicidal crisis, feeling helpless, hopeless, and totally alienated.

Research by P. A. Marks and D. L. Haller has shown that, as compared with nonsuicide attempters, adolescents referred for suicide attempts are characterized by sadness, emotionality, and a proclivity to react to frustration through inappropriate self-criticism. Male suicide attempters lack close rela-tionships with male peers. Female suicide attempters characteristically have few or no friends during childhood and are not able to talk about their personal problems with anyone. During adolescence, female suicide at-tempters are alienated from family and peers. They feel socially isolated and rejected by their parents. The fantasizing or planning of suicide among teenagers usually indicates that the youngster has reached such an extreme of depression that he or she has to reach out for someone to listen, understand, and assist in finding a new life direction.

A recent approach to the study of suicide among teenagers consists of performing "psychological autopsies" on adolescents who have committed suicide. The procedure consists of gathering a large amount of information from records, diaries, notes, and interviews with friends and parents regard-ing the adolescent prior to his or her suicide. The corresponding research is

Table 13.2. Sample Studied in Three Midwestern High Schools.

Subject	Surburban Teenagers (N = 294)		Urban Teenagers (N = 203)		Total
	Male	Female	Male	Female	
White	126	135	0	0	261
Black	6	7	101	99	213
Other	13	7	3	0	23
Total	145	149	104	99	497

Note: Two suburban high schools, $N = 294$; one urban high school, $N = 203$; total adolescents studied in 1987, $N = 497$.

ongoing, and the results, while promising to be of extreme interest, are not yet available.

A Recent Epidemiological Study

Recently, we carried out a study of disturbance among adolescents under the auspices of the Chicago Community Trust and the Center for the Study of Adolescence at Michael Reese Hospital and Medical Center, in Chicago. Its primary purpose was epidemiological: to determine the prevalence of disturbance among adolescents in several communities and how many disturbed adolescents had obtained help and, if they had obtained help, from what source. The subjects were drawn from three high schools. The high schools were located, respectively, in an all-white, upper-middle-class suburb of Chicago, an integrated middle-class suburb of Chicago, and an all-black, lower-middle-class to working-class area in Chicago. The final sample consisted of 497 adolescents. Some characteristics of these teenagers are shown in Table 13.2.

Research instruments administered to these adolescents included the Offer Self-Image Questionnaire (OSIQ), the Delinquency Checklist (DCL), the Symptom Checklist (SCL), and the Mental Health Services Utilization Questionnaire. The OSIQ is a self-report questionnaire that measures adjustment in eleven areas relevant to an adolescent's life. It inquires about areas of functioning such as relationships with parents, the adolescent's body, and how he or she copes with the internal and external world. The DCL is a self-report inventory of extent of delinquent behaviors engaged in. Examples of behaviors inquired about are running away from home, stealing, and problems with the police. The SCL covers a wide spectrum of psychiatric symptomatology. It inquires about symptoms such as palpitations, light-headedness, hopelessness, and phobias. On the basis of their OSIQ, DCL, and SCL factor scores, adolescents were defined as either disturbed or nondisturbed.

With the use of the OSIQ alone, 12 percent of the adolescent boys and 15 percent of the adolescent girls were found to be disturbed; with the use of the DCL alone, 4 percent of the boys and 6 percent of the girls were found to

Table 13.3. Percentage of Usage of Mental Health Resources in the Past Year by
Disturbed and Nondisturbed Adolescents in Three Communities.

Type of Mental Health Resource	Type of Community/Status					
	UMC[a] Suburban Normal (N = 145)	MC[b] Suburban Normal (N = 43)	MC Suburban Normal (N = 76)	MC Suburban Disturbed (N = 30)	LMC[c] Urban Normal (N = 165)	LMC Urban Disturbed (N = 38)
Mental health professional	14	33	5	33	1	5
Alcohol/drug abuse center	0	5	0	0	0	0
Teenage drop-in center	3	5	0	3	0	3
Crisis hot line	0	0	0	0	3	3
School counselor	6	12	15	13	21	32
Clergy	3	2	0	3	1	0

[a]UMC = upper-middle class
[b]MC = middle class
[c]LMC = lower-middle class

be disturbed; with the use of the SCL alone, 4 percent of the boys and 3 percent of the girls were found to be disturbed. When all three tests were used simultaneously, results showed that 18 percent of the boys and 21 percent of the girls were disturbed.

The Mental Health Utilization Questionnaire was used to identify the number of disturbed and nondisturbed teenagers who had visited mental health professionals. Since many adolescents have used school counselors or social workers in a therapeutic way, it was hard to differentiate between casual use of these professionals (for instance, to discuss low grades or choice of college) from actual treatment. As a result, the criterion used was that the adolescent must have had more than three visits to any mental source to be considered to have used mental health services.

Table 13.3 shows the extent of utilization of various types of mental health resources in the previous year by disturbed and nondisturbed adolescents in the three communities studied. Suburban children revealed the highest use of services of mental health professionals. One-third of the disturbed adolescents in the two suburban samples had used mental health services in the previous year, whereas only 5 percent of disturbed adolescents in the inner-city black community had used mental health services. In addition, an appreciable number (14 percent) of nondisturbed adolescents had used professionals' mental health services in the upper-middle-class white suburban community. This rate of utilization contrasts with that found among nondisturbed adolescents in the middle-class integrated community (5 percent) and in the black inner-city neighborhood (less than 1 percent). In contrast to results pertaining to mental health professionals, results show that disturbed urban teenagers use school counselors to a greater degree than do disturbed suburban teenagers (32 percent versus 13 percent). School counselors clearly play a greater role in treating disturbed urban teenagers than suburban teenagers.

One implication of these results is that many disturbed adolescents are not receiving treatment. Even in the suburban communities, two-thirds of the disturbed adolescents had not received any treatment in the previous year. Data show that 40 percent of the disturbed suburban teenagers had never received any mental health treatment. Among disturbed inner-city adolescents, the results are even more compelling. In that community, 95 percent of disturbed adolescents had not received treatment in the past year, and 79 percent had never received any treatment at all. These findings have strong implications for the effective use of mental health resources: it is clear that among the subjects studied here, most are not receiving mental health care.

Treatment and Prevention Implications

A minority of adolescents are disturbed in the sense of feeling bad about themselves. That minority, however, represents a very large number of teenagers when viewed nationally. In the United States, there are about nineteen million adolescents in school. If 20 percent of these adolescents are disturbed, there are nearly four million teenagers who may require some kind of help or intervention. At least two-thirds of these children are receiving no help or are not disturbed enough to attract attention. One could conclude that at least two million adolescents are quietly disturbed and are not receiving or have not been identified as needing help.

Theories describing unhappiness and turmoil as a normal and expected part of adolescence tend to militate against taking a particular interest in adolescents who are unhappy, particularly if they are unhappy in a nondisturbing way. Our research has shown that approximately 50 percent of disturbed teenagers—as shown by their having a negative self-image in a number of areas—remained disturbed when studied a year and a half later. Many studies show a persistence of emotional disturbance during the teenage years into adulthood. The clinical literature indicates that some lonely and withdrawn adolescents may end their lives through suicide. However, the vast majority of disturbed adolescents may never manifest a disturbance in any overt way. They may never reach out for or receive psychiatric help or counseling. If not helped, they may grow up to be disturbed adults, possibly showing pathology at a later stage of life or perhaps just passing their disturbance on to a new generation.

For disturbed adolescents, it may be necessary to offer help in innovative ways, be sensitive to sub rosa pleas for help, and to ask whether help is needed. For many disturbed adolescents, school counselors are the professionals most likely to be seen. These counselors, particularly in urban areas, should be given the resources needed to identify and encourage treatment for depressed or otherwise disturbed youth.

Disturbed adolescents attest to relatively poor adjustment in a number of areas. One conclusion is that these adolescents, male and female, want to relate to other people. They may be quietly unhappy, but they have not given up hope of relating to others.

Summary and Conclusion

The thesis of this chapter is that there is a relatively large group of adolescents who are deeply disturbed, many quietly. We contend that these teenagers are not simply manifesting transient, age-appropriate angst. Instead, persistent low self-esteem and depression are unusual in adolescence. Moreover, disturbed adolescents probably will continue to be disturbed throughout adulthood. It is possible that offering and encouraging these adolescents to accept help might save them years of anguish and in some cases may prevent suicide.

Many teenagers in need of psychiatric help or counseling do not receive it. Many of these unhelped adolescents probably are too shy and withdrawn to reach out for help and too lonely, quiet, and depressed to reach out for intervention. One definition of loneliness is a yearning for others that goes unfulfilled. The evidence is that most adolescents in need of help are not receiving it. Offering a helping relationship to disturbed adolescents may yield a surprisingly receptive response. It also may prevent considerable suffering.

Suggested Readings

Adler, A. *The Practice and Theory of Individual Psychology*. New York: Harcourt Brace Jovanovich, 1924.

American Psychiatric Association. *Diagnostic and Statistical Manual of Mental Disorders (DSM-III)*. (3rd ed.) Washington, D.C.: American Psychiatric Association, 1980.

Blos, P. "The Second Individuation Process of Adolescence." *Psychoanalytic Study of the Child*, 1967, *22*, 162–185.

Brenner, M. H. *Time Series Analysis of Relationships Between Selected Economic and Social Indicators*. Springfield, Va.: National Technical Information Services, 1971.

Brenner, M. H. "Mortality and the National Economy." *Lancet*, 1979, *2*, 568–573.

Crumley, F. E. "The Adolescent Suicide Attempt: A Cardinal Symptom of a Serious Psychiatric Disorder." *American Journal of Psychotherapy*, 1982, *36*, 158–165.

Czikszentmihalyi, M., and Larson, R. *Being Adolescent*. New York: Basic Books, 1984.

Douvan, E., and Adelson, J. *The Adolescent Experience*. New York: Wiley, 1966.

Easterlin, R. A. *Birth and Future*. New York: Basic Books, 1980.

Erikson, E. H. *Childhood and Society*. New York: Norton, 1950.

Farberow, N. L. "Adolescent Suicide." In H. Golombek (ed.), *The Adolescent Mood Disturbances*. New York: International Universities Press, 1983.

Freud, A. "Adolescence." *Psychoanalytic Study of the Child*, 1958, *16*, 255–278.

Freud, S. *A General Introduction to Psychoanalysis*. New York: Washington Square Press, 1935.

Goswick, R., and Jones, W. H. "Components of Loneliness During Adolescence." *Journal of Youth and Adolescence*, 1982, *11*, 373–383.

Graham, P., and Rutter, M. "Psychiatric Disorder in the Young Adolescent: A Follow-Up Study." *Proceedings of the Royal Society of Medicine*, 1973, *66*, 58–61.

Hall, G. S. *Adolescence: Its Psychology and Its Relation to Physiology, Anthropology, Sex, Crime, Religion, and Education*. New York: Appleton, 1904.

Hendin, H. *Suicide in America*. New York: Norton, 1982.

Holinger, P. C., and Offer, D. *Adolescent Suicide*. New York: Guilford Press, 1990.

Hudgens, R. W. "Suicide Communications and Attempts." In R. W. Hudgens (ed.), *Psychiatric Disorders in Adolescents*. Baltimore, Md.: Williams & Wilkens, 1974.

Kandel, D. B., and Davies, M. "Epidemiology of Depressive Mood in Adolescents." *Archives of General Psychiatry*, 1982, *39*, 1205–1212.

Kohut, H. *The Analysis of the Self: The Psychoanalytic Study of the Child*. Monograph no. 4. New York: International Universities Press, 1971.

Krupinski, J., and others. "A Community Health Survey of Heyfield, Victoria." *Medical Journal of Australia*, 1967, *54*, 1204–1211.

Langner, T. S., Gersten, J. C., and Eisenberg, J. D. "Approaches to Measurements and Definition in Epidemiology of Behavior Disorders: Ethnic Background and Child Behavior." *International Journal of Health Services*, 1974, *4*, 483–501.

Locksley, A., and Douvan, E. "Problem Behavior in Adolescents." In E. Gomerer and V. Frank (eds.), *Gender and Disordered Behavior*. New York: Brunner/Mazel, 1979.

Marks, P. A., and Haller, D. L. "Now I Lay Me Down for Keeps: A Study of Adolescent Suicide Attempts." *Journal of Clinical Psychology*, 1977, *33*, 390–400.

Mitchell, J. R. "Normality in Adolescence." *Adolescent Psychiatry*, 1980, *8*, 201–213.

Murphy, G. E., and Wetzel, R. D. "Suicide Risk by Birth Cohort in the United States, 1949–1974." *Archives of General Psychiatry*, 1980, *37*, 519–537.

Offer, D., and Offer, J. B. *From Teenage to Young Manhood: A Psychological Study*. New York: Basic Books, 1975.

Offer, D., Ostrov, E., and Howard, K. I. *The Adolescent: A Psychological Self-Portrait*. New York: Basic Books, 1981.

Offer, D., Ostrov, E., and Howard, K. I. "The Mental Health Professional's Concept of the Normal Adolescent." *Archives of General Psychiatry*, 1981, *38*, 149–153.

Offer, D., Ostrov, E., Howard, K. I., and Atkinson, R. *The Teenage World: Adolescents' Self-Image in Ten Countries.* New York: Plenum, 1988.

Oldham, D. G. "Adolescent Turmoil: A Myth Revisited." *Adolescent Psychiatry,* 1978, *6,* 267–282.

Ostrov, E. "Loneliness, Shyness, and Withdrawal in Adolescence." In R. A. Feldman and A. R. Stiffman (eds.), *Advances in Adolescent Mental Health.* Vol. 1, part B. Greenwich, Conn.: JAI Press, 1986.

Ostrov, E., Offer, D., and Howard, K. I. "Gender Differences in Adolescent Symptomatology: A Normative Study." *Journal of the American Academy of Child and Adolescent Psychiatry,* 1989, *28* (3), 394–398.

Peck, M. L. "The Loner: An Exploration of a Suicidal Subtype in Adolescence." *Adolescent Psychiatry,* 1982, *9,* 461–466.

Rabichow, H., and Sklansky, M. D. *Effective Counseling of Adolescents.* Chicago: Follet, 1980.

Rutter, M., Graham, P., Chadwick, O.F.D., and Yule, W. "Adolescent Turmoil: Fact or Fiction?" *Journal of Child Psychology and Psychiatry,* 1976, *17,* 35–56.

Westley, W. A., and Epstein, N. B. *The Silent Majority: Families of Emotionally Healthy College Students.* San Francisco: Jossey-Bass, 1969.

Wylie, R. L. *The Self-Concept Theory and Research.* (rev. ed.) Vol. 2. Lincoln: University of Nebraska Press, 1979.

14

Maltreatment of Adolescents

Joanne Oreskovich, M.A., Ph.D. candidate
Robert W. ten Bensel, M.D., M.P.H.

"The world is passing through troublesome times. The young people of today think of nothing but themselves. They have not reverence for parents or old age. They are impatient of all restraint. They talk as if they alone know everything." These words were written by Peter the Monk in 1274.

How do we as parents and as a society interact with and care for our adolescents in today's world? This chapter provides a framework to facilitate an understanding of the social construct of the issues of neglect and abuse. It examines the magnitude of the problem and some of the developmental and social factors that characterize the victimization both of and by adolescents. It reviews particular methodological issues and current theoretical debates in the study of abuse and neglect of adolescents, as well as implications for practical recommendations.

History

Our current conception of what constitutes neglect and abuse results from redefining and relabeling due to changes in society's consciousness and awareness of child-rearing practices that previously were accepted but now are considered unacceptable by the majority of society and according to law.

The authors wish to express their gratitude to Chris Dropik for her excellent secretarial support. This work was made possible by the support of the Bureau of Maternal and Child Health (Training Grant #MCT0100), Department of Health and Human Services, Washington, D.C.

As Herbert Blumer posited in *Social Problems*, "Society problems are not the result of an intrinsic malfunctioning of a society, but are a result of a process of definition in which a given condition is picked out and identified as a social problem. A social problem does not exist for a society unless it is recognized by that society to exist." Some basic human issues, such as abandonment, incest, and cruelty, remain and never vanish, but emerge or reemerge occasionally as social problems, though not necessarily as the same kind of problem with the same suggested solution.

What adult behaviors are considered neglectful or abusive depends on the particular culture's interpretation of the role of the child and youth, the limits placed on parental behavior, and various social and economic factors. Child neglect and abuse occur within a family and cultural context: a context that shapes our view of youth and how they should be treated in it. Circumstances that we now consider horrendous were considered normal ways of rearing children in earlier historical periods. Historically, religious and secular laws have been based on the concept of "reasonableness" and the development of a social order that fosters trust and consistency in the lives of children; thus, there has been some interest over time in determining when a person becomes "unreasonable" and, hence, abusive or neglectful.

In antiquity, the beating of children was widely condoned, especially in the name of discipline for the child's education. Yet limits were set by societies through written language such as the Talmud, which states, "If you must beat a child use a strand of straw." The book of Proverbs contains many statements about the care and instruction of children. Proverbs 2:15 states that "foolishness is bound up in the heart of the child, but the rod of correction drives it far from him." Yet Proverbs 19:18 says, "discipline your son while there is hope; do not set your heart on his destruction." Discipline implies direction and limits to correction. The "rod of correction" refers to "support" or a "walking stick," while the "staff" is to "lift sheep who have fallen off the path back on the path" and "give direction to get back to the flock." The directional implication of discipline is stated in Proverbs 22:6: "Bring up a child in a way he should go, and when he is old he will not depart from it."

Concern for the child was demonstrated in the fourth century A.D., when Constantine the Great (A.D. 280–337) introduced the concept of *parens patriae*, which is the precedent for the legal principle of the state's intervention in family life when the level of care falls below an established minimum. He articulated the principle of the government's role in providing for the vital needs of children—maintenance (food, clothing, and shelter) and education—and in setting legal standards to guard against exposure and infanticide. A child's needs stood in relationship first to the family and second to the state, but always with the caveat that "the state should not be a parent." The state's role was to provide appropriate caring parental substitutes when parents failed.

The concepts of boundaries within which parents can deal with their children and beyond which the intervention of other societal institutions is required was thus established in our language. When the Germanic tribes invaded the Roman Empire in the late fourth century A.D., they brought with them the Visigothic code and the concept of "reasonableness" in dealing with children. In the sixth and seventh centuries A.D., the Old German word *evil* meant "exceeding the boundary" or "causing harm," usually implying intent. *Wickedness* has meant evil that is intentional. Thus, through distinctions in language, the cultural limitations about appropriate behavior for the era can be observed.

The idea of "reasonable" limits was further established through subsequent developments in the law. In the thirteenth century, it was the law that "if one beats a child until it bleeds, then it will remember, but if one beats it to death, the law applies." During the Renaissance, the law admonished, "approval of beating judiciously applied, hit him upon the sides . . . with the rod, he shall not die thereof." The acceptance of physical punishment persisted throughout Western history, such that, as DeMause wrote in his book *The History of Childhood*, of the 200 surviving biographical statements prior to the year 1690, only three did not report beatings.

During the mid-eighteenth century, there was a gradual rise in the understanding of pain and suffering, and severe physical punishment of animals, women, and children began to decline. In the nineteenth century, the whipping of children started to diminish in many Western societies; however, it was not until 1986 that Britain, with a long tradition of school caning, ended this practice. Today, the United States remains the only "developed country" to allow corporal punishment of school-age children, at least in thirty-one of the fifty states as of 1989.

In a discussion of the victimization of and by adolescents, the emphasis on the sociocultural context is an ever present aspect of the scientific enterprise. The concepts of adolescence, discipline, and reasonableness in the treatment of youth have had different connotations over time. The concept of adolescence as a stage in human development is fairly recent in our history. While children's lives were once not considered to be distinct from the lives of adults, today we consider the onset of adolescence as a crucial period in which important developmental tasks are to be mastered. The establishment of one's own identity is one of these tasks, as is autonomy from parents. It is this period of self-absorption between childhood expectations and envisioned adulthood that has the potential of creating conflict between parents and youth. The perceptions and expectations of society, parents, and adolescents toward parental care influence what is reported as adolescent maltreatment. The images of adolescence contribute to the context in which the dynamics of maltreatment take place, as well as how we define what is normal and abnormal conflict in adolescence.

Thus, at various times in our history, distinctions have been made about which behaviors are considered neglectful or abusive, laws have been created regarding these behaviors, and some remedies have been suggested.

However, it is only recently that the maltreatment of adolescents has begun to attract serious public attention.

Contemporary Definitions of Adolescent Abuse and Neglect

A Chinese proverb states that "the beginning of wisdom is to call things by their right name." Herbert Blumer has reminded us that definitions such as those used in the study of adolescent maltreatment contain many ambiguities, and careful consideration of the sociocultural context is required before specific behaviors can be identified as harmful to the child or as social problems. As societies change, so do our definitions and conceptions of social problems. Cultures that must rely on oral history must by necessity have close-knit families for communication of cultural values and, therefore, place more stress on similar values than is the case in "more developed" societies. An oral tradition from Africa states that "a loving parent's hands must be soft as feathers and not cast iron and not break bones." The Havasupai Indians, who, in the 1920s, were the last Native American tribe to be "discovered," had an oral tradition that "a whipped child loses courage and his soul withers and dwindles away until he dies, for the soul of a child is a tender thing and easily hurt." In more traditional societies, taboos, rules of discipline, and maintenance of incest prohibitions are more inviolable than in Western settings. As societies become more complex, values become more diverse and less unified. Today, in America, organized "proincest" and "propedophilia" groups have values opposed to those of child protection advocates. The René Guyon Society, for example, believes that children need sex with compassionate adults to reduce delinquency, suicide, gang warfare, and assault. Their slogan is "sex by eight or else it's too late."

In contemporary America, there is a blurring of boundaries between acceptable and unacceptable behaviors. Close scrutiny by the state and others has been viewed as a violation of the family's sanctity or, at times, a violation of the exercise of one's religious prerogative. The failure to establish clear boundaries of reasonableness leads to what Alice Miller refers to as "poisonous pedagogy"—early conditioning of the child that is based in the belief that the child's behavior is bad and that the parent is motivated by good. This sets the stage for the parent to be always "right" and for parents and other adults to blame children for their behavior ("blaming the victim"). Miller extends this concept to explain why our society has such a difficult time in defining and dealing with child maltreatment.

Despite conflicting values, contemporary definitions of abuse and neglect have been adopted. Since the mid 1970s, definitions of abuse and neglect in the United States have been based on identifiable and documented harm to a child that can be attributed to acts of commission or omission by a caretaker. The primary conceptual model of neglect views it as an *omission* of care, usually combined with an unintentional *chronic behavior pattern* of the parent(s), either lack of availability or lack of parental skills. Abuse, on the other hand, is considered to result from acts of *commission* — an intentionally excessive punishment or sexual activity that leads to harm or threat of harm. The community standard of what is "reasonable" or "acceptable" has become the basis by which professionals judge adequate child care or maltreatment of children for purposes of reporting maltreatment. Culturally sensitive working definitions of child maltreatment are based on concepts of harm to children that result from human behavior that is prohibited, immediate, and preventable. Yet, to date, the focus of attention in child maltreatment is primarily on young children.

This age orientation stems from Kempe's landmark publication "The Battered Child Syndrome," in which he reported the results of a survey of district attorneys who reported the cases of more than 700 severely beaten children where the perpetrators were criminally prosecuted. "The syndrome may occur at any age," Kempe said, "but, in general, the affected children are younger than 3 years." Kempe's concern was for the protection of the very young child, who is more vulnerable to physical sequelae of abuse than older children. While that publication greatly heightened both the general public's and professionals' awareness of the problem of child abuse, the focus was on the plight of young children, and the concerns of neglected and abused school-age children and adolescents were largely neglected. However, the first laws passed as a result of Kempe's article, which were enacted in 1963, were designed to protect all children, including adolescents. And, in 1974, the Child Abuse Prevention and Treatment Act reiterated that protection from maltreatment applied equally to all children under the age of eighteen. But, since young children sustain the highest mortality and morbidity from abuse, the majority of intervention and prevention programs have remained focused on preadolescents.

In 1976, the first national conference on adolescent abuse was held at the University of Minnesota, and the concern for neglected and abused school-age children began to increase. Throughout the 1970s, professionals mandated to report abuse began to extend beyond physicians to include other professionals, especially schoolteachers. Since that time, school-teachers have become the largest group of professionals reporting child maltreatment, especially emotional neglect, which accounts for approximately 20 percent of total reports. There has been a move to include reporting by a broader range of professionals. For example, Minnesota became the fourth state to require clergy to report in 1988.

The Child Abuse Prevention and Treatment Act was amended in 1978 to add sexual abuse (pedophilia, incest, and child pornography) to the definition of child abuse. The inclusion of sexual abuse further increased the focus on sexual offenses against adolescents. Thus, with this expanded re-porting network, the scope of reported abuse began to expand. Not only was sexual abuse a concern in the adolescent age group, but so, too, was physical maltreatment. Grants became available for demonstration programs for physically abused children in the late 1970s and early 1980s. The current trend is a change from treatment to primary prevention.

The most practical way to look at definitions of child maltreatment is to know state laws and consult with appropriate professionals (for example, local child protective services or district attorneys' offices). In general, the concepts of physical abuse, neglect, and sexual abuse are defined according to whether they occur within or outside the family. Therefore, in order to assess maltreatment definitions, one should refer to individual state laws regarding intrafamilial abuse, institutional abuse, and so on. In addition, the federal guidelines have been changing throughout the years. For instance, in 1983, "Baby Doe" legislation was recommended for all state laws in which medical neglect was defined. States may broaden federal definitions in defining child maltreatment (including, for example, emotional abuse). Use of illicit drugs such as cocaine during pregnancy has been termed neglect by the states of Minnesota, Utah, Oklahoma, and Illinois. Thus, theoretical, practical, and political factors continue to affect definitions and their legal consequences. It is of interest that, since 1963, child abuse legislation has undergone the most changes of any type of legislation in the entire history of the United States. The only constant theme appears to be the fact that it is in the best interest of society to prevent harm to children under age eighteen and that the best way to protect and help children is to provide services for their families. Thus, for mandated reporters of child abuse and neglect, a yearly update of new developments in the state laws is strongly recommended, since there are penalties for "failure to report" in all states.

The Scope of the Problem

As Thomas Carlyle (1795–1881) said, "A judicious man . . . looks at statistics, not to get knowledge, but to save himself from having ignorance foisted on him."

The extent of adolescent victimization is significant, but incidence reports vary. Available data from the U.S. Department of Health and Human Services' Study of National Incidence and Prevalence of Child Abuse and Neglect (National Incidence Study) of 1981 indicate that adolescents account for 47 percent of known recorded cases of abuse and neglect. Of the cases reported in that study, 42 percent were substantiated. From 1984 to 1987, the American Association for Protecting Children (AAPC) indicated that 24 percent of reported cases from fifty states involved youth between the ages of twelve and seventeen. A statewide study in Minnesota in 1980 found that 42.3 percent of all confirmed cases of child maltreatment involved adolescent victims. Regional variations in maltreatment data are known to exist, but specific factors have not been identified to account for these differences.

The effects of adolescent physical abuse are moderate to severe. As Fisher and associates report, 41 percent of all serious injuries in reported cases of child abuse occurred in children in the age group twelve to seven-teen. The true incidence of abuse is probably far greater than these studies estimate from the reported rate, since the abused and neglected are fre-quently unrecognized and not reported in this age group.

A complete analysis of the 1976–1982 reporting years conducted by the AAPC (1984) showed that adolescent victims (ages twelve through seven-teen) were more often female (57.1 percent), while younger victims were more often male (52.1 percent). The National Incidence Study of 1981 showed female adolescent victims outnumbering males two to one, and the National Incidence Study of 1988 showed a four-to-one ratio. Both suggest that females appear more likely to be abused as they pass through adolescence than they are during childhood, while male abuse peaks at an earlier age.

There are three national organizations that collect data on child maltreatment. The AAPC has been collecting pooled national data from the states since 1976. The basis of this collection mechanism is that abstracts of cases referred to child protective services in the fifty states are forwarded to the AAPC national reporting center in Denver. The National Committee for the Prevention of Child Abuse (NCPCA) has performed an annual fifty-state survey based on cases reported. In addition, there have been two national incidence studies performed by a private research company (Westat, Inc.), one in 1980 (published in 1981) and the other in 1986 (published in 1988). The advantage of the national incidence studies is that they do not rely solely on cases known to social services but also include cases known to hospitals and other agencies. None of these surveys gives a truly accurate account of the incidence of maltreatment, and none deals with prevalence of maltreatment. Neither do the national data sets identify those cases known only to friends, relatives, or the victims themselves.

Further, the national incidence studies of 1981 and 1988 employed two different definitions of maltreatment. In 1981 abuse was limited to only those reported cases that involved observable harm as a result of abuse or neglect. In 1988, cases of abuse also included those where the victims were "en-dangered" but not necessarily harmed. In 1981, more than 1 million cases were reported; 16.3 per 1,000 children eighteen years old or younger were estimated to be abused or neglected annually. Applying the second set of definitions in 1988, the prevalence increased to 1.6 million, or 25.2 cases per 1,000.

During the first half of the 1980s, there was a consistent rise in the incidence of maltreatment of children eight years old and younger; however, a comparable increase after age eight did not emerge as statistically signifi-cant. Of interest is the fact that infants from birth to two years old were reported as significantly less abused than children in all other age brackets; three- to five-year-olds were reported as significantly more abused than the twelve- to fourteen-year-olds. Of children under age five, less neglect was reported than was reported for older children and adolescents.

Figures 14.1, 14.2, 14.3, and 14.4 present graphs of the original 1981 data, which are essentially the same as the data produced with the use of the 1988 revised definitions. Figure 14.1 shows the age differences between abused and neglected children from birth through age seventeen. There is an increase in reported cases with increasing age. Older children and adolescents have been given more permission to report maltreatment, whereas younger children still depend on adults to carry the message of suspected neglect or abuse to child protection authorities. Figure 14.2 shows age differences in type of abuse (physical, sexual, and emotional). The most common form of maltreatment is physical, and, as can be seen from the figure, its incidence rises steadily throughout childhood. On the other hand, child fatalities decline particularly over the first few years of life. Emotional abuse also demonstrates age-related differences, with a rise beginning at ages nine to eleven and a peak at ages twelve to fourteen. There was no difference among older children in the reporting of emotional abuse. The sexual abuse of children, while tending to rise over time, shows that those in the age group of birth through two years were significantly less likely to be sexually abused than older children, and older age groups did not differ statistically by age. Figure 14.3 reveals that children five years old and younger are less neglected; however, this finding proves largely to be an artifact of the weighting of older children with educational neglect, which is the largest neglect category. Neglect reporting shows that there is a dramatic increase between ages nine through eleven and fifteen through seventeen. Figure 14.4 shows that when the data are analyzed for moderate and serious physical injuries for different ages, there are significant differences between children five years old and under and those six years old and older. There were no statistical differences among the old age groups.

The summary of the National Incidence Study concludes that the 1988 abuse statistics have increased 66 percent over 1981. While not significant, there are increases in rates of fatal and serious physical abuse; all forms of emotional abuse; abandonment; refusal to provide a child necessary health care; educational neglect; and most forms of emotional neglect. However, it is still not clear whether there are more actual cases of abuse and neglect occurring, or whether there is simply greater recognition and reporting on the part of professionals.

The National Incidence Study of 1981 shows that only one-third of cases referred by medical personnel, educators, social service personnel, or police to child protective services were substantiated. The 1988 data show a significant variation between the number of cases of child maltreatment reported by various professional groups and the number of cases opened to services for the child and family. The percentages of cases reported that were opened for services are 16 percent for day care providers, 24 percent for teachers, 61 percent for police, and 66 percent for hospital personnel. Thus, it appears that the source of reporting influences services given in cases in which police or medical personnel are making the initial judgment to report. These data underscore the frustration that professionals continue to feel

Figure 14.1. Age Differences in Maltreatment (Original Definitions).

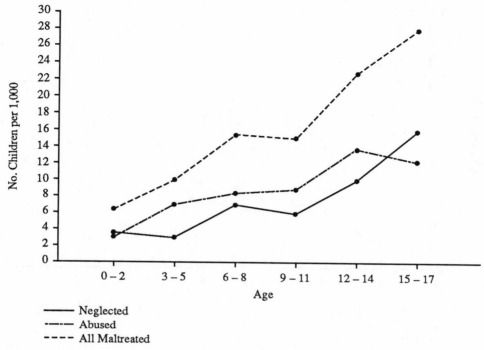

Source: U.S. Department of Health and Human Services. *Study Findings: Study of National Incidence and Prevalence of Child Abuse and Neglect.* DHHS Contract no. 105-85-1702. Washington, D.C.: National Center on Child Abuse and Neglect, 1988.

with respect to the manner in which cases are handled once they are reported. Most states allow for some feedback once a report is made, but this is usually limited to the name of a worker or a concise summary. There is no mandate that professionals making reports be involved in the case planning or follow-up management. Often reports are made by checklist, are impersonal, and tend to fragment continuity of care. Continuity of care is particularly important within the adolescent age group.

The 1988 National Incidence Study indicated that both physical and sexual abuse occurred to a disproportionately greater extent among adolescents than among other age groups. Family income was found to be a significant predictor of reported maltreatment. The rates of maltreatment were *five times* higher for all children living in families with annual incomes of less than $15,000. This association between poverty and abuse is particularly strong in relationship to child neglect, where poor children are twelve times more likely to be identified than those of middle and upper income. The only type of maltreatment with significant sex differential was sexual abuse, where girls are four times more likely to be identified as victims than boys.

Adolescent maltreatment is found in all types of families and crosses all social-class boundaries. However, lower-income people who are caught

Figure 14.2. Age Differences in Abuse (Original Definitions).

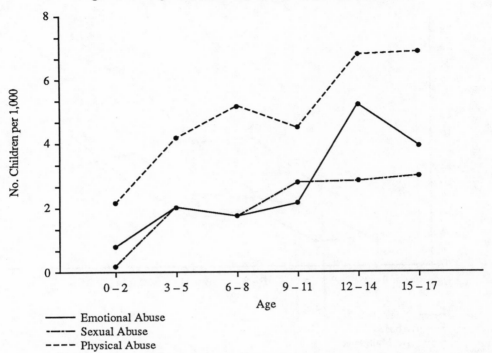

Source: U.S. Department of Health and Human Services. *Study Findings: Study of National Incidence and Prevalence of Child Abuse and Neglect*. DHHS Contract no. 105-85-1702. Washington, D.C.: National Center on Child Abuse and Neglect, 1988.

abusing their children are relatively visible and powerless. It is the low-income victimizers, rather than the well-to-do or middle-class, who are disproportionately identified, processed, and punished by police and the courts. Consequently, many cases of abuse by lower-income perpetrators become a matter of public record and produce biased data regarding the abuse of young children. For teenagers, however, the large social-class differences found to characterize child maltreatment cases are largely absent or attenuated. A 1980 study by Berdie and associates reported that adolescent-onset abusive families were four times (42 percent) more likely to earn incomes in excess of $11,000 (in 1978 dollars) than childhood-onset abusive families (11 percent). Other studies indicated that 59 percent of the families were in the middle to upper classes and only 12 percent were in the lowest socioeconomic classes.

A major limitation in understanding adolescent maltreatment is that there is no single comprehensive data base available on adolescent victims. Although several sources provide partial information, attempts to develop a composite picture are confounded by variations in definitions and reporting practices. Some sources provide only "snapshot," one-time views of victimization. Thus, the incidence, prevalence, and causative factors vary depending

Figure 14.3. Age Differences in Neglect (Original Definitions).

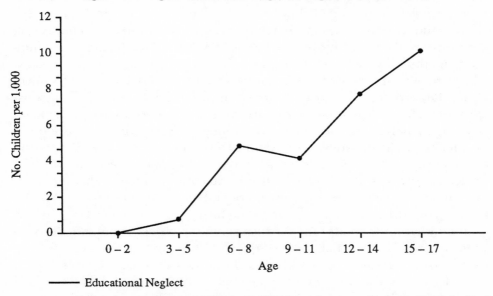

— Educational Neglect

Source: U.S. Department of Health and Human Services. *Study Findings: Study of National Incidence and Prevalence of Child Abuse and Neglect.* DHHS Contract no. 105-85-1702. Washington, D.C.: National Center on Child Abuse and Neglect, 1988.

Figure 14.4. Age Differences in Moderate Injuries (Original Definitions).

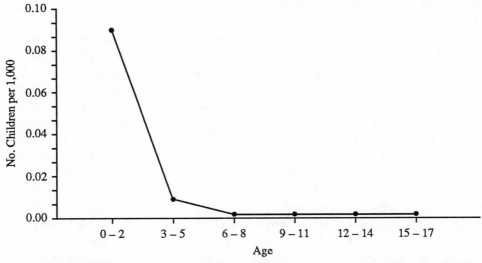

Source: U.S. Department of Health and Human Services. *Study Findings: Study of National Incidence and Prevalence of Child Abuse and Neglect.* DHHS Contract no. 105-85-1702. Washington, D.C.: National Center on Child Abuse and Neglect, 1988.

on when measurements are taken. In addition, sources of statistics on victimization define the end of childhood at different ages, varying from ten to sixteen and in some cases up to age twenty-one. Additionally complicating the statistics, the Child Protection Act of 1984 raised the legal age of childhood in the United States from age sixteen to age eighteen. The most complete official source of crime statistics in the United States, the Uniform Crime Reports (UCR), provides almost no information on crimes against children. The UCR contains data from 16,000 law-enforcement agencies covering 97 percent of the American population, yet, with the exception of murder, the UCR statistics do not report by victim age. Still, even if accurate and complete statistics could be gathered from law-enforcement or child protective services, the Bureau of Justice Statistics estimated that less than one-third of all crimes and 48 percent of violent crimes are reported to the police. Threatened by reprisals or the embarrassment of reporting, adolescents may handle their assaults as private events. Physicians and other professionals may fail to file official reports on adolescent maltreatment, preferring to refer troubled families to mental health or private social services.

Even so, the number of maltreated adolescents reported has increased steadily since 1976. There is no way of knowing, however, whether these statistics reflect increases in actual incidences, increases in reporting as the result of greater awareness of the problem, or changes in definitions in law or state policies. What is labeled as adolescent maltreatment may vary among reports. In the United States, there is currently much overlap of statutes concerning neglected, abused, and delinquent children. Many neglected and abused adolescents are treated as delinquent or status offenders by legal authorities. Labels such as "school adjustment problems," "acting out," "running away," and "truancy" may all mask adolescent maltreatment and make identification more difficult.

These definitional issues, of course, have implications for sampling procedures. Furthermore, much of the existing research on abuse and neglect is based on sample sources that are less likely to identify adolescents, such as hospitals and protective services. In addition, child protective agencies may be likely to give a higher priority to younger maltreated children than to adolescents. Such priority is due in part to the actual or perceived vulnerability of younger children compared with adolescents. Common perception holds that while younger children are seen to be helpless, adolescents have the ability to physically retaliate and influence conflict.

Gelles and Straus point out that "helplessness" is often a criterion for determining who is and is not considered a victim and thus that "it is not surprising that teenage victims are among the missing persons of the official child abuse reports compiled by each state." As does Alice Miller, they point out that teenage victims are often held responsible for the assaults that they sustain, while infants and young children cannot be held responsible for parental violence. It has been noted, however, by many observers that adolescents may participate in or provoke their own victimization through provocative behavior. The way in which a youth enters the child welfare system and the label given to an adolescent's behavior, whether abused, neglected, delinquent, and so on, will ultimately determine how a youth is treated and which services he or she will receive. Unfortunately, the labels given adolescent behavior also create a fragmentation in the literature designed to assess the causes, correlates, and consequences of abuse and neglect, making knowledge fragmentary and disjointed among the various disciplines.

Methodological Issues

In addition to collecting data about the amount of victimization of children and adolescents, child maltreatment research done in the past twenty-five years has steadily increased. This new research has led to new correlations and hypotheses of child maltreatment. But before reviewing the theoretical literature, one must recognize the methodological problems inherent in abuse and neglect research and the limitations for its findings.

Even though the term *battered child* was conceptualized more than twenty-five years ago, most researchers and other professionals would agree that solid knowledge of child abuse was not available to social workers or other professionals until only two decades ago. Most studies were descriptive in nature; few elaborated on methodology or used sophisticated statistical analyses; and most made only cursory attempts to relate their findings to theory, practice, or previous studies.

Within the past decade, there has been a sizable increase in the research on child abuse and neglect that is more empirically grounded and sophisticated. However, many reports of this work have been characterized by sampling difficulties and other research problems. In *The Dark Side of Families*, Gelles states, "there is no question that if we are to improve our understanding of child maltreatment, there are many research issues and problems that need to be addressed, overcome, and solved." While this review is intended to present an overview rather than a critique of the literature, it is nevertheless important to understand the way that the methodology employed can influence the outcome of research in child maltreatment. To begin with, one must keep in mind, as discussed earlier, that the words *abuse* and *neglect* have not been in our vocabularies, nor have abuse and neglect been recognized as "phenomena" or "social problems," for very long in our human history. Most studies that have reviewed the methodologies and literature in the area of maltreatment have mentioned the pervasive problem of a lack of precisely defined concepts and adequate definitions.

Most articles written on child and adolescent abuse begin with a discussion of the problems inherent in defining it. The broadest definition places it within a continuum of parental behavior that ranges from mild physical punishment to extreme violence. As Cathy Spatz Widom states in her 1988 article in the *American Journal of Orthopsychiatry*, "The complexity of the definitional issue is illustrated by the question of general cultural acceptance of physical punishment in child rearing practices. Few people object to the spanking of a child by a parent; reactions are likely to be quite different if the child is spanked by a stranger. To what extent is a particular definition of child abuse sufficiently discriminating to be useful?"

The question of how physical child abuse should be defined for research and treatment purposes remains unresolved. Operational standards often place the definition in terms of the outcome of parental disciplinary actions, such that if an injury has been incurred, the act is quantifiably abusive. This excludes many situations that involve no physical evidence of physical injury but that may be just as damaging developmentally to the child or youth. States also differ in the ways they define child or adolescent abuse and the relevant codes and statutes for making the child a dependent of the court. The distinction between child and adolescent varies qualitatively as well as quantitatively. When does a child become an adolescent, and when is an adolescent emancipated? The answers to these questions play a role in determining how a population is sampled and the subsequent research findings.

Furthermore, the lack of consistency in definition of concepts of abuse complicates research. In many studies, abuse and neglect populations are lumped together even though they are generally considered to have different dynamics. Decisions about how, when, and whether to include physical abuse, sexual abuse, and neglect influence the kinds of samples studied and, therefore, the results. Some studies distinguish between abused and neglected children; others combine them in the same category. Similar inconsistencies occur between the topics of sexual abuse and physical abuse. In the absence of clearer definitions, many children and youth who require protection will go undetected, and some children or youth who are not maltreated will be mislabeled and subjected to unnecessary treatment and intervention.

How the population under investigation is defined, of course, has an immediate impact on the sample selection. Essentially, there have been three data sources on child and adolescent maltreatment. A large portion of the research is derived from clinical (psychiatrists, psychologists, physicians, social workers, and counselors) studies. The clinical setting provides direct access to cases of maltreatment and a wealth of in-depth information about the dynamics of particular cases. Yet this source is suspect, because clinicians' samples are typically nonrandom and of small size, limiting their representativeness and generalizability. Further, the type of professional contacted and the personal qualities of the parents influence how a child's injuries are labeled; for example, whether they are accidental or intentionally inflicted. This also implies that the samples of abusive families that are produced are biased and unrepresentative, since a disproportionate number from the lower-class and poorly educated come to the public's attention through these professionals. As Bradley and Lindsay suggest in their 1987 article in the *Journal of Family Violence*, "Greater effort must be made to locate samples of abusive families from the middle class. Only then can we untangle the influence of factors such as socioeconomic class so that professionals working in this area can avoid the possibility of blaming 'the poor' for the problem, or conversely, blaming the abuse problem on situational characteristics that have more to do with the lack of education or poverty of the individuals under study than with the causes and treatment of abusive parents."

A second source of data is official reports made at the case-level and aggregate-level of states, all of which require mandatory reporting of suspected abuse. Official report data provide information on a large number of cases but are still limited to those cases known by service providers. Service providers such as child protective services, departments of social services, public welfare, and child welfare, and national agencies (such as the American Humane Association) and child registries provide statistical reports of abuse. Gelles found in 1983 that the status of the person making the report, not the nature of the reported injury, influenced whether the report would be found valid. If a reporter was a professional, a report was much more likely to be found valid even controlling for the nature of the injury to child or the social status of the alleged abuser. Hence, a major weakness of official reports is the selection bias of the reporter.

Further, as with most official report and clinical data, the poor and minorities tend to be overrepresented. Since community agencies are less likely to intervene in middle- or upper-class families, they tend to be underrepresented in official statistics. This, of course, contributes to the many cases of abuse that go unrecognized or unreported and, hence, makes the incidence of abuse artificially low in official reports.

A third source of data on abuse and neglect is social surveys. Prospective studies, of which there are few, attempt to follow families over time to compare the incidence of abuse and neglect between groups that are at low risk and those that are at high risk. Because the known incidence of abuse and neglect is low, prospective studies require very large samples if they are to produce groups that can be statistically compared. But to follow a large group over time is costly, and the accuracy of data collection is difficult to maintain. Retrospective studies, on the other hand, are less expensive and relatively easier than prospective ones. Yet retrospective studies lose some of the accuracy and ability to generalize about the incidences, correlates, causes, or consequences, as they are based on recall, and the time order of events is difficult to assess. Furthermore, self-report studies, as compared with official reports, have the advantage of being free of the biases of official reporting, as well as covering a wider geographical area. On the other hand, self-report surveys suffer from the problems associated with the unreliability of information based on recall, the interpretation of questionnaire items, and the social desirability of certain types of responses, as well as problems associated with one-time-only measurements and biases introduced in regard to nonrespondents. All said and done, few national surveys have been conducted that gathered data from a representative probability sample of families.

Regardless of the source of data, the research on adolescent maltreatment is characterized by inadequate and biased sampling, confounding variables, faulty inferences, and generalizations. Very few samples are truly random, and just as few employ any control or comparison groups in order to assess confounding influences or alternative explanations. Control groups are necessary to determine unambiguously whether a given factor is a cause; however, the majority of studies are conducted without attention to even the most elementary principles of experimental design.

Furthermore, the use of adequate statistical techniques for interpreting the relationships of child and adolescent maltreatment is lacking. For research in maltreatment to advance, post-hoc conclusions based on single-variable accounts need to be rectified. Prospective, longitudinal, quasi-experimental designs may offer the greatest promise for illuminating the etiology and consequences of child and adolescent maltreatment. Complex causal networks require commensurately complex statistical analyses, such as path analysis or cross-lag correlations. Finally, the importance of using multiple measures of social phenomena, such as triangulation, is widely recognized, since an increased diversity in measurement instruments and data-collection techniques aids in the evaluation of the validity of the study and the findings. It is hoped that these reflections will caution the reader to employ better models in systematic investigations that will, in turn, lead to incremental empirical support of them and greater understanding of the complex issues surrounding adolescent maltreatment.

Literature Review and Theoretical Models

Despite the methodological problems encountered in examining the literature in the area of abuse and neglect, it is useful to review the research on the correlates, causes, and consequences of adolescent maltreatment. We now summarize the major theories that exist in the literature, which range from the individual's developmental experiences and the influence of the family of origin to ecological models that include the influences of community and culture.

Correlates and Causative Factors in Adolescent Maltreatment

Many early hypotheses for the origins of child maltreatment focused on parental psychological characteristics, such as character defects resulting from a lack of inhibition in expressing frustration or other impulsive behavior. Many other attempts have been made to describe and document a personality type indicative of abusers. Several studies have used the Minnesota Multiphasic Personality Inventory (MMPI) to determine which characteristics are common to abusers. Yet no single homogeneous MMPI profile pattern characterizes the abuser. Other personality research findings characterize abusive parents as having low self-esteem, severely frustrated dependency needs, feelings of social isolation or loneliness, and emotional deprivation in their childhood. Research on parental psychological characteristics as a whole suggests that there is no single type of abusive parents, just as there is no single cluster of characteristics of adequate parents. To date, no studies have compared differences between parental characteristics of adolescent physical abusers and those of early child abusers.

Other research on abuse and neglect has examined the young child's role in abuse; certain child characteristics, such as prematurity, mental retardation, physical handicaps; and difficult family interactional patterns as a result of the child. These studies have shown a variety of factors that are not consistently present and that may reflect the study group and research methodologies used.

Despite the extent of the problem of adolescent maltreatment, only limited information is available in the literature concerning the characteristics of maltreated adolescents and their families. As previously mentioned, the National Incidence Studies of 1981 and 1988 report that adolescents receive less severe physical injuries, more psychological maltreatment, and more sexual abuse than do children. But empirical research on the causes of physical abuse and emotional neglect of adolescents is unduly sparse. Circumstances within the family as a whole that may result in adolescent abuse and neglect should be considered. Family interaction is in a state of disequilibrium as the adolescent discovers new identities, roles, and behaviors. Complicating family dynamics is the fact that the teenager and his or her parents are often at significantly different and potentially conflictual life junctures. The parents are often facing midlife readjustments as a consequence of a decrease in physical strength, attractiveness, and/or sexuality; a decline or leveling off of employment status; a decrease in parental responsibilities and established patterns of family life; and heightened awareness of the reality of death as a result of the death of their own parents. Conversely, the adolescent is only beginning to realize emerging physical, cognitive, emotional, and sexual potential. Such a parent-child mix is a setup for conflict and can contribute to the conditions precipitating abusive or neglectful behavior.

Within such family dynamics, adolescents may be more vulnerable than younger children. Their vulnerability stems from their stage of development, which simultaneously creates great dependence on family and a striving for separation from the family and one's own identity. As a consequence, "normal adolescents" may exhibit behaviors that are provocative, annoying, and destabilizing to parents.

The difference between parenting adolescents and parenting children is exemplified in the work of I. Lourie, which differentiates three patterns of abuse in adolescents: (1) abuse that begins in childhood and continues in adolescence, (2) abuse that occurs as a result of physical punishment and discipline from parents that increases significantly in quality and quantity during adolescence, and (3) abuse that has its onset only in adolescence and is directly related to it. Lourie believes that the second and third patterns predominate. In fact, he concludes that 90 percent of adolescent abuse cases have their onset during the teen years. Others validate Lourie's perspective; however, some report that 50 percent or more of adolescent maltreatment begins in adolescence. Some authors suggest that adolescent abuse is simply a result of the continuation of abuse and neglect in childhood, but that the abuse becomes qualitatively more severe in adolescence. No definitive research exists on these patterns.

Being a parent to an adolescent is, thus, different from parenting a child. Such differences arise from adolescents' capability to find flaws in their parents' reasoning, their greater capacity to retaliate and/or leave home, and their ability to seek autonomous relationships with others that the parents may perceive as threatening. Furthermore, the adolescent's power is much greater than that of the child. The adolescent not only has greater physical power to retaliate but also has the capability to stimulate family conflict, to harm self and others, and to embarrass parents. Patterns of parenting must be altered to accommodate the changing needs and development of "normal" adolescents. The families of adolescents are best characterized by parental confusion that leads to continuous crises.

Some researchers suggest that families in which there is adolescent maltreatment are often multiproblem families, with high rates of divorce and separation, financial stresses, and family conflict. Changing social relationships, not only within the family but also between the family and the community, are also cited as causes of family disorganization and dysfunction. There is widespread belief that disruptions in family functioning contribute to the excessive use of violence among family members, including adolescents. The Gelles and Straus 1980 study estimated that the American family has a 20 percent chance of becoming the arena for violence. In fact, family violence researchers assert that the family is the most violent of social groups, with individuals being more likely to be harmed by an angry family member than by anyone else. We live in a society that continues to advocate the use of "pragmatic" violence and sanctions its use in many settings (for example, "discipline in the classroom," police and youth conflicts, and, in general, the concept of "reasonable force to correct the behavior of a child").

Additional theory building has focused on sociocultural explanations. Variables such as the level of social support, parental availability to meet basic needs, and poverty-related stress and adjustment have been implicated. Still other research has considered social and cultural values, such as the norms of viewing children as possessions or the use of corporal punishment as an appropriate tool of training, as well as social policies in the larger environment that provide conditions in which abuse is likely to occur.

In an attempt to integrate these divergent hypotheses of the causes of child maltreatment, Belsky (1980) proposed a framework (Figure 14.5) that

Figure 14.5. Belsky's Ecologically Integrative Model of Child Abuse.

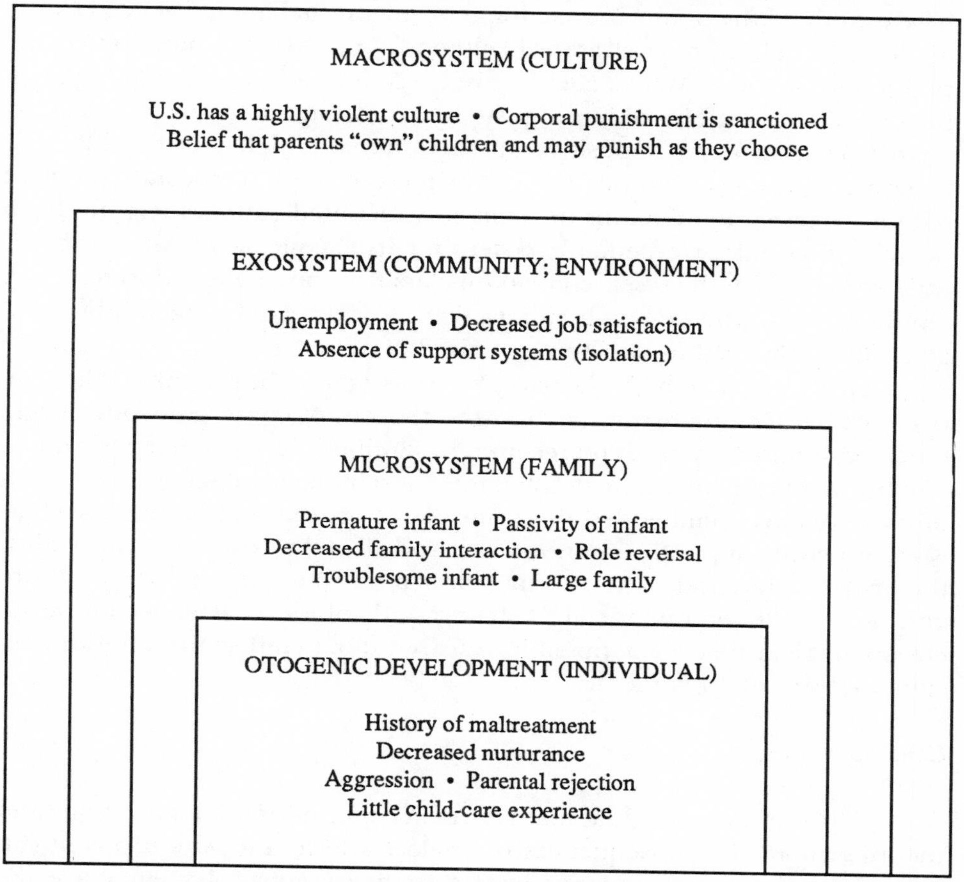

MACROSYSTEM (CULTURE)

U.S. has a highly violent culture • Corporal punishment is sanctioned
Belief that parents "own" children and may punish as they choose

EXOSYSTEM (COMMUNITY; ENVIRONMENT)

Unemployment • Decreased job satisfaction
Absence of support systems (isolation)

MICROSYSTEM (FAMILY)

Premature infant • Passivity of infant
Decreased family interaction • Role reversal
Troublesome infant • Large family

OTOGENIC DEVELOPMENT (INDIVIDUAL)

History of maltreatment
Decreased nurturance
Aggression • Parental rejection
Little child-care experience

Sources: Adapted from Hamilton, A., Stills, W. B., Milowsky, F., and Beal, D. G. "A Multilevel Comparison of Child Abusers with Non-Abusers." *Journal of Family Violence*, 1987, *2* (3), 215; Belsky, J. "Child Maltreatment: An Ecological Integration." *American Psychologist*, 1980, *35*, 320–355.

views abuse as a result of multiple forces within the individual (ontogenic development), the family (microsystem), the community (exosystem), and the culture (macrosystem). This model, which Belsky calls *ecological*, Burgess calls *social interactional*, and Parke and Collmer call *social situational*, does not focus on child abuse as a uniform phenomenon but offers a complex interaction of factors. Belsky argues that individual parent and child characteristics, family interactional patterns, situationally determined stress in both near and distant environments, and the values of the broader culture interact to produce child abuse and neglect. Yet a few authors are providing evidence that the correlates of abuse and neglect are not necessarily theoretically or practically equivalent.

The underpinnings of this ecological model, however, are that maltreatment results from a variety of factors. The microsystem has, perhaps, been given the most attention in both theory and practice. Some researchers have examined the family interactional problems that are influenced by the adolescents' behavior as well as the likelihood of maladaptive parenting in the prediction of abuse. Many articles have been devoted to assessing high-risk factors in families. Typical findings suggest that abusive families are characterized by lower levels of positive interaction and a higher probability that negative behaviors or interactions will be reciprocated. Yet the measurement of abusive parenting remains problematic. As stated earlier, there has been no reliable, valid, or acceptable system for its classification. Since there is little consensus in the research field on classification of abuse and high-risk families, much past research suffers from a lack of internal validity, and external validity is thus also compromised.

Further, research by Garbarino and associates has reported the connections between maltreatment and the amount of community and neighborhood support given to and received by families. Adolescents spend much of their developmental time in the family, at school, or in peer groups. Each of these groups is embedded in a complex of institutional settings, such as work or private or public organizations. And all of the groups operate within the broad ideological patterns that characterize our contemporary culture and how we define our social problems and solutions. It is becoming increasingly clear that, when possible, research should reflect this multidimensional view of maltreatment.

Consequences

The literature on child maltreatment contains many assumptions and theories about the consequences of neglect and abuse. Any problem can create both short- and long-term effects. In the case of adolescent abuse, the short-term effects obviously involve the trauma incurred from the physical and emotional distress. Most studies comment on the dysfunctional character of the adolescent victim of maltreatment. The victim characteristics often examined include acting-out or oppositional behaviors, such as arguing, disobeying, and provocative actions; depression and low frustration tolerance; helplessness and dependency; and generalized anxiety or emotional thought disturbances. Adolescents at high risk for maltreatment appear to be less socially competent and experience more developmental problems than their peers. Whether these characteristics are an outcome of or a contributor to adolescent maltreatment remains to be seen and requires longitudinal and prospective data.

The long-term effects are numerous and varied. Many researchers believe that untreated abused children become juvenile delinquents, murderers, and the next generation of abusers. The literature consistently includes assumptions that physically abused children exhibit violent behavior as adults, as well as that they have higher rates of drug and alcohol abuse, criminal behavior, psychiatric disturbances, including developmental delays, and more social and emotional difficulties. However, actual data that both meet the normal rules of empirical evidence and conclusively demonstrate the negative short- and long-term consequences of maltreatment are rare. The large majority of studies of the outcomes of maltreatment have one or more significant methodological flaws, as discussed previously. Research thus far has not differentiated among the effects resulting from maltreatment during childhood, effects resulting from maltreatment during adolescence, and effects resulting from the same family factors that may cause maltreatment.

Despite these flaws, there is consistency in research findings in a number of areas. Adolescents at high risk for maltreatment are often seen to be less socially competent and to exhibit more developmental problems than their peers. Most studies discuss, in one way or another, the dysfunctional character of the adolescent victim of maltreatment. The dysfunctional problems of adolescents who typically have been abused include such patterns of behavior as juvenile delinquency (theft, drug abuse, truancy) and other forms of aggressive and acting-out behavior; running away (for instance, to escape); depression and related behaviors, which have been described as withdrawal, wariness of strangers, fearfulness, and generalized anxiety; other emotional thought disorders; and feelings of helplessness and dependency. It remains unclear whether these consequences are short-lived or long-term, and the interaction of these consequences is still undetermined.

The literature has attempted to address maltreatment and delinquency, which remain two difficult social problems that seem to be closely linked. Research on the relationship between abuse and delinquency began in the early 1970s; since that time, numerous studies have been conducted in the various fields of medicine, sociology, social work, psychology, and other human service professions. To date, there is a lack of consensus regarding the precise causes of maltreatment and delinquency. Yet the link between abuse, neglect, and delinquency has been historically forged in the rise of the Houses of Refuge in the mid 1820s and the first juvenile court in Illinois in 1899. Houses of Refuge were developed first privately, then publicly, to deal with the "new urban poor" or "dangerous class" of children who wandered the streets during the period of rapid industrialization, urbanization, and immigration of the nineteenth century. States made little or no distinction between neglected and delinquent children, and both were confined in Houses of Refuge.

The development of the juvenile court institutionalizes the concept of legal immaturity of children and the weakness of the family to function adequately. The juvenile court processes not only delinquent youth but also neglected and dependent children. Thus, there is a de facto link between abused, neglected children and youth and delinquents and status offenders created by the juvenile justice system.

Some evidence also exists for an empirical link between maltreatment as a child and being involved in delinquent activities as a juvenile. Looking at incidence alone, data from the National Incidence Study of 1981 suggest that juvenile delinquents have experienced maltreatment at a higher rate than that of the general population. Others have assessed the relationship between child abuse and juvenile delinquency by retrospectively studying reports of child-rearing practices among delinquent populations. Typical findings suggest that childhood abuse is somewhat related to later delinquency and adult criminal behavior. But the lack of comparison groups in most studies makes the findings ambiguous. It is argued that a well-designed and controlled prospective longitudinal study may find such an association. And, indeed, a combination of available empirical findings and years of observation of practitioners does suggest some relationship. A relationship between abuse and delinquency may exist, if only as a result of the juvenile attempting to remedy the situation by running away or retaliation, either of which would be considered a delinquent act, despite the cause of the delinquency. As mentioned earlier, the juvenile justice system itself may not only create links between maltreatment and delinquency but may also do so disproportionately for the low-income adolescents who tend to end up in the system.

It is clear that child abuse and neglect are associated with a variety of negative outcomes other than subsequent delinquency, including death. It is unclear whether "violence begets violence," as in the cycle-of-abuse hypothesis, or if violent behavior decreases future violence and increases withdrawal. Both of these hypotheses may be correct under certain conditions, but the relative nature, importance, and strength of the links remain undetermined and require further investigation. Questions such as why some abused youth become abusers and others do not, why some abused youth become delinquent while others do not, and why some nonabused youth become abusers and/or delinquents need to be answered.

A further link to be explored is the extent to which delinquent behavior puts an adolescent at risk for abuse, be it in the home, on the street, or in an institution. Runaways often become victims of pornographers and pimps. Many reports have been written on the deplorable conditions of juvenile detention facilities and other institutional settings. The risk that children and youth incur as a result of the increasing number of them who are currently homeless in our country, whether because of family economic situations, running away, or being forced from the home, needs more investigation and intervention.

The endless abuse-delinquency-abuse cycle, if there really is one, requires intervention if it is to be broken or if abusive situations are to be prevented. The empirical evidence of the adolescent as a perpetrator of abuse is becoming more prevalent. Adolescent mothers who maltreat their own children or aggressive teenagers who assault their siblings and peers are at continued risk in our society. Why, under similar conditions and histories, some youth abuse and others do not needs to be assessed, with attention to the varying levels or combinations of events and situations. Our ignorance needs to be further challenged by researchers and policy makers alike in order for the risks to lessen. The next step is to determine what policies, programs, and procedures for maltreated children and youth need to be further modified, changed, or abandoned.

Intervention and Prevention

Intervention refers to confronting a "problem," such as child maltreatment, that is perceived as needing to be changed or modified. As with definitional questions of abuse, there is a debate in terminology regarding the use of the words *intervention*, *treatment*, and *therapy*. Intervention generally is applied by social services systems providing a range of services for the child and the family "in need of services." The beginning of intervention starts with the identification of maltreatment of children through age eighteen. This is the rationale behind the mandatory child abuse and neglect reporting laws that have been in existence in all fifty states since 1968. The purpose of these laws is to arrest the maltreatment that is occurring and to provide services for families. Penalties for failing to report by mandated reporters are provided in all states. Recently, there has been a trend toward penalties for making "false allegations" as a result of backlash against child abuse legislation and reporting laws.

As a result of the increased numbers of child abuse and neglect cases being reported, attempts are being made to set criteria based on the severity of cases. These strategies create a bias for the continuing focus on younger children. Adolescents who are maltreated are perceived as less vulnerable, because they have the ability to defend themselves by striking back or running away. This continues to create a lack of services for the adolescent maltreated population. The expansion of child abuse and neglect reporting laws has been more concerned with issues regarding infants and the health of the fetus ("fetal abuse") than with adolescent abuse.

The concept of the "battered child syndrome" focuses on the abuse of young children and pervades pediatric textbooks. Even more recent books that stress adolescent medical care omit or only briefly comment on adolescent maltreatment. In assessment of risk factors in child abuse and neglect, the adolescent is considered "low risk." Also, there is omission of the mention of alcohol and other drugs and family dynamics in discussions of youth with disabilities and maltreatment. These adolescents are probably at great risk for sexual or physical abuse.

Treatment modality interventions initially dealt with psychological or mental health models. In *Confronting Child Abuse*, D. Daro classifies intervention models as psychological, sociological, and psychosocial. These models tend to deal with some of the broad social system issues, such as unemployment, adequate support systems, and control of alcohol, as well as with the individual. The inability to achieve broad-scale system reforms in any one of these areas has pointed out a need for a more systemic approach, one that supports the Belsky model.

The focus of adolescent treatment centers on the adolescent perpetrator, the family, and society. To date, one of the best-designed studies, performed by N. C. Klein and J. F. Alexander, is aimed at both intervention and prevention. In this study, eighty-six delinquents were randomly placed into four treatment groups: a group that received a chat-centered family approach; a group that received an eclectic-dynamic approach; a group that received a behaviorally oriented short-term family systems approach; and a control group, which received no intervention. The only group in which there was improvement in the family system as well as in primary prevention (as measured by subsequent delinquency of siblings) was the one that received the family systems approach. Of those that received the family systems approach, 20 percent came to court in the next two-and-a-half to three-and-a-half years, compared with 40 percent of the control group. The other intervention groups had significantly higher court appearance rates of the youth involved. It appears that some intervention may, in fact, be harmful!

This family systems model is supported by Daro's description of the National Clinical Evaluation Study. This study involved nineteen national demonstration projects, all of which adopted a family treatment focus rather than an ontological or individual one. More than 80 percent of all families served by the nineteen projects received direct services for both the perpetrators and the victims of maltreatment. With this model, there were gains made in more areas of functioning in the lives of maltreated children than of controls — in areas of physical and emotional support systems, improved interactional family communication patterns, and improved parent-child interactions that helped the children through their developmental stages with less conflict. Even though adolescents were included in this project, most of the attention was given to the younger children. Other well-designed intervention programs for adolescents are in their beginning stages of evaluation.

It is difficult to differentiate intervention and prevention strategies as two distinct and separate processes. Both treatment and prevention interventions require a commitment from all parts of society. Each discipline that interacts with families and adolescents has a role to play. A recent study by Joffe and others indicates that adolescents and youth are largely neglected by health professionals. More than 75 percent of college freshmen reported that they received no counseling from health providers. The study's data suggest that adolescents receive little health counseling from personal physicians, whether they be internists, family physicians, or pediatricians. The authors recommend that pediatricians must increase the extent of their counseling if they are to meet the Academy of Pediatrics' goal of providing care to adolescents and young adults. Clearly, further awareness and education as to the need to reach out to maltreated adolescents are becoming more critical.

Recent programs have developed curricula designed to reduce impulsive and aggressive behavior in children and increase their level of social competency through empathy training, impulse control, and anger management. Programs representing the prevention model of personal safety and effective use of community resources are needed to counteract the increased violence in schools, especially harassment and physical attacks by peers. The concept of early intervention in peer relations for physically abusive adolescents parallels the model of early intervention models for juvenile sex offenders.

Educational systems are beginning to deal with the adverse effects of child abuse and neglect on learning and school behavior. Federal educational legislation (the School Improvement Act of 1987) states that "child abuse is another growing and serious problem which can adversely affect a child's performance in school." This bill provides for block grants for local or educational agencies for special programs and projects for "at-risk" and "high-cost" students and for development of curricula that would help children avoid potentially abusing situations. Questions that need our immediate attention for possible intervention and prevention include the following.

1. *Is there a relationship between teenage parenting and child abuse?* No statistical significance was found in a controlled study of teenage mothers by Kinard and Klerman, although other studies do purport to demonstrate such a relationship. The problem of separating the variables of poverty, teenage pregnancy, abusive backgrounds, and so on has not been resolved. Among various models of prevention are programs that provide home visitors and "total push programs," which enroll large numbers of teen parents in order to provide support services such as day care, support groups, and counseling. From the data on these programs, they appear very promising as ways to offer support in preventing child maltreatment during pregnancy and the first and second years of life for isolated teenage mothers.

2. *Are there data that provide documentation that our prevention efforts are working?* The data from the National Incidence Studies of 1981 and 1988 allow us to compare the statistics from two different points in time. Although this comparison does not enable us to determine whether prevention efforts have been successful, the data suggest that very young children have not experienced the same type of increase in neglect and abuse as noted in adolescents. This may be because the development of child abuse intervention and prevention has been focused primarily on the infant and younger child. There may be independent factors affecting the high rates of adolescent maltreatment, and these rates may also reflect secondary consequences, such as running away, engaging in delinquent behavior, use of illicit drugs (for example, cocaine) and licit drugs (for examples, alcohol), violence, and, in some cases, suicide.

3. *Is there any merit in further investigation of the concept that the victim becomes the perpetrator?* The number of children abused by adult sex offenders (pedophiles) is estimated to be at least fifty times greater than the number of

children abused by adolescent sex offenders. Our rapidly developing under-standing of the juvenile sex offender indicates that intervention with the juvenile sex offender may be an effective way of decreasing adult sex offend-ing. If this hypothesis is correct, early intervention strategies may prevent later sex offending. Community networking, prevention, and intervention with juvenile sex offenders offer some models that may also be effective in dealing with other types of violent juvenile offenders. Early childhood inter-vention programs may still offer the best hope for effective intervention and prevention.

The Future and Recommendations

The future for children will in large part depend on the commitment of our society to dealing with the entire developmental spectrum of maltreatment. This extends from preconceptional care to adequate prenatal care to care to ensure the health of the infants. Healthy infants have a greater chance to become healthy children who grow into healthy adolescents and adults. Child maltreatment occurs when our society and families neglect the basic needs of our children. The consequences and the symptoms play out across the life cycle and into subsequent generations. Adolescence represents an area of emerging concern for research and policy implementation because of high incidence and severity of maltreatment and its potential consequences.

There is a need for more definitive studies to determine the factors involved in adolescent maltreatment. Ideally, one would like to see multilevel research analysis into different subsets of the population to examine inter-vention more carefully. In the late 1970s, Ramsey County (St. Paul), Min-nesota, received a grant from the Law Enforcement Assistance Administra-tion (LEAA) and the National Institute for Mental Health (NIMH) for a three-year (1977–1979) study to broaden and improve services to adolescents who were physically abused. Researchers worked with schools for consulta-tion and identification of abuse. Eighty substantiated cases of adolescent physical abuse were identified and studied. The findings identified three major categories of intervention. The first of these categories, "situational," involved 50 percent of the cases. The children in this category required short-term treatment using community resources such as school, private agencies, and public mental health services. The second category involved total family therapy systems in cases of long-term abuse from childhood through adoles-cence; these cases included half of the study group. The third category involved a child protective element; in this category were children who were handicapped or judged to be vulnerable and required juvenile court inter-vention. This latter "vulnerable" group of adolescents was small (10 percent of the total) and reflects in part why adolescent abuse is not perceived as a greater problem as compared to abuse of infants and younger children, who are de facto vulnerable. Adolescents have more resources of power in phys-ical strength and the ability to ask for help and defend themselves.

The Ramsey County Adolescent Abuse Project revealed that physically abused adolescents need to talk when they have concerns and that their appointments should not be deferred for adults' convenience. It is true that adolescents who are physically abused do not require as much physical protection as do young children who are abused and that adolescents may contribute more to their abuse than younger children do. Yet adolescents need to be more involved in the treatment process than has been the case. A balance must be struck between the youth's desire to be independent and the professional's need to be careful not to destroy parental authority and to work with the entire family. The study also showed that there is a need on the part of professionals working with youth to diffuse the stronger, more violent feelings of the adolescents by helping them to learn anger control.

Another area of adolescent maltreatment that requires further investigation for possible intervention and prevention is the relationship between adolescent abuse and teenage pregnancy. Associations have been made between child maltreatment and the adequacy of adolescent parenting. It may be that abused and neglected children and adolescents perceive that having a child will increase their self-esteem and fill some of the void created by inadequate nurturing from their own parents. A number of studies suggest that the young adolescent parent who was isolated and without support is more at risk for early child abuse, increased accidents, and problems with parenting. What happens to these children over time when they become adolescents? Also, does maltreatment of adolescents contribute to the incidence of poverty and neglect by interrupting educational goals and limiting choices as well as the ability to make judgments? There are many unanswered questions.

Adolescents are common caretakers for children. J. Martin states that adolescents who baby-sit may take out their frustrations on other children. Normal adolescents report negative experiences while baby-sitting. In Martin's random sample of "normal" adolescent baby-sitters, 46.5 percent reported being very angry, 38.3 percent reported spanking the child with whom they were sitting, 13.3 percent called for parental help and advice, 8.3 percent had an attack of fear or panic, 7.7 percent struck the children, and 7.7 percent became frustrated and angry and cried. These data portray the need for parents to exercise caution in using adolescent baby-sitters and to assess their ability to deal with children and handle anger. The fact that calls for help are relatively infrequent indicates the need for further studies in this area to prevent maltreatment. Would the rates of anger, spanking, and hitting be even higher in adolescents who have been or are being maltreated? A broad vision is needed to engage our culture in the care of our youth. Our society is a violent one, and role models given to adolescents reflect that violence. A commonly held belief is that parents "own their children" and may punish them as they choose. Is adolescent maltreatment an extension of the lack of support to families in our society and a continued disregard for children and youth as human beings?

The 1960s and 1970s saw the emergence of concern for the legal rights of adolescents. In 1988, the U.S. Supreme Court, in *Thompson* v. *Oklahoma*, ruled that states cannot execute children under sixteen unless there are specific state laws that allow state execution. A divided Supreme Court decided in June 1989 to allow states to execute convicted murderers who were as young as sixteen at the time of the crime (*Wilkins* v. *Missouri*). This case suggests that the Supreme Court has in fact set sixteen as the minimum age for the execution of juveniles. There are only five countries in the world that now execute children under age eighteen. Americans, with all our ideals, still do harm to youth, a largely ignored segment of our population. Societal change is occurring, but the direction that it will take requires a constant vigil for youth advocacy.

Currently, more data on adolescent behavior are emerging that will bring more creative ideas, research, and interventions. Increased awareness by all professionals, especially health and mental health professionals who have a major role to play in documenting the physical and sexual injuries done to children and their psychological consequences, is important in providing preventive counseling as well as support and intervention. Health professionals can provide leadership roles in working with other disciplines through team efforts in their local communities. The community is the arena for solution. Linkages with the educational system, chemical abuse programs, family systems, and religious and other youth groups that provide support for adolescents and their families are part of the solution. Being available to meet the basic needs of adolescents affects almost every aspect of adolescent health. What will be the consequences of our efforts? To paraphrase the English author J. B. Priestley, our society will have the teenagers that it deserves.

Adolescence and youth lie mostly in the territory at the edge of our psychosocial and health systems map. Adolescent maltreatment is a largely unexplored terrain, and it is difficult to explore new issues that require much energy and resources in order to forge new knowledge. Who is responsible for the care of adolescents who have been maltreated? In the last analysis, we all are, and we must work together to ensure that our current philosophies for meeting the basic health needs of children extend fully to the adolescent. We can protect all humans against maltreatment by fostering the multilevel changes needed to overcome this social problem.

Suggested Readings

Belsky, J. "Child Maltreatment: An Ecological Interpretation." *American Psychologist*, 1980, *35* (4), 320–335.

For a complete bibliography, contact Robert W. ten Bensel, University of Minnesota, School of Public Health, Maternal and Child Health Department, Box 197, Mayo Memorial Building, 420 Delaware Street S.E., Minneapolis, MN 55455.

Berdie, J., and others. *An Empirical Study of Families Involved in Adolescent Maltreatment*. San Francisco: URSA Institute, 1983.

Blumer, H. "Social Problems as Collective Behavior." *Social Problems*, 1971, *18* (3), 298–306.

Bradley, E., and Lindsay, R.C.L. "Methodological and Ethical Issues in Child Abuse." *Journal of Family Violence*, 1987, *2* (3), 239–255.

Burchard, J. D., and Burchard, S. N. (eds.). *Prevention of Delinquent Behavior*. Newbury Park, Calif.: Sage, 1987.

Burgess, R. L. "Child Abuse: A Social Interactional Analysis." In B. B. Lahey and A. E. Kazdin (eds.), *Advances in Clinical Child Psychology*. Vol. 2. New York: Plenum, 1979.

Daro, D. *Confronting Child Abuse: Research for Effective Programs*. New York: Free Press, 1988.

DeMause, L. *The History of Childhood*. New York: Psychohistory Press, 1974.

Finkelhor, D., and others. *The Dark Side of Families*. Newbury Park, Calif.: Sage, 1983.

Fisher, B., and others. *Adolescent Abuse and Neglect: Intervention Strategies*. DHHA Publication no. (OHDS) 80-30266. Washington, D.C.: U.S. Department of Health and Human Services, 1980.

Garbarino, J., Schellenback, C. J., and Sebes, J. M. *Troubled Youth, Troubled Families: Understanding Families at Risk for Adolescent Maltreatment*. New York: Aldine, 1986.

Gelles, R. J., and Lancaster, J. B. (eds.). *Child Abuse and Neglect: Biosocial Dimension*. New York: Aldine DeGruyter, 1987

Gelles, R. J., and Straus, M. A. *Intimate Violence*. New York: Simon & Schuster, 1988.

Joffe, A., Radius, S., and Gall, M. "Health Counseling for Adolescents: What They Want, What They Get, and Who Gives It." *Pediatrics*, 1988, *82* (3), 481–485.

Kempe, H. C., and others. "The Battered-Child Syndrome." *Journal of the American Medical Association*, 1962, *181* (1), 105–112.

Kinard, E. M., and Klerman, L. "Teenage Parenting and Child Abuse: Are They Related?" *American Journal of Orthopsychiatry*, 1980, *50* (30), 481–488.

Klein, N. C., and Alexander, J. F. "Impact of Family Systems Intervention on Recidivism and Sibling Delinquency: A Model of Primary Prevention and Program Evaluation." *Journal of Consulting and Clinical Psychology*, 1977, *45* (3), 469–474.

Kourany, R.F.C., Gwinn, M., and Martin, J. E. "Adolescent Babysitting—a 30 Year Old Phenomenon." *Adolescence*, 1980, *15* (60), 939–945.

Libbey, P., and Bybee, R. "The Physical Abuse of Adolescents." *Journal of Social Issues*, 1979, *35*, 101–126.

Lourie, I. "The Phenomenon of the Abused Adolescent: A Clinical Study." *Victimology: An International Journal*, 1977, *2*, 268–276.

Martin, J. "Child Abuse by Babysitters." *Child Abuse and Neglect*, 1980, *4*, 15.

Miller, A. *Thou Shall Not Be Aware: Society's Betrayal of the Child.* New York: Farrar, Straus, Giroux, 1984.

Paperney, D. M., and Deisher, R. W. "Maltreatment of Adolescents: The Relationship to a Predisposition Toward Violent Behavior and Delinquency." *Adolescence*, 1983, *18*, 499–506.

Parke, R., and Collmer, G. "Child Abuse: An Interdisciplinary Analysis." In M. Hetherington (ed.), *Review of Child Development Research.* Vol. 5. Chicago: University of Chicago Press, 1975.

Pelcovitz, D., and others. "Adolescent Abuse: Family Structure and Implications for Treatment." *Journal of Child Psychiatry*, 1984, *23*, 85–90.

Smith, C. P., Beckman, D. J., and Fraser, W. M. *A Preliminary National Assessment of Child Abuse and Neglect and the Juvenile Justice System: The Shadows of Distress.* Sacramento, Calif.: American Justice Institute, 1980.

U.S. Department of Health and Human Services. *Study Findings: National Study of the Incidence and Severity of Child Abuse and Neglect.* DHHS Publication no. (OHDS) 81-80325. Washington, D.C.: National Center on Child Abuse and Neglect, 1981.

U.S. Department of Health and Human Services. *Study Findings: Study of National Incidence and Prevalence of Child Abuse and Neglect.* DHHS Contract no. 105-85-1702. Washington, D.C.: National Center on Child Abuse and Neglect, 1988.

Widom, C. S. "Sampling Biases and Implications for Child Abuse Research." *American Journal of Orthopsychiatry*, 1988, *58* (2), 260–270.

Part Four

Adolescents' Access to Care

PART EDITOR
Jeffrey C. Bauer, Ph.D.

Introduction

Jeffrey C. Bauer, Ph.D.

The successful evolution of adolescent medicine as a discrete specialty of medical practice will require much more than a solid scientific understanding of the special health needs and clinical characteristics of adolescents. Nonclinical dimensions of medical care delivery will also play a strong supporting role in the future of adolescent medicine and adolescent patients. Medically oriented social and behavioral scientists and specialists in health care management can offer observations and advice that will enhance clinicians' abilities to develop the full potential of adolescent medicine as a specialty practice. The diversity of academic backgrounds of this part's authors shows that leaders in the field have already recognized the need for a multidisciplinary approach that merges clinical and nonclinical perspectives. The nonphysician authors have long-standing affiliations with medical organizations, and several of the physicians have developed advanced expertise in nonclinical areas such as administration, interpersonal communications, sociology, and policy analysis.

The complexity that compels multidisciplinary approaches is first addressed in Chapter Fifteen by Judith S. Bensinger, a physician, and Abigail H. Natenshon, a social worker. Their chapter provides strong evidence of the need to address adolescent medicine from different perspectives as a precondition of successful clinical and programmatic intervention, and it offers numerous examples of the synergy created when clinicians recognize the diverse factors that underpin correct diagnosis and successful therapy. The chapter carefully addresses the complications created by the fact that many of the indicators of health problems are also normal signs of growing up. The multidisciplinary approach presented here will help clinicians distinguish between true pathology and normal development in the context of the ever changing culture of adolescents and their families.

Chapter Sixteen, by Kimball Austin Miller, helps bridge the gap between sound clinical practice and successful practice management. Miller, a specialist in adolescent medicine with a graduate degree in health administration and author of a book on feasibility analysis for medical practice, examines the development of adolescent-oriented clinics from the perspective of marketing. He addresses the business of health care from the viewpoint of the teenage patient and specifies practical considerations (for example, location, decor, advertising, and fees) that could be incorporated into the operation of an adolescent clinic. His chapter also presents a useful model for identifying practice opportunities and planning their implementation.

In Chapter Seventeen, medical sociologist and medical school professor Robert H. DuRant explores the health services that adolescents seek and where they go to get them. An epidemiological approach is used to match demands for services with socioeconomic classifications of patients. Special emphasis is placed on the barriers that affect adolescents' use of the health care system. Examples and lessons are drawn from case studies of actual adolescent clinics and the problems they have encountered in meeting the needs of this special patient population. Legal, economic, physical, and psychological barriers are also addressed in an instructive framework.

Marilyn Moon, an economist recognized as one of the country's leading experts in the economics of poverty, explores relevant financing and payment issues in Chapter Eighteen. She presents the latest available data on the economic status of adolescents, both as individuals and as members of families, and identifies special problems related to the large number of adolescents who live at or near the poverty line. She also presents information on the disposable income of adolescents, reminding us that many do have some economic power of their own. A careful analysis of insurance coverage for adolescent health services precedes concluding comments on the special needs of adolescents and programs to meet them. The need for more research on these issues is underscored throughout the chapter.

Robert H. DuRant, Carolyn Seymore, and M. Susan Jay explore adolescents' compliance with therapeutic regimens in the final chapter of this part. Sharing their own experiences as researchers and clinicians, they apply a model of compliance to some of the specific services that are provided most often to adolescents. The chapter offers considerable practical information for providers and administrators who want to enhance the effectiveness of intervention and provides specific illustrations of the general theme of this part: the importance of multidisciplinary approaches and their potential contributions to improved access.

❧ 15 ❧

Difficulties in Recognizing Adolescent Health Issues

Judith S. Bensinger, M.D.
Abigail H. Natenshon, M.A., L.C.S.W.

During adolescence, biological, psychological, and social changes occur at such a rapid rate that adjustments must constantly be made by the individual. The constant change of the adolescent development process makes pathological issues extremely difficult to recognize and track, especially in the sociological and psychological spheres. There is a question as to what constitutes normality and what characterizes pathology. At best, it is hard to clarify or define adolescent health, thus it is doubly difficult to define or recognize disease or illness issues of the adolescent. For the professional, it is difficult to know when to intervene.

Each major adolescent health issue involves a combination of factors; thus a multidisciplinary approach is required for diagnosis and treatment. Because of the complexity of the biopsychosocial etiology of adolescent issues, problems are often not understood and not recognized. There is good working knowledge of issues in the separate disciplines of medicine and psychology; however, the separateness of each discipline may preclude complete understanding or interrelated treatment of the adolescent issues. Anorexia, bulimia, drug abuse, sexuality, depression, and suicide all involve multidisciplinary diagnostic criteria. For the component problem areas to be accurately identified and the problems treated effectively, an interdisciplinary team of professionals must be involved and treatment plans and progress coordinated and discussed.

The very nature of these conditions is a source of embarrassment to most people. Societal norms and personal denial mechanisms motivate individuals to hide psychosocial signs and symptomatic behavior and to ignore the clues that are precursors to the medical problems. These are conditions that people traditionally "sweep under the rug" because they imply personal failure on the part of the adolescents or their parents in controlling themselves or their life circumstances. Thus, social stressors are manifested in psychological signs and symptoms that are often silent until they are finally expressed or erupt into dysfunctional behavior or physical symptoms.

The highly evolved, well-defined medical problem can be easily identified. The end-stage physical manifestations of certain nonresponsible behaviors become obvious. The sexually active teen is pregnant; the sixteen-year-old anorexic weighs sixty-two pounds; the seventeen-year-old party drinker is critically injured in an accident. At this point, problems are physically and medically apparent and easily identifiable; intervention is obvious along the lines of traditional medicine. The problem is in recognizing these issues while they are still in the early, hard-to-detect psychosocial stages. Intervention should be made before the issues become medically and emotionally apparent and before they compromise the future life of the adolescent. Intervention must be made with the sexually active young person before pelvic inflammatory disease and sterility occur. The drug abuser must be stopped before he or she has a seizure on cocaine or becomes a death statistic from a car accident because of alcohol intoxication. The depressed youth must be treated before he or she commits suicide.

If symptoms remain unrecognized and issues unresolved during the adolescent years, individuals will tend to perpetuate and recreate the unhealthy emotional environment of their youth when they marry and have families. Adolescent needs that go unmet often evolve into the untended needs of battered wives and otherwise abused and self-abused adults.

Many young people are involved with one or more major health issues during their adolescent years. Many behaviors start as normal experimentation; the teens' motivation for involvement will determine whether these behaviors become integrated into their emotional fabric and affect their lives. Problems need to be confronted and overcome. It is important to address these issues at the "hurdle level," before they become insurmountable brick walls that the adolescent cannot get over or around.

We know that 90 percent of high school seniors have tried alcohol and approximately 50 percent are sexually active. We know that the major causes of teen deaths are accidents and suicides due to a combination of emotional instability and alcohol. Yet adolescents typically do not reveal their involvement in such behaviors and rarely seek help in the early stages. They maintain a hidden agenda of concerns about the adult activities in which they are engaged. They may seek medical help for headaches, fatigue, mononucleosis, abdominal pain, or a sore throat, but rarely do they present with the statement "I'm thirteen and thinking of doing drugs" or "I'd like to see the social worker or psychiatrist."

They want the problems to be simple and medical, because they have learned that taking a pill can cure a pain. They have not been educated to talk to their doctor; thus, the physician must invite them into discussions of these issues. If the physician knows how to listen skillfully, he or she will often find deeper symptoms or clues to the "invisible diseases" and will be able to tap into that hidden agenda. How the physician does this is crucial; adolescents usually do not volunteer information.

Medical people must be able to recognize psychological and social symptoms, and psychologists and social workers must be able to understand the medical ramifications of these behaviors.

Traditional Professional Considerations

Because adolescent issues have only recently been identified, the biopsychosocial concept has not been part of the traditional medical educational process. Lack of awareness of adolescent problems on the part of the various professional disciplines is one of the major difficulties in recognizing adolescent issues.

Identification and treatment of adolescent problems require a multidisciplinary approach. Yet it is difficult for the professional person to think across the traditional boundaries of his or her field. Psychotherapists must look for medical issues of weight gain or loss, sexuality, and drug abuse; the physician must look for depression, loneliness, and changes in behavioral modes and must be aware of the psychosocial impact on the physical condition. Few professionals are trained to uncover pathology that is addressed by other disciplines.

Traditionally, medical professionals deal with adults. The pediatrician speaks with the parents—often in front of the child—and it is with the parents that the treatment for the child is established. The child remains the object of the discussions. When the person is over twenty years old, the professional is again dealing with an adult. It is only in the now-lengthening adolescent time frame of ten to twenty-one years of age that the doctor must deal directly with the young individual and his or her variable cognitive mind. Professionals must gain the confidence of their young patients and develop confidence in their own ability to relate to youth. They must begin to ask more in-depth questions of the adolescent, directly and in private, and then communicate appropriately to the parents; the communication should be handled in such a way that the facts are interpreted in the same way by both the parents and the adolescent.

The older traditionalists of medicine consider those between the ages of ten and twenty-four to be the "well population" and often do not recognize the problems of this age group. Young children are treated by pediatricians and as they enter school they receive legally mandated medical exams. From early adolescence, however, their medical care may be limited to health screening exams consisting of only five- to ten-minute physicals for sports participation or camp, in which deeper issues are often not uncovered.

Teenagers are usually very uncomfortable in a pediatrician's office. They are attempting to put the world of childhood behind them, and surrounded by infants, it is hard for them to consider their evolving adult life issues. Then where do they go? To the gynecologist, to sit with pregnant women? Or to the internist, to sit with geriatric patients? Teens rarely present with such obvious problems as chest pain or gout. As life expectancy increases, the traditional internal medicine practice is moving farther from the adolescent issues into geriatrics. The adolescent is afraid of illness and barely understands wellness. To sit in a roomful of patients with emphysema, colostomy bags, and heart failure is often difficult for them. They may be uncomfortable, shy, and embarrassed in these situations, and the result is that they are reticent to seek professional medical help.

There is no real medical niche for these teens. There is still very little in the way of problem recognition or services. There is a need for adolescent medical practices or clinics, where teens are comfortable and will feel that their concerns are understood. Pediatricians attempt to provide adolescent services, yet it is difficult for them to provide the necessary gynecological and psychological intervention services necessary to deal with the multifaceted adolescent issues and at the same time adequately address the newborn. Approximately 50 percent of seventeen-year-old girls are sexually active. How many pediatricians are set up to do pelvic exams for these patients?

Since 1975, there have been adolescent health centers established across the country, mostly in hospital centers or satellite clinics. There are few private practices dedicated solely to adolescents and young adults. These practices are more successful away from the hospital environment, because adolescents seem to be less threatened in noninstitutional settings.

Some university medical centers, usually located in urban settings, do recognize adolescent issues and often provide fine in-depth care. Traditionally, however, the community hospitals—primary and secondary hospitals—apportion only token space to eating disorders, adolescent drug abuse, and adolescent psychiatry. Adolescents and teens are low on the priority list for space in community hospitals; they are still in a stepchild category.

Adolescent health issues are not yet a part of traditional medical concerns. As a result, the insurance companies find many reasons not to cover these newly defined adolescent diseases. Insurance policies often exclude treatment for eating disorders and substance abuse and provide only very limited mental health benefits. Adolescent issues take professional time, and time is expensive. Physicians may be reluctant to deal with these issues because they do require a disproportionate amount of time and emotional expenditure. It is easier and economically more rewarding to practice traditional medicine.

Communication Barriers and Confidentiality

Adolescents often distrust adults and authority figures. They question the ability of adults to listen to and understand their feelings and behaviors. Young people often will not talk for fear of revealing their vulnerabilities and of being wrongly judged, and they typically are suspicious of adults asking questions. The professional needs to develop effective techniques for obtaining information. Privacy and a quiet atmosphere are important to set the scene. No one will talk confidentially when a nurse is bustling about or a receptionist is paging.

Listening with a "third ear" to hear the unspoken is essential. Active listening involves nonjudgmental, noncritical acceptance of the patient and indicates the listener's desire to know more. Adolescents understand and are attuned to body language and will stop talking if the professional seems bored or uninterested. Being attentive to what is being said, maintaining eye contact, nodding, repeating the last few words of the patient's phrase—all these are listening techniques that will help gather information.

The line of questioning can open or close a patient's mouth. The professional's tendency to provide a quick solution may cut off the patient's freedom to elaborate and prevent fears and anxieties from being expressed. Open-ended questions are a good place to start and will often elicit information. Usually, however, questions such as "How are you?" and "How's school?" precipitate answers such as "Fine," "Nice," or "Okay." Open-ended questions need to address deeper more specific concerns: "Is there anything that you might be worried or really concerned about?" Often the young person may not be aware that stress and psychosocial concerns are real issues, worthy of being considered problems that may have an impact on biological functioning and behavior.

The health care provider introduces the issues and communicates his or her concern. The more specific the questioning, the more precise the answers will be. Adolescents will not reveal that they are using drugs unless asked about use of specific drugs such as alcohol, marijuana, or crack. One needs to inquire about quantity, frequency, and incidence of use. Concerning sexuality, one needs to ask specifically about intimacy and intercourse. Teen pregnancy is a preventable high-risk condition, yet adolescents will not tell the professional that they are sexually active unless they are sure that he or she will keep it confidential. Some of the more personal, precise questions can be asked in the privacy of the examining room when the patient is alone and undressed. Young people are usually open and vulnerable in this situation, and may reveal much more than they originally intended to.

The professional must gain the confidence of the young person and ensure confidentiality if the adolescent is to reveal his or her personal concerns. Confidentiality is the cornerstone of a successful patient-professional relationship. Without assurance of confidentiality, many adolescents may not utilize the professional services available and may not reveal concerns about sensitive issues. Confidentiality allows the adolescent autonomy and the opportunity to be responsible for his or her own decisions. It permits an adolescent to rise above the dependency of childhood and move closer to the independence and responsibility of adulthood.

In life-threatening or extremely critical situations, such as possible suicide, teen pregnancy, or severe substance abuse, confidentiality may have to be broken and communication not left to the discretion of the young person if he or she is reluctant to disclose the problem. In these cases, in order to maintain trust, it is essential to discuss the violation of confidentiality with the adolescent before contacting the parents or authorities.

If the professional treats adolescents as young adults, they will usually respond by being honest and trusting. It takes time to establish a trusting relationship. Teens often have difficulty with trust on many levels; as part of their adolescent development, they struggle to establish and maintain some degree of trust within themselves. This complicates the trust relationship that is to be established with the professional.

Through this developmental life phase, adolescents need to establish varying degrees of separateness from their parents. Some communication breakdown between parents and the adolescent is usual. As parents often put it, "The silence is deafening." Often adolescents do not know how to communicate with their parents. Thus, it is often difficult for parents to recognize their concerns and problems.

Initially, most young people fear parental involvement because of the consequences that they may have to suffer for their actions. They often fear the authoritative and punitive role of the parent. Adolescent involvements can be serious and require understanding and intervention that go beyond punishment. Both parent and young person must be aware of the consequences of actions and realize that support and professional intervention are available and may be necessary. When an adolescent brings an issue to a professional, communication may need to be reestablished between the patient and the parent; they may need help to build bridges between them. Although the professional can facilitate communication between the parent and the adolescent, the young person must be encouraged to approach the parents with his or her concerns.

Parents need education, encouragement, and support in order to accept potentially threatening information. Parents may have closed ears and minds and may not be able to perceive what the young person is really saying. The diagnostician should encourage parents to be nonjudg-mental, which is crucial for effective communication. Young people are usually aware of parental values and know when they are defying them. Parental moralizing and lecturing cut off communication and interfere with the negotiation of mutual needs and the potential for effective problem resolution.

It is important to encourage adolescents to build these bridges and to open lines of communication at an appropriate moment when they feel in control and free to discuss the pertinent issues fully. Otherwise, issues could surface at inopportune times, placing the relationship and the opportunity for effective communication in jeopardy. Open and frank discussions are necessary between adolescents or young adults and their parents.

When parents have a hunch that a problem exists and are unable to communicate effectively or intervene, they may need to seek professional counsel. By learning parenting and communication techniques, parents can more affectively confront the young person appropriately and directly. Parents may need some professional support or intervention, and all parties (parents, professionals, and the young person) may need to be present in order for the confrontation to take place in peace—and not pieces.

Patients are often reluctant to communicate or are inarticulate, and a tool such as a questionnaire may be useful. Robert Brown of Children's Hospital in Columbus, Ohio, has developed a very good example of a "concern questionnaire" (Exhibit 15.1). The practitioner can help to uncover adolescent issues by giving the patient private time to fill it out and then reviewing it with the patient. If major issues are uncovered by the question-naire, it is of value for the practitioner to speak of his or her concern about those issues and ask the patient to make another appointment to discuss them in depth. Given the usual time span of the initial interview, it is often difficult to discuss many issues substantively, and a second or even third appointment may be necessary for an adequate evaluation, intensive and comprehensive enough to allow appropriate assessment of adolescent pathology.

Adolescent Development: Normal or Pathological

Adolescence may be thought of as youth trying to capture the essence of adulthood. Adolescence has been described by some as a "disease" in itself, an ongoing crisis state, a period of temporary insanity marked by ambiguity, personality disorganization, and the breakdown and reevaluation of old values, all forerunners to the eventual phoenix-like rebirth of a new identity from out of the ashes.

Exhibit 15.1. Adolescent Concern Questionnaire.

Circle Your Grade: 5   6   7   8   9   10   11   12   *Circle Your Sex:*   Male   Female

Circle Your Age: 10   11   12   13   14   15   16   *Circle Your Race:* White   Black
17   18   19   Biracial   Other

My grades at school are: (Check one)   ☐ above average   ☐ average   ☐ below average

Are you in a special education class?   ☐ Yes   ☐ No   Specify_____

I am here because_____

Things That Worry Me

Instructions: We are interested in any problems you might have and in any thoughts or feelings that bother you. These may be thoughts or feelings about things that have happened or that you think may happen in the future. That is why we've called this survey *Things That Worry Me*. Remember, there aren't any right or wrong answers to this survey and all of your answers are confidential. We just want you to place a checkmark next to the following things that you worry about.

THE THINGS THAT WORRY ME ARE:

☐ 1. Tests at school
☐ 2. Feeling sex is bad
☐ 3. Pressure to try drugs and/or alcohol
☐ 4. My parents' divorce
☐ 5. Going out on a date
☐ 6. New brother or sister
☐ 7. Trouble with the law
☐ 8. Going to a new school
☐ 9. Teacher problems
☐ 10. My parents' fighting
☐ 11. Venereal disease (VD)
☐ 12. Being alone
☐ 13. Getting bad grades
☐ 14. Handling stress and anger
☐ 15. Feelings about hurting or getting even with someone
☐ 16. My weight
☐ 17. Feelings that I'm a bad person
☐ 18. My parents' use of alcohol/drugs
☐ 19. Going to a new home
☐ 20. Not being treated my age
☐ 21. A.I.D.S.
☐ 22. The physical or mental health of my parents
☐ 23. Thoughts about sex
☐ 24. Breaking up with a boyfriend or a girlfriend
☐ 25. My own illness
☐ 26. Having sex
☐ 27. Making friends
☐ 28. Do I have the "right" clothes
☐ 29. Getting along with my brothers and sisters
☐ 30. My physical health
☐ 31. Being left back in school
☐ 32. The death or illness of a friend or relative
☐ 33. Getting special recognition at school

☐ 34. Needing help
☐ 35. Terrorism
☐ 36. Being unable to participate in sports or after school activities
☐ 37. Popularity with others
☐ 38. Death in family
☐ 39. Being hit by my parents
☐ 40. Taking my medication
☐ 41. Problems with classmates
☐ 42. How I do in sports
☐ 43. Using drugs/alcohol
☐ 44. My mental health
☐ 45. Rules at home
☐ 46. People not listening to me
☐ 47. My body
☐ 48. World hunger
☐ 49. My parents are too protective
☐ 50. Being asked out for a date
☐ 51. Increased absence of parent from home
☐ 52. Talking to my parents
☐ 53. My diet
☐ 54. Not enough exercise
☐ 55. Sexual abuse/rape
☐ 56. My sexual development
☐ 57. Losing a close friend
☐ 58. My appearance
☐ 59. Being made fun of
☐ 60. Getting along with the opposite sex
☐ 61. Not getting things that I want
☐ 62. Brother/sister leaves home
☐ 63. Change in family financial status
☐ 64. Pregnancy or getting someone pregnant
☐ 65. New stepmother or stepfather
☐ 66. Too much free time
☐ 67. Job/career
☐ 68. Homosexuality
☐ 69. Arguments with parents

Exhibit 15.1. Adolescent Concern Questionnaire (Cont'd).

☐ 70. Thoughts of killing myself		people
☐ 71. Graduation	☐ 78.	Discipline at school
☐ 72. Not having enough money	☐ 79.	My own death
☐ 73. Adult (parent, grandparent,	☐ 80.	Getting hurt
boyfriend, and so on) moving in/	☐ 81.	Having no friends
out of home	☐ 82.	Going to school
☐ 74. Others being afraid of me	☐ 83.	The possibility of war/nuclear war
☐ 75. Having an abortion or your	☐ 84.	Relationships with parents
girlfriend having an abortion	☐ 85.	Mother/father loss of job
☐ 76. My face	☐ 86.	My period
☐ 77. Wondering if I am like other	☐ 87.	Loss of a pet

Source: Brown, R. T., and Henderson, P. B. "Treating the Adolescent: The Initial Meeting." *Seminars in Adolescent Medicine,* 1987, *3* (2). Reprinted with permission.

Interpreting Adolescent Behavior

As "normal" adolescent behavior often is erratic, impulsive, and self-destructive, it is not uncommon for observers to inadvertently throw the teenager's serious demands for help into the generalized category of manipulations and attention-getting devices and therefore to consider them not worthy of recognition as viable pathology. An example concerns a bulimic teenager who, in response to rejection by her peers, cut her wrists. Since the cutting was superficial enough not to have endangered her life and happened only once, her father saw the behavior as an isolated incident and not worthy of being seriously addressed in treatment.

The adolescent may not perceive that he or she has a problem. "I don't have a problem, there is nothing wrong with me!" Or an adolescent may perceive that he or she has a problem but be unwilling or unable to change. Antisocial behavior or symptoms may be filling a critical need for that person. They may represent the individual's dysfunctional attempt to self-soothe or cry out for help. Individuals often may be willing to face a medical problem but reluctant to confront psychological issues. Making internal change is a very difficult process and may require more, emotionally, than a person is willing or able to give. Anyone who tries to convince an adolescent to change against his or her will is suspect and may get a reply of "It's none of your business." The doors will then remain closed to any therapeutic intervention.

There are many changes during this developmental time that render the adolescent particularly vulnerable to pressures. Coping with change is one of the most difficult life tasks of adolescents, because their coping mechanisms are just being developed. In today's world, the stressors on our young people are many and complex, including pressures that require early decisions about involvement in adult issues: At twelve, should he use drugs? At fifteen, should she become sexually active? Today's world requires adolescents to be mature, integrated individuals with adult coping and problem-solving skills even though they are still in the process of developing and are therefore vulnerable and unprepared.

Young people often become engaged in activities over which they have no control. Underlying, unresolved psychological pressures may be driving them, and their symptoms may be expressions of unresolved anxiety. Loss of control is often the basis of many pathological adolescent issues. Adolescents normally experiment briefly with all aspects of life; however, when they lose control or cannot take personal responsibility for their actions, the result may be the development of pathological conditions and problems such as anorexia, bulimia, drug abuse, or other addictive and maladaptive behaviors that may need professional intervention.

Adolescents may feel ashamed or guilty about having lost control. They may have personal moral conflicts or qualms, knowing that sexual behavior and drug use at an early age put them at high risk physically and emotionally. Their ambivalence or embarrassment about their behavior may inhibit honest communication with professionals.

Self-esteem is one of the essential ingredients in a developing sense of identity and contributes to the maturation of a responsible, independent, functional young adult. When this is challenged and the adolescent has little feeling of self-worth, then high-risk behaviors may occur. Through dysfunctional behavior, the adolescent attempts to produce a sense of identity and self-esteem, however temporary it may be.

Many adolescents view the health care provider as their parent. They may anticipate moralizing or lecturing if they reveal their inner secrets. Doctors and professionals are wise not to abuse their power as authority figures; however, it can be very comforting for the out-of-control youth to have limits and boundaries wisely set and sensitively put forth.

Stages of Adolescent Development

Adolescent development is a process over time during which young people explore and experiment with adult roles. This maturational process from childhood to adulthood incorporates dramatic physical, psychological, cognitive, social, moral, and ethical changes through which the adult evolves. In order to understand the pathology of adolescent disease, one must be aware of the normal variances of the adolescent developmental life stage. It can be difficult to determine whether erratic behaviors and mood variability are dysfunctional or normal adolescent developmental behaviors.

Those who work with adolescents must be aware of the psychosocial developmental phases of the adolescent as well as the physical changes of puberty so as not to miss potential problems. When a physician senses a change in behavior or in the physical appearance of the patient, then questions concerning high-risk behavior should be asked. For example, if the teen presents with a sore throat and changes have occurred, such as increased fatigue or use of eyeshadow, then the professional should tactfully discuss issues such as sexual and drug experimentation.

Early Adolescence. During early adolescence, the experience of the physical changes alone can mark the beginning of the young person's vulnerability and insecurity. When the pubertal changes take place, youngsters become self-conscious, withdrawn, and secretive. There may be changes in modes of communication. Withdrawal may indicate the need for privacy, which is normal, or the beginning of depression or marijuana use or otherwise addictive behaviors. Wide mood swings may be normal and hormonal or may be the first signs of substance abuse.

Middle Adolescence. Middle adolescence is often the highest experimental, risk-taking time. Drinking, drugs, smoking, and sexual experiences are of high interest to twelve- to sixteen-year-olds. This is the age when teenage pregnancies begin to occur, unless the young people have been informed about prevention and use of birth control. There is often a feeling of omnipotence and invulnerability at this time — "Nothing bad will happen to me." Adolescents also often have little concept of cause and effect. Thus, when they are sexually active, they do not consider sexually transmitted diseases or pregnancy. They often do not connect drinking with deadly car accidents, although they have been repeatedly warned through driver's education courses or even the death of a friend. When they experiment with alcohol and drugs, they are unaware of how the substance will affect their young bodies. They overdose easily because they do not know their own tolerance levels and they want to experience a changed state of mind. In today's world, the variety and types of experimentation have more serious consequences than in any previous decade.

Striving for independence and autonomy is greatly increased during this time, often resulting in parental conflicts that need to be confronted and resolved. The resolution process is necessary for growth, and denial of this process may lead to pathology. Teenage-parental conflicts are normal and necessary.

Peer relationships become important. Adolescents often confide in each other and not in those who can help. A peer may hear about a buddy who is thinking of suicide or may be the first to be aware of a friend's anorexic behavior. These are heavy burdens for youth, who often do not know what to do with the information and then feel guilty when their friends develop serious medical complications. "Why didn't we listen to him?" "Why didn't we take her seriously?" Yet they feel that, if they obtain help, they may risk the loss of the friend who is in trouble.

Late Adolescence. In late adolescence (high school, college), there is usually more acceptance of self, yet youth have a strong desire to belong to peer groups, some of which involve risk-taking behavior. The out-of-control adolescent does not know how or when to contain this behavior. Risk behavior can start very early, and the concept of cause and effect is late to develop.

The Family as a Factor in Disease Denial

One might expect the adolescent's family to be a primary and reliable resource in the identification of disease. However, the dynamics of the dysfunctional family often serve to obscure the recognition of pathology, promote disease denial, and reinforce symptomatology.

All families have problems. A significant distinction between the unhealthy and the healthy family is that the unhealthy family often copes with problems by denying their existence. By contrast, the healthy family confronts and copes with problems openly and constructively. Among dysfunctional families, it is a commonly held myth that what constitutes normality is the absence of problems, conflicts, and crises. Often these families openly emulate the stereotypical "Brady Bunch." In a therapy group for families of individuals with eating disorders, one patient asked the parents of a recovered family, "What was your family like before therapy?" The response was, "Perfect."

The erroneous notion of perfection in families does not allow for the normal conflicts inherent in the parent-adolescent relationship. In their struggle to establish or clarify their sense of self, adolescents often determine their own value positions and struggle to achieve autonomy in opposition to those around them. They determine who they are on the basis of what they know they are *not*; they determine what they think on the basis of how their thinking differs from the thinking of others. In the face of this turbulence, parents need to maintain consistency in imparting their own values. The unhealthy family, with its steadfast determination to preserve tranquillity and good will, denies the normal eruption of human differences and problem identification at all costs. Thus, the parents forfeit the opportunity to accurately assess and appropriately respond to their children's needs and problems. Anxiety resulting from unresolved conflict within families ultimately leads to the emergence of adolescent symptomatology or to the exacerbation of already existing pathology. The symptoms themselves, such as alcoholism, drug abuse, or eating disorders, are in turn denied and remain unacknowledged by the family. The family's desire to obscure problems makes it difficult for the physician to make an accurate diagnosis in the early stages before the symptoms have become clearly pronounced.

It is common for such families to feel that appearances must be maintained to avoid social stigma. They also sense and fear the risk of confronting crises that may ultimately be beyond their capacity to resolve and that may result in uncomfortable feelings of inadequacy, powerlessness, and lack of control. In an effort to maintain control, such families often opt for the assurance of magical thinking: What they don't see won't hurt them; what they don't acknowledge may disappear. These families often have difficulty grasping the reality that by not dealing with a problem, they forfeit their chance to remediate it, thereby achieving real control.

Parents often admit that they do not know what constitutes a problem and what actions would be appropriate in response. They often lack objective standards about what is and what is not healthy behavior, often not having been parented properly themselves.

Sometimes, in an effort to protect their fragile egos, parents may not acknowledge or deal with problems in their children for fear that confrontation might result in an intolerable counterattack. Parents who accept and tolerate abuse by overpowerful children were often abused children themselves who never learned that they have a right to be treated in any other way. One mother confided that she was reluctant to confront her child's flagrant out-of-control behavior for fear of incurring her daughter's wrath.

Other factors contributing to the family's reluctance to recognize and disclose adolescent pathology are the demands and the dynamics of the family system. The family is a dynamic network of emotional interdependencies, a system where all behaviors can be understood contextually in response and relation to all other behaviors. The family system's primary function is to strive to sustain its own existence, through the stability of a homeostatic balance. The dysfunctional family cannot risk the presence of conflicts, problems, or disruptions within its system for fear of jeopardizing the sometimes precarious equilibrium. Dysfunctional families manipulate and control situations and their members by superimposing an implicitly contracted structure of "shoulds" and "oughts," leaving nothing to chance. These families allow little opportunity for authentic, spontaneous, rational, situation-appropriate responsiveness and problem solving.

Parents of symptomatic adolescents often manage to sublimate similar problems and unresolved issues into constructive activities or life-styles. Dysfunctions around such issues of control, perfectionism, dealing with difficult feelings, are often hidden in adaptive behaviors that are appropriate to specific careers or hobbies. Therefore, such issues are typically not recognized as warranting concern in their children.

Attitudes and assumptions attributed to and displayed by the identified patient are often shared by the rest of the family, though they do not appear as symptoms in the other family members. An example of this occurred in a multifamily group session in a hospital eating disorders unit, where a mother of a bulimic teenager remained silent throughout a therapy session. After the session, she explained that her silence was in response to her fear that she would monopolize the session if she allowed herself to participate at all. The mother's issues of faulty internal controls and behavioral extremism paralleled those of her bulimic daughter. The patient's father concluded that the best way to handle conflict is "through humor, by making people laugh," paralleling his daughter's fear of openly engaging in conflict.

In return for bearing the symptom and for internalizing the family dysfunction, the adolescent is guaranteed the security of an intact family; the family ensures its balance and survival through the covert agreement "not to reveal the role of the child or the function of the symptoms." The mutually interdependent needs and hidden agendas of the family and the patient reinforce the collusion for nondisclosure. As an example, one may consider the child victim of incest who submits to the sexual compulsions of her father for fear of catastrophic consequences to father, family, and self if she resists. The mother's unspoken acceptance of the arrangement is implied in instances where the pathological behavior is ongoing. Despite the likelihood of emotional scarring, the child subconsciously understands the benefits of submission for the survival of the family. Her parents stay together despite their sexual dysfunction and she secures continuity and equilibrium within the structure of the family.

If the adolescent's troubled relationship with his or her family remains unrecognized and unresolved, it is not unusual for untreated teenagers to create mock families with peers, in which they reenact dysfunctional family themes and destructive interactional patterns. In the context of such mock families, it is not uncommon for teens to be emotionally abused, intimidated, or blackmailed into compliance with accepted peer norms and to risk ostracism as the consequence for any behavior that might threaten the equilibrium of the friendship system. Pathology is hidden within the peer structure.

Just as the functional family hands down a legacy of healthy values from generation to generation, the unhealthy family passes on its own legacy of dysfunctional coping to succeeding generations of offspring. This phenomenon is illustrated by the case of a seventeen-year-old boy who had functioned successfully at school, at his job, and within relationships but suddenly began to exhibit various dropping-out behaviors, truancy, quitting work, and alienation from people. He ultimately turned to alcohol and was hospitalized in total breakdown. Treatment revealed that the boy's emerging denial pathologies were a response to the impending, though covert, disintegration of his family and directly paralleled the behavior of his mother, who refused to deal directly with her imminent divorce and passively allowed her son to bear the heat of her husband's abusiveness. It took the seriousness of his symptoms to jog the family into acknowledging and dealing with its problems.

Problem denial within unhealthy family systems is extremely resistant to change because, very simply, *it works*. On many levels, it is adaptive and mutually beneficial to the patient and family and results in the systematic avoidance of intervention and change. For example, the father of a bulimic teenager confides that, as far as he is concerned, she is "healthier now than she's been for years" and does not need therapeutic help. The fact is that for two years prior to the onset of her disease, she had been stealing cars and harboring runaways. His daughter's self-abuse behind the bathroom door was certainly more palatable for the family than having to deal with the police department on a regular basis. Or consider a young bulimic woman just entering family treatment who questions the efficacy of taking a "perfectly happy" and conflict-free family such as her own and threatening its well-being with a focus on problem issues.

Major Adolescent Health Issues

Adolescent pathological syndromes are often addictive in character. Adolescents whose families cope with problems through manipulation and denial may turn to addictive behaviors that provide a further outlet for denial and avoidance of emotional pain. Thus, addictions provide the teen with a solution to personal problems that may be congruent with the family rules. Such compulsive syndromes include abuse of alcohol, drugs, nicotine, food, laxatives, or diuretics; sexual promiscuity; truancy; compulsive shopping; gambling; hedonistic fun seeking; workaholism; and others.

Addictive diseases have mechanisms that provide for the systematic anesthetizing of emotional discomfort. Thus, pain and the desire for symptom relief is absent. This is a significant element in the reluctance of the adolescent to identify his or her problem and reveal it to others. A case example is a twenty-year-old patient with severe addictive pathologies who alternated between her compulsive obsessions of cocaine abuse and bulimia. As soon as the cocaine supply was exhausted, she would order pizzas and begin binging and purging. Her anxieties were relieved as long as she could engage in either addictive behavior.

The irony in treating adolescent addictions is that the removal of symptoms tends to *cause* pain. Therefore, the decision to alter this behavior requires a great deal of courage, especially in light of typical preexisting feelings of inadequacy and a dearth of experience with productive problem solving. It is not easy to reveal and let go of behavior that has afforded consistent and reliable protection to the ego, which may otherwise be overcome by anxiety. Because of the emergence of pain caused by addressing the underlying issues, the patient may resist commitment to treatment or even terminate therapy and resume addictive behaviors.

Drug Use

Adolescence is above all a time of change — in relationships, in self-perception, and in body chemistry. When mood and behavior changes occur, they often present as natural, consistent developmental happenings. Resentment of authority, experimentation, obsession with privacy, and testing the limits of authority are rites of passage of young teenagers; they are also symptoms of drug use. It is hard to tell the difference, because the signs and symptoms of drug use often reflect other explainable or characteristic adolescent behavior symptoms.

It is particularly difficult for professionals to diagnose drug use, principally because the time spent with a teenage patient is very limited. How much of that time is really spent talking about personal experiences? Most of it is usually spent obtaining yes-or-no answers or looking at and listening to technical signs. The problems of drug use occur over time and are manifested over time. Is a sore throat caused by smoking, the flu, or marijuana? Is the redness of the eyes due to lack of sleep, personal problems, allergy, hay fever, a cold, or pot?

Drugs used currently by adolescents are different from those used ten or fifteen years ago. Today's marijuana is ten times more potent. Today's cocaine purity averages 16 percent — 40 to 50 percent higher than fifteen years ago. And crack is in fact a whole new ball game. When inhaled, it is 80 to 90 percent pure cocaine. Cocaine and crack, above all else, are fast acting, and the euphoria of this stimulant lasts one to two hours at the most. Adolescents who use cocaine or crack on a Friday or Saturday night and then see the doctor on Monday will not necessarily walk into the office either in a daze or hyperactive. The recognizable physiological effects will have worn off within hours. Smokable heroin is also now available.

Use of marijuana and cocaine, even recent use, may go unrecognized by those who know the users well and who have had an opportunity to see them at work or school. At first, they appear normal, even though function may be compromised. Cocaine and marijuana use can be confidently detected only after maladaptive behavior has occurred.

If cocaine and marijuana use goes unrecognized, its impact, of course, can be disastrous, particularly over time and with regular or chronic use. The immediate postuse signals of cocaine — hyperactivity, anxiety, mood swings, rapid eye movement, dry lips, and lack of interest in food and drink — erode within two to four hours. Marijuana-induced lethargy, ataxic gait, spaced-out attitude, redness of the eyes, and the odor of marijuana smoke all are reduced after a good night's sleep and a shower, although the marijuana metabolites are still in the system and function is compromised. There are more than 421 different chemicals and more than 60 cannabinoids in marijuana. These elements, which are fat soluble, stay in the body fat for more than twenty days and are slowly metabolized, thus continually feeding the brain. Marijuana, like cocaine, causes problems for both the diagnostician and the user.

Substance abuse is difficult to recognize because the user may appear normal long into the course of the addictive behavior, though his or her functioning is usually compromised. The typical adolescent spends most of his or her time with peers, not with adults. Time spent at home, including at meals, is minimal, as is time spent talking with either parents or the physician. Thus, neither parents nor physicians are able to observe the adolescent's behavior over an extended time, either for several hours in a row or even over a period of several days or weeks. This makes it difficult for the parent or physician to assess the adolescent's judgment and short-term memory.

Young people resist interaction with adults, and many teenagers who use drugs avoid contact with authorities when they may show signs and symptoms of recent drug use. Regular drug users develop the ability to mask their drug use. They delay appointments with physicians and make excuses for failing to appear for family meals or conferences. Like the adult alcoholic, they begin to sense situations where they might get caught and thus avoid them. This includes when and where adolescents take drugs as well as when and where they can be seen immediately after use.

The presence of drugs in teenagers' rooms is unlikely. If drugs are kept at home, they will often be secreted in an out-of-way location, far from where parents might come across them, even in the course of housework. Paraphernalia will not be left out in the open or even kept in desk drawers or under clothes. Drug use will probably be very private; it is usually scheduled in advance, for a time when parents are not home or when the youth is out—at someone else's home or, as is more often the case, at a beach, in a park, or at an unsupervised party. It is therefore difficult to observe drug use and difficult to diagnose it in adolescents. The greater the opportunity to be with the young person, to participate in conversation, to observe work, the better the chance for early recognition; but even then, problems resulting from use of the two most prevalent illegal drugs, marijuana and cocaine, are often not apparent.

This will remain a serious challenge, because drug availability will continue to be widespread, drug purity has continued to increase, and drug use by adolescents is a major health problem in America today. More than 25 percent of high school seniors use marijuana, 5.4 percent use cocaine, and more than 60 percent regularly use alcohol.

The one tool that is scientifically accurate for the diagnosis of drug use is urinalysis. It is an underutilized test that could be used preventively and informationally with adolescents. Traditionally, the drug test for the young person comes after the overdose, after the referral to treatment, after the loss of health. Making urinalysis a part of every physical examination for adolescents is not a common practice, but it could be done. Physicians test body fluids regularly. Taking a reading for marijuana and cocaine and other substances can be done accurately, economically, and promptly.

The legal questions regarding this practice are several, and by no means insignificant. Schools, for example, generally have not been able to sustain random drug tests for students unless as part of a drug-testing program for sports participation run by the schools themselves or outside agencies. Urinalysis to detect drug use as part of a teenage physical would most advisedly be done with the parents' and adolescent's knowledge. The physician can share the results with the teenager and discuss a plan of action with him or her. Parental knowledge, in our opinion, is appropriate but in some cases may be withheld if progress is satisfactory. For monitoring a teenager's progress toward becoming drug-free, the observations of the football coach, teacher, and parent will never be able to match the accuracy of a drug urine test.

In summary, physicians, teachers, and parents are not in a position, even under close living and school conditions, to recognize and to prevent at an early stage experimentation with or even regular use of illegal drugs. The problems are caused in part by the difficulty in recognizing the signs and symptoms of such use that results from the nature of the drugs themselves and the short-lived symptoms associated with them. Given the normal changes that accompany adolescence, the mood swings and unexplainable behavior often caused by illegal drugs may appear to be normal.

Some of the most effective scientific technology—urinalysis to detect drug use, for example—is not being utilized to monitor what is going on with the people most at risk. It is a challenge that is particularly significant in view of the devastating impact that drug use and abuse can have on the lives of adolescents.

Sexuality

Sexuality is a normal function of adolescence, and there is a thin line between normal sexuality and pathology. The appropriate expression of sexuality requires exercising the full depth and breadth of one's emotional capacities, which in adolescents are frequently variable and unformulated at best.

Adolescents often respond to emotional urges and become sexually involved without thinking of the consequences. They often do not connect the concept of cause and effect—the sexual act and the risk of pregnancy and disease. Their sense of omnipotence allows them to feel immune to sexually transmitted diseases, including AIDS, and confident that pregnancy will not happen to them; thus, most adolescents do not take precautions or use birth control in the first six months of sexual relationships, with the result that there are 600,000 births to teenagers per year and an equal number of legal terminations.

Because of unstable internal control monitors, adolescents are often subject to extremes in impulsive sexual behavior, varying from abstinence to promiscuity, which leave them at the mercy of the moment. Promiscuity often takes on the ameliorative function of an addiction, in anesthetizing emotional pain and distracting the individual from the chaotic force of inner turmoil; it is therefore not considered to be a problem by the acting-out adolescent.

Teens are often embarrassed to convey out-of-control feelings regarding sexual conduct and their feelings of inadequacy make them reluctant to divulge their questions and concerns. They are reluctant to speak about experiences such as rape, incest, homosexuality, and impotence because of societal taboos and the anticipation of judgment, criticism, and rejection by the adult listener. In many instances, especially with alcoholic or incestuous families, adolescents learn that sexual compliance and a general willingness to accommodate others are the important ways to ensure acceptance and the constancy of important relationships. Sometimes teens live with guilt arising from misconceptions about issues such as masturbation, which leave them fearful that they are perverse. In an effort to stave off condemnation, adolescents maintain a wall of secrecy.

Adolescents are reluctant to share their concerns about sexuality because this, like dieting, is one area in which the teen has managed to assume complete independence over his or her life. Sexual behavior, which takes place in seclusion, far from the probing eyes of the adult, launches adolescents into instant autonomy and the status of adulthood. It is no wonder that they are reluctant to divulge information that could jeopardize this precious position.

Depression—Overt and Masked

Depression is frequently found in adolescents and is often related to the mood swings that are natural consequences of hormonal surges or emotional adjustments involving peers or family. The duration of normal depression is usually short, ranging from a few days to a month, and behavior usually reverts to the nondepressive state after time has elapsed, circumstances change, or problems have been resolved. When adolescents cannot work through their situational turmoil or grief, they become increasingly depressed and often experience dysfunction in social and work performance. When this process lasts over a protracted period of time or when chronic depression is present, intervention is necessary.

Mildly depressed adolescents often go unnoticed. Teachers and parents find them likable because they do not cause trouble. They are quiet and unobtrusive—until more severe signs and symptoms begin to appear or suicidal ideations begin to occur.

In the depressive state, adolescents may alienate friends or withdraw from peer and family activities. They may retreat to their bedrooms, close the door, and isolate themselves behind a wall of music or television; their grades may deteriorate as concentration, initiative, and motivation decline. They may be tired as a result of sleep disturbances. Eating patterns may become irregular. These behaviors are believed by some to be extremes of normal adolescent adjustment. Because of human variance, it is difficult to determine the subtle line between normalcy and pathology.

Depression in adolescents is often masked by unsocialized, aggressive, disruptive, or erratic behavior. By camouflaging their depression in aggressive behavior, adolescents invite punishment rather than a sympathetic ear. Often, children who meet criteria for depression also meet criteria for other disorders—such as hyperactivity, conduct disorders, and anorexia nervosa or bulimia. These are the problems that most often bring them to psychiatric or medical attention and thus may divert attention away from the underlying depression.

Depressive symptoms can be understood in the framework of the adolescent stages of development. In preadolescence, irritability and regressive infantile behavior, such as whining, baby talk, and crying, may be the presenting depressive symptoms. Yet these also indicate changes and mood swings that typically occur with the onset of normal hormonal rushes. In mid-adolescence, depression may be manifested as delinquent behavior, learning difficulties, school phobia, drug abuse, sexual promiscuity, or eating disorders. As adolescents develop and are able to comprehend the future with more abstract thinking processes they may become increasingly frightened; feeling hopeless and out of control, they may therefore turn to thoughts of suicide as a solution. They may engage in "accidental" self-destructive activities such as drag racing or drugs. In late adolescence, failure to measure up to expectations and unresolved separation issues can precipitate the more classical depressive symptoms of low motivation, sleeplessness, or agitative depression.

Adolescent depression may be hidden behind somatic complaints that ultimately become real. The psychosomatic manifestations of depression are common and not difficult to discern: Many patients develop headaches, abdominal pain, fatigue, and nausea. Medical evaluation and pain relief are often sought for these ailments, and a major medical workup often ensues. The severity of symptoms requires a physician to evaluate whether a medically treatable illness is present or whether indeed the symptoms may be psychosomatic in etiology. It is much easier for a family to accept medical illness for which there may be a direct treatment; thus, they will typically pursue the medical evaluation and deny the psychological aspects of the problem. Even when the medical evaluation is negative for physical disease, both the family and the patient may continue to deny the possibility of depression.

Suicide

Suicide is the third leading cause of death among young adults age fifteen to twenty-four and the second leading cause of death in college students. Teen suicide has jumped 250 percent since 1965. Today, 12.5 out of every 100,000 fifteen- to twenty-four-year-olds actually do commit suicide, and there are as many as 120 suicide attempts for each completed act. Certain characteristics of adolescents make them more vulnerable to pressure and less emotionally available for help.

Suicidal tendencies are difficult to recognize for several reasons: (1) After adolescents have made the decision to take control of their problems by ending their life, they are often so relieved or euphoric that their depression seems to lift, and they appear to be out of danger. Intent on carrying their plans through to completion, they are not inclined to offer clues to others or opportunities to be saved. (2) Adolescents may not exhibit signs or clues because their intention with experimentation and impulse behavior is not to die, but merely to flirt with death or enjoy the excitement of misadventure. (3) Sometimes adolescents are so dissociated from their feelings that they do not experience any warning about their own intentions.

At least three out of four suicide victims do, however, state their suicidal intentions in advance. In cases where clues are presented, it is not uncommon for them to be misread or ignored. The adolescent life stage is normally punctuated by the kinds of feelings that could propel people toward self-inflicted death: helplessness, irrationality, impulsivity, risk taking, alienation, and so on. Teenagers typically act out in an effort to gain attention. In the throes of a chaotic emotionally wrought life stage, adolescents may normally tend to exaggerate or overstate their views and thus may not be taken seriously.

Certain types of behavioral changes can be recognized as indicators of suicidal ideation; often these changes occur so slowly as not to be noticed or considered significant. Sometimes, in the face of hearing a loved one threaten suicide, people tend to feel fear, helplessness, and inadequacy, which often give rise to denial and a refusal to accept responsibility for taking action.

Family life in cases where teens contemplate suicide is usually chaotic or systemically dysfunctional. Family members often need to deny the existence of problems and symptoms in their offspring in an effort to maintain the integrity of their family system and protect themselves. Parents often are too threatened to acknowledge information that might require them to take responsibility for making difficult changes that they feel unable to accomplish. The suicide attempt might be seen as one part of a long history of expressed or unexpressed needs that go unmet.

The suicide attempt rate for repeaters is 643 times higher than the overall rate of the general population. Myths, beliefs, and fears concerning suicide provide a smoke screen that tends to impair the observer's ability to predict and prevent subsequent attempts. Myths include such notions as (1) the offender will have "learned his lesson" and thus will not be in danger of repeating the act; (2) suicide attempts are manipulative attention-getting devices that do not warrant serious concern; (3) talkers are rarely offenders; (4) discussing past attempts may serve to reinforce the behavior; (5) only mentally ill people commit suicide; (6) suicide runs in families; (7) suicide occurs only among the poor and disadvantaged; and (8) if an individual wants to die, it is his or her choice, and no one has the right to interfere.

The social taboo regarding suicide reinforces the reluctance that physicians might feel in questioning patients about whether they are contemplating suicide or have ever attempted it. The doctor is thus deprived of vital data and the patient of the opportunity to ventilate feelings or be referred for help. Potential victims hide suicidal thoughts for fear of being perceived as crazy.

In the case of an adolescent who makes a suicide attempt and is admitted to an emergency room or to the hospital, the diagnosis on the admitting form will often be situational reaction, adolescent adjustment reaction, manipulative gesture, juvenile delinquency, personality disorder, suicidal gesture with no suicidal intent, or inappropriate behavior. Physicians are careful not to saddle people with a diagnosis that they may carry for the rest of their lives, which might render them unlikely candidates for future health insurance coverage. Thus, suicide attempts frequently go unreported.

Certain kinds of personality characteristics make it hard for people to ask for help. Adult children of alcoholics, typically having had to subjugate their own needs to those of the alcoholic parent, have learned to maintain silence about their own pain and to protect their family's secrets at all costs. An extremely high percentage of adolescent suicides occur in children of alcoholics.

It is critical that health professionals, parents, and school personnel attempt to anticipate and offset these events before they occur. If a teenager is reluctant to accept assistance, then directness, persistence, and tenacity on the part of the professional may result in turning the tide. Just knowing that someone cares and that there is a place for him or her somewhere is often sufficient to carry the suicidal adolescent through to the other side of the crisis.

Eating Disorders: Diseases of Denial

Anorexia nervosa and bulimia nervosa are addictive processes in which the primary abused substances are food, laxatives, diuretics, or diet pills. These are secretive and self-anesthetizing diseases of isolation, withdrawal, and denial. Cloaked by ambiguity and inconsistency, these diseases usually appear during the adolescent years.

Typically, the anorexic is a perfectionistic, diligent female student who excels in sports or dance and may exercise excessively. Obsessed with thoughts of food and the fear of being overweight, she may restrict her intake of food or fast for days on end. Though the anorexic is often slim or underweight, she experiences humiliation and shame because she thinks that she is fat and unattractive and may therefore wear layers of oversized clothing to hide her body.

The bulimic individual is typically of normal weight and is difficult to recognize. The bulimic may achieve comfort and relief from anxiety through the satiated fullness from binging and/or from the process of purging and becoming totally empty. She may spend large sums of money on food; she may steal or hide food. The bulimic often abuses diuretics, laxatives, or diet pills and may sustain a simultaneous addiction to alcohol or drugs or alternate between her eating disorder and other types of addictions.

Eating disorders allow the individual to mask feelings and maintain the illusion of adequacy and control over life situations. By engaging in these behaviors, patients avoid directly confronting and realistically coping with problems. What distinguishes an eating disorder from an otherwise benign distortion in eating behavior is the function that the eating disturbance serves for the impaired personality. When food is used for purposes other than refueling the body or satisfying hunger, abuse may be indicated.

Individuals with eating disorders present with such dramatic variation in symptoms as to almost defy consistent and reliable recognition and diagnosis. At the one extreme are individuals who vomit once a week to ward off "boredom" on a Sunday evening; and at the other extreme are those individuals who vomit twenty times a day and feel tyrannized by an internal monster dominating their every thought and sabotaging their daily functioning. While some individuals abuse themselves infrequently and irregularly, there are those who describe the compulsive intake of as many as 150 laxatives a day.

Effective diagnosis of eating disorders requires a dual diagnostic framework, which includes consideration of criteria that fall into the configuration of a double track: (1) the *behavioral track*, incorporating the individual's use and abuse of food, laxatives, diuretics, and exercise; and (2) the *emotional track*, concerning psychosocial considerations, intra- and interpersonal issues, and the emotional underpinnings of the affected individual. The pathological behaviors usually follow the emotional dysfunction, and it is the behaviors that precipitate the physiological signs and symptoms of the illness. It is often difficult to recognize the emotional precursors to the disease state.

In cases where behavioral symptoms are vague, unpredictable, and inconsistent, a focus on the emotional aspect of the dual-track diagnosis provides the diagnostician with access to criteria that are more inclusive of relevant factors than is the behavioral sphere alone. Thus, the emotional track is the consistent common denominator and the more accurate determinant of pathology for recognizing and accurately diagnosing this disease.

A recent study conducted at Northwestern University determined that the prognosis for the individual with the most severe symptoms could be more favorable than that for the individual exhibiting mild behavioral involvement. The significant factor in prognostic determination was the individual's personality structure, not the severity of her behavioral symptoms.

Failure to recognize eating disorder tendencies as indicators of disease is the most significant reason why early diagnosis is frequently missed. In a study at a midwestern university researching the incidence of eating disorders among women, 5.7 percent of female students were clearly diagnosable as having eating disorders. Even more significantly, 13 percent of those surveyed displayed eating disorder "tendencies," characterized by mild or infrequent symptom presentation. Thus, approximately one out of five, or 20 percent of, women on college campuses suffers from some degree of food preoccupation or abuse, which is a problem of significant magnitude. If eating disorder "tendencies" are not considered significant diagnostic criteria, then opportunities for early detection and intervention are forfeited.

Predisposing emotional factors for individuals with a definitively diagnosed eating disorder and for those who have significant tendencies are similar. Such factors include low self-esteem, feelings of being out of control, powerlessness, fear of facing conflicts, denial of feelings, inadequate coping skills, and a tendency to subjugate personal needs to the needs of others. These characteristics are usually associated with dysfunctional family systems.

Parents and educators fear that exposure to information about eating disorders will lead to symptom development. It is not uncommon for school professionals to exclude students with erratic eating behaviors from support groups for fear that these students could develop an eating disorder by association with hard-core symptomatology. However, an understanding of the dual diagnostic approach would allay their fears, for, even in the face of normal adolescent behavioral experimentation and curiosity, without the emotional predisposition for addictive denial and maladaptive coping, there would be no fertile ground for pathological behaviors to take root.

The Individual and Denial. The patient's reluctance to regard his or her symptoms as pathological contributes to the likelihood that the disease will remain undetected and untreated. The motivations for symptom concealment may be understood in light of the function that the symptoms serve: maintaining a sense of order and control in the patient's life and often in the life of the family. Symptoms may serve as coping tools, which provide mechanisms for anesthetizing pain and avoiding conflict. Purging typically rids the bulimic of anxiety and guilt, returning the psyche to a state of cohesion and relaxed reorganization. Often the patient maintains an unalterably predictable and nurturing "relationship" with the disease, which provides a sense of security not experienced elsewhere in her life.

Pain and the desire to reduce it are what generally motivates the patient to seek medical care. The demanding necessity of an inflamed appendix leaves the individual with little choice. For people with eating disorders, however, the behavior soothes and relieves pain albeit at the expense of emotional integration and versatility of personality function. For these people, it is the *absence* of the disease that causes pain; recovery entails unearthing dreaded feelings and walking headlong into potentially volative, conflictual, and hurtful situations. It is painful to give up the symptoms and face the underlying emotional issues. The bulimerexic's resistance to seeing a doctor often stems from the fear of confronting difficult realities related to her much-despised body, such as getting on a scale or having her body seen by the physician.

Many of the factors typical of the eating disorder personality, such as learned helplessness, low self-esteem, limited experience in self-expansion and problem-solving, a self-limiting fear of risk, failure, and conflict, and the tendency to view others (including professionals) as adversarial and judgmental, render the patient an unlikely candidate for voluntary disease disclosure, at best.

The patient's reluctance to disclose an eating disorder is consistent with lifelong tendencies to avoid and deny unpleasantness of any kind. For example, one patient, who had been abandoned by her father at an early age and relentlessly abused by her alcoholic mother throughout her youth, refused to allow herself to feel pain as a child. She coped with the abuse by attempting to swallow her feelings and accommodate her mother's cruel demands in order to survive. Similarly, in her adult life, prior to treatment, she coped with the remnants of her early experiences by continuing to deny herself access to her feelings, except for the sensations of food hitting her stomach followed by automatic expulsion, a process that took place as many as twenty times a day.

Cultural factors influence people to believe that weight and food control is synonymous with success, reinforcing their reluctance to see thinness as a problem. Fashion magazines entice readers with bold-faced advertising about techniques to lose pounds and inches and camouflage fat, implying the promise of happiness, romance, and personal fulfillment through the achievement of thinness. The double entendre in the Hershey's advertisement for a thin candy bar—"You can never be too rich or too thin"—was an effective ad that did not go unnoticed by the American subconscious. Far from subtle, however, this ad aroused enough ire on the part of parents and health professionals to warrant petitions against it, resulting in the company's ultimately withdrawing it.

Lack of education and misunderstanding about what constitutes an eating disorder are widespread. Clusters of teenage girls are overheard in high school corridors discussing pathological eating behaviors as normal, accepted techniques for weight control. A knowledgeable young psychology student, participating in an eating disorders support group as part of her research, disclosed facts about her own adolescence; she described being "ridiculously thin," exercising compulsively, fasting for days on end, and then breaking her fast with fifteen candy bars. It did not occur to her that she had ever had an eating disorder.

Myths and misconceptions about food consumption and weight control compound the lack of knowledge about the disease. Individuals erroneously assume that they will gain weight by eating normally and that the use of diet pills or diuretic or laxative abuse will result in weight loss. Teens with eating disorders, often victims of a distorted body image, feel fat despite the reality of their actual body weight and have no concept of the deleterious effect of starvation or binging and purging on metabolic function. One young woman felt she could gain 30 pounds from eating a piece of turkey and 50 pounds from consuming a dessert. The diagnostician must probe these misconceptions in order to bring them to light and correct them.

The tendency of individuals with eating disorders to tolerate extremes as a matter of course clouds their ability to determine what constitutes a distortion. Individuals engaged in drastic, unbalanced quick weight-loss regimens tend to see themselves as being "simply on a diet—isn't everybody?" Recently, there has been a surge of public interest and positive press around nonfood quick-weight-loss programs. Such unbalanced programs, if they do not systematically address or monitor the individual's problems with control, could be dangerous for participants prone to extreme behavior. If control issues were not addressed during the course of the program, once the weight-loss goal has been reached, overweight individuals with a history of faulty internal monitoring, who are thus deficient in their ability to know when they are full and when to stop eating, may develop recurrent obesity. Or they may not know when or how to *begin* to eat or develop a normal relationship with food; anorexia or bulimia may result. In tracing the etiology of eating disorders, one typically finds disease onset occurring simultaneously with a major dieting effort.

An important obstacle to detection of eating disorders is the fact that the primary substance of abuse is food; unlike alcohol, drugs, or other contraband, far from being toxic, lethal, or destructive to the body, it is an intrinsic part of everyday life, necessary for the health, well-being, and very survival of the individual. It is not uncommon for professionals to observe a parent's need to consider his or her child's eating dysfunction as a benign offense, especially in light of the dire consequences and illegal nature of alternative kinds of addictions. These same parents often take great pride in seeing their children looking thin and attractive. Many of them wish that they too could demonstrate the willpower and determination of their children.

The Family in Collusion Toward Denial. Families of adolescents with eating disorders are not necessarily dysfunctional or pathological. However, the issues that erupt as symptoms in the adolescent are often composed of threads interwoven throughout the emotional fabric of the entire family and may well have roots in previous generations. Because attitudes and values may be shared by the entire family, parents are often too intricately bound up in the pathological system to recognize their children's problems impartially or objectively. The family, in its efforts to survive and sustain its structure and functional equilibrium, has a vested interest in the individual's maintaining the pathology. The need for concealment of problems, from both themselves and the professional, is therefore a function of highest priority for the family of denial.

For example, in a multifamily group for eating disorders, one mother revealed that she had been beaten and abused during her childhood and had not been allowed to express her rage. Now she was afraid that if she were to express her still existent, though dormant, rage, she might lose control to the point of committing violence. Her daughter, a recovering anorexic, suffered from a congruent emotional paralysis based on her denial of feelings and her loss of self-control. Her symptoms, which were consistently reinforced by the family, reverberated in sympathetic overtones with the mother's unresolved emotional tasks.

   Professionals in Inadvertent Collusion Toward Denial. The dilemma of the health professional in recognizing eating disorders is real. In diagnostic work, the most substantive tools available to the practitioner are complaints from the patient. The eating disorder patient often does not recognize the symptoms as a problem, seeing them as basic requirements for coping with the difficulties of her life. Patients, especially if bulimic, often are of normal weight, and their concern about food consumption and weight control is certainly not atypical within society as a whole. Professionals are denied access to significant diagnostic information by virtue of the secretive nature of the pathological behavior. When taking the patient's history, the diagnostician is at the mercy of the patient's distortions in judgment and subjective perceptions of her reality.

   Even in the presence of definitive disease, however, there is wide variation in the severity of symptoms, which makes recognition and diagnosis difficult. Differing opinions about what actually constitutes disease further complicate diagnosis. Medical, mental health, and school professionals often overlook or fail to diagnose pathology in the presence of such varied diagnostic clues as an individual's fear of or obsessive thoughts about food, the regular or irregular incidence of vomiting, or evidence of empty suppository boxes hidden behind the adolescent's dresser.

   Even in the case of tracking down educated hunches, diagnosis in the case of eating disorders often evades the medical investigator. The physical exam in bulimics and bulimerexics usually reveals well-developed, well-nourished, attractive individuals. The pathology can go undetected for several years while the behaviors become habitual and ingrained into their life-style. Abnormal diagnostic lab test results do not appear until well into the disease process. Anorexics are typically more easily recognized because of rapid weight loss and acute electrolyte problems that may occur earlier in the illness.

   Though anorexia nervosa was documented in England as early as the seventeenth century, professionals trained prior to the last ten to fifteen years may not have had sufficient opportunity to learn about the nature and treatment of the disease, as pertinent literature and research have only recently become available. Because of the paucity of research into treatment techniques and long-term outcomes, professionals often approach treatment in diverse and arbitrary ways.

   On occasion, psychotherapists, because of their own discomfort with the idea of the patient's vomiting, taking enemas, and committing other compulsive self-abusive behaviors, have been known to avoid addressing such topics altogether, preferring to focus solely on more palatable emotional issues, such as low self-esteem or depression, to the exclusion of the necessary, systematic confrontation and management of food-related problems. In one case, a patient who had been involved for years with a psychotherapist with whom she shared a "good and productive relationship" was vomiting twenty times a day yet never felt that she had the therapist's permission to disclose the eating and purging behavior. She felt that her therapist would see this behavior as too "disgusting or obscene."

Therapists or physicians are often hesitant to recognize and handle the disease because of the overriding ambiguity surrounding it. Professionals who, like their patients, have a strong need for control may experience anxiety and reluctance to establish a definitive diagnosis because of the unpredictable and complicated realities of eating disorder disease management. One internist denied the existence of a youngster's disease despite her vomiting regularly. Only later did he admit his reluctance to diagnose and treat the case properly because of feeling at a loss for how to handle the child's extreme resistance and the "crazy parents."

The pathology of eating disorders is many-faceted, requiring monitoring by professionals in various specialties. Recovery requires input from (1) physicians, for blood chemistry and physiological and weight monitoring as well as symptom management; (2) psychiatrists, for psychotherapy and regulating medications in appropriate cases; (3) individual, family, and group psychotherapists, for handling ongoing intra- and interpersonal psychosocial dynamics; (4) nutritionists, for food planning and establishing control over food; and (5) school professionals, for environmental management. For the best chance of recovery, the entire treatment team needs to be in place.

In its complexity, *recovery may be difficult to recognize*. Pathological elements within the disease can change sporadically. Progress can wax and wane, sometimes in the behavioral sphere and sometimes in the emotional sphere. Setbacks, though discouraging, are a normal function of the recovery process; it is difficult to recognize recovery when these setbacks occur. It is essential that professionals comprehend the many facets and complex circularity of the recovery process and help patients contend with the setbacks and frustrations that typically characterize getting better.

Changes in eating behaviors are often the last to occur, trailing emotional and communication changes. Making hard-to-recognize successes apparent to the eating disorder family is a potent motivation for families to persevere in the difficult recovery process. When families and teens do choose to take risks and work together with professionals toward restructuring nonproductive interactional patterns, all members stand to gain in substantive ways.

Conclusions

Involvement in eating disorders, alcohol and drug abuse, early sexuality, depression, or suicide ideation is a significant diagnostic indicator of underlying emotional problems of the adolescent. The earlier the diagnosis is made, the better chance there is for recovery.

In light of the apparent difficulty in recognizing pathological involvement of the adolescent in high-risk behaviors and of the reality that it is the layperson—teacher, peer, parent, or sibling—who is at times in the best position to observe problems, community education may be one key to early assessment. Health classes and wellness assemblies can educate people and provide open forums for sharing information and offering techniques and suggestions for reaching individuals in denial stages. Confrontational intervention teams of school professionals and parents should include peers. The affinity for traditional approaches to diagnosis can be put aside as people open themselves to assistance from unlikely sources.

Professionals must approach adolescents with diagnostic acumen and knowledge about high-risk disorders. They must listen carefully for information that is not spoken. In assessing catastrophic elements in an adolescent's life, the diagnostician must investigate not only the teenager's experiences with depression, suicide, sleep disorders, alcohol, and drug abuse but his or her use and abuse of food, laxatives, diuretics, and exercise as well. Diagnosticians must be courageous and direct in confronting the patient with their educated hunches. Professionals should utilize the dual diagnostic approach in discovering and assessing the emotional component of the diseases associated with high-risk behavior and the team approach, which provide the components of the most effective treatment.

Because of the unique aspects of the phases of adolescent development it is difficult to recognize adolescent health issues. However, it is imperative that these issues are recognized as early as possible in order to accomplish the most effective treatment mode. When the adolescent is involved in high-risk behaviors to the extent that the behaviors become pathological, discovery, diagnosis, and treatment are an investment in the overall quality of the individual's present and future life.

Suggested Readings

American Psychiatric Association. *Diagnostic and Statistical Manual of Mental Disorders*. (3rd ed. rev.) Washington, D.C.: American Psychiatric Association, 1987.

Brown, R. T., and Henderson, P. B. "Treating the Adolescent: The Initial Meeting." *Seminars in Adolescent Medicine*, 1987, *3* (2).

Bruch, H. *The Golden Cage*. Cambridge, Mass.: Harvard University Press, 1977.

DuPont, R. L., Jr. *Getting Tough on Gateway Drugs*. Washington, D.C.: American Psychiatric Press, 1984.

DuRant, R. H., and Jay, M. S. (eds.). "Communication and Compliance Issues in Adolescent Medicine." *Seminars in Adolescent Medicine*, 1987, *3* (entire issue 2).

Garfinkel, P., and Gardner, D. *Anorexia Nervosa: A Multi-Dimensional Perspective*. New York: Brunner/Mazel, 1982.

Hofmann, A.D. (ed.). *Adolescent Medicine*. Reading, Mass.: Addison-Wesley, 1983.

Yesavage, J. A., Leirer, V. O., Denari, M., and Hollister, L. E. "Carry-Over Effects of Marijuana Intoxication on Aircraft Pilot Performance: A Preliminary Report." *American Journal of Psychiatry*, 1985, *142* (11), 1325–1329.

16

Analyzing, Planning, Implementing, and Sustaining Successful Interventions

Kimball Austin Miller, M.D., M.S.H.A.

This chapter extensively reviews the process used by health care service institutions to determine the product, service, or group of services that they will develop and provide for their patients. The format is a progression from global concepts to specifically defined steps, with examples from adolescent medicine. The analysis, planning, and implementation of successful adolescent health care interventions require an in-depth study of the wants and needs of the various consumers and payers. This chapter's in-depth review of service selection and resource determination is followed by a discussion of the strategic planning and marketing process used for implementation. Finally, the chapter reviews the process for sustaining the service intervention and monitoring procedures used in the modification of the service or product. This constant realignment with consumers and payers is needed for survival and growth in the rapidly changing health care market.

Overview

Successfully initiating and sustaining adolescent health care interventions requires the ability of the organizational unit to carefully analyze potential opportunities in its environment and to develop a strategic plan for intervention that is consistent with the organization's other functional areas and overarching or principal mission. The organizational unit can vary in size from a small section or clinic to a substantial division or department within a large organization. However, the unit must be specifically defined with regard to purpose and relationship with other organizational units.

Extensive analysis of potential opportunities is now considered a mandatory management function in the competitive, resource-limited health care market. It allows the institution or agency to review all segments of the internal (functional groups within the organization) and external (groups or coalitions not directly related to the organization) environments and to develop a service or group of services that fills the needs and wants of all consumers and payers of health services. Its overall value to the organization is determined by its ability to identify opportunities and threats. Once implemented, it requires scheduled, mandatory reevaluation and modification that reflect changes in environmental influences. Although biennial reviews were common until recently, the revolutionary change in health care now requires semiannual reviews to maintain a close alignment with all segments of the internal and external environments.

The effective management of adolescent interventions requires that the organizational unit relate to a broad and increasingly large spectrum of consumers and payers. These must include at a minimum patients, parents or guardians, physicians, nurses, regulators, employers, alternative health care delivery systems, public and private third-party payers, business health coalitions, and integrated hospital systems. All these participants of the external environment are integral to the development of a successful intervention or service and will determine whether a program has targeted the appropriate group of consumers and will be reimbursed for its services and, therefore, survive and prosper.

The traditional strategic intervention plan for designing the marketing mix for a service is appropriate for use in the health care industry. This model includes (1) definition of the specific product, service, or group of services that the subunit of the organization will provide to the consumers, (2) determination of the place and distribution channels for the service, (3) a pricing analysis to determine the elasticity of demand or the relationship between price and demand, the existence of substitutes, and the cost of complements that could affect the demand for the proposed service, and (4) determination of the appropriate mix of advertising and promotion that will inform the target market segments or consumers of the existence of providers that will perform the services that they want and need.

This intervention is based on a knowledge of the organization's physical structure and professional resources and capabilities. Institutional strengths and weaknesses and professional adaptability influence the choice of opportunities and resultant strategies that have a high probability for success. Each organizational unit must extensively analyze its own structure, areas of effectiveness and strength, and known vulnerabilities and weaknesses to be able to develop a successful intervention. In an adolescent health care intervention, the physical environment is crucial to the trend-conscious adolescent; therefore, organizational and staff member adaptability must be at a high level.

Although the strategic intervention model uses the four major instruments of intervention planning (product or service, place, price, and promotion), adolescent health care interventions must also conform to the values and mission of the organization's internal environment (that is, its corporate culture) and the norms and mores of society. Many governmental and non-profit health care organizations perceive that health care services are a basic right of the individual and therefore should not be looked on as subjects for intervention planning and strategies. However, in an increasingly competitive and resource-limited environment, the use of this model is appropriate because it allows for the efficient use of institutional resources to fill the needs and wants of all the consumers. Consumers must determine the best allocation of their limited financial resources and therefore must be informed of their options and the cost-benefit ratio of their service choice. Only an informed consumer and payer will force the health service provider to constantly evaluate and modify its intervention programs, resulting in the efficient provision of health care services and an organizational orientation toward consumer satisfaction.

Environmental Opportunity Analysis and Planning

In adolescent health care, an environmental opportunity analysis, followed by specific program planning, should be a group process where the service providers evaluate all segments of their internal and external environment to develop a finite group of steps that result in a plan for service implementation. To survive, succeed, and sustain institutional programs, the organizational unit must

1. Determine what specific services it will provide
2. Understand its target markets or groups of consumers
3. Evaluate and allocate the resources needed to produce and promote the product or group of services efficiently and effectively
4. Develop a cost-effective plan to distribute these services to the appropriate consumers in a timely and professional manner
5. Review the effect of future health care trends on the proposed new service

Identifying Service Opportunities

The first step in achieving the organizational objective depends on the identification of a range of adolescent health service opportunities that are congruent with the mission and goals of the institution. The mission or principal goal of an organization is molded by three elements: the history of the organization's aims, policies, and accomplishments; the current dominant preferences of senior management; and the institution's resources and areas of special competence. These three elements fuse into the determination of a principal mission. The global mission statement of the institution not only usually sets the organizational tone and views but also sets limitations on service provision and target populations or service groups. An intervention plan that does not consider organizational goals and the program objectives of other functional areas of the institution will be inefficient, possibly redundant or in conflict, and often short-lived.

Once the internal environmental evaluation is completed, the analysis of the external environment can proceed. This analysis attempts to determine the range of specific health services that fulfills the needs and wants of the adolescent, his or her parent or guardian, and the third-party payer. Health care institutions or agencies usually produce services, not products. Services are described by the variables time, energy, and skill. When deciding on the array of services to be provided, the provider must recognize that services are intangible, inseparable, and perishable. The output of the organizational unit cannot be stored and is totally dependent on the provider, since the production and consumption of the service occur simultaneously. However, if the appropriate mix of services is chosen and the other instruments of intervention planning are accurately determined, these services will be accepted in the marketplace by the consumers with minimal promotion.

Determining the range of services by such an analysis, rather than according to personal or organizational beliefs, is essential, because the imposition of the providers' or administrators' views of service needs when they are not consistent with those of the consumers will likely cause the failure of the endeavor. Both the adolescent patients' perspectives and their adult parents' views must be considered and combined in a single, uniformly acceptable manner. Effective methods for determining consumer interest include direct surveys, focus groups, and reviewing complaints and suggestions made in correspondence. A common measurement technique for determining consumer views is semantic differential analysis. With this technique, a random sample of adolescents and their parents or legal guardians who complete the surveys or participate in the focus-group discussions are questioned about their interest in specific health care topics and health-related problems, in addition to demographic and socioeconomic determinants. Within each potential service area, the adolescent and adult consumers are asked to rate their interest on an ordinal scale in terms of their view of the service (positive versus negative) and the potency of their view (strong versus weak). From the data generated by this instrument, the planner can select potentially promising services for further evaluation to align the organizational unit with environmental opportunities.

Targeting Markets to Be Served

The next stage of this determination is the selection of which services should be targeted toward each potential specific segment of the population.

Target marketing analysis allows for three general methods of segmentation. With product/market concentration, the organizational unit focuses on one specific service in only one segment of the adolescent population; for example, sexually transmitted disease treatment for urban male adolescents or weight control programs for senior male high school students. With product specialization, the unit focuses on one specific service but designs the program to provide this service to several segments of the adolescent population; for example, sports medicine for all adolescents between the ages of thirteen and nineteen years. With the market specialization model, the unit focuses on a specific population segment and provides all or most available services to that population. An example of this demographic segmentation model in the field of adolescent medicine is a teenage women's clinic with services ranging from general medicine and gynecological care through weight loss programs, sports medicine, and personal counseling. Each market segment must be not only of adequate size but homogeneous within and heterogeneous between groups. Focusing on specific segments of the population to serve, rather than attempting to provide selected services to all portions of the population, will help the organizational unit survive by providing it with potential flexibility to modify its portfolio of services and targeted market segments.

Planning the Service Program

Once this segmentation has been completed, the organizational unit can proceed with planning a service program for the specific segment or group of segments of adolescent consumers that it can effectively and competitively serve. This planning must include an analysis of buyer and competitor behavior. Buyers include three major categories: patients (usually legal minors able to give assent but unable to be legally responsible for their actions and give consent except in specific medical situations), parents or legal guardians (legally and financially responsible parties), and private third-party or governmental payers. The buyer behavior characteristics of all three types of consumers must be analyzed if the adolescent health care service is to be successful and sustainable. Traditionally, such analysis has focused on the behavior characteristics of the patient and parent or legal guardian. However, with the rapid development of alternative health care systems, business health coalitions, and managed health care forms of medical insurance, the wants and goals of the private and governmental payers must be thoroughly considered.

Competitor behavior also should be evaluated at this stage of analysis. Competitors' market share, current profitability, and cost of service provision must be documented and customer satisfaction assessed. If possible, trend analysis should be completed to determine the responsiveness of these competitor health care organizations to demographic, economic, regulatory, reimbursement, and social value changes that have affected this consumer segment.

Evaluating and Allocating Resources

The first three parts of the environmental opportunity analysis are oriented toward groups outside the provider unit to determine the current feasibility and need for development of the service. Once this foundation is completed, the fourth step is to look within the organizational unit to identify its strengths and weaknesses and to determine whether the professionals within the unit have the ability and resources to develop, maintain, and distribute the specific health care services. This analysis must be objectively completed through the use of a self-study model and perhaps an experienced outside consultant. The unit must identify its current allocation of physical facilities, financial resources, and professional time and determine whether this is appropriate for delivery of the new service. This is especially important if the new service is a vertically integrated activity rather than a diversified venture. Both backward vertical integration (control of sources of supply) and forward vertical integration (control of distribution channels) must be configured for smooth interactions and transitions for optimal service provision, cost efficiency, and provider satisfaction.

At this stage of planning, it is useful to evaluate the product/market opportunity matrix (Figure 16.1). This matrix forces the organizational unit to look at different opportunities and the resources needed to achieve each option. When implemented, new services can be promoted in new (total innovation) or current (product innovation) market segments. In general, it requires fewer resources to introduce a new service to an old or current market than to a new market. Therefore, in the planning stage, the total resources necessary for each choice should be calculated, and the impact on the total resource allocation of the organizational unit should be evaluated. In adolescent medicine, an example of product innovation is the initiation of outpatient counseling services to the current patients of a general adolescent medicine practice; an example of total innovation is initiating such services for residents of a juvenile detention center located near the general adolescent medicine practice.

If integration or diversification strategies would result in reallocation of resources, leaders must determine whether such reallocation would have detrimental effects on current programs and whether the professional and support staff agree with the new priorities of the service-providing unit. It is usually appropriate to develop a collective ownership of the new priorities through the provision of a mechanism for staff input and feedback. Further, if it is determined that new staff would be needed to implement this service program, then there should be a clear understanding of the responsibilities of these new team members and their direct and indirect interactions with the current staff. The time and effort expended during this phase will yield

Figure 16.1. Product/Market Opportunity Matrix.

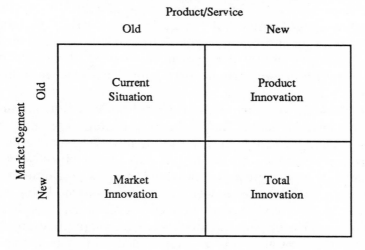

substantial benefits by producing a unified and goal-oriented team, inclusive of administration and clinical staff, focused on the established priorities. With this collective focus and use of participative management, the group is able to progress to the final step of the environmental opportunity analysis.

Analyzing Future Trends

The last step in opportunity analysis and planning forces professionals to evaluate future adolescent health care trends within and outside their organization. The previous four steps will have resulted in organizational agreement on the specific service that will be provided, determination of the targeted adolescent consumer segments that will be receptive to the defined services, and identification of the resource allocations that will be required to develop, maintain, and distribute the service. Before developing the strategic intervention plan, the organization must evaluate predicted influences (social, economic, demographic, technological, governmental, and competitive) that would change the marketplace characteristics or needs and wants of the adolescent consumers and health care payers.

Planning at this stage must attempt to prevent "future shock" during the implementation and maintenance stages. Data from future trend analysis and Delphi study extrapolations are important for this selected service because of the revolutionary changes taking place in the health care marketplace. This analysis should predict opportunities viable in the current environment and with a growth potential in the future. Accurate data from future trend analysis allow the adolescent health care provider to foresee not only potential changes in the external environment that could result in new problems but also situations that could create new opportunities. Health care

variables that could affect the future of adolescent medicine include changing reimbursement policies, changing and expanding health education programs, decreased governmental regulation, dwindling philanthropic
sources, changing grant-funding emphasis, increased managed health care
protocols, a changing supply of allopathic and osteopathic specialty physicians, and the effect of long-term health promotion and disease prevention
campaigns.

Given these factors, the provider of adolescent health care must consider potential environmental changes in the planning stage and determine
whether these changes would affect the adaptability and survivability of the
specific proposed service and the institution's global objectives (survival,
growth, quality of service, profit or increased reserves, consumer good will,
management flexibility). Multiple-scenario-construction modeling with com-
puters should be generated to predict the effects of assumed future environmental changes on economic factors and segment population size. The
proposed service must allow for management flexibility to realign with a
change in the environment. The organization cannot react to the changes,
threats, and opportunities with denial or opposition. Only through modification and adaptation can it react successfully to environmental challenges
and flourish.

In summary, there are multiple dynamic forces that interact in a
complex manner to affect the outcome of the adolescent health care opportunity analysis (Figure 16.2). In addition to internal and external environmental forces and resources, management flexibility must be taken into
consideration and incorporated into the planning analysis. The overall
objective of the environmental opportunity analysis and planning program
is to define for the targeted groups all consumer needs, wants, and interests
and to develop a service delivery model that effectively delivers this mix of
services for the optimal benefit and satisfaction of the consumers, the providers, and the organization.

Strategic Intervention Plan

The final result of the environmental opportunity analysis and planning
stage is the information foundation needed to design the specific intervention plan for the implementation of the adolescent health care service
activity. The type of information available has been transformed from broad
global views to specific finite statements regarding new products and target
market or consumer segments. The function of the marketing-mix intervention analysis is to obtain an objective decision process to implement a service
activity on schedule, within budget forecasts, and with ongoing evaluation
protocols. The traditional four P's of the analysis mix are product or service,
place, price, and promotion. However, for health care in general and
specifically for adolescent medicine, since the output of the organizational

Figure 16.2. Organizational Unit Service Variables.

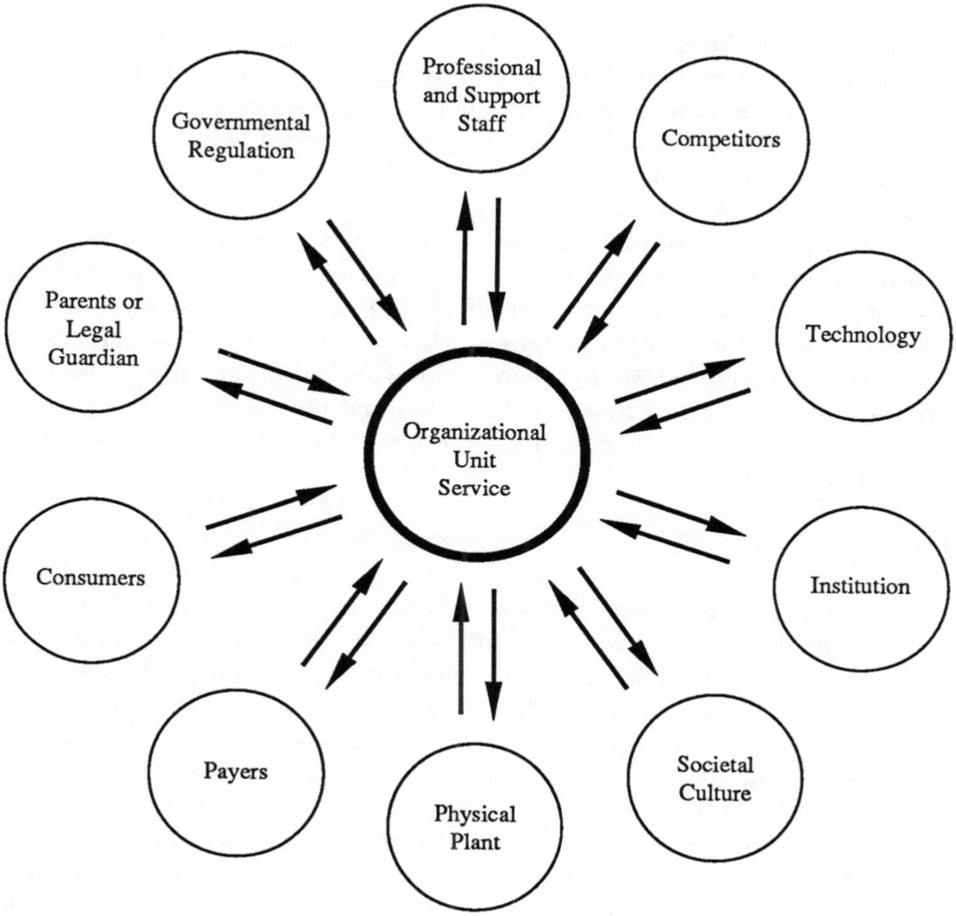

unit is usually a service, a fifth P — for people — must be added to the intervention plan.

People

Because the character and quality of adolescent health care services are inseparable from the provider that delivers them, the fifth P must be the first area of the analysis. Health care services are an interactive activity that depends on the personal relationship between the health care provider and the adolescent. The service is produced and consumed concurrently and is highly variable depending on the provider of the service and integral support staff team members. Therefore, at this stage of the analysis and planning, the organizational unit must specifically determine the members of the team that will interact and deliver the services to the target population. This team selection must include all professional and full- and part-time support staff that will interact with any consumer segment, be it patient, parent, or payer. Personnel budget determinations must be planned, and staff compatibility must be evaluated. In order to promote the chosen behaviors and activities of the team members throughout the implementation and maintenance stages, the organization should specify objective behavioral and performance goals and rewards, in writing, at the outset, as well as implementing a method of regular assessment.

The team philosophy must reflect a customer-oriented emphasis and culture. Each individual member of the service team must look at the provision of the service as a team effort and must coordinate his or her activities with those of other members. This service focus can be achieved if the members are chosen so that there is congruence between the goals of the organizational unit and those of the individual members. This alignment philosophy must be evident within all levels of the clinical, administrative, and support staff.

Product

The products of adolescent health care organizational units usually include health status assessment, acute medical illness evaluation and treatment, chronic illness management, behavioral assessment and treatment, preventive health services, and health education. These activities, which benefit one party in the interaction, are often intangible and usually do not result in the physical transfer of an object from one party to the other. However, while services cannot be packaged, counted, and stored, the product is measurable in terms of the physiological and psychological benefit obtained by the adolescent patient and his or her family. Although there is a benefit to the consumer, the demand for the service can be negative or positive. There is a negative demand when the consumer dislikes the product and will avoid it if even though it will result in a personal benefit. Examples of negative-demand services from adolescent medicine are immunizations, dental work, and chemical usage evaluations. There is a positive demand for a service when the consumer has an active interest in obtaining it. Interventional medical examples such as acne treatment and acute respiratory illness management typify services provided to adolescents that are both desired and beneficial. Therefore, in the intervention planning analysis, there must be a quantitative determination of the specific service product of the provider team that measures and documents the magnitude of demand and benefits derived from the service.

Specific resource utilization necessary to provide the individual service must also be determined. This cost will depend on the volume of services provided; therefore, a determination must be done for different volumes of service, and the marginal cost per service must be calculated. Since a major determinant of the volume will be the service's position on the product life

Figure 16.3. Product Life Cycle.

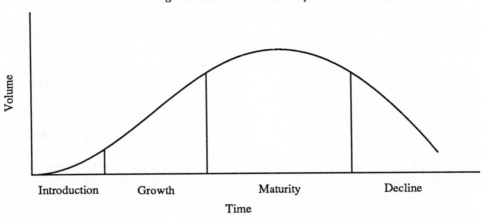

cycle (see Figure 16.3), its current position should be located on the curve, and a prediction of the rate of change should be estimated. Product-life-cycle theory views the service or product as having an expected growth and decline cycle. In the typical S-shaped curve, there are four stages of product life: introduction, growth, maturity, and decline. During the introduction stage of the cycle, volume is typically low and costs per unit high. This is the time when the staff must work out technical and information systems problems, because the next stage is growth. During the growth stage, there is a rapid increase in the volume of service provided and a drop in the cost per unit as the organizational unit benefits from the economies of scale generated by the increased volume. Just as there is a decline in the rate of growth in late adolescence, there is a drop in velocity of growth as the service unit goes into the maturity stage of the product life cycle. During the long maturity stage, there is minimal or no growth in the volume of service provided by the organizational unit. The volume is at its maximum, and the average cost and marginal cost per unit (additional cost to produce the next unit of service) are at their minimum. The service being provided is well developed and vulnerable to challenge from newer service methods. When this occurs, the service is in the decline, or final, stage of the product life cycle.

Price

When the average and marginal costs projections have been calculated for the growth and maturity stages, the organizational unit can address the issue of service price. In determining the price of the service, the unit must address three areas of analysis: pricing objectives, pricing strategy, and market segment differential pricing. The determination of price objective uses the basic microeconomic concepts of supply and demand and elasticity of demand while taking into consideration the organizational objective of ideal consumer usage. Surplus or profit maximization is achieved when there is maximum difference between price and costs. According to the micro-economic supply and demand equation, this would occur when the volume is such that per-unit costs are minimal and the price is such that demand is equal to or greater than the supply. This determination depends on the elastic nature of supply and demand. In an ideally elastic situation, there is a proportional decline in demand with an increase in price. However, in health care, inelastic demand sometimes allows for an increase in price without a proportional decline in volume, resulting in greater profit or surplus max-imization. This inelastic nature of some adolescent health services is a result of the consumers' positive view toward life and good health and aversion to death and disability, plus the lack of consumer options with regard to providers of services in specific situations. For example, in adolescent medi-cine, consumers have greater discretion in determining whether to accept a given price when they are considering routine health maintenance care than when they must use emergency care as a result of accident or trauma.

Once the cost per unit of service or break-even price and the max-imum price are determined, the organizational unit must look at other factors that will affect the determination of the final fee or charge. There are two primary methods for determining price strategy: price differentiation and quality differentiation. With price differentiation, the organizational unit attempts to become the price leader in the market segment. By offering the lowest unit price, it achieves a rapid increase in volume to realize the optimal cost-per-unit volume; it can then redetermine price according to demand. With the quality-differentiation approach, a "going-rate" pricing strategy is used: The price is set according to the usual and customary charges of the community, and the organizational unit does not attempt to maintain a fixed relationship between price and cost or to maximize profits. With this method, no institution has a competitive price advantage in the market, and, therefore, the organizational unit must offer services that con-sumers perceive as higher in quality than those offered by competitors if it is to have a competitive advantage. Quality emphases with this approach are on service providers, physical environment, and consumer convenience.

While the approaches of price and quality differentiation are available to providers in the open fee-for-service marketplace, the increasing role of managed health care blunts their effects. A third approach, market differen-tial pricing, acknowledges the existence of external environmental control-lers of pricing in specific market segments. Health care service charges in certain areas are regulated by rate-setting agencies and determined through negotiation with large commercial insurance companies and alternative health care delivery systems. The price for a particular service is usually cost plus a finite percentage or a specific negotiated price unrelated to cost. The price charged can differ for each market segment and payer. In summary, pricing is set through an analysis of cost, demand, and competition, though the final price will likely be influenced by mandated regulation and/or negotiation with third-party payers and alternative health care delivery systems.

Place

The third P — place — is especially important to the image-conscious adolescent. Therefore, when doing strategic intervention planning, the organization must evaluate how the services will be made available to the targeted adolescent market segments. This evaluation has two components: (1) physical plant location and structure and (2) time management. Determination of targeted adolescent consumer traffic and activity patterns will indicate opportunities for location of the organizational service unit if new construction is contemplated. Other options include a single-tenant office building, a high school–based facility, a leased area in a shopping mall, a multispecialty office suite, and a mixed-use office building. Factors that must be considered in the choice of location include the current and predicted competition in the area, the location of major educational and recreational facilities, the projected demographic composition of the area, and the proximity to needed medical inpatient and laboratory facilities. The structure must be distinctive, but it must also conform to the norms, mores, and values of adolescent patients, their families, and the community. Convenience of access to multiple modes of transportation must be considered as well as vehicle parking and structural lighting for security. Knowledge of the needs and desires of the selected segment of the adolescent population cannot be overemphasized at this point in the planning process. For example, availability to public transportation could be important to one group and the availability of valet parking mandatory to a different segment.

If a new physical structure is not being considered, then the location or relocation of the unit within the institution must be evaluated in terms of access, confidentiality, and potential signage. The internal physical environment of the service-providing unit should be coordinated by a professional interior designer cognizant of current design trends and fads among the adolescent population. Office furnishings and written and video materials in the waiting room should be appropriate for the age and educational level of the selected adolescent population. The dimensions of the service unit should also be appropriate for the predicted volume during the early growth phase and easily expandable for expected utilization during the mature phase. Surveys of primary care health providers document that a space of approximately 1,400 to 1,600 square feet is typically needed for each health care provider. The internal design should promote efficient patient flow while allowing for adequate waiting areas, examining room space, and counseling offices. Overall, the environment should promote a professional atmosphere that reinforces the feeling of quality of care and comfort. The design and structure should promote a positive mood for the staff, adolescents, and their families.

Time-management aspects of the intervention planning process include the hours and days of operation, office waiting time, and waiting time to schedule an appointment. Health care service programs in general and adolescent medicine providers specifically must be sensitive to barriers to service that can be created by limited hours of operation and lengthy waiting time: Services should be provided in a timely manner and available during times of easy access for adolescents and their parents. Constant monitoring of consumer satisfaction is important, and responsiveness to consumer feedback is essential. Every effort must be made to promote access and convenience to families with diverse life-styles and time schedules.

Promotion

The last *P* in the intervention plan is promotion. This aspect of intervention has undergone significant changes over the last two decades, from the use of professional referral networks, word-of-mouth communication, and general public topic awareness methods to sophisticated multimedia advertising campaigns integrated with rebate and reward programs. All new service units use open-house events and basic informational advertising to appropriate medical and health care professionals in the community, announcements in professional publications and newsletters, and visibility at professional educational meetings. Further, it is customary to provide basic descriptive service-oriented material to various health professional and community groups. In adolescent medicine, these groups include educators, mental health counselors, school counselors, chemical abuse counselors, public health nurses, social workers, juvenile justice case workers, and members of school and church parent associations.

The choice of promotional activities in addition to this basic advertising depends on the norms and values of the organization and the professional societies in the region. What might be considered appropriate in one area could be seen as trivial or overzealous in another. Examples of successful adolescent advertising range from simple radio and newspaper informational messages and rebates to coordinated efforts with other adolescent-oriented service providers, such as athletic equipment stores and fitness centers. These activities can be coordinated with current news topics or can be related to a local or regional adolescent-oriented activity. Typical examples include a teen-oriented health column in a community newspaper and cosponsorship of a health run with a nonprofit community agency. Further, it is now customary for health professionals to be guest speakers at school and community functions, in-service programs for allied health professionals, and community governmental meetings.

A philosophical dichotomy seems to exist between selling and marketing in promotional planning. With the selling mode of promotion, the major emphasis is on creating consumer awareness of the product or service and willingness to purchase it. There is no tailoring of the product or service; all research and promotional time is devoted to the process of selling it. The assumption is that there is purchaser inertia or minimal interest that must be aggressively stimulated by multiple informational avenues.

With the marketing mode, in contrast, the organization attempts to define the exact needs and interests of the consumer and then to design the most efficient method of meeting them. The emphasis is on quality production, product availability, and consumer satisfaction. The basic assumption is that when opportunity analysis and intervention planning are thoroughly implemented, selling is superfluous. With this method, the process is constantly in flux and requires adaptability of the organizational unit. However, the close alignment of provider and consumer results in a promotional synergy that should result in satisfaction for both parties. Most new adolescent health care programs use a combination of the selling and marketing methods of promotion; over time, all successful programs use some aspects of the marketing philosophy in order to flourish and survive the assault of new competitors.

The final result of the sequential opportunity analysis and strategic intervention plan is a specifically defined intervention strategy for the proposed adolescent health care service in the targeted market segments (Figure 16.4). All constituencies of the internal and external environments have been analyzed, and relevant needs and desires have been addressed and satisfied. Participative management systems and adaptability to environmental changes have been implemented to promote long-term survival and growth, and the organizational unit is ready to deliver the desired service more effectively and efficiently than its competitors. The final test for an intervention lies in its ability to survive and succeed in the targeted consumer-driven market.

Sustaining and Monitoring Interventions

Strategic planning must play a critical role in the management of an organization. All institutions must look beyond their current situation and develop short- and long-term strategies to fit the rapidly changing health care environment. Every health care provider has strengths and weaknesses and is presented with opportunities and threats. Although much of the institutional energy and resources is expended on the analysis and implementation stages, for survival and growth, the organization must allocate effort and resources to monitoring the intervention and its interaction with the multiple domains of the internal and external environments. The monitoring system must give direct feedback on all aspects of the intervention and all members of the staff. This function can be divided into four areas: scheduled time-frame analysis, profitability determination, compatibility assessment, and strategic positioning (Figure 16.5).

Figure 16.4. Analysis/Intervention Process Algorithm.

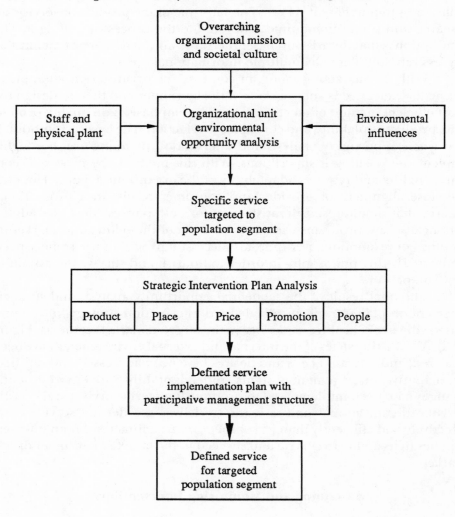

Scheduled Time-Frame Analysis

Scheduled time-frame analysis compares management goals and projections for the current time period with the results actually achieved. A crucial part of this process is a volume–cost variance analysis, which determines whether failure to meet a specific service goal is related to volume or to cost per unit of service. (For example, the process appropriate for correcting a projected cost overrun within a family planning clinic would depend on whether the cause of the overrun was higher than projected patient volume, with cost per patient at or below the projected level, or higher cost per unit, with patient volume at or below the projected level.) The second part of this process is market-share analysis, which compares the relative market shares

Figure 16.5. Monitoring Interventions.

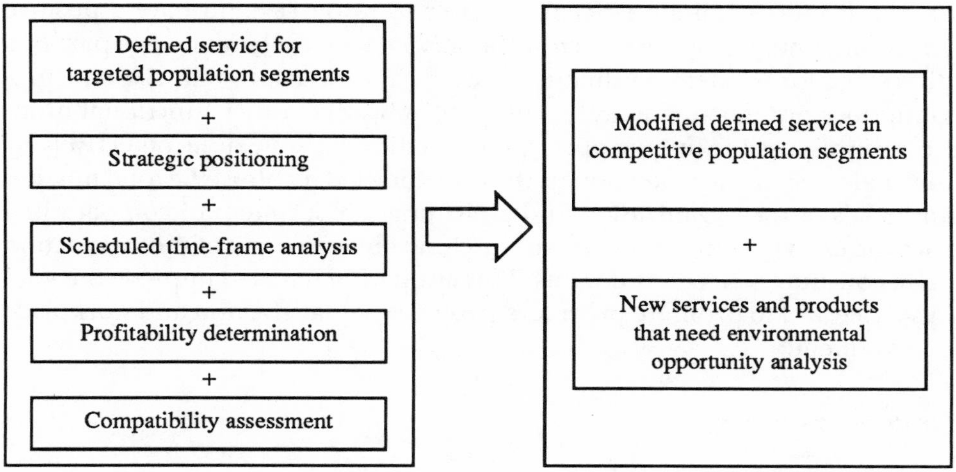

Defined service for targeted population segments
+
Strategic positioning
+
Scheduled time-frame analysis
+
Profitability determination
+
Compatibility assessment

⟹

Modified defined service in competitive population segments
+
New services and products that need environmental opportunity analysis

of the organizational unit and its competitors. This comparison of market shares must take into account both the current situation and the trends that have evolved since the service was implemented.

Analysis of these three factors — volume, cost per unit, and market share — allows the organization to evaluate its ongoing performance and deviations from model projections. It forms a clear objective data base for higher levels of the organization to compare different organizational units, allows for appropriate allocation of total institutional resources, and forms the foundation for projections that will be used during the next evaluation period.

Profitability Determination

The second area of monitoring is the overall profitability of the primary service and auxiliary services. The profit-or-loss determination must be undertaken for each target segment and analyzed in comparison to prior time periods. Institutional standards of minimum profitability are usually used as a basis for comparison, and pruning of unprofitable population segments can allow for survival of selected target segments or groups of segments. Although a service might be provided efficiently to a large segment of the population, overall direct and indirect profitability must be achievable for survival. In adolescent medicine, for example, an unprofitable, resource-draining satellite clinic might be eliminated in order to allow for the survival of the core program.

Compatibility Assessment

Compatibility assessment is important for internal environmental harmony and for promoting the overarching or principal mission that is central to the existence of the organization. If the service is vertically integrated, it must facilitate efficient transfer of resources and have a positive effect on contiguous units. Even if the service was implemented as part of a diversification strategy, evaluation is necessary to ensure that the new program does not detrimentally or competitively affect other functional units. Because of possible unit myopia, this evaluation must be done objectively by internal or external professionals who are knowledgeable of the total mission and goals of the organization and all its units. Assessment of compatibility with the external environment must include measurement of the satisfaction of all consumers' needs and wants. This evaluation tends to improve the level of service and to promote providers' professional satisfaction and workplace contentment.

Strategic Positioning

The final area of intervention monitoring, strategic positioning, is an extension of the systematic measurement of compatibility with the external environment that allows for the prediction of future service needs and resource allocations. Assessment of the adolescent consumers' satisfaction with currently provided services provides information that enables the organization to select new products and services to provide and to choose new market niches where it can competitively operate and prosper. For example, comments from participants in a sports medicine program might identify a consumer desire for a weight control program.

In summary, the final aspect of implementation monitoring is most crucial to the continued health of the organization. Strategic positioning allows for the continuing evaluation of the unit's performance in meeting the opportunities and threats presented by the targeted segments. With the current revolution in health care, obsolescence of policies and strategies is inevitable. The adaptive organization is constantly repositioning to promote efficiency and performance and actively reviewing new services that meet adolescent wants and needs.

Conclusions

The analysis, planning, implementation, and sustaining of successful adolescent health care interventions require an in-depth study of the internal and external environments. Emphasis must be placed on the analytical procedures of opportunity analysis and intervention planning. The organizational unit, whether a small clinic or a section of a large organization, must identify opportunities and risks in terms of the consumer, the organization, its competitors, and society. Once the unit determines that there is a need and want that it can effectively and competitively satisfy, then it must evaluate this opportunity in terms of the issues of people, place, price, product, and promotion. All organizational units that pursue consumer needs and interests find that innovations designed to promote consumer satisfaction create opportunities for growth, image enhancement, and alignment of provider and consumer desires. However, any plan, no matter how well thought out and implemented, must adapt to the responses of the target population segments and maintain constant evaluation of the service and its congruence with the current and future desires of the target population segment. The entire concept can be summarized as "find wants and satisfy them rather than create products and sell them."

Suggested Readings

Albrecht, K., and Zemke, R. *Service America!* Homewood, Ill.: Dow Jones–Irwin, 1985.

Alsop, R., and Abrams, B. *The Wall Street Journal on Marketing.* Homewood, Ill.: Dow Jones–Irwin, 1986.

Altman, S. H., Brecher, C., Henderson, M. G., and Thorpe, K. E. *Competition and Compassion.* Ann Arbor, Mich.: Health Administration Press, 1989.

Augustine, N. R. *Augustine's Laws.* New York: Penguin Books, 1987.

Bolman, L. G., and Deal, T. E. *Modern Approaches to Understanding and Managing Organizations.* San Francisco: Jossey-Bass, 1984.

Bradford, D., and Cohen, A. *Managing for Excellence.* New York: Wiley, 1984.

Califano, J. A. *America's Health Care Revolution.* New York: Random House, 1986.

Coddington, D. C., and Moore, K. D. *Market-Driven Strategies in Health Care.* San Francisco: Jossey-Bass, 1987.

Doeksen, G. A., Miller, K. A., Jacobs, P. S., and Miller, D. A. *A Systematic Approach to the Planning and Development of a Practice.* St. David, Pa.: Argus Press, 1989.

Doeksen, G. A., Miller, K. A., Jacobs-Shelton, P. S., and Miller, D. A. *Family Medicine: A Systematic Approach to the Planning and Development of a Community Practice.* Oklahoma City, Ok.: The University of Oklahoma College of Medicine Press, 1990.

Drucker, P. *Innovation and Entrepreneurship.* New York: Harper & Row, 1985.

Dyer, W. G. *Team Building: Issues and Alternatives.* Reading, Mass.: Addison-Wesley, 1977.

Kotler, P., and Clarke, R. *Marketing for Health Care Organizations.* Englewood Cliffs, N.J.: Prentice-Hall, 1987.

Kotter, J. *Organizational Dynamics.* Reading, Mass.: Addison-Wesley, 1978.

Lazarus, G. *Marketing Immunity.* Homewood, Ill.: Dow Jones–Irwin, 1988.

Ouchi, W. *The M-Form Society.* Reading, Mass.: Addison-Wesley, 1984.

Peters, T. J., and Waterman, R. H. *In Search of Excellence.* New York: Harper & Row, 1982.

Raffia, H. *The Art and Science of Negotiation.* Cambridge, Mass.: Harvard University Press, 1982.

Seay, J. D., and Vladeck, B. C. *In Sickness and in Health: The Mission of Voluntary Health Care Institutions*. New York: McGraw-Hill, 1988.

Thompson, A. A., and Strickland, A. J. *Strategy Formulation and Implementation*. Homewood, Ill.: BPI/Irwin, 1989.

Wolinsky, F., and Marder, W. *The Organization of Medical Practice and the Practice of Medicine*. Ann Arbor, Mich.: Health Administration Press, 1986.

❧ 17 ❧

Overcoming Barriers
to Health Care Access

Robert H. DuRant, Ph.D.

Health care professionals outside the area of adolescent medicine have traditionally viewed teenagers as a relatively healthy population. This impression has been reinforced by the observation that adolescents show relatively low rates of conventional health care utilization and are rarely hospitalized. Yet an increasing number of studies are documenting significant unmet health needs among all groups of adolescents in this country. Although young people between the ages of eleven and twenty have the lowest rate of visits to physicians of any age group, the Children's Defense Fund reports that they have the highest rate of medical conditions requiring immediate care. Most of the health problems experienced by adolescents that require immediate care are related to risk-taking behavior. Many of the same factors that are associated with risk-taking behavior by adolescents are also associated with their reluctance to utilize conventional health care services. Adolescents often live for the moment, responding to immediate life situations and not considering the long-term consequences of their actions or decisions. Perceived inaccessibility of health care services, whether due to physical, economic, psychological, social, or legal barriers, can seem an insurmountable obstacle to many youths. Even when suffering from significant medical or psychosocial problems, adolescents may not seek help if they perceive that the immediate "costs" associated with seeking health care outweigh the long-term benefits.

Adolescents' Utilization of Health Care

The 1980–1981 National Ambulatory Medical Care Survey (NAMCS) reveals that the overall rate of physician visits by eleven- to twenty-year-old adolescents (165 per 100 population) was substantially lower than the rate of 281 per 100 population for all other age groups (Table 17.1). Fifteen- to twenty-year-old youths visited physicians more often (179/100) than eleven- to fourteen-year-olds (140/100), partially as a result of the greater number of visits to physicians by fifteen- to twenty-year-old females. Although there were virtually no differences in the rates of visits by eleven- to fourteen- and fifteen- to twenty-year-old males (138 versus 139/100), fifteen- to twenty-year-old females visited physicians at a rate of 219/100, compared to only 142/100 for eleven- to fourteen-year-old females. These age differences are consistent for both black and white adolescents. However, black adolescents visited physicians significantly less (111/100) than white adolescents (177/100). The magnitude of the difference in the utilization rates for black and white adolescents was also greater than has been observed between blacks and whites in all other age groups (291 versus 239/100). This suggests that black adolescents may perceive greater barriers to conventional health care than are encountered by white adolescents.

The NAMCS also found different utilization patterns among adolescents of other races than among black and white youth. While the rate of visits among eleven- to fourteen-year-old other-race youths (95/100) differed little from that for black eleven- to fourteen-year-olds (89/100), there was a substantial drop in the utilization rate (51/100) by fifteen- to twenty-year-old other-race teens. When this decrease in physician visits by other-race adolescents is compared to the increase in the utilization rate from ages eleven to fourteen to ages fifteen to twenty among black and white youth, it appears that significant barriers to health care may also exist for fifteen- to twenty-year-old Hispanics, Asians, Native Americans, and so on.

Providers of Health Care to Adolescents

Adolescents' utilization of specific types of physicians from the NAMCSs conducted in 1980–1981 and in 1985 are recorded in Table 17.2.

Table 17.1. Average Annual Office Visit Rate per 100 Population by Sex, Race, and Age.

	Age			
Sex and Race	11–14	15–20	11–20	All Others
Sex				
Both sexes	140	179	165	281
Female	142	219	191	326
Male	138	139	139	231
Race				
White	151	192	177	291
Black	89	124	111	239
Other	95	50	67	127

Source: Cypress, B. K. "Health Care of Adolescents by Office-Based Physicians." *National Ambulatory Medical Care Survey, 1980–1981.* Advance data, no. 99. Hyattsville, MD.: National Center for Health Statistics, U.S. Department of Health and Human Services, Sept. 28, 1984, pp. 1–8.

Table 17.2. Percent Distribution of Adolescents'
Utilization of Physicians by Age, 1980–1981 and 1985.

Physician Specialty	1980–1981		1985	
	11–14 Years	15–20 Years	11–14 Years	15–20 Years
General/family medicine	34.1	35.8	30.8	37.6
Pediatrics	29.3	8.3	33.3	9.9
Dermatology	6.4	11.1	3.7	7.8
Ophthalmology	4.9	3.9	4.9	4.5
General surgery	3.3	4.7	2.1	4.5
Internal medicine	2.8	5.8	4.0	5.7
Otolaryngology	2.6	2.1	2.8	2.4
Psychiatry	1.7	2.3	1.8	2.1
Obstetrics/gynecology	0.9	13.9	1.3	11.4
Other	14.1	12.1	15.2	14.1

Source: 1980–1981 data from Cypress, B. K. "Health Care of Adolescents by Office-Based Physicians." *National Ambulatory Medical Care Survey, 1980–1981.* Advance data, National Center for Health Statistics publication no. 99. U.S. Department of Health and Human Services, Sept. 28, 1984, pp. 1–8. 1985 data provided by the National Center for Health Statistics.

These surveys indicate that between 1980 and 1985, family physicians and general practitioners delivered most of the primary health care to adolescents in this country. Pediatricians saw the second-largest proportion of adolescents, although there was a significant drop in the number of adolescents who went to pediatricians after they reached fifteen years of age. Obstetrician-gynecologists and dermatologists saw a greater percentage of the older adolescents than of the younger ones. However, when 1980–1981 data are compared to 1985 data, several changes in health care utilization appear. Among eleven- to fourteen-year-olds, there was a drop in the percentage using family physicians and general practitioners and a corresponding increase in the proportion of these adolescents receiving primary care from pediatricians. While the reasons for this change are unclear, it may be due partly to the increased emphasis that the American Academy of Pediatrics and the Society for Adolescent Medicine placed on adolescent health care during this time. For economic and other reasons, many pediatricians who previously referred their patients to other specialists when they reached adolescence may now be expanding their delivery of care to these older youth.

Among fifteen- to twenty-year-olds, a greater proportion received primary health care from family physicians, general practitioners, and pediatricians in 1985 than in 1981. In turn, there was also a decrease in the amount of health care delivered by most of the other specialties from 1981 to 1985. These changes may be a result of family physicians and pediatricians taking care of some of the dermatological and gynecological problems that they previously referred to other specialists.

Sex differences in adolescents' utilization of physician specialties are recorded in Table 17.3. Among eleven- to fourteen-year-olds, females tended to utilize pediatricians more than family physicians, while little difference existed between these categories of physicians in the utilization pattern of younger males. Younger teenage males tended to utilize the services of orthopedists, dermatologists, general surgeons, and psychiatrists more than did their female counterparts. In contrast, eleven- to fourteen-year-old females sought care from ophthalmologists, internists, otolaryngologists, and obstetrician-gynecologists more often than did younger males. Apart from the smaller percentage of fifteen- to twenty-year-olds seeking health care from pediatricians, similar sex differences in physician utilization were found among older adolescents. The additional exceptions were that older males utilized ophthalmologists and otolaryngologists slightly more frequently than did older females. Most of these patterns of physician utilization are related to specific health problems associated with gender differences in physical and psychosocial development and in risk-taking behavior. However, this is reflected more clearly in the types of problems for which adolescents seek health care and the principal diagnoses made by physicians during office visits.

Reasons Adolescents Seek Health Care

Although the major health problems of adolescents are covered in more detail earlier in this book, it is useful to examine the reasons teenagers go to physicians for health care. Among eleven- to fourteen-year-old males, physical examinations for extracurricular activities, such as athletic, and general medical examinations accounted for the largest (12.4 percent) proportion of their physician visits (Table 17.4). Coughs and other symptoms related to the throat accounted for the most frequent medical problems (9.3

**Table 17.3. Percent Distribution of Adolescents'
Utilization of Physicians by Age and Sex, 1985.**

Physician Specialty	11–14 Years		15–20 Years	
	Male	Female	Male	Female
General/family medicine	31.3	30.2	37.5	37.7
Pediatrics	29.8	36.8	10.6	9.4
Orthopedics	9.5	6.5	11.2	4.3
Dermatology	4.5	2.8	9.4	6.8
Ophthalmology	4.7	5.1	5.1	4.1
General surgery	3.3	0.9	5.7	3.7
Internal medicine	2.6	5.4	5.5	5.8
Otolaryngology	2.3	3.4	2.8	2.1
Psychiatry	2.6	1.1	2.6	1.8
Obstetrics/gynecology	0.2	2.4	0.1	18.6
Other	9.0	5.3	9.5	5.6

Source: Data provided by the National Center for Health Statistics.

Table 17.4. Percent Distribution of the Most Frequent Principal Reasons for Office Visits by Adolescents, by Age and Sex, 1985.

Symptoms	11–14 Years		15–20 Years	
	Male	Female	Male	Female
Physical examination for extra-curricular activities	6.5	2.1	1.6	(0.7)
General medical examination	5.9	8.4	4.2	3.6
Throat problem	5.3	11.4	5.7	7.3
Cough	4.0	3.8	1.6	1.9
Allergy	3.1	1.7	(1.4)	(0.5)
Knee	2.8	1.7	1.9	(1.4)
Skin rash	2.6	3.2	2.2	1.7
Acne	2.4	(1.1)	7.1	4.2
Allergy medication	2.3	(1.4)	3.1	(0.9)
Progress visit	2.0	(1.0)	1.6	(1.2)
School examination	2.0	(0.9)	(1.3)	(0.7)
Earache	1.9	3.6	2.5	1.9
Vision dysfunctions	1.8	(1.3)	(1.2)	(0.8)
Head cold (URI)	1.8	(1.0)	1.5	(0.9)
Nasal congestion	1.5	1.5	(0.5)	(0.6)
Warts	(0.9)*	2.2	2.5	1.1
Headache	(1.4)	1.7	(1.3)	1.9
Abdominal pain/cramps	(1.0)	1.6	(1.2)	1.7
Suture insertion, removal	(1.4)	(1.0)	2.1	—
Postoperative visit	—	—	1.6	(1.3)
Eye examination	(1.2)	(1.0)	1.6	(1.1)
Physical examination for employment	—	—	1.6	—
Upper extremity	—	—	1.6	—
Prenatal	—	—	—	14.0
Residual	48.2	48.4	49.1	50.6

*( ) percentage below 1.5%

Source: Data provided by the National Center for Health Statistics.

percent) for which they sought care. Cosmetic problems such as skin rashes, acne, and warts accounted for 5.9 percent of younger males' physician visits. Medical problems possibly associated with athletics (knee problems or injuries) or risk-taking behavior (suture insertion or removal) accounted for only 4.2 percent of the physician visits of this age group of males. Although eleven- to fourteen-year-old females received physical examinations for extracurricular activities less often than did males, when their higher percentage of physician visits for general medical examinations is taken into account, their overall rate of preventive health care appears to be similar. Unlike males, the younger females sought medical care most often for coughs and throat problems (15.2 percent). However, in a finding similar to that for younger males, cosmetic problems accounted for 6.5 percent of the physician visits by the younger female group.

Among fifteen- to twenty-year-old males, cosmetic problems such as acne, rashes, and warts accounted for the largest proportion (11.8 percent) of

physician visits (Table 17.4). Older adolescent males visited physicians significantly less often for preventive health care than did the younger males but
demonstrated little difference in their physician visits for other medical
reasons. Older adolescent females also sought general preventive health care
less often than did younger females (Table 17.4). Yet 14 percent of the older
females' visits to physicians were for prenatal care. Similar to the younger
females, fifteen- to twenty-year-old females sought medical care for coughs
and throat problems during 9.2 percent of their visits and made 7 percent of
their physician visits for cosmetic problems.

When the physicians' primary diagnoses for adolescent visits were
examined, several different patterns emerged (Table 17.5). The ICD-9-cm
code (*International Classification of Diseases*, Ninth Revision, Clinical Modifications) for "certain adverse effects not classified elsewhere" was the single
most frequent diagnosis for eleven- to fourteen-year-old male patients (ex-
cluding general medical examinations). While it is unclear what specific
problems were included in this classification, it is quite possible that many
problems resulting from risk taking may be included in this category. Injuries possibly due to risk-taking behavior or sports participation accounted
for an additional 6 percent of the diagnoses. The younger male adolescents'
primary diagnoses for other medical conditions were fairly evenly distributed among ICD-9 categories. The primary diagnoses made among
eleven- to fourteen-year-old females included acute pharyngitis (4.9 percent),
infectious diseases (virus or chlamydia) (3.4 percent), otitis media (3.3 percent), and acute upper respiratory infection (3.2 percent). Problems related
to risk-taking behavior accounted for few of the principal diagnoses in this
age group of females.

As was consistent with the findings for the primary reasons older
adolescents seek care from physicians, cosmetic problems accounted for 10.6
percent of the principal diagnoses for fifteen- to twenty-year-old males (Table
17.5). Allergic rhinitis and common infections accounted for many of the
other diagnoses among older males. Problems associated with either risk-
taking behavior, athletic injuries, or other accidents that required immediate
care accounted for 18.7 percent of physician diagnoses among older adolescent males. Normal pregnancy accounted for 14 percent and other gynecological problems made up an additional 12.5 percent of the diagnoses for
fifteen- to twenty- year-old females. Unlike the case with older males, only 6.5
percent of the females' diagnoses were for cosmetic problems. When pregnancy and sexually transmitted diseases were excluded, diagnoses associated
with injuries or problems associated with risk-taking behavior or athletics
were also much lower (3.6 percent) than were observed among older male
youth.

Theoretical Models of Physician Utilization

Because of the complexity of the problem of adolescents' poor utilization of health care, multivariate models are often needed to help delineate

Table 17.5. Percent Distribution of the Most Frequent Principal Diagnoses for Office Visits by Adolescents, by Age and Sex, 1985.

Diagnoses/ICD-9 Codes	11–14 Years		15–20 Years	
	Male	Female	Male	Female
General medical exam	8.8	6.0	6.3	4.0
Certain adverse effects	4.0	1.8	2.0	(0.7)
Acute URI	3.4	3.2	2.7	3.1
Allergic rhinitis	3.0	2.7	3.1	(1.3)
Diseases of sebaceous glands	2.6	—	8.1	5.1
Fracture (hand)	2.6	—	(0.6)	—
Contact dermatitis	2.5	2.4	1.8	(1.0)
Health supervision	2.5	3.0	(0.9)	(0.8)
Acute pharyngitis	2.4	4.9	2.1	3.3
Disorder of refraction accommodation	2.3	—	2.4	1.7
Asthma	1.9	(1.2)	(0.9)	(0.5)
Noninfectious GI	1.7	(0.7)	(0.6)	—
Fracture (radius and ulna)	1.6	(1.0)	—	—
Otitis media	1.5	3.3	1.9	1.5
Head and neck symptoms	1.5	(0.6)	—	—
Open wounds	1.8	(1.4)	2.8	—
Other viral diseases/chlamydia	(1.3)	3.4	3.1	2.0
Streptococcal sore throat	—	2.6	(0.9)	—
Acute tonsillitis	(0.8)	2.4	(1.3)	1.6
Curvature of spine	(1.2)	2.1	—	—
Influenza	(0.7)	1.8	—	—
Conjunctiva disorders	—	1.8	—	—
External ear disorder	(1.0)	1.6	(1.0)	—
Osteochondropathies	(0.9)	1.5	—	—
Normal pregnancy	—	—	—	14.0
Urinary tract infection	—	—	—	2.2
Contraceptive management	—	—	—	2.1
Special examinations	—	(0.8)	—	1.6
Inflammatory disease of cervix/ vagina	—	—	—	1.6

Source: Data provided by the National Center for Health Statistics.

the multiple interrelationships among factors associated with health care utilization. A model that has received considerable attention and study is the Health Belief Model. Based on a well-established body of social and psychological theory, the Health Belief Model postulates that health behavior is a function of:

1. The person's perceived susceptibility to a particular illness
2. The degree of severity or the consequences (physical and/or social) that might result from contracting the condition or illness
3. The perceived benefits or efficacy of preventing or reducing susceptibility if health action is taken
4. The physical, psychological, financial, and other barriers or costs related to the particular health behavior
5. A stimulus or cue to action to initiate a particular health behavior

The model uses a rational approach to explain preventive health behavior, health maintenance behavior, and help seeking associated with specific illnesses. For example, the model assumes that if an unprotected sexually active adolescent female experiences a cue to action such as a friend or sibling becoming pregnant or experiencing a pregnancy scare because of a late menstrual period, then her perceived susceptibility to becoming pregnant following unprotected intercourse will increase. Once the adolescent female perceives that she is susceptible to becoming pregnant, she will evaluate the positive and negative consequences that would occur if she were to become pregnant. If she determines that the negative consequences of pregnancy outweigh the benefits, then she will evaluate the benefits or the efficacy of preventing the pregnancy by acquiring birth control. This evaluation will include a cost-benefit analysis weighing the costs versus the benefits of pregnancy compared to the costs versus the benefits of going to a physician to acquire birth control. These include the physical, psychological, and financial barriers or costs associated with making an appointment and going to a physician, having to relate to the physician that she is sexually active, possibly having to undergo a pelvic examination, and then having to purchase the particular contraceptive method. If the adolescent determines that these costs or barriers are less significant than the consequences of pregnancy, then she will engage in preventive health behavior.

David Mechanic has developed a physician utilization model that is based on the contention that illness behavior is a culturally and socially learned response. Mechanic's approach stresses that social, cultural, and psychosocial factors interact to explain physician utilization. These factors are broken down into ten separate determinants: (1) visibility and recognition of symptoms; (2) the extent to which the symptoms are perceived as dangerous; (3) the extent to which the symptoms disrupt family, work, and other social activities; (4) the frequency and persistence of the symptoms; (5) the amount of tolerance for the symptoms; (6) available information, knowledge, and cultural assumptions; (7) basic needs that lead to denial; (8) other needs competing with illness responses; (9) competing interpretations of the symptoms once they are recognized; and (10) availability of treatment resources, physical proximity, and the psychological and financial costs of taking action.

One advantage of Mechanic's model is that it depicts a detailed and systematic explanation of the perceptual processes involved in individual decision making about one's symptoms or illness. The approach is consistent with other models of seeking medical care in that the perceived severity of symptoms is shown as a major factor in the health-seeking process. Another advantage is that it takes into consideration the psychological costs of taking health action. For example, low-income patients in public health care systems (general hospital outpatient clinics or emergency rooms, public health clinics) often experience long waits, relatively poor patient-physician relationships, and perceived high costs of certain items and services not fully covered by public benefits. Mechanic's model assumes that this situation is a significant barrier that discourages these patients from seeking medical care and that it operates above and beyond the detrimental effects of inadequate financial coverage and the cultural barriers that foster negative attitudes toward professional health care. With this approach, low utilization of health care is seen as a normal response to an unpleasant experience. Although Mechanic's model has not been tested as extensively as the Health Belief Model has been, both models provide us with a framework for understanding the barriers that prevent adolescents from adequately utilizing appropriate health care.

Previous research has found significant discrepancies between what adolescents said they actually did in various situations regarding the seeking of health services and what they will actually do when confronted with hypothetical health problems. What has emerged from this research is that the factors described by the Health Belief Model and Mechanic's model on health care utilization are highly associated with adolescents' utilization of health care.

Types of Barriers

Although adolescents' reluctance to utilize health care services may be influenced by a variety of social, psychological, economic, and structural factors, of primary importance are the adolescents' perceptions of the appropriateness of health care services available to them. Traditionally, most of the health services available to adolescents have been offered in private-practice settings or in public health facilities. Private-practice settings are more likely to attract financially secure, socially advantaged, or chronically ill adolescents. Although public health facilities tend to reduce the financial barriers for disadvantaged youth, the format and the types of services offered often do not attract high-risk youth. Innovative, alternative, or nontraditional settings are often needed to reduce the barriers perceived by high-risk, disadvantaged adolescents. Significant differences exist in the health information and beliefs and the medical concerns of adolescents from different socioeconomic backgrounds and geographical locations. The health needs of adolescents also vary with ethnic background, age, and gender. In order to reduce access barriers, alternative health services should be based on the health concerns that are relevant to the target population.

The perceived quality, style, and expertise of the physicians and staff members treating adolescents can also act as a significant barrier to access to health care. M. Resnick and others have reported that many teenagers perceive health care providers from traditional settings as being cold, aloof, and inconsiderate. These youth express resentment toward impersonal or condescending treatment and inconsiderate, inappropriate behavior (for example, sexual advances, violations of privacy, rudeness, or moral indignation over a presenting symptom, condition, complaint, or situation). Adolescents tend to desire health care professionals who express caring and concern in regard to their health problems. Factors that tend not to be as important are the age of the professional, use of teen jargon, and dressing in youthful styles. Adolescents expect physicians and other health professionals to dress and act in an appropriate professional manner. They expect warmth, compassion, and a willingness to communicate in a straightforward, understandable fashion.

Also of importance are the adolescents' perceptions of the physicians' and health care professionals' expertise in areas that are of concern to them. High-risk youth are very reluctant to seek health care unless they think that the professionals have special expertise in the particular problem that they are concerned about. Even if an adolescent does seek health care from a professional without knowledge of his or her expertise in a particular area, it usually does not take long during the initial encounter for the patient to determine the health professional's level of knowledge and interest in the problem area. A negative experience during the initial visit will practically guarantee that the high-risk youth will not return for follow-up care. This principle applies not only to problems such as substance abuse or suicide but also to less traumatic problems, such as athletic injuries or dysmenorrhea.

Physical Barriers

The setting in which health services are offered can also serve as a significant barrier to access to health care. Many traditional pediatric waiting rooms are decorated in a manner that is appealing to mothers and young children. Usually, the decor of the office, the magazines and other reading material available to the patients, and the numerous mothers, young children, and babies in the waiting room are very unappealing to the average adolescent. For the adolescent with multiple high-risk medical, social, and/or psychological problems, the impact of the lack of appeal of the traditional pediatric waiting room may be enhanced.

Other factors that may serve as significant physical barriers to the adolescent include the location of services or clinics, the time at which special teen clinics are offered, the length of time it takes to get an appointment, and the amount of time the adolescent has to wait to see the health care professional after arriving at the office. There has been much debate concerning the degree that offering clinics only during the hours of nine to five acts as a significant barrier to adolescents. Some investigators have found that even low-income, minority adolescents prefer to come to teen clinics during the day, especially during the hours that school is in session. Other health care providers have found that after-hours, evening, and Saturday morning clinics were very successful. They provide access to care for youth who do not want to miss school or who have a job. However, the success of these alternative clinic times has been found to vary considerably among different adolescent patient populations. For many adolescents, the afternoon and evening hours and weekends are times set aside for their own activities and are not times they want to "waste" sitting in a waiting room to see a physician. Related to this is the fact that having to sit for even short periods of time in a waiting room without appropriate entertainment can also become a significant barrier to seeking health care. Adolescents often live for the moment, responding to immediate life situations and not considering the long-term consequences of their health actions or decisions.

Once adolescents decide that they need to seek medical care for a particular problem, long appointment and waiting times increase the chance that the adolescents will not be compliant with the appointments. Among teens, even relatively minor conditions, such as a mild case of acne, may be perceived as a significant life-changing problem. The manner in which the health care professional responds to the teen's request for health care, in terms of sensitivity to the problem and understanding of appropriate treatment, and the length of time it takes to be seen for that problem can have a substantial impact on whether the adolescent will seek health care from the same source for more significant, life-changing problems in the future.

Economic Barriers

Most adolescents do not have the financial resources, independent of their parents, to pay for traditional health care services. Resnick and others have reported that teens were unequivocal about their belief that the high cost of medical care and their own lack of financial resources act as barriers to service utilization. While many adolescents acquire the financial resources necessary to pay for health care from their parents, this often requires that they inform their parents of their reasons for seeking medical care. When they desire confidential health care, they may be forced to seek low-cost or free health services from places such as public health department clinics. The perceived physical and psychological barriers often associated with these types of clinics may outweigh the decrease in the economic barriers, resulting in the adolescent's failure to acquire appropriate health care for health problems with possible significant consequences.

Many physicians have found that establishing contracts with parents to pay for confidential services for their adolescent children has been very successful in private-practice settings. Adolescents also may be able to pay for part of the services they receive. It is reasonable to surmise that it is the magnitude of the cost and not the lack of willingness to pay the fee for service that is perceived as the barrier by adolescents seeking appropriate health care.

Psychological Barriers

Fear of and anxiety with the physical examination and medical procedures can also become a significant barrier to adolescents seeking health care. For example, with the high rate of adolescent pregnancy and sexually transmitted diseases, the pelvic examination has become an essential part of the physical examination and health maintenance of adolescent females. However, many adolescents are reluctant to have a pelvic examination because of embarrassment about breast and genital exposure during the examination, feelings of loss of control of one's body and vulnerability when in the lithotomy position, pain from the examination and the insertion of the speculum, and fear that some disorder will be discovered. However, these psychological barriers are not limited to females. Adolescents of both sexes express significant anxiety about having to undergo a physical examination or other medical procedures by a physician or health professional of the opposite gender.

Fear and anxiety associated with the possible treatment of problems found during an examination may also be viewed as a barrier to seeking care. For example, the adolescent may avoid seeking care to receive birth control because of perceived adverse side effects associated with certain contraceptives. Adolescents may also avoid seeking care from a physician concerning lumps in the breast or testicle because of fear that "something really might be wrong" and surgery might be necessary to cut off the affected body part. Such perceptions may contribute to delay in seeking necessary medical attention for health problems with significant long-term consequences, such as sexually transmitted disease, pregnancy, or breast or testicular cancer.

As mentioned briefly above, adolescents' perceptions of the quality of the patient-physician relationship can have a significant effect on their utilization of appropriate health care services. Initially, many adolescent patients may have a negative perception of health care providers in authority roles because of their developing independence and difficulty in separating the authority of the physician from that of their parents. If this perception is reinforced by the physician during the health care encounter, the patient may be reluctant to seek care from the physician for future problems.

What factors contribute to the patient-physician relationship? As mentioned earlier, a willingness to listen and to be available to the adolescent when needed is essential. Also, the physician must be an advocate of the adolescent patient. This is especially true when the adolescent is accompanied by his or her parents to the physician's office. The physician must remember that the adolescent, and not the parent, is the patient. During encounters that include the adolescent, his or her parents, and the physician, if the physician focuses most of the conversation and attention toward the parents, this will serve to reinforce barriers that the patient perceives in regard to the patient-physician relationship. Six factors have been proposed that help develop a therapeutic alliance between the physician and the adolescent: honesty, respect, expediency, simplicity of education offered, involvement in the therapeutic modality, and encouragement of responsibility for self. Such characteristics will often reduce many psychological barriers that hinder adolescents from acquiring appropriate health care.

Even when physical, economic, and other psychological barriers are minimal or nonexistent, the degree that adolescents feel that services are provided confidentially can be a determining factor in their health care utilization. Adolescents are often embarrassed to answer questions and to discuss issues related to their body development, sexuality, or personal hygiene. Knowledge and assurance that these issues will be kept in confidence will often reduce adolescents' discomfort with discussing them. In a survey conducted by Resnick and others, adolescents expressed a great deal of concern that friends might find out if they sought medical care for sensitive, personal problems such as sexually transmitted diseases, chemical dependency, or pregnancy. This threat to reputation is crucial for the adolescent, because it is during this period of life that self-esteem and personal identification are developed primarily from the perceived judgment of significant others. Since confidentiality of services is so highly associated with maintaining both reputation and self-worth, the perceived lack of confidentiality of a particular health facility may be seen as an overwhelming barrier by adolescents.

Confidentiality was also seen as a means of avoiding potential abuse, punishment, or retribution from parents who, from the adolescent's standpoint, would be unwilling or unable to understand the adolescent's perspective on the health problem. Consequently, confidentiality is not merely a means of saving face by the adolescent but also a pivotal determinant in the assessment of what constitutes appropriate health care. Resnick also argues that confidentiality serves as a means of enhancing an adolescent's problem-solving capabilities by facilitating the utilization of services where the social cost of self-disclosure may otherwise appear to be too high.

Cross-cultural issues can also develop into significant barriers to adolescents' access to health care. The failure to consider health beliefs and behaviors associated with an adolescent's cultural background, particularly when it differs from the physician's, may lead to misdiagnoses of illness, lack of cooperation, noncompliance, poor utilization of health resources, and a general alienation of the adolescent patient from the health care system. For example, M. E. Felice has pointed out that Southeast Asian cultural and religious beliefs encourage females to be shy and modest and never to permit discussion of personal matters with males. Because of cultural taboos, these women are unable to share information or seek medical care for issues related to sexuality, family planning, pregnancy, sexually transmitted diseases, or sexual-physical abuse. If the physician is unaware of these cultural taboos when questioning the female Southeast Asian adolescent concerning sensitive issues, he or she is likely to receive inaccurate data, as well as increasing the patient's anxiety over the health encounter.

J. F. Nidorf and M. C. Morgan argue that if the physician wishes to facilitate communication, mutual respect, and understanding within the cross-cultural patient-physician relationship, he or she must make every effort to elicit the adolescent's perspective about certain issues (for example, what caused his or her problem; the meaning of the symptoms; how the problem should be handled; and what the expected roles of both the adolescent and the physician are). For the physician to become sensitive to cultural factors, the introductory interview with the patient should involve a "cultural assessment" of such factors as ethnic affiliation, religious beliefs, standard diet, customs regarding communication, family patterns, grieving, assignment of the sick role, and so on.

Cross-cultural issues affect not only health care delivery to adolescents from different ethnic, socioeconomic, and religious groups but also the health behavior of adolescents from rural versus urban areas or adolescents with different sexual orientations. For example, the health beliefs and the corresponding health behavior of rural adolescents vary significantly from those of adolescents living in large urban areas. Health care providers who do not take these urban-rural differences into account may encounter problems in delivering adequate health care to these patients similar to those encountered with adolescents from a different ethnic or cultural background. Similarly, the same cultural and ethnic biases that may interfere with a white, middle-class physician providing adequate health care for low-income Hispanic youth in south Texas may also interfere with providing health care to a homosexual adolescent.

Adolescents are usually very astute at perceiving biases or preferences of the health care provider. Such perceived prejudices may act as significant barriers to access to future health care. Nidorf and Morgan have suggested that the physician caring for adolescents from different cultural and ethnic backgrounds confront his or her attitudes concerning (1) patient etiquette regarding appointment keeping, communication styles and appropriate body language, cleanliness, and so on; (2) parental discipline; (3) alternative health practices; (4) sexual conduct and drug use; (5) tolerance for ambiguity; (6) involvement of family members in the treatment decision; and (7) responses to pain. In addition, the physician should also conduct a self-assessment of his or her own beliefs and values concerning appropriate health and sexual behavior. In most cases, clinicians who embrace a cross-cultural perspective in the provision of health care to adolescents will find themselves rewarded with patient loyalty, respect, and gratitude.

Legal Barriers

Most states have passed laws providing the adolescent the right to seek health care and the physician the right to provide some forms of care without parental consent. Although laws vary considerably among states, they usually include access to medical care for reproductive health issues and substance use or abuse. However, they usually do not allow physicians to provide health care to nonemancipated adolescents for other health problems. The fact that adolescents' parents must give informed consent to provision of health care for other issues may act as a barrier to health care utilization for some teens.

Some states have enacted specific laws that correspond with the American Academy of Pediatrics' "mature minor doctrine." This doctrine states that minor individuals sufficiently mature to understand the benefits and risks of a medical evaluation and treatment are legally able to give valid informed consent. This valid consent allows physicians to provide care for adolescents if parents are not available, if there is a need for immediate treatment, or if the health care problem falls within a number of sensitive areas. These laws vary considerably, so the physician needs to check with the appropriate state agencies for information on the statutes.

In contrast to mature-minor or emancipated-minor laws, some states have enacted parental notification laws covering adolescents receiving certain types of treatment, such as abortions. In general, these laws state that a minor must demonstrate that one or both biological parents, if living, have been notified of her attempt to terminate the pregnancy. In some states, court "bypass" provisions have been added whereby minors who are unwilling to notify one or both biological parents may seek court certification of maturity so as to provide informed consent for abortion on their own. Studies conducted after the passing of such a law in Massachusetts suggest that the law has served as a barrier to adolescents receiving abortions in that state and that many adolescents are going to other states to receive their abortions. However, a report from Minnesota suggests that the law is having little effect in regard to adolescents leaving Minnesota to go to Wisconsin to receive abortions. Although based on a small sample size, the Minnesota study also suggests that the parental notification law may have a slight effect on the number of adolescents notifying both parents. However, when the Minnesota youth were compared to teens receiving abortions in Wisconsin, it was found that more than 60 percent of the youth in both states notified at least one parent of their decision to receive an abortion.

Although it is still not clear to what extent statutes such as parental notification laws serve as barriers to health care, physicians can take a number of steps to reduce the degree to which adolescents perceive these laws as barriers. As was stated earlier, the physician can establish a contract with the adolescent's parents that all care will be provided confidentially, except in cases where the life or safety of the adolescent is in jeopardy. The physician should assure adolescents that he or she will also gain their consent before sharing confidences with their parents. However, the physician should help and encourage adolescents to increase their communication with their parents concerning issues related to their health. The more the physician can help adolescents talk with their parents about sensitive issues, the less legal and ethical factors will act as barriers to the adolescents' receiving appropriate health care.

Overcoming Barriers: Alternative Health Care Approaches

Although the attitude of the personnel in the office or clinic is more important than the decor of the physical setting, adolescents are attracted to those settings that are not oriented toward younger children. While posters of rock music stars and strobe lights are not necessary, a more adult setting with appropriate decorations and activities will enhance the attractiveness of the clinic setting for the adolescent patient. Just as the design of health services should take into consideration the specific characteristics of the target population, the design of the waiting room and examination areas of an adolescent clinic should be appropriate to the interests and backgrounds of the adolescents for whom care is being provided. For example, the decorations and the type of background music that are chosen for the waiting room may be very different for lower-income minority adolescents in a large urban area than for a private-practice office treating predominantly white middle- and upper-middle-class adolescents. In a similar fashion, the choice of appropriate books, other reading material, and educational pamphlets should take into account the ethnic, racial, religious, educational, and socioeconomic backgrounds of the target population. Video games and computer-based health education stations have practically universal appeal to adolescents. Both microcomputers and software can be purchased at relatively low cost and can greatly enhance the appeal of the office and waiting room from the adolescent's perspective. Regardless of the choice of decor, the physician should remember that a relaxed and pleasant environment creates a comfortable feeling that carries over to the examining room.

A number of innovative approaches can be used to reduce the financial barriers to adolescents' access to health care. In some adolescent populations, it is appropriate to establish contracts with the parents to pay for confidential care when the adolescent desires to see the physician without informing the parents. These contracts can be tailored for each family, providing assurances to both the adolescent and the parents that services will not be provided that compromise the religious or moral values of the adolescent or the parents. The contract should include provisions that the physician will not break the patient-physician confidentiality relationship unless the adolescent's life is in danger. Provisions also need to be made that the adolescent will not be cross-examined when the bill is received. However, such contracts can be used to increase the communication between the adolescents and his or her parents about sensitive issues.

Because of their desire for privacy, some adolescent patients may choose to bear the cost of their own health care. Therefore, a nominal fee and/or a structured reimbursement schedule can make the clinic more financially acceptable and facilitate utilization. The staff should also be knowledgeable about financial resources such as Medicaid, Title X, Title V, and Early and Periodic Screening, Diagnosis, and Treatment Programs (EPSDTs) in their state and community. The office staff should help the adolescent to qualify and to file any third-party payment forms. The willingness to work with the adolescent in dealing with the cost of health care can significantly reduce the financial barriers that adolescents perceive to their acquiring appropriate care.

Peer Counselor Programs

In addition to the design and the decor of the adolescent clinic, a number of other innovative approaches can be taken to help reduce barriers to access to health care. Peer counselor programs have been found to be very successful in increasing some adolescents' access to health care. A group of investigators from Montefiore Medical Center in the south Bronx of New York City have successfully used peer counselors as health screeners in a high school setting to reach students who would be unlikely to interact with routine health care systems. A large number of similar programs have also been established throughout the country. In these programs, adolescents are trained to play several roles, including those of information provider, referral agent, and counselor. Peer counselors have also been used successfully in health care clinics to reduce some of the structural and psychological barriers to health care. Susan Jay and others experimentally compared the influence of peer counselors and of nurse clinicians on compliance with oral contraception by adolescent females. They found that peer counselors can be easily incorporated into the multidisciplinary team approach to adolescent health care. The peer counselors acted not only as health screeners but also as educators of the adolescent patients.

Peer counselors are often more aware of and sensitive to the social status and health concerns of other adolescent patients than are adult practitioners. They provide a necessary link between the adult health community and the adolescent patient population. Although the peer counselor's ability to act as a liaison between the adolescent community and the health care system can help reduce a number of barriers to health care, the use of peer counselors can potentially threaten the health care provider's ability to provide confidential services to adolescents. Some adolescents may not trust their peers' ability to keep sensitive health information confidential. Yet adequate training and supervision of peer counselors usually reduce the chance that they will break the rule of confidentiality. Proper education of adolescent patients will also decrease their distrust of the peer counselor's ability to keep information confidential. The use of peer counselors requires the organization of a system that encourages students to want to help one another. It also requires a structure that clearly delineates for peer counselors what aspects of health care delivery they can legitimately perform. When used properly, a peer counselor program can significantly reduce many of the structural and psychological barriers to adolescents' access to health care.

Adult Mentor Programs

More recently, health care providers have experimented with using adult mentor programs to reduce access barriers for some high-risk youth. One example is the use of an adult mentor program to reduce second-time adolescent pregnancies among high-risk urban adolescent females. Adult women from the community are trained and assigned to adolescents who have already had one child. The mentors help teen parents and their families achieve agreed-upon goals for positive life options and improvement in their current situations. The mentor serves as a role model and resource guide, spending a specified amount of time with the teen and her family on a weekly basis over a period of two years. These contacts take place in a variety of settings and include interaction with the teen mother and her child, the teen father, the parents of the teen mother, and her siblings. The initial results suggest that the use of adult mentors helps facilitate high-risk teens' utilization of health and social resources by reducing many of the physical, economic, structural, and legal barriers that they normally encounter.

School-Based Health Clinics

The use of school-based health clinics has also been proposed as a method for reducing many of the barriers that adolescents perceive to exist to their acquiring health care. The concept of school health programs providing primary health care to adolescents is not new in the United States. However, the school-based health clinic model that exists today has been developed primarily over the last twenty years. The first school-based health clinic was established in a Dallas, Texas, elementary school in 1968, and the first high school clinic opened in 1970. The widely publicized St. Paul High School Clinic opened in 1973, but few additional clinics were established until 1979. To date, there are more than a hundred school-based clinics operating in the United States.

School-based clinics are usually primary health care centers located on or near the campuses of junior and senior high schools. They usually offer a variety of health and social services to students, using a multidisciplinary professional team approach. The advantage of school-based clinics is that they provide excellent accessibility, reduce most of the economic barriers, and provide a method for channeling adolescents into appropriate traditional health care settings. However, they still require that students receive informed consent from their parents to receive care for such sensitive issues as family planning and contraceptive services. Although a majority of parents give formal permission for their adolescents to receive services, school-based health clinics are not without controversy. Many opponents express concern about program management of adolescent sexuality and reproductive health, especially easy access to contraception; fear that parents will lose control over the medical and reproductive health care of their adolescent children; and an economic threat to community physicians in the form of loss of their adolescent patients to school-based clinics.

While many professional organizations, such as the Society for Adolescent Medicine and the American Academy of Pediatrics, endorse the concept of the school-based health clinic initiative, it is recognized that school-based health clinics' efficacy at improving the health status of adolescents has not been fully evaluated. However, most agree that school-based health clinics offer a promising addition to existing service systems and that they reduce many of the barriers that prevent adolescents from acquiring adequate health care.

Shopping-Mall-Based Clinics

It has been proposed that primary health care clinics similar to school-based clinics but located in shopping malls may also reduce some of the health care barriers to adolescents. Over the last few years, shopping malls have become a primary location of social interaction for younger teens. This assumption can be substantiated by going into any shopping mall in this country on a Saturday or Sunday afternoon. Shopping malls have been found to be excellent locations for health promotion programs for both adults and adolescents. Shopping malls also may provide excellent locations for clinics that provide care for problems that state laws allow adolescents to be treated for without parental informed consent. While many of the structural, psychological, and legal barriers to health care access may be reduced by shopping-mall-based clinics, the economic barriers may in fact be increased as a result of the high cost of leasing space within most shopping malls. However, the economic problems associated with mall-based clinics are not unresolvable, especially for nonprofit organizations that are attempting to reduce significant public health problems such as adolescent pregnancy.

Athletic Examination Programs

The preparticipation health screening programs that have been established in communities around this country provide another example of how alternative approaches can be used to reduce barriers to health care access. Working in conjunction with the local county medical society and board of education, the Medical College of Georgia developed a model program for providing comprehensive preparticipation athletic examinations for all student athletes in Augusta (Richmond County), Georgia. All public high school students in the county who plan to participate in a scholastic sport are required to undergo a physical examination at the beginning of the sports season. Students may choose between an examination by their own physician or a free examination provided by groups of volunteer physicians, dentists, and physical therapists from the local community and the medical school. On scheduled evenings, groups of athletes are transported from their school by their coaches to the outpatient building of the local community hospital. Groups of 50 to 150 students are evaluated through the use of a station examination approach. The students rotate through seven examination stations, each designed to assess or evaluate a different area.

At present, students are charged $5.00 apiece for the examination. For students who cannot afford to pay the $5.00, the fee is paid by the school system. All examinations are recorded on a standardized form that is currently recommended by the American Academy of Pediatrics. This approach to the preparticipation examination of athletes is both comprehensive and effective. The station examination has been found to detect more abnormalities that would place the student athlete at risk of injury than are found by individual physicians. The approach reduces most structural, economic, psychological, and legal barriers usually experienced by student athletes. It also provides a mechanism to channel adolescents found to have specific problems back into the traditional health care setting for follow-up care or treatment.

Alternative Comprehensive Health Care Approaches

Teen-Link: Lincoln Community Health Center. Mary Vernon has developed a health promotion–disease prevention program in Durham, North Carolina, that serves adolescents between the ages of ten and eighteen. The goal of the program is to provide disadvantaged inner-city adolescents with the knowledge, skills, and alternative sources of social and medical support necessary to develop positive attitudes and behavior. Along with the development of health maintenance skills, the program is designed to develop health-promoting behaviors that have lifetime significance. The Teen-Link program is located in the Lincoln Community Health Center, a family-oriented community health facility. The program accomplishes its goal through a network of agencies such as Duke University Medical Center, the county health department, the department of social services, the public and private school systems, the county recreation department, the public housing authority, churches, civic organizations, and businesses. Additional strategies include special-interest groups in such areas as swimming, karate, and computer literacy to recruit adolescents; a health-risk-appraisal questionnaire to identify high-risk adolescents; and psychosocial support groups for adolescents at high risk for problems such as pregnancy, obesity, alcohol and drug abuse, violence, juvenile delinquency, poor physical fitness, school dropout, and stress-related disorders. Teen-Link also provides comprehensive primary health care maintenance, including family planning, dental services, prenatal care, nutrition and WIC services, mental health services, and specialty medical services. To reduce access barriers, transportation is also provided free of charge to those who need it.

Services are provided by a multidisciplinary team of health professionals with special training in adolescent health issues. In addition to the health care providers, the staff includes outreach workers to conduct home visits and follow-up and a community health facilitator who lives in the community and recruits adolescents to the program through personal contact with the adolescents and their families. The health care team also includes a nutritionist who provides exercise programs and diet counseling for the adolescent patient.

Teen-Link has been found to be an effective program in reaching high-risk youth with multiple health care problems. It was recently chosen as a model program by the American Medical Association's Congress on Adolescent Health.

The Door: A Center for Alternatives. The Door provides comprehensive services to adolescents between the ages of twelve and twenty-one through a community-based facility located in New York City. Programs include social, medical, and psychological services provided at no charge or for nominal fees. Health care ranges from physical examinations and treatment for minor problems to family planning and contraceptive counseling. Other services include weight control and food budgeting counseling by a nutritionist, remedial studies and vocational training, and high school–equivalence workshops conducted by educators. The Door also provides counseling for drugs and alcohol problems, legal matters, and crisis intervention. Programs including exercise, crafts, and creative arts are provided to help adolescents develop additional skills and self-confidence. In addition to the medical services that are provided, the Door also has established prevention programs aimed at reducing adolescent pregnancy and alcohol and drug abuse. Special family programs for targeted groups, such as the handicapped, the male adolescent, adolescent parents, and very young patients, are also components of the program.

The Door serves approximately 200 adolescents per day and has been reported to have over 13,000 visits per year. Ninety percent of the women seen at the Door are at or below the poverty level. Because of the Door's ability to reduce the economic barriers for these adolescents, it has fulfilled the needs of many New York teens who have not been reached through the city's varied health resources.

Bridge over Troubled Water. The Bridge over Troubled Water is a free mobile medical van that serves runaways and street youth between the ages of twelve and twenty-one in Boston. Many of the youth served by the Bridge are depressed, alienated adolescents who are referred by concerned individuals, community agencies, and police officers. Since 1970, the goal of the Bridge has been to provide health and social care to runaway youth and to help them leave the street. Services include medical care, drug and alcohol counseling, vocational education, family planning counseling, dental care, and laboratory screenings for hepatitis, sexually transmitted diseases, other infections, and pregnancy.

The Bridge over Troubled Water has been evaluated on a number of occasions. Its success has been attributed to its use of a multidisciplinary approach to assist the runaway adolescent in a friendly, trusting manner by reducing many of the barriers that these high-risk youth perceive to access to traditional health care settings. It offers acute care to street youth who otherwise would not receive health care. The Bridge over Troubled Water is a model program for reaching the one million adolescents who run away each year and take refuge on the streets of metropolitan areas.

Conclusion

Many adolescents in this country are not utilizing existing health care resources because they perceive significant physical, social, psychological, financial, or legal barriers to access to care. Yet it appears that certain subgroups of adolescents, such as those from minority or ethnic groups, runaways, and so on, encounter more significant barriers than other adolescents. This chapter has described the sources of these barriers and offered suggestions concerning how health care facilities can be reorganized or restructured to reduce barriers. However, increasing adolescents' access to health care is not solely a structural or organizational problem. Health professionals must always remember that reducing barriers to health care depends predominantly on the attitudes, beliefs, behavior, and expertise of the people who deliver care to adolescents.

Suggested Readings

Anglin, T. "Position Paper on School-Based Health Clinics. Society for Adolescent Health Care." *Journal of Adolescent Health Care*, 1988, *9*, 526–530.

Becker, M. H., and others. "Patient Perception and Compliance: Recent Studies of the Health Belief Model." In R. B. Haynes and D. W. Sockett (eds.), *Compliance in Health Care*. Baltimore, Md.: Johns Hopkins University Press, 1979.

DuRant, R. H., and Jay, M. S. (eds.). "Communication and Compliance Issues in Adolescent Medicine." *Seminars in Adolescent Medicine*, 1987, *3* (entire issue 2).

DuRant, R. H., Seymore, C., Linder, C. W., and Jay, S. "The Preparticipation Examination of Athletes: Comparison of Single and Multiple Examiners." *American Journal of Diseases in Children*, 1985, *139*, 657–661.

Felice, M. E. "Reflections on Caring for Indo-Chinese Children and Youth." *Journal of Developmental and Behavioral Pediatrics*, 1986, 7, 124–128.

Giblin, P. T., and Polen, M. L. "Primary Care of Adolescents: Issues and Program Development and Implementation." *Journal of Adolescent Health Care*, 1985, *6*, 387–391.

Mechanic, D. (ed.) *Handbook of Health, Health Care, and the Health Professions*. New York: Free Press, 1983.

Nidorf, J. F., and Morgan, M. C. "Cross Cultural Issues in Adolescent Medicine." *Primary Care*, 1987, *14*, 69–82.

Resnick, M., Blum, R. W., and Hedin, D. "The Appropriateness of Health Services for Adolescents: Youths' Opinions and Attitudes." *Journal of Adolescent Health Care*, 1980, *1*, 137–141.

18

Economic Issues Affecting Health Care Access

Marilyn Moon, Ph.D.

The patchwork system of health insurance and the varying economic status of families may severely limit access to health care for many adolescents in the United States. Gaps in insurance coverage are increasingly receiving attention as employer-related coverage has declined rather than increased during the past decade. Today, the majority of those without insurance live in families with at least one worker. These are often lower-income families, and lack of insurance may mean that needed health care is simply inaccessible.

Access to health care for adolescents depends on a complex interaction of financial resources and family dynamics. Unlike younger children, who are fully dependent on their parents, adolescents often have at least some resources of their own and in some cases may be fully independent from parents or other family members. Dependence on insurance coverage or out-of-pocket support from parents will vary with the family's internal relationships, the adolescent's willingness to discuss sensitive health issues, income levels, and insurance availability. Adolescents from well-to-do families may still lack access to care for drug, pregnancy, or family planning activities, for example. Thus, although this chapter focuses on the economic issues affecting access to care, these important sociological factors ought always to be kept in mind.

First, we separate adolescents into two groups: those in households headed by others (usually a parent) and those who head their own households. Young women in this latter group are likely to be pregnant or mothers of young children. In addition, this chapter emphasizes two different types of access problems. First, the overarching issue of availability of economic resources (including insurance coverage) influences the general availability of health services for adolescents. Second, care initiated by adolescents beyond parents' wishes or knowledge—such as pregnancy counseling services or substance abuse programs—may create special access barriers.

Economic constraints and special barriers can reduce access by adolescents to needed medical care. This chapter concentrates on the economic barriers. The next section offers some basic statistics on the economic status of adolescents and their families. Income is the most important determinant of health care use aside from basic health status.

The second major section surveys public and private insurance coverage. Usually closely related to income is the availability of third-party payment for covering the costs of health care. Insurance coverage also strongly affects use of care—an issue examined in the third section of the chapter. Just how strong is the impact of financial resources on the use of services?

The last section of this chapter considers the special types of barriers erected by the combination of financial and sociological factors facing adolescents. In this case, teenagers may seek care without the financial support of families when the problems that require care may be a source of tension within the family.

The Economic Status of Adolescents

The income and wealth of families in the United States usually determine the affordability of health care. Generally, there is a close correlation between economic status and health insurance coverage. Moreover, those with high incomes and no insurance may have decided to "self-insure" if they can afford to pay out of pocket for their own care. Thus, before looking at insurance coverage, it is important to consider the overall economic status of adolescents.

Our knowledge of the financial status of adolescents is limited, largely because many published statistics lump all children together in reporting income or insurance coverage. When children are differentiated, it is often only into two groups: generally those below school age and those age six to eighteen. This is troubling for our purposes, since we wish to concentrate on the particular problems of adolescents (whom I define here as young persons age twelve to eighteen). In some cases, relatively crude assumptions about economic status and coverage have to be made in the analysis that follows.

Income of Adolescents in Larger Families

Nearly thirteen million children reside in households with incomes so low that they cannot afford the basic necessities of life, according to the U.S. Bureau of the Census. In the year 1980, poverty among children in the United States reached a higher level than had been seen since the mid 1960s and remained there for a decade. Although the proportion of persons under age

Table 18.1. Rates of Poverty Among Children by Race and Age, 1988.

	Number in Poverty (in Millions)	Poverty Rates			
		All Races	White	Black	Hispanic
Under 3 years	2.6	23.3%	17.5%	50.4%	43.6%
3 to 5 years	2.4	21.9	16.7	48.6	42.7
6 to 11 years	4.3	19.9	14.8	44.8	37.1
12 to 17 years	3.3	16.3	11.6	38.0	32.2
All children	12.6	19.7	14.6	44.2	37.9

Source: U.S. Bureau of the Census, *Money Income and Poverty Status in the U.S.: 1988.* Series P-60, no. 166, U.S. Department of Commerce. Washington, D.C.: U.S. Government Printing Office, 1990, p. 66.

eighteen in poverty peaked at 22.3 percent at the end of the recession in 1983, the decline has been quite slow, with the rate standing at 19.7 percent in 1988. Between 1966 and 1979, in contrast, poverty rates for children ranged between 14.0 and 17.6 percent. Thus, the economic status of children in the 1980s remained consistently below the levels of the 1970s.

Poverty rates tend to be higher in families with very young children. Their parents also tend to be younger or have larger families, both factors that are related to a greater chance of being poor. Young workers have higher rates of unemployment and lower rates of pay overall. For adolescents still residing with their parents, the chances of being in poverty are thus somewhat lower than for other children. (But as we shall see below, adolescents who are very young household heads are particularly vulnerable to poverty.)

Table 18.1 indicates the numbers and proportions of poor children. In 1988, 3.3 million adolescents were categorized as poor. And although they are less likely to be poor than younger children, at least one in every seven adolescents lives in a household that receives a less than subsistence level of income. The picture for minority children is considerably bleaker. More than a third of black and Hispanic teenagers live in poverty households. And the high rates of poverty among younger children indicate that many of those who becomes adolescents in the near future will have lived for at least some period in poor households, where they may have received inadequate nutrition and health care.

Statistics from the major welfare program to benefit nonelderly families, Aid to Families with Dependent Children (AFDC), indicate that in 1986 almost a quarter (24.3 percent) of all recipient children were age twelve or over. This figure was down from 31 percent in 1969. While the concentration of children in poverty is shifting to the younger age range, a substantial number of those receiving AFDC are still teenagers. Indeed, most of this shift is attributable to demographic changes rather than to increased average incomes for such families. The cohort of teenagers is a small one; relatively, there are more very young children than there were ten years ago.

Broader-based statistics on income and well-being also indicate that many families with children are struggling—particularly as compared to childless families. One in every five families with children has an income below 125 percent of the poverty threshold (about $13,800 for a family of four in 1988). Again, more families with children have incomes below 125 percent of poverty than do families without children. Families with no children have median incomes above that for all families, and median incomes tend to fall as family size increases. Also, the lowest incomes are associated with families headed by a woman. The median income in 1988 was $32,191 for all families and $31,770 for families with children, but only $11,865 for female-headed families with children. Children growing up in families headed by women are seldom in strong financial positions. At least half of such families are at or near the poverty level.

The statistics indicate that younger children live in the most disadvantaged families as measured by median income. While the average family in which all children are under the age of six had an income of $29,275 in 1988, the median rose to $34,849 for families in which all children were between the ages of six and seventeen. This latter figure is above the overall median. Children in female-headed households display the same pattern.

Older children who reside in above-poverty-level families thus seem to be relatively well-off. Their older parents are able to generate reasonable income, although we do not know how their economic status would compare to that of childless families if adjusted for differences in family size.

Thus, it appears that adolescent children at the bottom of the income scale are greatly disadvantaged and their numbers remain high. In contrast, for those in the middle class and above, considerable resources are available. Compared with younger children, most adolescents (about two-thirds) are probably in economically secure households. But the income disadvantages facing many younger children must also raise concern about the resulting health problems that may be carried over into adolescence and beyond. Poor nutrition and inadequate medical care for the very young are likely to create health problems in later years. Thus, even if families do better over time, their children may suffer lingering consequences from the early deprivation.

What are the actual discretionary resources available to adolescents? While statistics are unavailable on how much parents give to their children, nearly two-thirds of adolescents age fifteen to nineteen had some income in 1987. But the numbers also indicate that these incomes were skewed, meaning that the average income was well above what the average teenager actually had. That is, the overall average of $3,112 would rise to an average of $4,624 for those teens who actually had any income (see Table 18.2). And the median amount, indicating what the average adolescent had in income, was a much lower $1,905. Only 7.3 percent of all the fifteen- to nineteen-year-olds worked full-time, year around. Nonetheless, a substantial number of adolescents have at least some discretionary income. Also, the small current cohort of teenagers means that a greater proportion may be able to find part-time work

Table 18.2. Income of Adolescents, 1987.

	Number Age 15 to 19 (in Thousands)
Without income	5,885
With income	12,111
Less than $2,000	6,359
$2,000 to $3,999	2,584
$4,000 to $9,999	2,441
$10,000 and above	727
Median income	$1,905
Mean income	$3,112

Source: U.S. Bureau of the Census, *Money Income of Households, Families, and Persons in the United States: 1987,* Series P-60, No. 162, U.S. Department of Commerce. Washington, D.C.: U.S. Government Printing Office, 1989, p. 132.

now than were able to in recent years. The high expenditures on goods aimed at the youth market also attests to discretionary income for at least some in this group.

Thus, at least some teenagers should be able to pay for some health care services on their own without asking permission and perhaps without the knowledge of their parents. On the other hand, teenagers with substantive incomes from part-time employment (likely to be a large share of those with incomes) may be less likely to need mental health services or substance abuse programs, for example. The mismatch between need and ability to pay may be substantial.

Income of Adolescents on Their Own

Only a very small percentage of adolescents live on their own, and often the numbers in survey samples are statistically insignificant and hence not reported separately. For example, the Current Population Survey (CPS) finds that only about 0.1 percent of children under eighteen in the United States are householders or spouses of householders (although the CPS arbitrarily places a lower bound of age fifteen on classification of those persons). About 0.8 percent of all people age fifteen to seventeen fall into that category. Consequently, poverty statistics are not listed for these individuals. Most of these teenagers are spouses of householders—most likely young women who have married older men.

A major reason that teenagers create separate households is the birth of a child. Teenage mothers are very likely to be poor and dependent on welfare programs. We can thus look at figures from the Aid to Families of Dependent Children program to provide some additional information. Only a small share of teenagers show up on the AFDC rolls as parents. In 1986, only 3.3 percent of all female AFDC recipients were under the age of eighteen— down from 6.6 percent in 1969. But, at the same time, a mother under the age of eighteen has a higher chance of being on AFDC than do older mothers.

More than 950,000 women age fifteen to nineteen gave birth to children in 1983, about 60 percent of them unmarried. A recent survey from the National Longitudinal Survey of Youth has estimated that more than one-fourth of such women will receive AFDC for at least one month within twenty-four months of giving birth.

Of adolescents of their own and not dependent on welfare, a relatively large proportion will be employed in industries not likely to offer health insurance. Youth are often employed in service-sector and other low-skill jobs — often with low pay and few fringe benefits. These and other insurance concerns are raised in the next section.

Public and Private Insurance Coverage in the United States

Health insurance coverage in the United Sates stems from two sources: public programs such as Medicaid (for low-income, categorically eligible persons) and private insurance, usually offered and sometimes subsidized by employers. For families not poor enough for Medicaid, but still poor or near-poor, private insurance coverage is often not affordable. Adolescents in these circumstances may be without coverage and hence, at least to some degree, lack access to care. Overall, in 1986, about eleven million children in the United States had no health insurance from either the public or the private sector. Effectively, one in every five children had no insurance protection, and, among poor children, the total rises to one in every three (even after accounting for Medicaid coverage).

The extent to which children are covered for health care in the United States depends on several factors, including whether and where their parents are employed and the state in which they live. Many children whose parents are in the work force are still outside the work-based health system. Their only alternative is to apply for coverage under Medicaid. But the United States has made it very difficult for even minimum-wage workers to qualify for AFDC — and therefore for Medicaid. The United States stands virtually alone among industrialized nations in segmenting its youth population for purposes of health care assistance in this way.

Medicaid and Other Public-Sector Coverage

In the United States, children are subject to a social policy that distinguishes between "deserving" and "undeserving" recipients of aid. While most Americans consider children as deserving of assistance, dollar transfers to children depend on public judgments of the worthiness of their parents. In most states, poor adolescents will not be eligible for Medicaid if they live in an intact family where the father is employed, no matter how little he makes.

And for those who are categorically eligible (usually in female-headed families), income of the family must be considerably below the poverty line before the family qualifies. For example, a teenager living with his or her mother and another child will qualify for Medicaid in Texas only if their monthly income is below $368. In 1988, this amount was about a third of the poverty level. While other states offer more generous coverage, families must usually have income substantially below the poverty level before they qualify.

Medicaid eligibility for adolescents can be extended beyond AFDC recipients in some states and circumstances. A majority of states now have programs for the medically needy that offer coverage to families who have "spent down" to eligibility by virtue of having very high medical expenses. Such coverage is by its nature, however, restricted to those with major health problems and would not offer help for preventive care.

The U.S. Congress has also recently expanded coverage to some individuals, particularly pregnant women and infants. The Omnibus Budget Reconciliation Act of 1986 permitted states to offer Medicaid coverage to categorically needy pregnant women and children. But few states moved rapidly to expand this coverage. The Catastrophic Health Act of 1988 mandated such coverage for all such persons with incomes at or below 75 percent of the poverty level by July 19, 1989, with the limit to move up to 100 percent of the poverty level by July 1, 1990. Thus, teenage mothers at least will be better covered than before, and not subject to the stringent income limits imposed now in many states. Nonetheless, a large number of the poor will remain without Medicaid coverage, and, with the exception of pregnant teenagers, many poor adolescents will lack such public-sector coverage. In fact, in 1986, only 49 percent of poor children in the United States were covered by Medicaid.

In addition to the question of coverage is the issue of how well Medicaid's coverage and benefits fit the needs of adolescents. Designed primarily to offer health care coverage once problems arise, Medicaid does not have a good record of providing preventive services or "frills" such as basic mental health services and counseling. Moreover, the low reimbursement levels offered physicians in many states sometimes make physician participation in Medicaid spotty at best. Medicaid recipients are thus likely not to have a regular physician but to use instead hospital emergency rooms or walk-in clinics. Maternity coverage has been particularly troublesome under Medicaid, with many providers unwilling to treat such patients. These types of environments are not conducive to encouraging reluctant adolescents to obtain care for emotionally sensitive problems.

Less organized public-sector programs may actually have a better chance of success in attracting teenagers. But the past decade has not been a period in which services such as family planning, adolescent pregnancy services, or mental health programs have been generously funded. For example, Title V Maternal and Child Health Block Grant funds and the Title X Family Planning Program have served many young women. But such funding has been subject to budget cuts and/or freezes in recent years. For example, the president's budget for 1989 proposed a funding level for Maternal and Child Health 18 percent below its 1981 level after controlling for inflation. Proposed spending on family planning in the federal budget for 1989 would be 43 percent below its 1981 levels.

The Title XX Social Services Block Grants sometimes cover substance abuse programs, counseling, and pregnancy programs. But in 1989, substance abuse services were offered in only twelve states (down from fourteen states in 1982), family planning in twenty-seven states (down from forty-seven in 1982), counseling in three states (as compared to forty-eight in 1982), and services for unmarried parents in thirteen states (down from fifteen). In 1988 dollars, funding declined from a high of $5.5 billion in 1977 for these social services to $2.8 billion in 1990.

Finally, public support through the schools may also offer a source of access to medical care for adolescents, or at least health and sex education. Adolescents are likely to be exposed to programs designed to reduce drug and alcohol abuse and to discourage sexual activity. Counseling services are also offered, some of which may provide mental health programs or referrals to community-based services. A few schools have experimented, amid considerable controversy, with actually providing on-site family planning services. A mismatch between availability of such programs and need will occur, however, if poorer inner-city schools cannot offer such services to students who can ill afford to go elsewhere.

Private Health Insurance Coverage

For most Americans, health insurance comes through the private sector, often subsidized by employers (and indirectly supported by the public sector through tax breaks). This fringe benefit had come to be viewed almost as a right by many middle-class Americans and has been taken for granted by many of those in the labor force. But the last decade has seen a major change in employer-sponsored health insurance. The increasing costs of such insurance (related to rising health care costs in general), the severe recession of 1982–1983, which disrupted many workers, and the shift of many workers in the labor force to the relatively lower-paying service sector and away from manufacturing jobs have all reduced employer support for health insurance.

When insurance costs rise each year, many employers look for ways to cut the costs of this commitment to employees, citing the need to remain competitive in the marketplace. Many workers lost their jobs and their insurance during the 1982–1983 recession. But researchers were surprised to discover that although the recovery reduced unemployment rates, the number of people with health insurance did not show a corresponding rise in the period 1983 through 1986. Some workers changed occupations; others returned to their old jobs to find that employers no longer offered the same benefits as before; and still others were able to find only part-time work. In fact, the proportion of the population covered by employment-based health insurance fell from 67.4 percent to 64.8 percent.

In certain industries and occupations, the lack of health coverage is widespread. For example, in 1985, 52 percent of all uninsured workers were employed in either retail trade or services. Of women working full-time in 1984 in jobs paying less than $10,000 per year, 57 percent lacked job-related health insurance; fully 87 percent of women working part-time in such jobs lacked group health coverage. (Most of these working women are *not* receiving Medicaid.)

For many who do have employer-sponsored insurance, deductibles, premiums, and coinsurance costs have increased substantially. For example, if costs of premiums for family coverage had remained constant after accounting for inflation since 1977, they would have averaged $148 per family per month in 1987. Instead, the average in 1987 was $201 — a 36 percent increase. And costs are expected to increase rapidly in coming years. Of particular concern for children is the fact that many employers now subsidize only the employee's insurance. Before 1983, 40 percent of employers paid the full cost of dependent coverage. By 1987, that figure dropped to about one-third. A low-income family may find that although dependents' benefits are offered, they are too expensive. Other family members in these cases go without coverage.

Only about two-thirds of all children are covered by private insurance. In families headed by full-year workers, one in five does not have employer coverage (see Table 18.3). Our expectation that full-time workers cover their children causes us to ignore serious coverage gaps. For poor families, having a full-year worker in the family helps very little; fewer than a quarter of children in such families receive coverage from the parent's employer. For these families, coverage is the exception and not the rule. This statistic is particularly troublesome because such children are almost always categorically ineligible to receive Medicaid.

If teenagers are proportionately represented among this group of uninsured children, then about three million adolescents have no insurance. Adolescents tend to live in families with higher incomes than do younger children, so they may be somewhat more likely to have insurance coverage from a parent's employer. But the number of uninsured teenagers is probably well above two million. A study using 1980 data found that while 21.7 percent of all children were uninsured for all or part of the year, the proportion dropped to 20.8 for children age twelve to eighteen. Teenagers did fare better, but not by any great degree.

A considerable number of adolescents can be termed as having inadequate coverage. Employers and Medicaid often limit what is covered and pay only part of the actual costs of care. For example, hospital inpatient care is relatively well covered by most insurance, but children are considerably less likely to use such services than are adults under the age of sixty-five. Physicians' services, which are used heavily by children, are less well insured.

Moreover, employer-sponsored health plans are not required to offer maternity care to dependent daughters of the insured. And in 1985, more than a third of employer plans excluded such coverage, affecting an estimated 2.7 million teenagers. Drug abuse treatment is also less likely to be covered. The U.S. Department of Labor has found that only two-thirds of employer plans cover drug abuse treatment. The rapid rise in the costs of such treatment may mean further limitations in the future.

Young adults, including some adolescents, are also the most likely family heads and spouses to have no insurance. Data from the 1980 National Medical Utilization and Expenditure Survey show that the fifteen-to-twenty-four age group has the highest rate of uninsured in the population. And a more recent study by the Congressional Research Service found that young workers age fifteen to seventeen almost never have health coverage (only 2.1 percent do). For workers age eighteen to twenty-one, 24.3 percent obtain insurance through their employers.

Insurance Coverage and Use of Services

Insurance coverage is directly linked to the amount of care received by Americans. People not covered by public or private insurance are much less likely to receive care, particularly physician's services. Emergency or inpatient hospital care does often seem to be available to the uninsured, however. The findings for children are no exception. Analysis of data from the Rand Experiment, which looked at variations in use of care by insurance coverage, also noted that less-well-insured people reduced their use of necessary services as well as those that might be deemed inappropriate. Cutbacks in use of care are thus likely to be associated with forgoing needed services.

The effectiveness of treatment such as immunizations and prenatal

Table 18.3. Private Health Insurance Coverage for Children, 1986.

	Number of Children (Millions)	Total Private Coverage	Employer-Provided Coverage
Total	55.7	67.5%	62.7%
Headed by full-year worker	47.0	77.5	72.9
Two-parent family	38.5	84.1	79.7
Single-parent family	8.5	47.6	42.3
Children in poverty	12.5	16.3	11.3
Headed by full-year worker	5.3	29.2	23.2
Two-parent family	2.9	36.3	29.4
Single-parent family	2.4	20.5	15.8

Source: Charles Betley, "Public and Private Issues in Financing Health Care for Children." *EBRI Issue Brief* no. 79. Washington, D.C.: Employee Benefit Research Institute, June 1988, p. 5. Reprinted with permission.

**Table 18.4. Average Number of Physician Visits for
Children and Young Adults by Insurance Coverage, 1980.**

Age	Medicaid Only	Private Insurance	No Insurance	All
Under 4 years	4.97	4.93	3.06	4.66
5 to 14 years	3.51	3.85	1.82	3.58
15 to 24 years	5.36	4.15	2.27	4.02

Source: Garfinkel, S., Corder, L., and Dobson, A. *Health Services Utilization in the U.S. Population by Health Insurance Coverage.* National Medical Care Utilization and Expenditure Survey, Series B, Descriptive Report no. 13. Washington, D.C.: U.S. Government Printing Office, 1986, pp. 174–179.

care makes such access even more critical for children. Preventive services, which may well be forgone, are particularly effective for young people—and may affect health and health care needs for years to come.

John Butler and his colleagues found that children up to age eighteen without insurance coverage of any sort have substantially fewer medical care visits than those who do have coverage (averages of 2.1 and 3.4, respectively). Significant differences also occur in the overall level of charges incurred; spending on the uninsured was less than half as high, but the uninsured had considerably higher out-of-pocket spending for those services. The lowest levels of spending on medical care were also associated with the near-poor and low-income families—those least likely to have private insurance or Medicaid coverage. Figures on the effect of insurance were not presented separately for adolescents in this study, but the overall patterns of service use that were shown seemed to be in line with those for other children, so the findings would also likely hold for the 27 percent of the sample who were age twelve to eighteen. And, as reported above, the share of adolescents lacking insurance in that sample corresponded closely to the totals for all children.

A second study, using these same data, had similar findings and did present some finer age breakdowns, as shown in Table 18.4. Again, the data do not correspond directly to the adolescent population, but it is possible to see that the results of fewer physician visits for the uninsured hold for both very young children and the age group five to fourteen years. The differences are even greater for the fifteen- to twenty-four-year-old group, indicating that young adults are also susceptible to the same problems of lack of insurance and lower use of care.

Findings from a Medicaid study also substantiate these differences in access to care. The data shown in Table 18.5 focus on children age six to seventeen who have fifteen or more restricted-activity days per year, disaggregated by poverty status and access to Medicaid. At least to some extent, this study has some controls on level of health status. Nonpoor children and those with Medicaid used about the same level of physician services on average, while poor children ineligible for Medicaid (and unlikely to be covered by

Table 18.5. Use of Health Services by Persons Under Age Eighteen
with Fifteen or More Restricted-Activity Days, 1980.

	Mean Number of Physician Visits	Mean Number of Prescribed Drugs
Under age 6		
With Medicaid	7.3	5.2
Without Medicaid		
Poor	6.7	4.8
Nonpoor	7.4	5.5
Ages 6–17		
With Medicaid	6.2	3.2
Without Medicaid		
Poor	5.4	2.8
Nonpoor	6.3	3.9

Source: Kasper, J. "Health Status and Utilization: Differences by Medicaid Coverage and Income." *Health Care Financing Review,* 1986, 7 (Summer), p. 9.

private insurance) had fewer such visits. Use of prescription drugs was also lower for poor children who lacked access to Medicaid.

Special Needs and Programs for Adolescents

Beyond basic health insurance coverage, adolescents may have special needs for access to health care in such sensitive areas as substance abuse, mental health, and pregnancy and family planning services. Adolescence is a time of life when major physical, mental, and emotional changes are taking place. Preventive and less traditional health care services are likely to be more in demand than coverage of major medical expenses, irrespective of what parents or their insurance coverages offer. Not only are such services less likely to be covered than inpatient hospitalization, for example, but also teenagers may be unwilling or unable to discuss the need for such services with their parents. In this way, adolescents may be on their own for affording care and finding where such services may be available to them.

Although little hard statistical information is available on this subject, some relatively powerful anecdotal evidence does exist. One study tried to determine whether adolescents are able and willing to pay for confidential health care through a survey conducted in New York City. The sample was drawn from 180 middle-class adolescents who were patients of the Adolescent Health Service—a clinic offering general medical, gynecological, and counseling services free of charge and without requiring parental consent. Nearly all (94 percent of continuing patients) indicated that they would be willing to pay something, and two-thirds said that they could afford $10 per visit. Most would have been unable to pay the full costs, however. Three-quarters of the respondents indicated that they would pay without any help from parents, indicating the importance of confidentiality to these patients.

Youth from more modest families would be even less likely to be able to afford such care on their own. A large number of adolescents may thus be dependent on free or subsidized clinics.

What is not known from this study, moreover, is whether patients would have forgone some or all treatment if they did have to pay; nor do we know the consequences of such forgone care. And, for the most part, it is not possible to separate the specific roles of ability to pay or knowledge of availability of such services in determining whether care is delivered. Given the emotional barriers, any financial or organizational impediments may have an exaggerated effect. If so, fewer adolescents will have access to needed care.

Take first the case of teenage pregnancy. Many studies have shown the efficacy and cost-effectiveness of prenatal care, particularly for the adolescent mother. As indicated above, adolescents on their own and in families may have trouble getting access to insurance coverage. And even if it is available, young women may delay notifying their parents when they learn that they are pregnant. To what extent then do teenagers have access to such services elsewhere? As noted above, federally supported health services for young adults do not exist in many states. Much less is known about local programs funded by government or charitable organizations. Youth in rural areas are likely to be particularly vulnerable, since many urban areas offer walk-in health clinics of a more general nature.

Some improvement in coverage for teenagers has already been noted above in the discussion of the Medicaid expansions of 1988. In addition, a study of the effects of Medicaid on children has discovered that the coverage of poor children otherwise ineligible for AFDC through a program often referred to as Ribicoff kids has been effective in giving teenagers early access to health coverage. Although the program was designed for young children, teenagers in four states were found to benefit from the provisions largely because, under the Ribicoff provisions, young people under the age of twenty-one do not have to prove pregnancy before they are covered.

Conclusions

While a large number of studies concerned with access to health care have focused on the plight of all children under the age of eighteen, little analysis has been targeted on adolescents. Indeed, nearly every study reported here that breaks down children by age uses different age groupings and almost never focuses solely on adolescents. But what we do know is disturbing. One in seven adolescents in the United States is poor, and a substantial additional number have family incomes just above poverty. If you are a member of a poor family, your chance of adequate coverage is minimal. Your needs may be greater than those of a richer adolescent, but you will not have the same access to care. Medicaid is largely restricted to the very poor and is often inadequate; employer-based insurance does a poor job of filling in, even for adolescents in families with full-time workers.

The middle class also have some access problems, as employer coverage is less available and less generous than in the late 1970s. Gaps in dependent coverage and perhaps some decrease in services covered represent alarming trends for adolescents' access to care. Not surprisingly, families with very high incomes tend to be well insured and can afford to supplement that coverage.

Adolescents who are economically independent from their families are also likely to face serious economic constraints and difficulties in getting access to health care. The primary exception is pregnant teenagers, who have better opportunities for access than other teens. Ironically, this may be a case of offering assistance, which is certainly needed, where the outcome might have been considerably different if counseling and family planning information had been available.

Adolescents from any economic class may have access problems for other sensitive health issues that they may wish to handle on their own, without benefit of family resources. In these cases, economic concerns are an issue but are not the primary barrier.

Suggested Readings

Alan Guttmacher Institute. *Financing Maternity Care in the United States*. New York: Alan Guttmacher Institute, 1987.

Anderson, R., Aday, L. A., and Chen, M. "Health Status and Medical Care Utilization." *Health Affairs*, Spring 1986, pp. 154–172.

Brook, R. H., and Lohr, K. *Use of Medical Care in the Rand Health Insurance Experiment*. Santa Monica, Calif.: Rand, 1986.

Butler, J., Winter, W., Singer, J., and Wenger, M. "Medical Care Use and Expenditure Among Children and Youth in the United States: Analysis of a National Probability Sample." *Pediatrics*, 1985, *76*, 495–507.

Children's Defense Fund. *A Children's Defense Budget*. Washington, D.C.: Children's Defense Fund, 1988.

Chollet, D. *Uninsured in the U.S.: The Nonelderly Population Without Health Insurance*. Washington, D.C.: Employee Benefits Research Institute, 1987.

Congressional Research Service. *Health Insurance and the Uninsured: Background Data and Analysis*. Washington, D.C.: U.S. Government Printing Office, 1988.

Employee Benefits Research Institute. *Public and Private Issues in Financing Health Care for Children*. Issue Brief no. 79. Washington, D.C.: Employee Benefits Research Institute, 1988.

Fisher, C. "Differences by Age Groups in Health Care Spending." *Health Care Financing Review*, 1980, *2*, 65–85.

Fisher, M., Marks, A. , Trieller, K., and Brody, R. "Are Adolescents Able and Willing to Pay the Fee for Confidential Health Care?" *Journal of Pediatrics*, 1985, *107* (Sept.), 480–483.

Garfinkel, S., Corder, L., and Dobson, A. *Health Services Utilization in the U.S.*

Population by Health Insurance Coverage. National Medical Care Utilization and Expenditure Survey, Series B, Descriptive Report no. 13. Washington, D.C.: U.S. Government Printing Office, 1986.

Kasper, J. "Health Status and Utilization Differences by Medicaid Coverage and Incomes." *Health Care Financing Review*, 1986, 7 (Summer), 1–18.

Leppert, P., and Namerow, P. "Costs Averted by Providing Comprehensive Prenatal Care to Teenagers." *Journal of Nurse-Midwifery*, 1985, *30* (Sept.–Oct.), 285–289.

Manber, M. "Adolescents: They Seek Care Outside the System." *Medical World News*, Apr. 2, 1979, pp. 39–51.

Meyer, J., and Moon, M. "Health Care Spending on Children and the Elderly." In J. Palmer, T. Smeeding, and B. Torrey (eds.), *The Vulnerable: America's Young and Old in the Industrial World.* Washington, D.C.: Urban Institute Press, 1989.

National Institute of Medicine. *Preventing Low Birthweight.* Washington, D.C.: National Academy Press, 1985.

Reischauer, R. Testimony before the Subcommittee on Social Security and Family Policy, Committee on Finance, U.S. Senate, Feb. 23, 1987.

Rymer, M., and Adler, G. "Children and Medicaid: The Experience in Four States." *Health Care Financing Review*, 1987, *9* (Fall), 1–20.

U.S. Bureau of the Census. *Money Income of Households, Families and Persons in the United States: 1987.* Series P-60, no. 162, U.S. Department of Commerce. Washington, D.C.: U.S. Government Printing Office, 1989.

U.S. Bureau of the Census. *Money, Income, and Poverty Status in the United States: 1988.* Series P-60, no. 166, U.S. Department of Commerce. Washington, D.C.: U.S. Government Printing Office, 1990.

U.S. Department of Labor, Bureau of Labor Statistics. *Employee Benefits in Medium and Large Firms, 1986.* Washington, D.C.: U.S. Government Printing Office, 1987.

U.S. General Accounting Office. *Prenatal Care: Medicaid Recipients and Uninsured Women Obtain Insufficient Care.* Washington, D.C.: U.S. Government Printing Office, 1987.

U.S. House of Representatives, Committee on Ways and Means. *Background Material and Data on Programs Within the Jurisdiction of the Committee on Ways and Means.* Washington, D.C.: U.S. Government Printing Office, 1987.

U.S. House of Representatives, Committee on Ways and Means. *Background Material and Data on Programs Within the Jurisdiction of the Committee on Ways and Means.* Washington, D.C.: U.S. Government Printing Office, 1988.

U.S. Office of Technology Assessment. *Healthy Children: Investing in the Future.* Washington, D.C.: U.S. Government Printing Office, 1988.

19

Adolescents' Compliance with Therapeutic Regimens

Robert H. DuRant, Ph.D.
Carolyn Seymore, M.D.
M. Susan Jay, M.D.

Patient noncompliance has always been a problem for health care professionals. Hippocrates advised that the physician "should keep aware of the fact that patients often lie when they state that they have taken certain medicines." However, it is only during the last fifteen years that the problem of noncompliance with therapy has been studied systematically. This increased focus on the reduction of noncompliant behavior has paralleled medicine's shift in emphasis toward the reduction in diseases associated with life-style choices. Diseases with significant behavioral components (for example, heart disease, cancer, and stroke) account for approximately 70 percent of all deaths among adults. These problems could be reduced to a large degree through a modification of the public's health behavior.

Among adolescents, health behavior plays an even larger role in many of the medical problems experienced. For example, risk-taking behavior is often involved in accidents, suicide, and homicide, the leading causes of death among adolescents. Substance abuse, sexually transmitted diseases, and unplanned pregnancy are also often the direct result of life-style decisions. Even our ability to treat diseases not associated with life-style can be complicated by adolescents' health behavior. Practitioners are often frustrated with their inability to manage chronic diseases such as diabetes, cancer, asthma, and cystic fibrosis because of adolescents' noncompliance with therapeutic regimens.

In this chapter, we first define compliance, describe the degree to which adolescents are noncompliant, and discuss the various methods for measuring compliance and noncompliance. We next describe the theoretical approaches that have been developed to explain compliant and non-compliant behavior and discuss the factors that are generally associated with adolescents' noncompliance with therapeutic advice. We then discuss four areas of adolescent health care in which health behavior plays a significant role: contraception, treatment for substance abuse, treatment for chronic diseases, and treatment for sexually transmitted diseases. We conclude with a description of methods that can be used to increase compliant behavior among adolescent patients.

Definition of Compliance

Compliance has been defined as the extent to which a person's behavior (in terms of taking medications, following diets, or executing life-style changes) coincides with medical or health advice. The terms *adherence* and *conformity* may be used interchangeably with the term *compliance*. Health care providers often view adolescents' compliance behavior in dichotomous terms, defining it as either absolute conformity or nonconformity with medical advice. In reality, compliance behavior is a continuous variable ranging from total noncompliance to partial compliance to absolute adherence to medical advice. For example, several types of noncompliance can be observed in adolescents. The first is the complete failure to take the prescribed medication. This includes patients who continue to see their physician but take little or none of the medication, as well as the greater number of adolescent patients who drop out of treatment or are lost to follow-up. Partial compliers include patients who may take their medication, but not as instructed, or patients who miss several doses of medication. These adolescent patients may increase or reduce the dose or number of doses of medication, take a prescribed medication for the wrong purpose, or take medicines that are out of date or have been discontinued by the physician. Each of these behaviors represents different patterns and levels of noncompliant behavior and results in varying degrees of treatment outcomes.

The rate of noncompliance reported in research varies considerably with the age of the subjects studied, the disease and the type of treatment regimen, and the experimental or study design used. In general, approximately one-third of adults either do not get their prescriptions filled or take none of the medication, one-third usually fill their prescriptions but do not adequately comply with the dosage regimen, and one-third take almost all of the medicine as prescribed. Depending on how compliance is measured, noncompliance among children ranges from 30 to 60 percent. The similarity between adults' and children's rates is due to the fact that most children are given their prescribed medication by their adult parents.

Studies of adolescent patients have also reported varying levels of compliance behavior. Adolescents with juvenile rheumatoid arthritis have been found to be more compliant than younger children when salicylate levels were used as a measure of noncompliance. In contrast, studies of renal transplant patients and patients taking steroid medication for the treatment of malignancy reported that adolescents were less compliant than younger children. In studies of adolescent patients with chronic asthma, only 10 percent were found to have serum theophylline levels in a therapeutic range. However, each of these studies assessed compliance among adolescents who were undergoing long-term therapy for chronic disease. Higher levels of compliance are usually found among adolescents being treated for acute conditions with short-term therapies.

Methods of Measuring Compliance

Direct Measures

Whether the purpose is to detect noncompliance among all patients in a clinical setting or to determine whether noncompliance is the reason for the absence of the clinical effect from the prescribed medication, the measurement of compliance is a challenging problem for practitioners treating adolescents. Quantitative or qualitative analysis of body fluids to determine the presence or absence of a prescribed medication, its metabolites, and/or an added marker substance provides the most objective measure of compliance. Determinations of serum levels of anticonvulsants, salicylates, and theophylline are frequently used in clinical settings. However, direct measures of compliance are limited by the bioavailability of the drug resulting from interactions with other medications, interference by food, or individual differences in rates of metabolism. These factors may inadvertently lower the serum level of the drug and result in an incorrect assessment of the patient's compliance. Also, the technology to determine serum levels of many drugs may not be available for physicians in private-practice offices or public health clinics. In addition to these methodological limitations, the use of blood samples to measure compliance is further limited by the necessity of performing a venipuncture. Adolescent patients often find this procedure painful, time consuming, and esthetically unacceptable. Alternative methods utilizing other body fluids that can be more readily obtained are more attractive for the adolescent patient. For example, acceptable reliability levels have been reported for procedures measuring anticonvulsants, theophylline, and digoxin levels in saliva. The clinician should keep in mind, however, that the routine quantitative analysis of body fluids for monitoring compliance may be economically prohibitive in many health care settings.

Qualitative assessments of compliance may be more practical and cost-effective in private-practice office settings or in public health clinics. For example, bioassays for determining a patient's compliance with medication such as penicillin are readily available. Certain substances, such as mefenamic acid, flufenamic acid, and riboflavin, fluoresce when present in urine exposed to fluorescent light. We have found that riboflavin combined with oral contraceptives can be used as an effective measures of adolescents' compliance with their birth control regimen.

Indirect Measures

Health care providers treating adolescents may be forced to measure compliance indirectly. When used alone, methods utilizing any approach other than the analyses of body fluids provide only clues about compliance. However, when several indirect measures are combined, they may provide as much information as more objective measures. The most commonly used indirect measures of compliance include pill counts, self-report, physician estimation, and outcome assessment. Although pill counts are a commonly used measure of compliance in research settings, they lack practicality in many clinical settings. This method requires the patient to return the medication bottle at the subsequent visit so that the remaining pills may be counted, and the discrepancy between the number remaining and those that should have been taken is documented. Using this method to assess adolescent compliance in an office or clinic setting is no more accurate than simply asking the patient whether he or she has taken the medication, since non-compliers often fail to bring their pills to the follow-up visit or alter the amount of medication in the container to reflect better than actual compliance. The use of pill counts may have higher utility when taken during "surprise" home visits. After making an appointment with the parent, a physician or a nurse can make a home follow-up visit with the adolescent patient to assess his or her response to treatment. During this follow-up visit, the health care provider can ask in a nonthreatening manner to check the medication bottle. A situation in which a home visit for pill count may be indicated is that where a patient with a seizure disorder or asthma denies missing or forgetting medication and continues to have significant symptoms in spite of adequate prescriptions for the appropriate medication.

Direct inquiry about the patient's compliance with the medication is yet another measure of his or her adherence to the treatment protocol. If this is accomplished in a nonthreatening, nonjudgmental manner, approximately half of noncompliant patients will admit to missing at least some of their dosages. The inquiry may include statements such as "We all have difficulties at times remembering to take our medications. To what degree is this true for you?" We recommend that adolescents who are beginning a regimen be asked to estimate their compliance with medications that they have been prescribed in the past. This will provide the practitioner with an important indicator of how compliant the adolescent will be with the present medication. When questioning the adolescent about his or her adherence to the treatment regimen, the health care provider should remember that teenagers tend to respond in socially desirable ways and will try to please the provider by indicating that they are compliant when they are not. Even patients who have confessed that they have not taken their medication will overestimate the extent of their compliance by approximately 20 percent. Thus, the admission of any noncompliance should be taken as an indicator for implementing strategies to improve compliance. Since half of non-compliers will deny that they are not following a prescribed medication, it may be necessary to employ more sophisticated methods for determining noncompliance when the provider suspects it. Despite these limitations, direct inquiry from the patient has advantages; it is easy, and there is much better correlation between reported and actual compliance than between therapeutic response and compliance. In a previous study of oral contraceptive compliance, we found that adolescents' self-reports correlated well with both serum norethindrone and urinary riboflavin measures.

The patient's response to treatment as a measurement of compliance lacks reliability and validity, since for most therapies the correlation between drug dosage and therapeutic response is far from perfect. However, monitoring a patient's response does help narrow the search for the noncomplier. Although noncompliance should always be considered when a patient fails to respond to the usual dosage of a drug, we must remember that patients may fail to display clinical improvement for reasons other than failure to take prescribed medication as directed.

The physician's clinical judgment or estimate of compliance is probably the most common method used in clinical situations. It is usually assumed that experienced physicians will be adept at estimating compliance among their established adolescent patients. However, most studies have not supported this assumption. In one study, medical students were found to be better than attending physicians at identifying patient noncompliance. In a study of private-practice pediatricians, the investigators found that these physicians' predictions of compliance were no better than would result from chance alone and that compliance tended to be overestimated by the pediatricians. Physicians who have established a mutually trusting relationship with their patients usually demonstrate a low index of suspicion concerning noncompliance behavior. Thus, in most situations, the physician's estimate of the patient's compliance cannot be relied on as an accurate measure of his or her adherence to the treatment protocol.

Theoretical Approaches to Compliance Research

The most common approach to the study of nonconforming health behavior has been to identify individual factors that are associated with various forms of noncompliance. The assumption has been that noncompliant patients possess a unique set of characteristics that differentiate them from those who are compliant. On the basis of this assumption, much research has been directed at discovering individual factors that identify compliant and non-compliant patients. Studies that have attempted to look at individual predictors of compliance have often been atheoretical in nature and have produced inconsistent findings.

One of the problems with the individualistic model's approach to explaining conforming health behavior has been its failure to take into consideration the possible interactions among behavioral, psychological, environmental, structural, physical, and medical variables. A second weakness of the individualistic model is that it places too much emphasis on patient characteristics and too little on the health provider. Studies that have used well-established theoretical models to test their hypotheses have been more successful in consistently predicting noncompliant health behavior.

A number of different theories have been proposed to explain noncompliant health behavior. For example, cognitive-oriented psychologists have hypothesized that noncompliance is due to patients' inability to comprehend and remember what practitioners tell them to do. Other psychologists have emphasized the patient's lack of motivation and other attitudinal orientations, such as locus of control, future orientation, and concept of self. Multivariate theoretical models have been more successful in predicting conformity with medical advice. Among these, the model that has received the most attention and study has been the Health Belief Model. The Health Belief Model postulates that health behavior is a function of (1) the patient's perceived susceptibility to the particular illness, (2) the degree of severity or the consequences (physical and/or social) that might result from contracting a condition, (3) the perceived benefits or efficacy of preventing or reducing susceptibility if a specific health action is taken, (4) the physical, psychological, financial, and other barriers or costs related to the particular health behaviors, and (5) a specific cue to action or stimulus to trigger the appropriate health behavior by making the individual consciously aware of his or her feelings about the health threat.

The Health Belief Model assumes that in order for an adolescent patient to be compliant with the prescribed medication, he or she must perceive a high level of susceptibility to the particular illness if the prescribed medication is not taken. This includes a cost-benefit analysis in which the degree of severity or consequences that may occur from the disease if the medication is not taken as prescribed are weighed against the perceived benefits or efficacy of reducing susceptibility to the disease or preventing the disease if the patient were compliant with the medication. The adolescent patient must also weigh the costs of or the barriers to compliance, such as the physical side effects of the medication, the financial costs of purchasing the medication, the inconvenience of taking the medication, and psychological costs, such as embarrassment if a significant other discovers that the patient is taking the medication. This cost-benefit analysis is continually activated by certain stimuli, such as physical symptoms or encouragement from others, such as a partner, parent, or friend. While there is empirical support for several components of the Health Belief Model, it does have some limitations.

The model tends to neglect the possibility that noncompliance can be unintentional. Adolescents who may be motivated to take their medication may not take it correctly for reasons such as not remembering or not

Figure 19.1. The Health Communication Model.

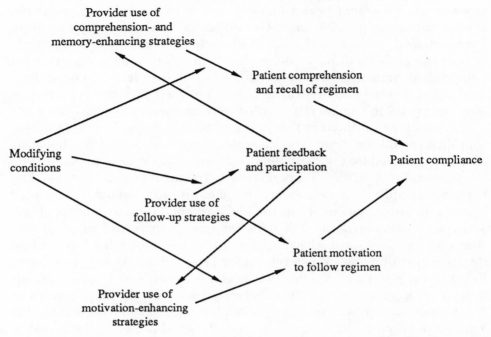

Source: From "Patient-Practitioner Relations and Compliance with Prescribed Medical Regimens" by Bonnie L. Svarstad in APPLICATIONS OF SOCIAL SCIENCE TO CLINICAL MEDICINE AND HEALTH POLICY, Linda H. Aiken and David Mechanic, editors. Copyright © 1986 by Rutgers, The State University.

understanding the physician's instructions. Second, the Health Belief Model does not clearly specify the determinants of the patient's motivation. The model hypothesizes that various social agents or cues to action, such as a health care provider, can affect patient motivation, but it does not specify how such social influences operate or why they may fail. Also, like the individualistic models, the Health Belief Model places too much emphasis on the patient and not enough emphasis on the process by which health care providers transmit their expectations in an attempt to motivate their patients.

B. L. Svarstad argues that none of the traditional approaches to compliant health behavior provides a complete picture of the problem. She states that a broader perspective, which places more emphasis on the quality of practitioner-patient communication, is necessary to adequately understand compliance behavior. She has developed a Health Communication Model that assumes that compliance is primarily, although not entirely, determined by the nature and the quality of practitioner-patient communication. The main components of this model are described in Figure 19.1.

The Health Communication Model assumes that adolescents' compliance with therapeutic regimens is primarily a factor of the level of comprehension and recall of the regimen, as well as motivation to follow the health advice. This suggests that the patient's compliance behavior is linked to the practitioner's behavior in several ways. The health care provider can influence an adolescent's adherence to the treatment protocol by using more effective techniques for enhancing patient understanding and recall and by using more effective ways of motivating the patient. The model assumes that the adolescent's experiences with a variety of problems and concerns will interfere with his or her willingness and ability to comply. However, these patient characteristics can be modified by the physician's monitoring of the patient's behavior, asking the patient about problems with the medication, and using follow-up strategies. These actions by the physician are likely to reveal misunderstandings that the adolescent patient may have and thus enable him or her to clarify any health advice. These follow-up strategies also allow the health care provider to determine any adverse drug reactions and the patient's specific fears, doubts, and hesitations about the diagnoses and treatment. If problems are detected, then the practitioner can individualize the regimen and resolve any concerns that may be undermining the adolescent's desire to be compliant. Follow-up strategies also reinforce the importance of the therapy and thereby directly affect the motivation of the adolescent patient (Figure 19.1).

The Health Communication Model also assumes that several factors have an indirect influence on the patient's willingness to adhere to medical advice. These include the patient's readiness to learn, willingness to provide accurate feedback and to cooperate during the encounter, and receptivity to the practitioner's problem-solving efforts. On the basis of her model, Svarstad has proposed seven strategies for enhancing patient comprehension and recall and thereby increasing adherence with medical advice: (1) providing more explicit directions; (2) explaining the purpose or importance of therapy; (3) supplementing oral counseling with written instructions; (4) presenting information in categorical form; (5) repeating important points; (6) amplifying instructions; and (7) providing consistent advice. A limitation of this model is that it has been based primarily on research with adult patients. However, we believe that communication issues have an even more profound effect on adolescent compliance than has been observed in adults.

Psychological Modifiers of Compliance

In order to communicate effectively with the adolescent patient, the practitioner must be aware of the social and psychological characteristics that may affect his or her ability to modify the adolescent's health behavior. A primary factor that can influence provider-patient communication is the adolescent's level of cognitive development. Adolescents in the transition from concrete to abstract thought often have a sense of uniqueness and invulnerability. At this stage, youths often lack the ability to perceive cause-and-effect relationships between preventive health behavior and certain later outcomes.

These cognitive characteristics decrease the adolescent's perceived suscep-tibility to contracting a certain disease if the specific health action is not taken. The younger adolescent's cognitive development also inhibits the physician's ability to reason with the patient on an abstract verbal level, such as appealing to future consequences of present behaviors.

For the adolescent in cognitive transition, it is often necessary to provide practical, simplistic analogies that clearly illustrate the need for the adolescent to comply with the medical advice and the short-term as well as future consequences to the patient if he or she fails to adhere to the physi-cian's recommendations. As the adolescent develops the ability to think abstractly, he or she is better able to evaluate the likelihood that present actions will have an impact on future events. Thus, if a positive provider-patient relationship has been established, the physician will be better able to elicit the older adolescent patient's cooperation with treatment.

A second factor that is associated with the adolescent's cognitive devel-opment is his or her level of locus of control. Locus of control is the degree to which a person feels that he or she is in control of the events or circumstances that affect his or her life. Similarly, health locus of control is the degree to which the adolescent feels that his or her health is influenced by internal rather than external forces. Adolescents with a high level of internal health locus of control will believe that they are in control of the events that affect their health and will be more likely to be compliant with the medical regimen. Those with a high level of external health locus of control will tend to believe that their health is the result of luck, chance, fate, or other external forces that are out of their control. Such adolescents may reason that their health behavior will have little or no impact on their health outcome and thus will be more likely to be noncompliant with the treatment regimen.

Health locus of control is easily measured in clinical settings. B. S. Walston has developed an eighteen-item instrument that measures three components of health locus of control: internal health locus of control, powerful others health locus of control, and chance health locus of control. This instrument can be easily administered and scored to classify adolescents according to whether they feel that their health may be a result of external forces, are more likely to be influenced by powerful others, such as a physi-cian or a nurse, or are likely to take chances with their health. Once an adolescent's cognitive development and personal sense of control over his or her health are better understood by the clinician, appropriate educational intervention can be instituted.

The adolescent's self-esteem and self-concept may also have an impact on the provider's ability to communicate effectively with the patient, as well as the adolescent's willingness to adhere to medical advice. For example, adoles-cents with low self-esteem and a fragile body image may suddenly become noncompliant with a medication if they perceive that the drug may be having an adverse effect on their physical appearance. This is a common occurrence among adolescents experiencing the side effects of weight gain or cushingoid appearance from taking immunosuppressants. Since the side effects may be perceived as a significant alteration in their appearance and a disruption of their social relationships, they may be unreceptive to the physician's attempt to counsel them about their noncompliant behavior. It is difficult to convince these adolescents that the cost to their personal life at the present time may result in positive future outcomes. Formal support or encounter groups made up of adolescents with similar chronic diseases often help these adolescents to accept the side effects of their medication.

Compliance with Contraceptive Regimens

A particularly frustrating problem for those caring for adolescents is the issue of noncompliance with contraception, which is an important antecedent of adolescent pregnancy. Unintended pregnancies among unmarried adolescent females continue to be a formidable health and social issue in this country. Despite the availability of effective contraception, the pregnancy rate among sexually active adolescents in the United States remains higher than in any other Western nation. This is a result of the failure of many sexually active adolescents to practice birth control consistently. Data from several surveys suggest that the proportion of adolescent pregnancies among contraceptive users rose substantially during the 1970s. This increase in the rate of pregnancy among adolescents who apparently initiated the use of contraception was partly due to noncompliance with contraceptive regimens.

Although the increased risk of pregnancy associated with noncompliance with contraceptives is well documented, social and medical scientists have not been successful in identifying the social, cultural, and psychological antecedents of this risk-taking behavior. One reason is that there have been few coherent and logically based theoretical models of adolescent contraceptive behavior from which to derive and test hypotheses. In an effort to better understand contraceptive behavior, we developed a social-psychological model of adolescent females' contraceptive risk-taking behavior. The model postulates a series of direct and interactive associations between variables leading to the prediction of four highly interrelated forms of contraceptive behavior: the decision to use birth control, the choice of method, contraceptive compliance, and continued use or contraceptive method switching (Figure 19.2).

Premarital Sexual Standards and Past Sexual Experiences

The model proposes that frequency of sexual intercourse is the "initiator" variable in the adolescent's decision whether to use contraception. As frequency of intercourse increases, the female becomes more aware of the possibility of pregnancy, which is directly associated with her likelihood of using birth control. Sexual frequency is largely influenced by two factors: the

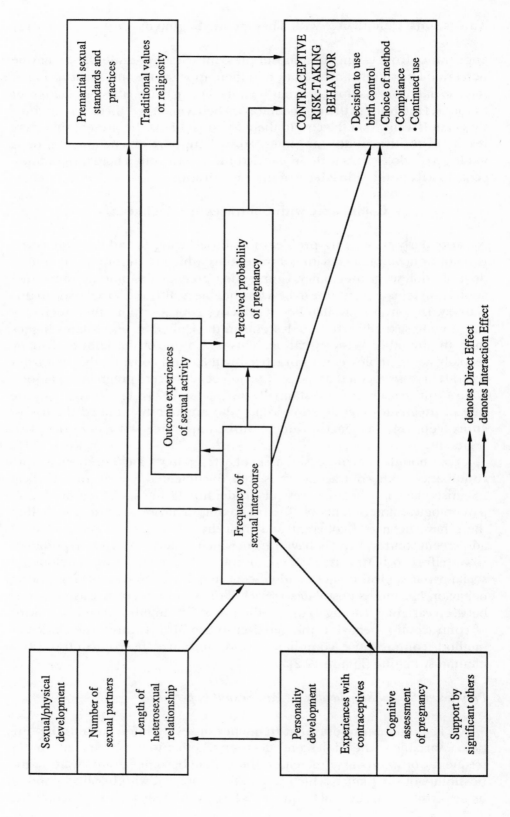

Figure 19.2. Compliance with Contraceptive Regimens.

individual's premarital experiences and standards and the emotional inti-macy of the heterosexual relationship. In general, there must be congruence between the adolescent's premarital sexual standards and actual sexual be-havior before sexual frequency will increase to a level at which she will rationally consider the risk of pregnancy.

Many sexually active adolescent females are not compliant with effec-tive methods of birth control because they do not fully acknowledge sexual intercourse as morally acceptable for themselves and, therefore, are unable to rationally prepare for it. Adolescent females may initiate sexual activity even if they believe that premarital sexual intercourse is not morally right. When it occurs, they may feel guilty about their sexual activity and tend to deny their sexual behavior. As long as there is incongruence between sexual standards and sexual activity, they will either not use contraceptives, use less effective methods, or be noncompliant with their regimen. This is because compliance with more effective contraceptive methods requires planning before sexual activity occurs. The process of acquiring and learning how to use a birth control method necessitates that the person acknowledge sexual activity and plan for future sexual activity. If sexual standards are not in congruence with behavior, then conflict will occur until either the behavior or the sexual standards change.

The model proposes that adolescents' perceptions of what significant others (for example, parents, peers, and sexual partners) think about sexual intercourse and contraceptive use affect their contraceptive behavior. If adolescents perceive that significant others' sexual standards differ from their own sexual behaviors, then they are less likely to be compliant with effective contraception.

Length of Sexual Relationship

Our model also specifies that as the length of time over which sexual intercourse has taken place increases, sexual attitudes and values generally shift to become consistent with behavior. American women typically are socialized to believe that premarital coitus is morally wrong. Thus, when an adolescent female initiates sexual activity, she will be in a state of "moral ambivalence," unable to accept her own sexual activity. Initiation and com-pliance with birth control are assumed to require the resolution of am-bivalence by acceptance of oneself as a sexually active person.

The degree of intimacy with the sexual partner in a monogamous relationship plays an important role in the resolution of moral ambivalence. The first step in this resolution is falling in love, which provides a rationale for coitus. However, women may not initially use birth control at this stage. As intercourse continues over time and increases in frequency, the adolescent may come to accept her sexual behavior as appropriate for that relationship and begin to use contraception. Thus, the quality of the relationship is directly related to the frequency of intercourse and indirectly related to contraceptive compliance. However, this relationship may be influenced by factors such as chronological age, postmenarchial age, and the number of years an adolescent has been dating.

Religiosity and Traditional Values

A variable that often receives little attention from scientists involved in adolescent health care issues is the impact of religious involvement on the adolescent's behavior. In general, frequency of coitus is inversely associated with religiosity. Religiosity may incorporate traditional values or standards of a society. It is an indicator of conventional behavior or proneness to behave in a socially approved, normatively expected fashion. Frequency of attendance at religious services is also an indicator of the amount of time during which the adolescent is exposed to social influences that generally do not support premarital sexual activity. Thus, the more that sexually active adolescents participate in religious groups that believe that premarital sexual activity is morally wrong, the less likely it is that their sexual norms and values will agree with their sexual behavior. As long as there is not congruence between an adolescent's sexual values and her sexual behavior, coital frequency will remain low and sporadic, and the likelihood of being compliant with effective birth control will remain low. If during counseling the health care provider attempts to help the adolescent resolve her moral conflict, care must always be taken not to undermine her value structure.

Physical and Sexual Development

Another factor that directly influences sexual frequency and indirectly affects contraceptive compliance is the adolescent female's physical and sexual development. An adolescent female must reach a certain level of emotional and sexual maturity before she can accept her adult role as a sexually active individual and cognitively deal with the realistic possibility of pregnancy. If an adolescent female is not emotionally mature enough to realistically assess the possibility of pregnancy, she is less likely than others to initiate birth control. Even if she does, she probably will not be compliant with her contraception.

Frequency of Sexual Intercourse and Perceived Risk of Pregnancy

The model proposes that as the sexually active adolescent female begins to reformulate and accept her sexual identity, resulting in a congruence between her premarital sexual standards and her sexual behavior, there will be an increase in her acceptance of continuing coitus. With this change in sexual identity, the frequency of intercourse will increase. As frequency of coitus increases or decreases, awareness of the possibility of pregnancy will vary correspondingly. It has been suggested that in the process of initiating and correctly using contraceptives, there are three distinct stages that are related to sexual frequency. In the first, or "natural," stage, sexual intercourse is infrequent and unpredictable. The adolescent perceives that her risk of becoming pregnant is low, rationalizes that it will not occur, and is unlikely to use contraceptives. This is followed by the "peer" stage, during which an ongoing relationship is associated with more frequent sexual intercourse. This produces a moderate awareness of the risk of pregnancy and results in the female seeking birth control information and devices from her partner or peers. During the peer stage, she will use nonprescription methods, such as condoms, foam, or suppositories. The third stage, labeled "expert," is characterized by a high frequency of intercourse, resulting in a higher awareness of the possibility of pregnancy. The expert stage is characterized by a higher motivation to use and be compliant with more effective contraceptive methods and an increased likelihood of seeing a health professional to acquire a prescription method, such as oral contraceptives.

Outcome Experiences of Sexual Activity and Perceived Probability of Pregnancy

The hypothesis that unmarried sexually active women will become more compliant with effective contraceptive methods as their frequency of sexual activity increases is based on an unstated assumption that single women view pregnancy as negative and will take action to avoid it. We know that this may not always be a correct assumption; some adolescents may view pregnancy as a positive possibility. Before deciding that pregnancy may be undesirable and initiating the use of birth control, a woman must first perceive that she is at significant risk of becoming pregnant. Even if an adolescent is highly motivated to avoid pregnancy, she is unlikely to use birth control if she believes that she has a low risk of becoming pregnant. For example, many younger adolescents believe that pregnancy cannot happen to them. They may believe that they are too young to get pregnant or that they or their partner are infertile, or they may never have considered pregnancy a possible outcome of their sexual activity. Such beliefs often occur when the adolescent has insufficient knowledge of when during her menstrual cycle she is at risk of becoming pregnant. Adolescence is characterized by a type of cognitive egocentricism labeled "the personal fable." Personal fables are beliefs that adolescents have about their lives that have a common theme of invulnerability. Adolescents typically reason that bad things such as auto accidents and pregnancy may happen to others but cannot happen to them. Thus, adolescents often assign a probability of zero to their risk of becoming pregnant. If an adolescent feels that pregnancy will never happen to her, she has little or no reason to use birth control.

The subjective probability that adolescents assign to their risk of becoming pregnant will depend partly on their own experiences or those of their peers, siblings, or parents. If an adolescent has been sexually active for a long time and has not become pregnant, she is likely to assign a low probability to that outcome. Similarly, if close friends have been sexually active without using birth control and have not become pregnant, this will also influence the adolescent's subjective perception. However, previous pregnancies or pregnancy scares will increases a woman's awareness of her risk of possibly pregnancy in the future. Although an adolescent female may perceive that she is at risk of pregnancy, she will not use birth control if she has determined that pregnancy would not be a negative experience for her. This partially explains why adolescents who have previously had a child are at higher risk of a second pregnancy during the teen years.

It is usually difficult for the health care provider to accurately measure an adolescent's perceived risk of becoming pregnant. However, previous research suggests four types of variables from which one might infer an adolescent's perception of her risk of pregnancy: (1) knowledge of risk variations during the menstrual cycle; (2) previous pregnancy experiences (for example, scares or actual pregnancy); (3) early contraceptive behavior (for example, length of time after first coitus before birth control is first used); and (4) previous family planning behavior (for example, going to a family planning clinic).

Support by Significant Others

During the last two decades, much of the research directed at the problems of adolescent sexuality, contraceptive behavior, and unwed pregnancy has been conducted outside the social context in which they normally occur. Instead of examining these behaviors in terms of the dynamics of interpersonal and sexual relationship development, researchers have tended to study various structural, social, psychological, and demographic factors thought to be predictive of premarital coital and contraceptive behavior using samples of predominantly older adolescent females. Until recently, peer and friendship networks were rarely studied, although it was assumed that such relationships were important in adolescent sexual socialization.

Previous research suggests that parental support may positively affect an adolescent female's compliance with contraceptives. Similarly, the degree of support provided by the girl's boyfriend may also influence her contraceptive compliance. If an adolescent female perceives that her boyfriend is in favor of birth control, she may be more compliant with her contraceptives. The influence of an adolescent's peers on her contraceptive behavior is also of significance. In a test of peers' effectiveness in clinical settings we found that adolescent peer counselors significantly enhanced adolescent females' contraceptive compliance.

Early studies found a strong positive relationship between adolescents' sexual attitudes and behaviors and their peers' sexual attitudes and behaviors. However, more recent research has revealed that after race and school grade were controlled, males neither influenced one another's sexual behavior nor selected each other as friends on the basis of whether they had sexual intercourse. Yet there was a relationship between adolescent females' sexual behavior and their friends' sexual behavior. In follow-up studies on a separate sample, these same investigators found no similarity in sexual behavior between adolescents and their same-sex friends for black males or females. Only white adolescents established same-sex best friendships on the basis of similarities in sexual behavior.

Although we have hypothesized that such a relationship exists, the question of what impact the adolescent female's boyfriend has on her sexual attitudes and behavior remains unanswered. As a heterosexual relationship develops, the female's boyfriend may evolve into the most significant reference individual in her life with regard to her sexual and contraceptive behavior. This may be especially true for black females, who are influenced less by same-sex friends than are white males or females. Although the male partner is very important in the dynamic social process that results in adolescent pregnancy, there is little information regarding the effect of the male partner on sexual and contraceptive behavior. We have previously hypothesized that the establishment of a long-term monogamous relationship will result in changes in both sexual attitudes and behavior. As the length of time of the heterosexual relationship increases, there will be a corresponding increase in the frequency of sexual intercourse and more consistent use of birth control.

In a recent study, we found that black female adolescents involved in stable heterosexual relationships characterized by more open communication expressed more negative feelings about the possibility of having a baby, had higher previous contraceptive compliance, used more effective contraceptive methods, and were more likely to state that their use of birth control was due to their plans to continue their monogamous sexual relationship. These findings support the hypothesis that the character of the heterosexual relationship may be associated with black female adolescents' sexual and contraceptive behaviors and attitudes.

When we compared this group of females' sexual and contraceptive behavior and attitudes with the behavior and attitudes of their boyfriends, the males reported more risky sexual and contraceptive behavior than their girlfriends. We also found that the females felt more pressure from their boyfriends not to use birth control than the males felt from their girlfriends. Part of this may have been due to the fact that the males also felt more positive about their girlfriends becoming pregnant and having a baby than was reported by the females. These gender differences in attitudes about having a baby are significant, considering that the self-esteems of the males and females were moderately inversely correlated. This would suggest that the risk of poor contraceptive behavior would be greatest among those couples where the male has higher self-esteem and a positive attitude toward pregnancy and the female has lower self-esteem and perceives a great deal of pressure from the male not to use birth control.

Although the mean scores of several of the attitudinal and behavioral variables differed significantly between the males and females, for many of these factors the males' and females' scores were moderately correlated. For example, although the males had less negative attitudes about the possibility of their girlfriends becoming pregnant and more positive attitudes toward their girlfriends' having a baby, the couples' scores on these scales were moderately positively correlated. These findings suggest that the establishment of these relationships may have been based partly on these adolescents' similarity in attitudes and behavior. The longer the relationship existed, the more opportunity the couples had to discuss their attitudes and beliefs about sex and birth control, and the more likely that congruence would occur in their sexual attitudes and behaviors.

Our research supports the assumption that characteristics of the heterosexual relationship are associated with the sexual and contraceptive behavior of some black female adolescents. Although our sample was representative of the population from which it was drawn, the fact that the target group was from a black lower-socioeconomic population from a southeastern city limits the national generalizability of the findings. However, this study reinforces the need for clinicians to inquire about the characteristics of an adolescent's sexual relationship during contraceptive counseling. Our findings also suggest that future research directed at adolescent sexuality, contraceptive behavior, and unwed pregnancy should continue to focus on the dynamics of interpersonal and sexual relationship development.

Personality Development

The degree to which adolescent females are influenced by others partly depends on their personality development. Formation of a stable self-image, sexual identity, and the concept of oneself as separate from parents is a final goal in the maturation process of the adolescent female. However, these developmental stages may occur long after biological and sexual maturity occurs. Also, an adolescent female may not always integrate the perception of herself as capable of procreation at the same time that she becomes physically capable of doing so. Therefore, the association between physical development and contraceptive compliance may be affected by the female adolescent's emotional maturity.

Factors such as self-concept, locus of control, future time perspective, and autonomy may also be associated with a female adolescent's contraceptive compliance. For example, among adolescent females with lower self-concept, childbearing may be perceived as a way to feel loved by the baby and/or the father or to be fulfilled and thus may increase the mother's feelings of self-worth. Adolescent females with high self-esteem may be happier with their lives and more motivated to maintain their life patterns by not becoming pregnant. Adolescent females who tend to have an internal locus of control and a high level of autonomy may be less influenced by peers or boyfriends to become sexually active and more likely to initiate action to prevent pregnancy.

Low expectations of a quality life-style outside of parenthood among lower-socioeconomic and minority-group adolescent females can also precipitate pregnancy. Contraception is a form of personal investment. For an adolescent female to be compliant with her contraceptive regimen, she must be able to conceptualize the future and see herself in a positive role. Since successful contraceptive behavior requires investing in inconvenient and possibly embarrassing behavior in order to obtain the future reward of nonpregnancy, the adolescent female must possess a positive outlook about future life. Among adolescent females with no hope for the future, pregnancy does not appear to threaten future life-styles and thus may be an acceptable alternative.

Experience with Contraceptives

The model presented above assumes that contraceptive behavior is a dynamic process and that contraceptive decisions made by adolescents vary over time in response to changes in any component of the model. If an adolescent experiences unpleasant physical or psychological side effects from a method, she is likely to reassess her choice. Similarly, if she becomes pregnant while using a particular method, she is likely to switch methods following the pregnancy. Experiences may also affect her feelings about sexual behavior or her sexual identity, which, in turn, may influence the frequency of intercourse. In contrast, if a woman's contraceptive experiences are positive, she may feel more confident about her sexual behavior and increase her coital frequency, which, in turn, would influence the other components in the model.

There are several variables not included in this model because of inconsistent empirical findings. One is the level of knowledge about birth control. Some investigators have asserted that adequate knowledge about birth control methods is a prerequisite to their use. In contrast, we have found that knowledge is not positively associated with birth control usage, since most adolescent women possess the basic information needed to acquire and use birth control. The model also does not include variables such as age, educational level, race, and the socioeconomic status of the adolescent's family. We believe that the specific components of the model may be associated with demographic background characteristics. However, it is the model's components that actually account for the impact. Any research that tests hypotheses derived from the model should also control for the effects of these demographic factors.

The theoretical model described in Figure 19.2 is derived from an accumulation of empirical studies over the last two decades. It has also undergone two tests since its development. It can be used to develop additional hypotheses that can be tested through multivariate analytical techniques. This paradigm can be used to justify the ordering of variables in statistical models, as well as the inclusion of interaction terms. The clinician can also use the model to anticipate and organize the multiple inter-relationships among factors that influence an adolescent female's compliance with birth control methods. The model can be used to help develop an appropriate sexual history when assessing an adolescent's risk of being noncompliant with her birth control regimen.

Compliance with Treatment for Substance Abuse

Adolescents have been identified as tending to be users of nonprescription drugs and nonusers of prescription medication. They tend not to adhere to the societal norm that involvement with illicit drugs or the use of harmful legal substances constitutes inappropriate behavior. Previous research indicates that by the time adolescents reach their senior year in high school, 92 percent have used alcohol, 69 percent have used tobacco, and 54 percent have experimented with marijuana. Although the majority of young people will not progress beyond the early or experimental stages of substance abuse, there is no absolute method for predicting which adolescents will progress to more advanced stages. Consequently, every young person who experiments with drugs needs to be identified, counseled as to the risk of involvement, and continuously monitored for further involvement.

J. M. Sanders points out that provider-patient communication is paramount in identifying, diagnosing, and treating the adolescent with a substance abuse problem. Although the diagnosis and treatment of substance abuse are beyond the scope of this chapter, a brief summary of the process is necessary to provide the framework for an adequate discussion of compliance issues. The initial step is to establish an effective trusting relationship in which confidentiality is ensured. Once this relationship has been established, most adolescents will be willing to express their concerns about involvement with drugs to the health care provider. Physicians treating adolescents should always have a high index of suspicion concerning substance abuse and should keep abreast of the common risk factors that may identify an adolescent with a substance abuse problem. When encountering adolescents who are unable or unwilling to honestly discuss their use of or experimentation with illicit substances, a physician can use a variety of screening methods. To date, there have been no screening questionnaires that have proved reliable and valid measures of drug use among adolescents. Some situations may warrant the use of the laboratory screening of body fluids, such as urine, to confirm the health care provider's suspicion that a problem exists.

If an adolescent patient is identified as having a substance abuse problem and a method of therapy has been established, the evaluation and enhancement of compliance with therapy are a major challenge. *Compliance* usually refers to a patient's adherence to a prescribed course of treatment. Paradoxically, in many cases, compliance with substance abuse therapy requires that the adolescent not use a medication. Although many of the methods discussed earlier for identifying compliant patients may not directly apply to the area of substance abuse, the principles used to assess conformity with treatment are the same. Drawing on health program evaluation terminology, the assessment of compliance with substance abuse therapy can be divided into process evaluation and program impact or outcome evaluation.

Process evaluation is usually defined as a documentation of what is going on in a program; it confirms the existence and availability of the essential elements of the program. Basically, this documentation describes the specific program activities and whether they are being accomplished efficiently. An essential element in assessing adolescent compliance with substance abuse therapy is evaluation of whether the adolescent is adhering to each component of the treatment regimen. During the initial (and, usually, the more intense) phases of treatment, the frequent interaction between the patient and the therapist facilitates this evaluation. As the adolescent patient begins to reintegrate into the social environment, the opportunities for monitoring the patient's progress decrease. During this reintegration period, the patient is usually confronted with the same social influences that initially precipitated the problem. The practitioner can measure compliance with a process evaluation approach by assessing the degree of success with which this reintegration occurs in terms of return to school or work, the level of communication with the family network, and the ability to successfully meet the demands established by the therapist. The reinstitution of stable family relationships and the establishment of peer relationships in which drug usage is not an inherent feature are also indicative of compliance. Thus, the return to a life-style in which the individual is able to function effectively represents evidence of continued compliance with the prescribed treatment program. Continuous positive reinforcement of the initiatives established during the intense therapeutic period is necessary for successful adherence to the therapeutic regimen. This includes regular opportunities for interacting with the therapeutic staff and other recovering patients, as well as continuous and appropriate social support from significant others, such as parents and peers.

Outcome evaluation usually involves an objective assessment of the overall effectiveness of a program in producing favorable cognitive, attitudinal, and behavioral effects or in improving morbidity, mortality, or other health status indicators. Several technologies are available for objectively evaluating compliance with substance abuse therapy. Body fluids such as urine can be analyzed for relatively minute traces of substances or their metabolic by-products. These laboratory tests have been refined to a point where they possess a high degree of sensitivity and specificity and can be performed at a reasonable cost. Immunoassay and chromatography techniques are also available to detect a wide variety of substances. There are also laboratory tests of more limited scope that can be used to monitor continued abstinence from specific substances.

Routine screening for drugs invokes a variety of legal and ethical concerns. When used to assess compliance with substance abuse therapy, routine screening produces less of a problem if certain approaches are taken. Experiences from military, corporate business, and university athletic programs suggest that random urine testing can serve as a significant deterrent to future drug usage. This same principle applies to a recovering adolescent patient. Random testing serves not only as a measure of noncompliance but also as an indirect motivator to increase compliance with therapy. However, the health care provider will be unsuccessful unless certain precautions are taken. Many substance abusers are aware of methods for invalidating urine test results. If they know that they are going to be tested at a certain time, specific chemicals can be consumed before the testing that can significantly alter the pH or specific gravity of the urine or change the physical properties of the specimen enough to produce unreliable test results. The substitution of urine from a drug-free person or some other liquid that has the appearance of urine is another method used to deceive the screener. To be successful, collection must be done randomly and without significant warning to the adolescent patient. Urine collection must also be accomplished under vigilant circumstances, including (if needed) disrobing and producing the specimen while being observed. Prior to screening, a protocol needs to be established specifying what actions will be taken if the patient is found to be noncompliant with the treatment regimen. This protocol needs to be developed specifically for each patient, addressing his or her unique social, psychological, and medical needs and characteristics. It is imperative that this protocol be enacted swiftly and effectively after discovery that the adolescent substance abuser has been noncompliant with therapy. Such an approach will have a greater chance of altering the noncompliant behavior.

Compliance and Chronic Diseases

Compliance with any treatment regimen is difficult, particularly when the duration of treatment lasts longer than several days. It is well recognized that even in acute illnesses, compliance with a treatment plan drops off as the patient improves. For complex or chronic diseases, the number and frequency of medications may make the therapeutic regimen too complicated for the average adolescent to follow. All too frequently for those youths with chronic illnesses, the treatment plan may entail dietary and activity manipulations as well as multiple medications. The ability of the adolescent to adhere to such a regimen over a long period of time is limited by the same factors that affect adult compliance and will only worsen over time. Even simplifying a treatment plan to the bare essentials may not change adherence if the treatment is to last the remainder of the adolescent's lifetime.

The developmental processes of adolescence may also aggravate the problem. At a time when many of their peers are seeking autonomy and developing a sense of self, adolescents with a chronic disease such as cystic fibrosis or diabetes may still find themselves relying on their immediate families for help and support. The perceived failure of adolescents to grow and mature creates conflicts within themselves and with those trying to help them follow the treatment plan. These conflicts may give rise to rebellion and noncompliance; for example, adolescent diabetics who fail to give themselves insulin because they are tired of following the same routine. In some instances, rebellion and noncompliance with medical therapy may also be the youth's way of "punishing" his or her family for the disease.

With the teenager with a chronic illness, other psychosocial modifiers may affect compliance. During the early transition from concrete thinking to abstract operations, peers play an increasingly important role. The perception of being different from their friends will make most adolescents feel that they are outcasts. A male adolescent with cancer may have no outward sign of his disease except alopecia yet may be extremely noncompliant with his antineoplastic regimen in order to prevent the hair loss that makes him "different."

As discussed earlier, another psychosocial factor that may play an important role in the compliance of adolescents with chronic diseases is their health locus of control. Adolescents who have an internal health locus of control seem to reason that they can influence the disease process by their beliefs and actions. Such individuals have been found to have a greater likelihood of adherence to medical therapy, presumably because they understand both the benefits and the costs of the therapeutic regimen and think that they can affect the outcome of the disease. On the other hand, adolescents who perceive that their illness happened to them because of external forces beyond their control may not feel that the benefit of adherence to a therapeutic plan is worth the effort. Adolescents with such an external health locus of control are difficult to motivate and monitor.

Having discussed the multiple negative factors affecting adolescent compliance, let us turn to those factors positively associated with compliance. Among adolescents with chronic diseases, positive family support and communication, expectations of positive outcome by the family, and family involvement have been correlated with medical compliance. The social support system of the patient and expectations regarding outcome seem to be crucial components of the treatment schedule. Although the adolescent's natural growing away from the family may conflict with the positive effect of family support, if the support given is appropriate to the youth's development, it can greatly enhance compliance. The lack of family support has been associated with medical noncompliance in epileptic adolescents. Harmonious family relationships and a sense of personal autonomy have been found to enhance an adolescent's self-esteem and improve compliance, not only with the anticonvulsant treatment but with the compliance-monitoring regimen. Adherence by these patients, and perhaps those with other illnesses, can be improved by inquiries about the interrelationships within the family and periodic discussions of the issues of family support throughout the treatment time.

Several additional factors also affect adolescents' compliance with their treatment for specific chronic illnesses. R. B. Haynes has developed a ranking of life-style changes that are associated with decreasing compliance, and this can easily be illustrated by the diabetic treatment plan. It is easier to acquire new habits, such as learning to self-administer insulin, than to alter old habits by complying, for example, with dietary restrictions or scheduling exercise at an appropriate time during the daily schedule. Although diabetes is a disease with which it is difficult to enhance compliance because of the life-style changes required, it has been documented that interventions that affect health beliefs can influence the health behavior of patients. Confidence about one's ability to carry out the regimen plays an enormous role in adherence; interventions that enable an adolescent to reach that level of confidence may be the most successful. Perceived severity of and susceptibility to disease and its complications are also important health beliefs to include in compliance-enhancing programs. Providing an appropriate support environment in addition to the social support of the family may contribute to an adolescent's compliance.

Asthma is another common ailment of adolescents that frequently requires long-term therapeutic intervention. Although many adolescents will state that they have taken the theophylline or other medicine as prescribed, as few as 10 percent may actually have therapeutic drug levels. Metabolism of theophylline in adolescent patients does not vary enough to account for all the variation in serum drug levels; noncompliance is the assumed mechanism. Education programs that increase short-term knowledge have been known to affect patient compliance with bronchodilator therapies and, along with serum drug monitoring, may improve patients' adherence.

Other methods of improving compliance have been developed for adolescents with such conditions as cystic fibrosis. The Medical Compliance Incomplete Stories Test was developed in an attempt to discriminate between compliant and noncompliant cystic fibrosis patients. The instrument uses five incomplete stories that follow a character through decision-making situations involving medication. Strong correlations between the scale and compliance suggest that it can be used to identify compliers and noncompliers.

Adolescents with chronic diseases represent a formidable challenge in terms of enhancing their compliance with treatment. While many of the instruments and methods described above were initially used only for a specific disease, it is likely that modifications of these methods may increase their applicability to adolescents with other chronic illnesses. Perhaps the most significant factors that may enhance medication compliance among adolescents with chronic diseases are the technological advances in medication delivery such as injection pumps and drug implants. However, these technological devices will need to be cosmetically appealing to be accepted by adolescents.

Compliance with Treatment for Sexually Transmitted Diseases

An area in which little research has been conducted is adolescents' compliance with therapy for sexually transmitted diseases (STDs). One reason for the scarcity of research is the long tradition in venereology of administering single-dose treatment to adolescents under direct supervision. With the increased frequency with which such STDs as *Chlamydia trachomatis*, penicillin-resistant *Neisseria gonorrheae*, genital warts, and pelvic inflammatory disease are being diagnosed in adolescents, compliance with treatment has become a more important issue.

Several factors specific to STDs have been identified that have an impact on adolescents' compliance with treatment. Although most STDs are common treatable diseases, they are socially stigmatizing. Because STDs carry the stigma of engaging in a socially unacceptable behavior, many adolescent patients are reluctant to seek health care if they suspect that they have an STD. If these adolescent patients perceive that the health care practitioner shares society's view of STDs and if the practitioner reflects this attitude during interaction with the patients, they will be less likely to be compliant with therapy and follow-up appointments.

A second factor that affects compliance with treatment for STDs is that treatment is often at public expense and/or in public facilities. A common public health approach used to address the increased frequency of STDs has been the creation of specialized STD clinics in public health facilities. Although the creation of STD clinics concentrates expertise and interest, the clinic usually operates on an appointment basis and restricts its hours of operation to 9:00 to 5:00. Having to wait for an appointment or come to a clinic during normal school or working hours can be a significant barrier for some adolescents. In some cities, public STD clinics remain open until 8:00 or 9:00 P.M., thus reducing structural barriers to care. An additional barrier to compliance is that the adolescent patient is often subjected to a long wait once he or she arrives at the clinic and usually does not see the same health care provider at each visit. STD clinics in public health facilities are often esthetically unappealing or staffed by health care providers who are unenthusiastic about treating adolescents. Adolescent patients attending an STD clinic are also clearly identified to each other and to clinic staff as possibly having a stigmatizing disease. Although adolescents may initially come to a clinic to be treated for a possible STD, if they encounter someone that they know in the waiting room, they may be less likely to return for follow-up treatment. One remedy for this dilemma is to establish clinics that deal with both STDs and more socially acceptable problems, such as urinary tract infections or contraception.

Inadequate training in venereology makes it difficult for practitioners to enhance compliance through education. Previous research suggests that high levels of motivation by the clinic staff enhance adolescent patients' compliance with treatment regimens and follow-up visits for tests of cure. However, several factors appear to influence the level to which the clinic staff are willing to motivate adolescent patients. Health care providers working in public health programs and in some prepaid health care organizations may unconsciously fail to provide a high level of motivation to patients to return for follow-up visits because of the increased work loads or financial costs involved in providing follow-up tests of cure. In contrast, practitioners in fee-for-service systems, as well as those engaged in compliance research, stand to benefit from return visits and may inspire a greater degree of motivation from the patient. These findings suggest that the provision of direct incentives to practitioners for providing a high level of motivation to adolescent patients might enhance their compliance.

Although the research directed at adolescents' compliance with the treatment of sexually transmitted diseases is limited, research conducted in other areas offers several recommendations for enhancing compliance: (1) diagnostic procedures for detecting STDs should be as atraumatic as possible; (2) single-dose treatment should be utilized and be administered in the clinic whenever possible; (3) STDs should be treated in clinics staffed by practitioners with special interest in venereology; (4) clinics should provide continuity of care and visits by appointment; (5) in health care facilities staffed by several practitioners, their ability to achieve compliance in terms of persuading patients to return for tests of cure and bringing sexual partners for evaluation should be monitored; (6) patient education concerning all aspects of the particular STD and treatment should be provided at each visit; and (7) STD clinics should be combined with other services relevant to reproductive health, such as contraception, where the similarities of issues and procedures will allow both an economy of effort and the opportunity to integrate prevention of STDs with that of unintended pregnancy.

Conclusion: Strategies for Enhancing Patient Compliance

Compliance behavior among adolescents is complex and incompletely understood. In this chapter, we have discussed adolescent noncompliance in general, as well as factors that affect adolescents' compliance with contraceptives, treatment for substance abuse, treatment for sexually transmitted diseases, and treatment for chronic diseases. While a large number of interrelated behavioral and cognitive factors are associated with whether an adolescent will be compliant with therapy, the clinician should keep in mind that the health care provider's behavior is often more important than the adolescent's behavior in determining what level of compliance the adolescent will achieve. Consequently, we conclude with a list of strategies that the health care provider should employ to increase adolescent patients' compliance with therapy:

1. Work to establish a good relationship with the adolescent patient.
2. Consider the possibility of noncompliance. Clinicians tend to over-estimate compliance, especially among patients who are socially, economically, and ethnically similar to themselves.
3. Reduce barriers to noncompliance, such as long waiting times, inconvenient hours, and embarrassing situations.
4. Ensure that instructions are clear, structured, and written so that they may be posted in a convenient place at home. The health care provider's expectations as to anticipated outcomes should be explicit. However, education and knowledge do not necessarily imply or increase patient compliance; therefore, do not assume that a knowledgeable patient will be compliant. Remember that the adolescent patient needs to be provided with explicit directions, to have the purpose or importance of therapy explained, to have oral counseling supplemented with written instructions, to be presented information in categorical form, to have important points repeated and amplified, and to be given consistent advice by all staff in the clinic.
5. Simplify the drug regimen as much as possible and cue compliance to specific times of the day and/or to a daily activity.
6. Increase the amount of attention paid to the patient and, by careful follow-up, ensure that therapeutic regimens are carried out. The level of monitoring of patient compliance should be inverse to the symptom relief anticipated; the greater the relief, the less monitoring required. Also, the adolescent should be an active partner in developing the therapeutic plan. The use of therapeutic contracts is a good way to include the adolescent patient in the treatment plan.
7. Reward and reinforce good or improving compliance, especially by giving encouragement. Remember that fear is an ineffective long-term motivator. Rewards and praise are often better methods to motivate adolescents to participate in their care.
8. Avoid judging compliance with the entire regimen on the basis of compliance or noncompliance with only one aspect of it. If noncompliance is detected, effective intervention should be instituted as quickly as possible.

Suggested Readings

Blum, R. W. "Adolescent Substance Abuse: Diagnostic and Treatment Issues." *Pediatric Clinics of North America*, 1987, *34*, 523–537.

DuRant, R. H., and Jay, M. S. (eds.). "Communication and Compliance Issues in Adolescent Medicine." *Seminars in Adolescent Medicine*, 1987, *3* (entire issue 2).

DuRant, R. H., Sanders, J. M., Jay, S., and Levinson, R. "An Analysis of the Contraceptive Behavior of Sexually Active Adolescent Females in the United States." *Journal of Pediatrics*, 1988, *113*, 930–936.

DuRant, R. H., Sanders, J. M., Jay, S., and Levinson, R. "Adolescent Contraceptive Risk-Taking Behavior: A Social Psychological Model of Females' Use of and Compliance with Birth Control." In A. R. Stiffman and R. A. Feldman (eds.), *Advances in Adolescent Mental Health*. Vol. 4: *Childbearing and Childrearing*. London, England: Jessica Kingsley, 1990.

Freidman, I. M., and Litt, I. F. "Promoting Adolescents' Compliance with Therapeutic Regimens." *Pediatric Clinics of North America*, 1986, *33*, 955–972.

Haynes, R. B., Taylor, D. W., and Sackett, D. L. (eds.). *Compliance in Health Care*. Baltimore, Md.: Johns Hopkins University Press, 1979.

Jay, S., Litt, I. F., and DuRant, R. H. "Compliance with Therapeutic Regimens." *Journal of Adolescent Health Care*, 1984, *5*, 124–136.

Svarstad, B. L. "Patient-Practitioner Relationships and Compliance with Prescribed Medical Regimens." In L. H. Aiken and D. Mechanic (eds.), *Applications of Social Science to Clinical Medicine and Health Policy*. New Brunswick, N.J.: Rutgers University Press, 1986.

Part Five

Improving the
Health of Adolescents

PART EDITOR
William A. Daniel, Jr., M.D.

Introduction

William A. Daniel, Jr., M.D.

This part proposes specific approaches for improving the health of adolescents and explores ways in which health care professionals, social services, and social networks can work separately and together to develop and implement these approaches.

As discussed in Chapter Twenty, societal etiologies have replaced infectious diseases as the chief causes of morbidity and mortality in adolescents. Risk-taking behaviors and emotional difficulties are increasing and often receive little or no attention. Often, parents and adolescents believe that physicians are uninterested in the problems of youth or unqualified to help. Not infrequently, the responsibility for addressing these problems and dealing with health care in general is left to the adolescents themselves. Most adolescents have not learned to be responsible health care consumers and are ill equipped to cope with the health care system. The number of handicapped adolescents is increasing as technological advances increase their chances of survival. Their complicated, often unmet needs constitute another responsibility to provide health care. Many adolescents have complex physical and emotional problems that require services from professionals in several disciplines. These needs increase the responsibility to coordinate services and share information.

Chapter Twenty-One points out that the erosion of family constraints, changes in societal influences, and increases in risk-taking behaviors of adolescents have dramatically increased the responsibilities of health care professionals. These providers should have a core body of knowledge about adolescent development and an awareness of the influences of family, society, and peers. They should also be familiar with the scope and value of a variety of health disciplines. Health professionals cannot solve all the problems of adolescence or provide appropriate care for all adolescent illnesses and aberrations. If adolescent health care is to be a high priority of the nation, improvements in its delivery must be made at all levels. The roles and responsibilities of health professionals must change in response to this priority. Increasing the awareness of health care professionals about the health needs of adolescents and becoming involved with forces outside the health care system in meeting these needs are responsibilities of all those involved in the health care system. Community involvement to provide social alternatives that promote health and reduce risk-taking behaviors is already increasing in importance in our society. Health professionals can help catalyze this involvement.

Attachment and social bonding are critical in human development. Societal changes have fractured many family relationships and often expose adolescents to life-threatening activities, technologies, and substances that can compromise their ability to thrive and to experience healthy development. In the last chapter in this part, ways are considered to restore social support and social networks that have been eroded by profoundly transformed conditions of contemporary society. Restructuring means of support and providing new social networks during critical periods of development would help foster the development of healthy adolescents and have a constructive effect on the entire course of their lives.

20

Meeting the Health Service
Needs of Adolescents

William A. Daniel, Jr., M.D.

Although adults assume that adolescence is a healthy period of life, data showing that adolescents are the only group with no decrease in the mortality rate in the past thirty years challenge this assumption. Increased numbers of violent deaths among adolescents have offset the lower death rate from infectious diseases. Adults also are dazzled by youth itself, ignore the stresses and dangers of growing up today, and are unaware of new morbidities that increase health needs.

Many risk-taking behaviors of adolescents can be precursors of chronic health problems or even death. There are new morbidities that affect psychosocial development, mental well-being, and, sometimes, physical health. Major social changes that have occurred exert powerful influences on the psychosocial development of adolescents. Until we address these multiple etiologies and changes for the better occur, health professionals must cope with the resultant problems and unmet needs of adolescents.

Health care is unavailable or unaffordable for some adolescents. There are reasons why those needs are unmet, but in many instances, adolescents do not avail themselves of convenient, free, or affordable services. Teenagers usually do not believe that they need health supervision, advice about the growth process, or visits with a physician for counseling. Friends and peer groups are the common sources of information, and much of that is erroneous. Doctors and other health professionals continue to devote their attention and energy to conventional health problems and illnesses. Health professionals and parents must become more aware of the deficit in care for the new, unmet health needs of adolescence and help adolescents recognize its value.

Physicians and the family form the cornerstone for educating adoles-cents about health. How the doctor defines health care can affect the type of care that teenagers will expect and continue to seek during adulthood. If parents and physicians regard risk-taking behaviors and new morbidities as deserving consideration and treatment, adolescents and young adults will be more likely to obtain available services. Many illnesses are complex. No physician is likely to be proficient in all areas of care, and physicians often simply lack sufficient time to deal with all aspects of a complex illness. To be responsible for comprehensive health care, doctors must have competent and available resources for referral, collate the findings, prescribe therapy, and ensure continuing supervision.

Previous chapters of this book have considered trends and major physical and emotional health problems, the influence of society and pov-erty, and risk-taking behavior. This chapter considers adolescent health needs that receive inadequate attention, considers why adolescents do not use the health system, and explores ways to increase our understanding of adolescents and improve their health care.

Unmet Health Needs

Physicians are primarily concerned with the maintenance of health in well patients and the diagnosis and treatment of acute and chronic illnesses. Other health professionals provide similar functions in their specific disci-plines. Physical illnesses or discipline-specific disorders usually receive the most time and attention. While this concentration of effort has produced progress in the quality of care, it does limit consideration of many conditions that are not included in the boundaries of traditional medical care but affect the health of adolescents. We need to increase our awareness of this area of adolescent health needs.

New Morbidities

New morbidities, and some that are not new but now receive greater attention, increase the anxiety of parents or adolescents. Although adoles-cent behaviors can have inherent risks, they are also functional responses to the environment. Teenagers usually choose behaviors that they believe will help them in their development, even though many of these can lead ulti-mately to illnesses. Adolescents are motivated by the discomfort that they feel about the changes that they are experiencing and are likely to choose behav-iors that enhance their feeling of well-being. Young people rarely consult a physician or other health professional about nonphysical difficulties, includ-ing behavioral disorders, school underachievement, sexual activities, grow-ing disengagement with the family, environmental effects, violence, eating disorders, and mental health.

Social changes, technological improvements, and new fads or activities can have undesirable side effects. For example, driving recreational vehicles, riding skateboards, or scuba diving can be associated with significant injury or death because adolescents do not consider them dangerous. Social changes are implicated in many of the disturbing morbidities. Moving to a new geographical location, living in a ghetto, coping with a new life-style brought about by divorce or remarriage of a parent, or having two working parents can cause behavioral difficulties or emotional problems. Risk-taking practices, substance abuse, and early sexual activity, for example, are frequently adopted by adolescents under stress and become important considerations for society and health professionals.

Many of the morbidities mentioned above are not age-specific. Risk taking can begin in childhood and be exacerbated in adolescence. Intervention in the disorders and behaviors of preadolescents can often help to prevent more serious difficulties during the ensuing years of rapid physical and emotional change. It is not unusual for these activities to affect the growth and development of adolescents. If risk taking begins during early adolescence, additional types of risk may appear, and harmful effects and consequent needs for health care may increase in the future.

With technological progress, more handicapped children are living to become adolescents. It is not unusual for physicians to concentrate their attention on a complex disease or handicap and neglect its effects on the psychosocial development of an adolescent. Insufficient research has been done to learn the biopsychosocial relationships between chronic disorders and adolescence. For example, how does rapid growth affect the treatment of diabetes in a child who developed the condition before the onset of puberty? How does that individual cope with adolescence? Conversely, are there psychosocial differences in the effects of diabetes whose onset is during adolescence? Is adjustment to the condition easier or more difficult in early or late onset of disease?

Surveys have shown that a handicapped or chronically ill adolescent may have more than one physical or associated behavioral disorder. The existence of mental or emotional difficulties can be greater than reported in some surveys because they were not specifically included in the questionnaires. Chronically ill adolescents often have more emotional disorders than do able-bodied persons. Further study is needed to determine the etiological role of chronic illnesses in emotional problems. A significant relationship probably exists, especially if the physical disorder begins during the early psychosocial development of the adolescent.

Significant correlation of behavioral problems with school achievement is also evident. Educational achievement is a high priority of most parents of adolescents, and there are many things that affect learning or motivation. Schools now attempt to detect learning disabilities in adolescent students and provide special methods of teaching for different types of disability. These efforts have identified many associated problems. Teenagers

with learning disabilities, for example, have more difficulty in social adjustment and a higher than average incidence of behavioral disorders. Data also
show a greater than average range of specific types of learning disorders in
adolescent juvenile offenders, who commonly have poor educational
achievement.

Major Morbidities

Adolescents invariably must experiment and test themselves and the
world around them. Unfortunately, many teenagers begin a sequence of
activities that are potentially dangerous to their health and development.
Society and health professionals often are unable to prevent these behaviors
and must daily cope with the consequences. Most major morbidities affect
individuals, but if large groups are involved, society may look to the health
professions for guidance and solutions. For adolescents, the risky actions
may result in significant illnesses or injuries that affect their maturation and
future adult capabilities. Medical problems caused by these actions are well
known. Effective methods of treating the physical consequences of these
behaviors are available, but psychosocial and emotional components are
difficult to assess and treat. As with lesser morbidities, the tendency to
concentrate on the physical aspects can lead to less awareness of the many
effects of risk taking.

Harmful behaviors rarely occur in isolation, and one commonly leads
to another, though this is not always the case. Age, developmental stage of
adolescence, gender, and local culture all affect young people's patterns of
behavior. In the United States, most seniors in high school have had at least
one drink of alcohol. One survey found that 40 percent of tenth-graders had
been drunk at least once during the school year. One in seven twelfth-grade
students became drunk at least once a week. Research has shown that
adolescents who abuse alcohol have several characteristics in common that
differentiate them from their non-alcohol-abusing peers: less tolerance of
social differences, less interest in school, and greater family tolerance of
drinking. They are usually male. Most adolescents who use alcohol during
their high school and college years do not become alcoholics but gradually
decrease their consumption as they become older. A significant number of
adolescents who drink alcohol try other chemical substances or engage in
other harmful behaviors. There is a high correlation between use of alcohol
and vehicular injuries and death in adolescents.

Accidents cause the largest number of teenage deaths and are responsible for most nonfatal injuries. The largest number of hospital days for
adolescent males and females is attributed to accidents, even if pregnancy-
related days are included. Boys are especially vulnerable to accidents at
school and from sports, with the highest incidence during early adolescence.

Tobacco use has begun to decrease with the greater social pressure against smoking. However, use of smokeless tobacco (snuff or chewing to-bacco) has increased. Thirteen percent of male students coming to the Adolescent Unit of the University of Alabama School of Medicine for prepar-ticipation physical examinations had begun to use tobacco before they were eleven years old. The percentage of initial users increased with age. Use was chiefly by white male students and almost nonexistent among black adoles-cents. The percentage of continued use greatly decreased with age. For most boys, chewing tobacco or dipping snuff was part of a temporary period of youthful experimentation. Of the users, 4.8 percent had early evidence of leukoplakia, and this finding showed a high correlation with the duration and quantity of use.

The use of marijuana and cocaine by adolescents has not decreased, and the age of initiation has become younger. The availability of "crack," an especially dangerous cocaine product, has greatly increased and begun to spread to smaller cities and rural areas. Many surveys show that adolescent users of marijuana and cocaine often experiment with additional drugs. Adolescents also inject chemical substances and run the risk of many ill-nesses transmitted by the sharing of infected needles. As with alcohol, there appear to be patterns of use by adolescents that are related to developmental stages and to gender.

In the past three decades, there has been a marked increase in sexual activity of girls fifteen to nineteen years old and an earlier age of onset of sexual activity by younger boys. Earlier sexual intercourse puts adolescents at increased risk of pregnancy and sexually transmitted diseases. There are many thousands of homosexual or bisexual male adolescents, and their sexual activities pose a great danger of contracting or spreading HIV infec-tion. The disease is also transmitted to both sexes by infected needles. Heterosexual male adolescents who inject drugs can sexually transmit the infection to teenage girls, many of whose babies also have AIDS.

An examination of the prevalence, age of onset, and gender differ-ences associated with specific risk-taking behaviors of adolescents reveals clear relationships between substance abuse, sexual activity, and accidents. These findings prove that different categories of behavior usually do not occur in isolation. In fact, one risk-taking behavior usually leads to others and increases the need for health care. Most physicians take a history and seek signs and symptoms that lead to a single diagnosis, but this style is not always appropriate. In treating adolescents, health professionals, particu-larly physicians, find great value in discussing with adolescents the psycho-social factors that may have led to their illness.

Increasing the Use of Health Services

Adolescents and their parents most often seek health care for acute illnesses and accidents or continuing care for handicaps. Because adolescents are generally healthy, they and their parents give little consideration to preventive care or seeking help from health professionals for nonphysical problems. Physicians have generally not stressed the value of help for these conditions and unfortunately are perceived as being uninterested in them or unqualified to deal with them. We must change our receptivity to adolescents and address these unmet needs.

Changing Ideas

Parents and adolescents believe that physicians are capable of providing quality care for most physical ailments. However, the chief priorities of parents and teenagers are now those of the new morbidities. Although health care priorities of physicians and adolescents may differ, changes in the attitudes of parents and adolescents are needed to improve preventive health care.

The value of health maintenance and the willingness of health professionals to help with both physical and behavioral problems should be communicated first to parents of small children and later directly to adolescents. Asking about family functions, school, peers, and other possible problem areas helps teenager and parents to know that physicians and other professionals are interested in and willing to discuss topics important to them. If this is done routinely, most parents and patients feel free to raise questions and will expect discussions to be a regular part of a visit. Physicians in particular are reluctant to do this, because discussions take time. Anticipatory guidance and informational handouts can establish education as one of the functions of health care. Pubescent boys and girls should be more directly involved in consideration of why they came to the health professional. Parents should be encouraged to promote the acceptance of responsibility for health by their adolescent children. Parents also need to take an active part in encouraging teenagers to discuss problems with health professionals other than physicians. Adolescents should gradually become the primary source of information about themselves and their health. Most contacts of adolescents with health professionals are on a one-to-one basis. Attitudinal changes can be a part of the visit and lay the foundation for more responsibility. The objective is for the teenager to think of and promptly use the health care system when biopsychosocial problems occur. Unfortunately, most early adolescents are incapable of anticipating the effects of their actions and do not seek more mature opinions before initiation of the actions.

Health professionals tend to think in terms of disciplines and priorities of care in specific areas. We, too, need to change our ideas about health needs of adolescents and become more aware of the priorities of young patients. Health care for adolescents has become increasingly complex, and often the skills of several professionals are required. Changes in attitudes about responsibility, scope of care, and the developmental stage of individual adolescents are also needed.

Sources of Health Care

Most adolescents receive health care from private physicians, but many of them go to ambulatory centers or health department specialty clinics. Teenagers, especially those living in rural areas, may receive care from a single physician who is usually competent to treat most physical illnesses and injuries but has little time, and perhaps limited interest or skill, to deal with the new morbidities. The consequences of early sexual activity, for example, may not be discussed until pregnancy or sexually transmitted diseases demand attention. There may be little time in which to ask about an adolescent's opinions on sexuality, to provide counseling, or to identify and assess harmful behaviors. Unfortunately, there are physicians who do not discuss these subjects during visits to assess adolescent development. Anticipatory guidance should be part of each office visit, particularly when addressing areas identified as potentially dangerous.

Group practice in cities is common. Individual members of a group often have special interests, and many patients receive services from more than one physician. Multiple care can be beneficial or confusing to adolescents, who often attempt to establish close ties with a single doctor. Physicians and other health professionals in group practice should select areas of special interest and evaluate their ability to meet the comprehensive needs of teenagers. Some physicians are uninterested in the psychosocial problems of adolescents and their families or do not have time for counseling. Those physicians should at least detect the need for services and refer the adolescents to professionals who can help. There are many sources for referral, and it is necessary to learn which ones are available, capable, and interested in teenagers. Sometimes, for example, a psychologist or psychiatrist may be skilled in adult care and ineffective or uninterested in working with teenagers.

A member of a group practice may develop a special interest in adolescents and gradually come to provide care for most teenagers who come to the group. In time, the other members of the group usually become more familiar with the psychosocial problems of adolescents and begin to apply their new interests to younger children.

Many adolescents do not obtain care from physicians in private practice. Ambulatory care facilities often have general and specialized clinics, but only a few are specially designed to provide comprehensive care to adolescents. A major criticism is lack of attention given to psychosocial problems and anticipatory guidance to prevent risk-taking behaviors. If a psychosocial problem is identified, referral is usually made to another clinic, thereby sometimes disrupting the feeling of trust in the adolescent. Often there is little follow-up information or sharing of findings among several health professionals who provide services to an adolescent. Agency facilities, health department clinics, or crippled children's services, for example, may provide categorical care and be limited in their scope of services. Their care is valuable, but it may be incomplete. Greater attention to the stress and emotional effects of a specific handicap or illness on adolescents and families often is needed. Chronic illness in a child or adolescent may lead to new family problems in several areas and demand greater attention for continuing care of the patient. Agencies and clinics also need to know where to refer adolescents to complement their own services.

Many practicing physicians, including those in ambulatory clinics, state that the number of patients cared for is so large that they have limited time to spend with each one. Another reason for not caring for adolescents in private practice is the belief that the physician cannot charge enough per visit. Some doctors have solved that problem by charging for units of time or scheduling repeat visits. Referral to another health professional would entail additional cost. It is difficult to understand why the primary physician or other practicing health professional is reluctant to charge for more time and services but feels free to refer patients. Usually, ways can be found to treat adolescents if there is a desire to do so.

It is paradoxical that the children of our nation are recognized as the most valuable resource for the future but that we are not willing to provide comprehensive health care for those who cannot pay for it. As an example of this, many states and cities have programs for alcoholism that do not accept adolescents. There is a great need for additional treatment centers for young abusers of chemical substances. Methods of preventing pregnancy may be unavailable for teenagers who wish to use them. Many mental health programs have limited education and counseling services for adolescents. The unmet health needs of adolescents will not be adequately cared for until ways to pay for those services are developed.

Educating Adolescents for Health Care

Meeting the health needs of adolescents depends on the cooperation of health professionals and adolescents. Teenagers should be educated about their responsibility to learn the value of health, to avoid behaviors that damage it, and to know how to obtain health services.

Value of Health

The idea of seeking care only for physical problems is established during the years before the onset of puberty and continues in adolescence. Parents accept the belief that routine examinations and answering questions are necessary during the first year or two of a child's life. After that, the purpose of visiting physicians and other health professionals has less relation with growth and development and more with illnesses and preschool immunizations. Continuity of care is an objective of all physicians. Parents can understand this and learn that adolescents, even those who appear healthy, should visit physicians at recommended intervals to ensure optimal physical and psychological progress toward adulthood.

Physicians and other professionals can assist parents in educating young people about the value of health, means of staying healthy, and being responsible for themselves. Adolescents need experience in making decisions because they will become adults who have to take charge of their lives. Among the many educational objectives, three stand out: understanding the scope of care available, the value of health, and the expectations of therapeutic care.

Scope of Services

Physicians and other health professionals should be interested in adolescents as persons, not as illnesses or disorders. This interest should extend to how teenagers feel about themselves and their relationships with family members and peers. Knowing the plans, hopes, and fears of individual adolescents is part of comprehensive health care. Above all, adolescents should understand that they can come to the physician or clinic for help with nonphysical problems and should be encouraged to do so. Practitioners' willingness to spend time to discuss their problems proves that there is a source of care for physical, cognitive, and psychosocial changes and disorders of health.

Adolescents may receive most of their health care from a single physician. Complexities of care increase with age. As the scope of health needs increases, it is likely that the number of health professionals involved in care will increase. Families and teenagers need to know about the health care system, the roles of various professionals, and the value of a wide range of services. If we expect adolescents to become capable of seeking their own health care, we must teach them how to do it. Education of teenagers about what the health system offers and how to obtain services is a great unmet need. Large numbers of adolescents have no families to help, many live in families that cause emotional or behavioral disorders, and all will enter the job market or go to college, where they will be responsible for themselves. The first lesson they should learn is the value of preventing illnesses and injuries.

Preventive Care

Preventive health care for adolescents often is inadequate. Many adolescents and adults do not, for example, keep current with recommended immunizations or accept valuable nutritional information. With health costs rising at an astounding rate, prevention is of value financially; however, the chief benefit is the continuation of health. Anticipatory guidance can some-times prevent potential harmful practices and reinforce family stability. This guidance should be appropriate for the developmental stage of an adoles-cent, and reinforcement is usually necessary at future visits. Discussions about the future can also teach problem solving and may enable an adoles-cent to evaluate a course of action more wisely before adopting it.

Care for Change or Cure

Not all afflictions can be cured, nor can anyone solve all problems. Adolescents rarely think about physical or mental disorders that may affect them until they occur, and they can have great difficulty in coping with illnesses or psychosocial disorders.

Some catastrophic events may cause disequilibrium in the develop-mental progress of adolescents. Injuries can bring a long, difficult period of adjustment to someone who is permanently handicapped. There are many purely medical problems, but the psychological needs can be more impor-tant and should be addressed from the beginning of therapy. Para- or quad-riplegia, for example, is incurable at the present time, and it is necessary to help an affected adolescent to restructure his or her self-image to achieve the developmental tasks of adolescence and a new life-style.

Other, less major conditions may be incurable, but therapy can bring great relief and an almost normal life. As an example, epilepsy initially may be a severe blow to an adolescent who cannot drive an automobile until a seizure-free period of time has passed. Control of seizures with medication is only a partial solution to the new problem, and many adolescents with epilepsy test the need for therapy before finally accepting it. Even then, they have many questions, and the answers must be tailored to their stage of adolescent development. Young teenagers may exhibit poor compliance with medication because they are unconvinced of its worth. Middle adolescents more often are eager to take medication in order to get a driver's license. Late adolescents may worry about how having epilepsy will affect their chances of getting a job. They may fear having a seizure in public or with a date. They may wonder whether they will marry, and many older teenagers ask whether the condition can be passed on to children. Effects of the medication can also produce difficulties in school or sports. Questions about conflicts with alcohol and other chemical substances should be addressed. The physician should consider how the condition and its management affect the person's life. Psychological difficulties may require greater attention than adjustment of the medication in order to prevent serious social maldevelopment.

Meeting the health needs of adolescents with disorders that can be ameliorated but not cured demands attention to tangential problems. Early prevention of future difficulties or intervention in existing maladaptation can be of great value.

Hospitalized adolescents have different reactions to diagnostic and therapeutic procedures. Anxiety is a frequent component of being hospitalized, especially for the first time, because the unknown and unexpected are always fearful. Other reactions—anger, crying, denial, intellectualization, regression, and acting out, for example—are common, particularly among early and middle adolescents. Many teenagers expect miracles from doctors and hospitals. Receiving a bottle of electrolyte solution may be expected to produce a cure, and confusion or distrust may result when this does not happen immediately. Involving an adolescent in making plans for treatment and explaining what is expected from the medication or procedure may prevent uncertainty and unwarranted expectations and create confidence in the people who provide care.

Adolescents receiving health care need to accept appropriate responsibility. Cooperation of the adolescent is valuable for maintenance of health, prevention of illness or injury, and compliance with prescribed treatment. Adults rarely comply with all directives, and it is probably too much to demand of adolescents to do so. As children, adolescents depended on their parents and other adults for guidance and care. It is hard for adolescents to take complete responsibility for their own health. Practitioners can help adolescents to take charge of their own health by discussing with them why tests are done, what the results mean, why selected medicines are used, and what is expected. Most adolescents accept the obligation to carry out instructions if they believe that there will be benefits. Early and most middle adolescents are not proficient in abstract or hypothetical thinking, and demonstrable results from anticipatory guidance do much to convince them of its worth. Young teenagers usually wish to please the physician or health professional. Middle and late adolescents may believe that medications or instructions are unnecessary. In those instances, the physician must try to get the attention and cooperation of the patient. There are many times when an adolescent or family cannot be responsible for personal health care because the health system is a confusing bureaucracy.

Using the Health System

One objective of adolescent health care is to help young people to function independently in obtaining health services. Reaching that objective is influenced by the developmental stages of adolescence and the results of teaching. Giving explicit instructions with explanations is appropriate during early adolescence, because cognitive development is then at an early stage. Information must be clear and specific; it may include written and oral directives. Middle adolescents are more capable of understanding the need for appointments, attending a specialty clinic, or returning to the doctor for follow-up care. Parents usually understand and work with the physician or other health professional to teach adolescents how to decide when health care is needed and how to develop the determination to get it. This independence should be fully developed by late adolescence, before the young person leaves home for independent living.

Personal decisions can be made and services of health professionals obtained more quickly and efficiently if the older adolescent assumes greater responsibility for health care and has learned the sources, barriers, and financial or eligibility requirements. Older adolescents should know how the system works. Getting health care is usually not a problem for young people who go to private physicians, because those physicians provide care for many conditions and make referrals for others. Ambulatory health facilities typically have many specialty clinics. In some ambulatory clinics, however, it is necessary to attend a general clinic first. If indicated, referral to a specialty clinic is made. In other facilities, an adolescent can obtain help more quickly and cheaply by knowing where to go initially. For example, a teenager may get an initial appointment with the orthopedic clinic and bypass the general clinic.

Counseling and other psychological services are of great value to adolescents and should be used by them more often. Teenagers generally do not think of the possibility of professional help in solving psychological or emotional problems. Health professionals should be alert to the needs of patients for services from other disciplines and refer adolescents to these disciplines for additional care. As they become older and more experienced, teenagers ought to be able to recognize a need for care in disciplines other than medicine and, with family help, seek it out. Increasing the awareness of available services is a responsibility of all health professionals, as is teaching adolescents about the health care system.

Summary

Deaths and morbidities of adolescents are major concerns of society and the health professions. Risk-taking behaviors and their consequences receive the most attention, but there are other morbidities that affect the lives of adolescents and continue in adulthood. Professionals tend to pay less attention to these morbidities, and adolescents often flounder in trying to cope with them.

Unmet needs are related to stages of adolescent growth and development and are the end products of personal and societal influences. Adolescent behaviors can be risky, but they are functional. Teenagers act in ways that they believe will make them more independent or popular with their peers or establish a sexual identity. The newer morbidities, many of which are associated with aberrant behaviors, rarely exist in isolation, and they can lead to additional biopsychosocial disruptions. Coping with these problems requires that professionals be aware of the possible associations between behaviors and illnesses. Young people must learn to recognize their emotional and behavioral needs and know that help for them is a legitimate part of health care. In addition, adolescents need to be taught to become responsible for their personal health. Young people are interested in their health, but if adolescents think of health services only in terms of physical ills, they will experience difficulty when it becomes necessary to obtain care for other types of health needs.

Suggested Readings

Fisher, M., and others. "Health Care Needs of Suburban Youth." *Pediatrics*, 1988, *81*, 8–13.

Giblin, P. T., and others. "Effects of Social Supports on Attitudes and Health Behaviors of Pregnant Adolescents." *Journal of Adolescent Health Care*, 1987, *8*, 273–280.

Haggerty, R. J., and others. "The New Morbidity." In R. J. Haggerty, K. J. Roghmann, and I. B. Pless (eds.), *Child Health and Community*. New York: Wiley, 1975.

Hamburg, D. A., and others. "Facilitating the Transitions of Adolescents." *Journal of the American Medical Association*, 1987, *257*, 3405–3406.

Irwin, C. E., Jr., and Millstein, S. G. "Biopsychosocial Correlates of Risk-Taking Behaviors in Adolescence: Can the Physician Intervene?" *Journal of Adolescent Health Care*, 1986, 7 (supp.), 82S–96S.

Marks, A., and others. "Assessment of Health Needs and Willingness to Utilize Health Care Resources of Adolescents in a Suburban Population." *Journal of Pediatrics*, 1983, *102*, 456–460.

Offer, D. "In Defense of Adolescents." *Journal of the American Medical Association*, 1987, *257*, 3407–3408.

Orr, D. P., and others. "Adolescent Health Care: Perceptions and Needs of the Practicing Physician." *Journal of Adolescent Health Care*, 1987, *8*, 239–246.

Remafedi, G. "Adolescent Homosexuality: Psychosocial and Medical Implications." *Journal of the American Medical Association*, 1987, *257*, 331–337.

Sobal, J., and others. "Health Concerns of High School Students and Teachers' Beliefs." *Pediatrics*, 1988, *81* (2), 218–223.

Zeltzer, L., and others. "Psychological Effects in Adolescence: II. Impact of Illness in Adolescence—Critical Issues and Coping Styles." *Journal of Pediatrics*, 1980, *97*, 132–138.

21

The Responsibility of Health Care Professionals Toward Adolescents

William A. Daniel, Jr., M.D.

In the best of all possible worlds, adolescents would be responsible for their health, know how to use the health care system, receive services from superbly trained professionals representing many disciplines, and have no financial worries. In such a world, severely ill adolescents would enter a hospital area dedicated to them, and a competent staff would quickly and correctly diagnose their needs and treat them. Young people with psychosocial problems would be cared for by highly trained, experienced psychiatrists, psychologists, and counselors who could quickly change adolescent behaviors, wants, and goals. Runaways and juvenile offenders would alter their beliefs and actions and pursue life-styles that contribute in positive ways to the betterment of society. Education of children would be so successful that they would avoid risk taking and develop habits to promote health. Unfortunately, we do not live in such a world, and we do not have solutions to many of the health problems of adolescents. However, we do have adolescents, and they do have health problems.

Adolescents became a high-risk population group in the mid 1960s, a time of great social turmoil in the United States. Many thousands of young people experimented with drugs, became sexually active, and left home to seek locations thought to be more exciting and free of adult restrictions or supervision. Health needs rapidly increased. Free clinics of varying quality, often staffed by untrained people, appeared and often replaced health facilities administered by what was called "the Establishment." In the intervening decades, there has come to be greater acceptance of the traditional health care system. Health problems that arose twenty years ago persist;

others, unknown or unanticipated, have emerged to challenge society and health professionals for solutions. The primary morbidities of adolescents are no longer infectious diseases but those with societal etiologies.

Two major trends complicate the provision of health care to adolescents and increase the responsibilities of health care professionals. First is the increasing number of young people in the population. The rising birthrate following World War II reached its peak in about 1970 and then decreased. Now, the birthrate is increasing again, and estimates suggest that there will be more than twenty-five million children age twelve to seventeen and forty million between ten and twenty-one years of age by the year 2000, these figures equaling those of 1970. Second is the increasing proportion of minority children, primarily as a result of higher birthrates among Hispanics and nonwhites. Estimates for 1990 show one-third of the population of the United States under twenty years of age to be Hispanic or nonwhite and one-fifth of all adolescents living at or below the poverty level.

Families have also changed in the past two decades. Almost half of the children born today can expect to spend several years in a single-parent family because of divorce or nonmarriage. Many children will cope with the effects of multiple divorces. About the same number of children have parents who both work outside the home. The probability of less supervision, greater permissiveness, and increased physical and sexual abuse, violence, homicide, suicide, and number of runaways complicates the tasks of health care professionals.

Appreciation of the societal changes and greater risk-taking behavior of adolescents illustrates the complexity of providing comprehensive health care. Adolescents commonly receive services in several disciplines. Much study and knowledge of the interrelated parts of adolescent health care are necessary for professionals to understand how to provide it, to counsel adolescents and families, to teach entry-level professionals, or to conduct research. A major responsibility of health care professionals is to be effective with all patients, including adolescents. To be effective, one must be competent, and competency embodies attitudes, knowledge, and skills.

Attitude

Adolescents are not a homogeneous group. Like adults, teenagers are people, the products of innate abilities and the perceptions of, adaptations to, and reactions to the culture in which they live. Each person is unique, but the behavior and beliefs of young people often reflect those of other young people with whom they associate. These similarities are more evident among adolescents than in other age groups.

It is the responsibility of health care professionals to have a genuine feeling of acceptance of adolescents for what they are individually and to enjoy working with them. This does not mean approving all that they are or all that they do. A common task of adults is to help adolescents change. Most adolescents are capable of becoming responsible adults and contributing to the world in which they live. Positive attitudes in adolescents can be fostered in many ways. Tolerance of mistakes, different standards, and the consequences of adolescent behavior, a genuine attempt to understand their problems and views, and commitment to help adolescents in decision making are valuable. In essence, we must like adolescents if we are to help them.

Knowledge

Knowledge is the product of information and experience. Health professionals represent many disciplines, most prominently medicine, nursing, psychology, nutrition, and social work. Specialized help in legal affairs, community services, vocational training, special education, substance abuse, and other areas is often needed by adolescents. Education in a specific discipline provides a foundation for services, but training may provide minimal information or experience about adolescence, which may require graduate or postgraduate education.

All professionals caring for adolescents should have a core of information that serves as the basis for understanding the process of adolescence. This information must cross disciplines and relate to teaching, research, delivery of health care, advocacy, and the development of community resources for adolescents.

Growth and Development

Understanding the process of puberty and its correlation with the social and psychological tasks of adolescence is fundamental. Physical, cognitive, and psychosocial growth proceed in sequential but rarely synchronous patterns. Disruption in one developmental area, whether temporary or permanent, can affect progress in others. The age of onset of puberty and the velocity of change vary for individual adolescents. It is imperative that in thinking about and working with young people, practitioners take into consideration the developmental stages of adolescence, because chronological age is a poor reference point.

Study of normal adolescent growth and the great range of normality is basic for developing screening skills. These skills are used to detect major deviations from the norm and to identify conditions requiring prompt intervention. Entry-level professionals are not expected to identify subtle deviations that should be addressed in graduate training. For example, school failure may occur because of a learning disability. Young professionals may be incapable of identifying the type of handicap or outlining a method of treatment. When that occurs, they should refer the adolescent to someone more competent. A young physician may be skilled in caring for a teenager who has diabetes but may lack the experience to help with the additional problem of substance abuse.

Families, peers, local cultures, and other social features can affect psychosocial development. External influences may change with time, and information about them, applied to individuals or groups of adolescents, can be important. Family dynamics deserve much consideration. Divorce, single-parent or blended families, and families with two working parents can affect growth and development of adolescents and bring new social problems.

An understanding of major physical and social morbidities of adolescents is essential. Professionals need to be aware of factors affecting the growth and development of handicapped youth. These young people often accomplish the tasks of adolescence through a series of detours rather than by regular sequential progress. It is necessary to become familiar with conditions that predispose adolescents to risk-taking behaviors. These morbidities highly correlate with the stages of adolescent development, and each can affect the other. Having this basic information permits health professionals to apply it, and the experience gained increases overall education.

Experience

Each professional providing care to adolescents should have had sufficient experience to be competent to deliver quality discipline-specific services. Special competency in adolescent health care can be achieved in many ways. Formal training programs, working in facilities or agencies caring for adolescents, and developing skills through independent practice are usually acceptable. However, the latter mode may be unsatisfactory, because experience is handicapped by meager learning about adolescence, and mistakes and inappropriate practices may continue because of the lack of evaluation or comparison with others. This possibility can be lessened or eliminated by extensive reading, attendance at seminars and conferences, and recognition of the need for improvement in specific areas. People who interact with adolescents should assume the obligation of learning more about them through active pursuit of information and experience. It also is important to understand and appreciate the cultural milieu and values that adolescents grow up with today and how they differ from those of times past.

Training programs in adolescent health are available, and several offer advanced academic degrees. Experience in these programs directs, evaluates, and supplements further education. Trainees learn the value and functions of many disciplines. Working with other professionals in a medical clinic for adolescents can provide experience of varying quality and scope.

It is almost always necessary to obtain additional education and experience if a health care professional plans to work with adolescents. Experience enables one to use what has been learned and to develop skills in its application.

Skills in Adolescent Health Care

Improving one's skills in health care delivery is a major responsibility of professionals working with adolescents. Young people do not grow in a vacuum, and the evolving times and situations complicate the changes in the physical, cognitive, and psychosocial growth of individual adolescents. It is necessary to establish rapport quickly with these young people and to develop a sense of mutual trust. It is important for an adolescent to regard the professional as friendly but not as an intimate friend. Adolescents need a friendly adult, not an adult friend. Few adolescents need another friend. There is a difference between the values and authority of health professionals and those of an adolescent. This difference should be recognized and tempered by trust, respect, and mutual understanding.

Communication

To help adolescents achieve optimal development, it is necessary to be able to communicate with them and their families and to help them develop problem-solving skills. Communicating well is the application of one's attitude, knowledge, and skills. An adolescent must understand what is said, and the professional must understand the adolescent and what he or she says. The meaning of words used by both parties has to be comprehended by both. Professional jargon and adolescent slang can seem to be part of a foreign language and need clarification. Although proficiency in communicating is something of an art, it can be developed, and the professional can learn much by being alert and perceptive to oral and nonverbal messages.

Health professionals need to help adolescents learn how to clarify and consider options and the effects of choices and to make decisions suitable for their developmental level. The objective is for health professionals to use their skills to facilitate the decision-making and social maturation of the adolescent. The average physician may have insufficient time or interest to assume all these obligations in caring for adolescents. Other health professionals may be needed to complement the medical services of the physician.

Interviewing

Interviewing is both an art and a skill. Some adults seem to communicate well with young people, putting them at ease, quickly establishing trust, and projecting empathy and understanding. For others, interviewing is difficult and the results unsatisfactory. Practice, recognition of mistakes and successes, and awareness of the perceptions of the adolescent can improve success in obtaining information from teenagers and helping them to mature. Adults must be flexible.

Most lengthy interviews occur at the first visit, and future information builds on the previous contacts. Later visits most often require little more than eliciting facts related to the present reason for visiting the office or providing follow-up information. The interview usually requires less time if the teenager is known to the health worker and has routine needs. On the other hand, behavioral or developmental problems may require much time and many visits.

The first interview can be difficult. It is not unusual for parents to force an adolescent to come to a health professional, and the initial reaction may be hostile and tax the skill and art of the interviewer. Many adolescents subtly test adults, and only after successfully establishing trust will they provide accurate information about themselves. Adolescents coming to a health facility should understand that information they give will be confidential within stated limits. They need to know that the interviewer will not take sides with the teenager, parents, or other adults. All of us are a bit anxious when we first visit a doctor or other person of authority. We also expect that person to give us full attention and have an interest in what we have to report. Adolescents in particular have difficulty presenting information, choosing words, or expressing exactly what they mean. Teenagers often give information circuitously or in bits and pieces. They may be reluctant to speak openly because they fear criticism, punishment, or rejection. Most adolescents feel rejected if the listener is inattentive, is interrupted by telephone calls, or reads reports during the interview.

One goal of the first interview is to determine the levels of development: physical, cognitive, and psychosocial. It is, for example, common for adults to relate differently to very small or very large early adolescents of the same age, although the smaller one may have greater cognitive growth. Unfortunately, there no rapid means of accurately assessing the mental ability of an adolescent, but rough estimates can be made. Communication with adolescents should be at their developmental levels. Early adolescents are unsure of themselves, of what they will be, and of how they appear to others and cannot appreciate the future. Middle adolescents have adjusted somewhat to their bodies and have developed a greater interest in the world around them. Late adolescents usually have developed the beginnings of abstract thought, can compare and contrast, and can appreciate the future; still, they are often immature and unskilled in decision making. Interviewing an adolescent is more productive when it is conducted along developmental lines than when it is based on chronological age.

Adolescents are amazingly frank in presenting information to an attentive health professional. Some very young teenagers may be embarrassed by sexual questions because they do not know how to express themselves. They may fear that the information will be given to parents, or the interviewer may represent a parent figure. With trust, even early adolescents will usually give accurate information, but some will lie in an attempt to deny an action or to assume greater perceived status. Experience helps to detect these ploys and guide the interview to get the truth.

Rarely, an adolescent will ask what to do about a problem. It is usually best for the teenager to make decisions on the basis of facts and discussions, but there are times when the boy or girl cannot do this and genuinely needs professional advice. In these rare instances, specific directives can be given.

Doing this may set up the professional to take the blame for an adolescent's actions or future unhappiness. The young patient may also use the directive to oppose parents. Nevertheless, there are times when an adolescent is incapable of making a decision and needs immediate professional help to cope temporarily with stress. It can be difficult to give advice without appearing authoritative to an adolescent, but discussion of a problem and options for solving it are useful.

Ending an interview is also something of an art. Teenagers generally resent an abrupt cessation of a visit and may interpret it as evidence that the physician or other professional considers time more important than they are. Usually, reviewing information obtained, clarifying important aspects of problem areas, and asking the adolescent to consider several questions before the next visit will end the interview in an acceptable manner. This gives the teenager a specific task and helps to set the purpose of the next visit. Ending the visit should also include telling the adolescent that he or she is free to call or come for help if the need arises. This final statement suggests that the relationship is continuing and not limited to the purpose of the present visit.

Responsibility to Parents

Most parents worry about their adolescent children who are ill or have psychosocial problems. They expect to receive information about the interview, evaluation of the condition, and plans for management. Parents usually accept the policy that information is confidential. They do not expect to learn all the details but wish to know about the seriousness of the problem and how they can help. If, for example, a psychologist counsels an adolescent, the parents want to know if progress is being made and whether they should be included in the counseling or advised about family relationships. Some parents are very hesitant to ask about the progress of treatment; they are often confused, but they do want and need to be informed about their children. There are health care professionals who refuse to provide any information, but this is unwise. Parents may be unable to understand the problems, a few do not care about the teenager, and others are overly concerned and make the treatment more difficult. All health professionals have a major responsibility to parents.

Interdisciplinary Skills

Comprehensive health care for adolescents is a complex process demanding the skills of many disciplines. This complexity is affected by many things: whether care is given by one person, in private practice, or in an ambulatory center; whether the staff members are competent; and whether there are qualified people in several different disciplines. Solo practitioners have the obligation of building a list of competent people in other disciplines to whom an adolescent can be referred when necessary. Multi- or inter-disciplinary ambulatory health centers for adolescents vary greatly in their structure and operation. Some clinics have specialists who work part-time, with the potential danger of overloading the professional with patients. As a result, attention may be given only to a major complaint, an adolescent's total health needs may not be met, and the quality of care may be deficient. All health professionals have the responsibility of providing high-quality care in a specific discipline. They should have knowledge of the value and function of other specialty areas and be aware of the competency of people providing services to adolescents. Multidisciplinary health centers often have turf problems and bureaucratic barriers that decrease the efficacy of care delivery. Working together requires much tolerance, skill, and leadership.

Interdisciplinary programs in which each new adolescent has a session with members of all disciplines can be excellent for training. However, the method can be unnecessary or time-inefficient in caring for adolescents. If the interdisciplinary function is rigid, obtaining consensus can sometimes be difficult or impossible. Usually, one professional skilled in interpersonal relationships and knowledge must be in charge and, if necessary, decide on a course of management.

Multidisciplinary participation is more typical of clinics providing health care to adolescents. These clinics can be efficient while providing continued supervision and evaluation. In this model of care, the adolescent is referred to a professional in another discipline who can provide better care for a specific problem. There is the danger of having multiple objectives that may conflict in desired sequential stages of care. Sometimes diagnostic or therapeutic opinions of professionals are not shared with others working with the adolescent. These difficulties can be minimized; nevertheless, communication is very important in these models of health programs. There is also the need for one person to be responsible for ensuring follow-up care and compliance with referrals to the other professionals in the health center.

The attitudes, knowledge, and skills of those who provide care affect all systems of delivery. Working together harmoniously is a major responsibility that each health care professional must cultivate.

Problems in Health Care Delivery

Even superbly trained professional staff members may have difficulty caring for adolescents. External forces can help or hinder caring for any population group, and adolescents often seem to have low priority for consideration. Some of these circumstances are significant barriers, but others can be changed or eliminated. One significant question is "What do adolescents expect?"

Perceptions of Adolescents

Adolescents often have strange perceptions of health care providers. For example, pediatricians are baby doctors, internists are physicians for the aged, psychiatrists and psychologists "see you if you're crazy," and nutritionists "want you to eat stuff that doesn't taste good." Many adolescents believe that they do not need health care. Teenagers with risk-taking behaviors or other psychosocial problems commonly profess that it is their parents and not they who have a problem. Other adolescents have unrealistic expectations and become angry when desired changes do not quickly occur. Young people often expect miracles and cannot understand explanations because of their immature cognition.

Research has shown that adolescents from middle-class families want help for personal (nonillness) problems but do not seek it from their private physicians because they believe that the physicians are uninterested or incapable of helping. Many of these misconceptions can be altered by discussions appropriate for the developmental level of the adolescent. Teenagers may be unable to comprehend the results of risk-taking behaviors or the likelihood that harm could come to them personally. Though their general health may be good, they must be educated to assume responsibility for maintenance of their own health and establishing habits for ensuring good health. Conversely, an adolescent may recognize the need for health care and seek it only to encounter many barriers. Health professionals have the responsibility to help educate adolescents and guide them in learning about the health system.

Confidentiality

Confidentiality, discussed in detail elsewhere in this book, can be a significant barrier for optimal health care delivery. Each professional or program establishes principles of confidentiality, including exceptions, and these should be discussed with adolescents at the time of the first visit.

It is difficult for adolescents to trust adults completely, especially those whom they have just met. Early adolescents are often afraid to disclose highly personal information, and older ones may purposefully give misinformation because they do not believe that confidentiality will be kept. Runaway adolescents rarely trust anyone, because they have been used, abused, betrayed, and tricked many times. Attitudes of runaways or throwaways can be important negative aspects in receiving or responding to efforts to provide health care.

Information frequently is needed from schools or psychological testing facilities. This information is confidential and may be unavailable because requirements for its release cannot be met. Lack of data can be a handicap in providing comprehensive care and can increase the cost of care by requiring duplication of procedures to obtain similar information.

Financial Factors

Thousands of adolescents live below the poverty level and are dependent on free health care. Financial qualifications for access to health care programs vary, but almost all plans require tests for eligibility and other information. For example, a health program may be limited to a specific geographical area of a city and have its own eligibility requirements. A dental program may have a different catchment area and set of criteria for inclusion in the program. A family planning project and a mental health program may geographically overlap parts of the other programs and have diverse requirements for acceptance. It is easy to imagine the time spent and the frustration developed in having four different interviews and trying to meet four sets of eligibility criteria. The adolescent may be ineligible for services from one program because home is across the street from the border of the catchment area or because only children in a certain age range are served.

Some health programs funded by federal, state, or local governments limit the number of visits per year regardless of the health need. Other approaches are categorical: Care is available only for a certain list of conditions, and complications arising from the primary illness are not included. For example, orthopedic care may be available to treat deformities caused by hemophiliac bleeding, but funds may be unavailable to treat an acute episode of bleeding to prevent orthopedic handicaps. Health professionals are usually skilled in adapting the guidelines of care to the needs of the patient; however, this ability is diminished as new cost constraints become increasingly rigid.

Care from private practitioners can be uncertain for adolescents belonging to families with incomes slightly above the poverty level. Third-party payers also have lists of approved services. Often, prior approval must be obtained before care can be given. In some instances, payment simply will not be made. Many physicians believe that finances are determining the type, quality, and quantity of health care. Teenagers rarely have sufficient funds to pay for their own health care. There are situations (for example, when they have a sexually transmitted disease) when they do not wish their parents to know about their problem or receive a bill for treatment. School health clinics sometimes are available, but funding, staffing, and the scope of services vary greatly.

There are chronic illnesses for which there is no support other than the family's income, and costs often exceed the ability to pay. Catastrophic illnesses can quickly ruin a family and be a great deterrent to health care delivery.

Ethnic and Racial Features

It is not unusual for a member of a health care team to differ racially or ethnically from the majority of adolescent patients seen in an ambulatory care unit. Health care professionals have the responsibility to be reasonably familiar with different racial or ethnic cultures and to respect their cultural heritages. Many adolescents feel more comfortable if the health professional is of the same race, but this is not always true. Team members of other races can be effective if they are skillful in communicating, show their awareness of cultural differences, and express interest in the adolescents. It would be wise, for example, to have staff members who speak Spanish in a center providing care for a predominantly Hispanic adolescent population or some black professionals on the staff if large numbers of adolescent patients are black.

Legal and Ethical Considerations

In most states, adolescents have the legal right to give consent for diagnosis and treatment of sexually transmitted diseases and for the diagnosis of pregnancy. State laws vary regarding the age when an adolescent can give consent for other forms of health care. Some states permit care when an adolescent is fourteen or fifteen years of age. Other states do not allow consent until the young person has left home and is self-supporting or has met specific legal requirements. Health professionals have the responsibility to know the laws of the state in which they work.

Ethical issues are often complex and influenced by ethnic, racial, religious, and cultural beliefs. These considerations may vary from one part of the nation to another. There are people who believe that certain legal health care practices are unethical, immoral, or contrary to particular religious beliefs. Familiarity with laws, ethics, and cultural differences can help professionals provide the best health care.

Community Responsibility

Health professionals working with adolescents usually have greater knowledge than the public in assessing health needs. These professionals have the responsibility to increase awareness and advocate changes. There are few integrated community-based health delivery programs; if these are to come about, health professionals must be involved in their design and function.

It is impossible for people in the health care field to solve all social problems, but community participation and cooperation can make a difference. Health professionals often have little appreciation of the limited information about adolescents available to the general public. What is common knowledge among professionals is often news to other people in the community. Many health projects now have professional community health workers on their staffs.

Community health workers can be effective in promoting services and nonhealth programs for adolescents, detecting unmet health needs, and obtaining changes and support. Communities are composed of people with many talents, and using their abilities in a cooperative effort is easier if needs and issues are understood. Risk-taking behaviors of adolescents are major morbidities, and community awareness can lead to participation in many different areas designed to provide less risky alternatives or preventive measures. Efforts to increase awareness and stimulate community action should not be limited to community health workers; they require input from professionals in all disciplines providing care for adolescents.

Health professionals may request, even demand, changes and have no idea about the difficulties involved in accomplishing these changes. Communities have "personalities," laws, and policies, and there are financial restrictions. Some professionals are out of touch with a community or have limited vision of a problem and may advocate changes that the community does not want. In these instances, a community health worker can educate and advise the health professional.

Cooperative Research

The complexity of adolescent health care has increased. There are many unanswered questions, for example, about the onset of puberty. Determinants of the velocity of growth, the interrelationship of biological changes and psychosocial actions, and genetic markers that may predispose individuals to certain harmful conditions are all poorly understood. Although fundamental biopsychosocial research is done in academic institutions, many findings need to be tested by clinical experience.

The primary morbidities of adolescents are behavioral and have social etiologies. Professionals in health care disciplines are more familiar with risk taking and other psychosocial problems of adolescents than are those in the basic sciences. Behavioral research will require the cooperation of clinical and basic sciences and include cross-disciplinary participation. The study of problems of adolescents requires knowledge of research methods and may be broad-based or limited in scope.

All professionals working with adolescents can contribute to research, some by designing studies and others by implementing them or evaluating results. Ambulatory health facilities and professionals in private practice have the opportunity to engage in longitudinal research and make significant contributions. It is common for private practitioners or members of a health team to believe that they are too busy providing services to consider doing research. In truth, they are conducting research with every adolescent they see. Plans for collecting information, evaluating the results, and trying different methods of intervention and prevention are needed. Often these efforts can be shared with representatives of several disciplines. Findings from the studies can lessen the time and stress associated with health care delivery and promote prevention of illnesses and disabilities.

Summary

Competency is the major responsibility of professionals providing health care. Attitude, knowledge, and skill affect how well they contribute to the total health and maturational growth of adolescents. Special training in adolescent health is desirable, but extensive reading and attending seminars and conferences can be of great value if additional training is unavailable. There is a core of knowledge unique to adolescent growth and development that is essential for members of all disciplines who provide health care for adolescents. Having specialized knowledge, skills, and the ability to communicate well with adolescents improves the quality of care.

The primary morbidities of adolescence have changed from communicable diseases to those having social etiologies. Health needs are more complex and comprehensive than in the past. More than one health discipline may be involved in adolescent health care. Groups of professionals working together or a solo practitioner who refers patients to other specialists familiar with adolescents can provide these services. There are many barriers to adolescents seeking health care. Perceptions of teenagers and parents, availability, finances, restrictions imposed by laws, customs, or beliefs, sponsored programs, and third-party payers can affect the delivery of care.

Health professionals have the responsibility to advocate means of improving adolescent health care, preventing risk-taking behaviors, and working with the community to provide integrated community-based health delivery programs and social alternatives that promote health. In addition, collaborative research benefits from having professionals in clinical areas, because they have more contact and experience with adolescents than do others in more basic sciences.

Adolescents are a distinct population group in the United States; they vary greatly in race, ethnic origin, levels of education, religion, beliefs, moral standards, goals, and actions. This diversity of characteristics taxes the skills of all who care for them. In spite of the vagaries of adolescents, giving help to young people changing from children into adults is important and can be very satisfying.

Suggested Readings

Bearinger, L. H., and McAnarney, E. R. "Integrated Community Health Delivery Programs for Youth: Study Group Report." *Journal of Adolescent Health Care*, 1988, *9* (supp.), 36–40.

Blum, R. "Contemporary Threats to Adolescent Health in the United States." *Journal of the American Medical Association*, 1987, *257*, 3390–3395.

Haggerty, R. J. "Behavioral Pediatrics: A Time for Research." *Pediatrics*, 1988, *81*, 179–185.

Haggerty, R. J., and others. "The New Morbidity." In R. J. Haggerty, K. J. Roghmann, and I. B. Pless (eds.), *Child Health and Community*. New York: Wiley, 1975.

Hickson, G. B., Altemeier, W. A., and O'Connor, S. "Concerns of Mothers Seeking Care in Private Pediatric Offices: Opportunities for Expanding Services." *Pediatrics*, 1983, *72*, 619.

Irwin, C. E., Jr., and Millstein, S. G. "Biopsychosocial Correlates of Risk-

Taking Behaviors in Adolescence: Can the Physician Intervene?" *Journal of Adolescent Health Care*, 1986, 7 (supp.), 82S–96S.

Marks, A., and others. "Assessment of Health Needs and Willingness to Utilize Health Care Resources of Adolescents in a Suburban Population." *Journal of Pediatrics*, 1983, *102*, 456–460.

Parcel, G. S., Muraskin, L. D., and Endert, C. M. "Community Education: Study Group Report." *Journal of Adolescent Health Care*, 1988, *9* (supp.), 41–45.

22

The Role of Social Support and Social Networks in Improving the Health of Adolescents

David A. Hamburg, M.D.
Allyn M. Mortimer, M.A.
Elena O. Nightingale, M.D., Ph.D.

Attachment and social bonding are crucial in human development. The formation early in life of a durable attachment to at least one experienced and competent adult is fundamental in human adaptation to the social environment. Early attachment gives an infant a secure, supportive base for exploration and thus for learning. This adaptive attachment behavior can be considered a precursor of social support. A growing body of scientific literature suggests that human beings have a need for sustained relationships and contact with others under satisfying circumstances. Socially isolated people are less healthy and more prone to physical and psychological illnesses and are more likely to die than people who are socially integrated. Throughout most of human history, small societies provided durable networks, familiar human relationships, and cultural guidance for young people, offering support in time of stress and skills necessary for coping and adaptation, including avoiding health-compromising behaviors.

Human and nonhuman primate offspring have a prolonged immaturity that lasts many years. One of the fundamental aspects of human social development is attachment of the infant to the mother or caretaker. Over the course of human evolution, infants who formed close attachments to their mothers (and whose mothers reciprocated) were usually healthier and less likely to be caught by predators, to get lost, to suffer from severe exposure, or to be injured by other members of their own species than those who did not. In the context of a secure environment and valued adult models, a child can learn certain prosocial behaviors, such as taking turns, sharing with others, cooperating, especially in learning and problem solving, and helping others, especially in times of stress.

During this immature period, the youngster is physically dependent on adults for survival. Historically, the parents, particularly the mother, have been governed by the necessity of keeping the baby close at hand, taking care of it, and seeing that it does not get into excessive danger. In the vulnerable years of growing up, human young can operate in a protected, guided milieu and learn what is required for adaptation — how to cope with dangers, how to make sense of the environment, how to take advantage of opportunities — in short, how to survive, flourish, reproduce, and pass genes along to subsequent generations.

This attachment behavior has emerged over millions of years of human evolution. A sense of cooperative behavior is foreshadowed in nonhuman primates and is found in all human societies. From belonging to a group, an individual develops a sense of personal worth and is able to interact within a mutually supportive environment and develop attachments that endure for the whole life cycle.

During the past few hundred years, changes in human society have in some circumstances fractured familial relationships. Mass migrations and the shift from small communities to massive cities have disrupted the previous pattern of evolution. Unfamiliar values and requirements have uprooted long-standing patterns of interaction and mutually supportive behavior. Changes since the Industrial Revolution — especially in this century — have drastically altered the experience of childhood and adolescence in ways that make it more prolonged and perplexing than ever before, even though there are also many new opportunities.

For adolescents, in particular, these changes are far-reaching and often expose the adolescent to potentially life-threatening activities, technologies, and substances. Adolescents are exposed not only to alcohol and drugs but also to smoking (cigarettes and marijuana), vehicles, weapons, and a variety of other temptations to engage in health-damaging behavior. A significant number of adolescents from many social groups engage in unprotected sex, attempt suicide, or die or become disabled from injuries. Although physically mature in early adolescence, young people age ten to fifteen years are able to and do make many fateful decisions that affect the entire life course, even though they are immature in cognitive development, knowledge, and social experience.

The lengthening period of adolescence, which for a great many people introduces a high degree of uncertainty and stress into their lives, coupled with an undeveloped sense of the future, frequently results in confusion in young minds about adult roles. In premodern times, children had abundant opportunity for direct observation of parents and other adults performing the adult roles that they would ultimately adopt when they matured. Skills necessary for assuming an adult role were gradually acquired. The end of puberty coincided with the development of an adult body and capabilities. Early adolescence today is less traditional and structured, more ambiguous and complex than in the past. What constitutes preparation for effective adulthood is less clear than was ever the case before.

The longer and more complex the transition from childhood to adulthood, the more the adolescent experiences uncertainty and ambiguity in meeting fundamental human needs that are crucial to survival and healthy development. These are the needs to (1) find a place in a valued group that provides a sense of belonging, (2) identify tasks that are generally recognized in the group as having adaptive value and that thereby earn respect when skill is acquired for coping with the tasks, (3) feel a sense of worth as a person, (4) establish reliable and predictable relationships with other people, especially a few relatively close relationships, (5) find constructive expression of the curiosity and exploration that strongly characterize adolescence, (6) find a basis for making informed, deliberate decisions, particularly decisions that have lifelong consequences, and (7) accept respectfully the enormous diversity of this society, the individual differences among adolescents in size, shape, color, and rates of body and behavior change.

The erosion of family and social support networks, therefore, has left young people in many cases without the support they need in time of stress, and without durable networks, familiar human relationships, and cultural guidance. Nevertheless, most young people do cope with the pressures to engage in high-risk-taking behaviors and weather the transition to adult life healthy and with opportunities for a rewarding life.

The importance of social bonds and relationships continues throughout childhood and adolescence and into adulthood. The literature on social networks has examined children's status with respect to peers and found, for example, that status among peers is a strong predictor of outcomes such as physical and psychiatric health, behavioral problems, learning difficulties, and delinquency. During adolescence, the nature and function of peer relationships change. Adolescents are frequently more dependent on peer relationships than younger children, because relations with parents become more variable as adolescents gain their independence. Adolescence is a time when pressure to conform to the values, customs, and fads of the peer group becomes intense. In some cases, adolescents lack the skills to meet society's demands for social independence and for assuming an adult role and all that it entails. Attempts to assist young people in mastering these skills and in establishing and fostering basic attachments have relied on social support.

In many contemporary societies, the needs of large numbers of adolescents, particularly with respect to their health, are not being met. Is it possible to provide teenagers with the basis for making wise decisions about the use of their own bodies, about how to plan for constructive futures, about how to care for others? Trying to build such capability through social support networks is one approach to helping adolescents with the transition to adulthood, especially in pursing education and protecting their health.

Because many young people no longer have access to traditional social support networks, there is an urgent need to improve society's capabilities for dealing with adolescents during their transition to adulthood. A recurrent theme throughout this chapter, therefore, is how to restore the functions served in less complex societies by family, friends, and communities that have been eroded by the profoundly transformed conditions of contemporary society. Which contemporary institutions, for example, can be restructured or institutions invented to meet basic human needs, particularly those that foster healthy adolescent development and thereby have a constructive effect on the entire life course?

Adolescent Health and the Social Environment

Social networks and social support are discrete and complex concepts. The personal social world of an individual is composed of family members, friends, acquaintances, and institutions or organizations such as schools, churches, social clubs, medical care facilities, and mental health and social service agencies. Within this context, an individual defines self and acquires a frame of reference for making decisions that affect the life course.

Social Networks

One's social network is characterized by a number of dimensions, including the quality of the interaction and its frequency, intensity, durability over time, and strength. In addition, a social network can be measured by the number of people in the network, the extent to which supports and obligations are shared among members, geographical proximity or dispersion, the extent to which network members are homogeneous (that is, similar in terms of age, social class, and religion), the ease with which other members of the network may be contacted, and the extent to which members of an individual's network are acquainted with and interact with each other.

An individual's pattern of social contact changes with age. As children mature, both biologically and socially, corresponding changes occur in their social networks in response to their evolving needs and competence. Gender and cultural differences in one's social networks also provide distinct patterns of social connections among young people who are situated in different environments. For example, social patterns among groups of children from single-parent households are different from those among children from two-parent households.

Social networks commonly have mutual aid functions. These are particularly important in self-help groups and increasingly used in health-oriented interventions.

Social Support

Social support is a concept that involves a set of personal contacts through which the individual maintains his or her social identity and receives emotional support, material aid and services, information, and new social contacts. Social support is also defined as involving instrumental aid, such as help to care for a child; informational support, such as information about how to take care of a child; appraisal support that involves information relevant to self-evaluation; and emotional support that expresses love and concern. Social support usually involves an exchange or validation of mutual obligation from one's social network. Social support improves both physical and mental health and is a factor in moderating the effects of stress. The essence of social support is in its personal relationships, and it is reflected in the ingenious ways that people enlist the aid of others.

Health Problems in Adolescence

The social support system that is fundamental to human life is now in jeopardy, especially in poor and seriously disadvantaged communities, where social networks are often weakened. Today, there are a variety of major indicators reflecting failure to provide avenues for the affirmation of fundamental needs to large numbers of adolescents. The historical recency of drastic technological, social, and cultural changes has outpaced our understanding and institutional capacity to adapt.

It is now generally recognized that adolescents are not as healthy as they were once thought to be. Overall mortality rates, while decreasing for other age groups, remain high for certain subgroups of the adolescent population. The formulation of the causes of morbidity and mortality in adolescence has expanded to consider not only the leading causes of death and disability but also other important categories of disability. These include accidents, suicide, homicide, substance use and abuse, teenage sexuality, contraception, teenage childbearing, sexually transmitted diseases, AIDS, social isolation, and chronic handicapping conditions. The physical, social, and economic consequences of adolescent childbearing, for example, are well documented.

Early adolescence is a time of particular vulnerability. The combined physical, social, and emotional changes of that period intersect with the new intellectual tasks imposed on youngsters in junior high school. The pressures to experiment with sex and drugs are hard to withstand for some. A significant number of adolescents from many social groups drop out of school, commit violent or otherwise criminal acts, become pregnant, take up smoking, abuse drugs or alcohol, succumb to mental disorders, attempt suicide, or die or become disabled from injuries. It is important, therefore, to orient supportive interventions toward early adolescence, because this is a time when behavior patterns are not yet cast in concrete. An important recurrent observation in the research on early interventions against smoking is that alcohol and other drug use tends to decrease along with a decrease in smoking.

One component of adolescents' desire to smoke or drink or engage in other potentially harmful practices is their desire to acquire credentials for entry into adulthood. Health-compromising behavior may be a way for the adolescent to gain control over the environment or achieve an alliance with peers. In some cases, adolescents are just not well equipped to enter the adult world and tend to behave in an inexperienced way with respect to risky behaviors such as using drugs, drinking, unprotected sexual activity, or smoking.

As an example, although most adolescents are not problem drinkers and are not likely to become problem drinkers, there is a core of young adolescents who are already heavy drinkers. The long-term abuse of alcohol is associated with a number of adverse health effects. Alcohol is an important contributor to motor vehicle accidents and assaultive behavior. For teenagers and for adults, alcohol use and abuse may have serious consequences for their unborn children. Over the past two decades, alcohol use has become a more serious problem among ten- to fifteen-year-olds. Teenagers now have their first drinking experiences earlier, drink larger quantities, and report more frequent intoxications. In 1984, 59 percent of adolescents thirteen to eighteen years old who were polled were at least occasional consumers of alcohol, and an additional 17 percent had tried alcohol at least once. Two-thirds of those polled had used alcohol before their sixteenth birthdays.

At-Risk and Disadvantaged Adolescents

A disproportionate burden of disease, disability, and mortality is found among people from lower socioeconomic conditions within a given population. In addition, it is generally recognized that there are an increased prevalence and severity of all of the major pediatric diseases among children in the United States of lower socioeconomic status.

The research literature also indicates that, in the first few years of life, family climate has a strong influence on emotional, social, and cognitive development; it can counteract the disadvantages of poverty. The commitment, support, encouragement, and practical help of a cohesive, resourceful family are indeed of fundamental importance to healthy child development. In very poor, disorganized, and socially disadvantaged settings, there tend to be certain patterns of parent-child interaction that are associated with impaired intellectual development, social responsibility, and motivation for later education. In addition, family discord and disturbance adversely affect learning. It is clear from human and animal experimentation that an environment of severe restriction either of sensory input or of active exploration is detrimental to cognitive development. Excessive stimulation, such as very noisy, crowded living conditions, may also increase distractibility and induce biological stress responses.

In addition to a supportive family environment, community-based support is important, especially in disadvantaged communities. In his book *The Truly Disadvantaged*, William Julius Wilson describes how the dramatic social transformation of the inner city has left a core of groups of families and individuals who are more socially isolated than previous urban black residents, and thus more susceptible to physical and mental health problems. The "social buffer"—that is, the working- and middle-class professional families—that sustained the neighborhoods by absorbing the economic fluctuations that affected inner-city neighborhoods does not exist in many of today's inner cities. Because these families have moved, the adequacy of institutions that supported neighborhoods and individuals, including churches, schools, stores, and recreational and health care facilities, has declined. According to Wilson, "the presence of stable working- and middle-class families in the ghetto provides mainstream role models that reinforce mainstream values pertaining to employment, education, and family structure. . . . A far more important effect is the institutional stability that these families are able to provide in their neighborhoods because of their greater economic and educational resources."

At-risk young adolescents may be most in need of social support interventions, because they are frequently susceptible to a number of risk factors. At-risk adolescents include children in communities in chaos or in violent or dangerous environments; children who are members of racial and ethnic minority groups and usually suffer discrimination; black males who are fatherless; adolescents in foster care; pregnant and parenting teens; and school dropouts. In addition, a variety of adolescents tend to need specialized support systems, including those that contribute to health maintenance and disease prevention. These include adolescents from single-parent families or highly mobile families, such as those in the military or those that are homeless; young people who are caregivers with "adult" responsibilities for others; adolescents who are recent immigrants and those for whom English is a second language; detained youth; war-traumatized refugees; and young people who have handicapping conditions or chronic illnesses.

In addition to problems faced by at-risk youth and young people for whom special support systems are needed, adolescents face a number of general problems that involve health-related behaviors and may have lifelong consequences. These include coping with blended families; transitions to school, work, or the military; and balancing academic, work, and social lives. Lack of social contacts outside the immediate neighborhood is a particular problem for disadvantaged minority youth. This social isolation may lead to low self-esteem, loneliness, a sense of isolation, and low expectations.

Opportunities to Support Healthy Adolescent Development

Social supports have been shown to have direct effects on health outcomes and buffering effects in the presence of major stressors. In addition, positive effects have been demonstrated on illness and health from a range of social supports. Although much of the social support literature does not specifically address adolescents, support interventions such as support groups, peer counselors, and home visitor programs are being widely used among various adolescent populations. Research from other contexts can be adapted to accommodate adolescence. In addition, research on adolescent development may also contribute to the social support knowledge base during this period of life.

Social networks can influence physical health status through four potential pathways. First, individuals with dependable relationships may obtain better medical care than others through the transmission of advice, services, and access to new social contacts. A second possibility is the direct provision of aid, economic assistance, or services by members of a particular social network. A third mechanism that may influence the health status of an adolescent is the peer group. Peer pressure can be either health-promoting or the opposite. During adolescence, there is a strong tendency to maintain a group or network identity. Finally, a biological response to a stressful condition may influence one's general susceptibility to illness by altering physiological functioning. For example, loss of intimacy or sense of belonging may result in depression, which can lead to a poor health outcome, or, alternatively, people who are depressed already may not be able to maintain or seek out the social contacts that can help to alleviate their depression.

In a discussion of support interventions, the large variability among adolescents needs to be taken into account. These differences are important in the receptivity to supportive interventions as well as the risks to which adolescents are exposed. Gender, ethnic, and cultural differences are the most striking disparities, although there is much individual variability within each group.

Elements of Successful Interventions

Interventions that support young people's healthy development are nonstigmatizing, are frequently multifaceted, and convey a sense of growing competence. The point of entry tends to be most useful if it captures the attention and sympathetic interest of adolescents. Such programs emphasize opportunities and visibly provide a chance to build on knowledge and skills that an individual already has. Ideally, comprehensive services are available in one place to meet adolescents' multiple needs so that they do not have to fight their way through bureaucratic obstacles.

Today, there are a number of programs addressing the complex physical and psychological needs of adolescents. Some target specific health and behavioral problems of adolescents, such as unprotected sexuality, unwanted pregnancy, or substance abuse, while others take a comprehensive approach to adolescent health and well-being. An example of an effort designed as a comprehensive approach to providing services for adolescents is the School

Based Youth Services Program in New Jersey. This program is designed to bring services for teenagers age thirteen to nineteen together and break down the barriers between the state departments that provide services for young people. In addition to offering health services, the program offers mental health services, employment counseling, family counseling, sub- stance abuse programs, information and referral services, and recreational activities. Some centers offer additional services, such as family planning services, day-care services, and instruction in parenting skills for adolescent parents.

Two other programs that deal with the multiple problems of adoles- cence—the Door and Teen-Link—are described more fully in Chapter Seventeen of this volume. The Door in New York City offers health, educa- tion, and cultural services for adolescents. A comprehensive program, in- cluding educational and prevocational preparation, creative and physical arts, mental health and social services, legal services, and primary medical care, is provided. The health center offers prenatal care and education, nutrition and food services, and sexual awareness education. Teen-Link, in Durham, North Carolina, provides primary health care, health promotion and disease prevention activities, and community outreach and health educa- tion to teens participating in the project. There is also a church connection project in which participating churches provide a prevention program based on assistance from trained adults and teen volunteers who keep the con- gregation informed about adolescent pregnancy and other teen health issues.

Family-Based Support

In considering current institutions and settings in the lives of adoles- cents, one must pay particular attention to the primary support rendered by the family. When adolescents lack family support, there is a good chance that the support available to their parents is also deficient. Young children and adolescents are at risk of inadequate parental support for many different reasons. Their parents may not be well enough themselves to meet their children's needs for care, as in the case of parents who suffer from major mental illnesses or alcoholism. Parents may be preoccupied with their own personal problems, making them less available to their children or causing them to behave inappropriately with their children. A separation or divorce may not only entail the loss of a parent's support but can result in parents making demands on adolescents that are impossible for them to meet given their level of developmental maturation. Other stressful family situations for which social support might be needed include dealing with stepparents, the death of a parent or sibling through illness or suicide, chronic unemploy- ment or repeated episodes of job loss, and the diagnosis of a serious illness in a family member.

Stressful family situations arise in all families but are particularly intense in many black, Hispanic, and Native American families, which have a disproportionate share of severe economic stress, social isolation, low self-esteem, and low levels of educational attainment. Familial problems can become deep-rooted and strongly influence learned behavior that is passed from one generation to the next. It is crucial, therefore, that families get the support and parenting skills that they need to rear their children effectively, especially during the early childhood and adolescent years.

Family support programs to address this problem are emerging throughout the nation. These programs, exemplified by AVANCE in San Antonio, Texas, are designed to strengthen families under stress and to provide the knowledge and skills necessary to nurture and supervise their children. AVANCE is a center-based parent support and education program serving low-income Mexican American families. Parents enroll when their children are anywhere from birth to three years of age, and all families in the community are welcome. The emphasis of the program is on the parents' own development, especially of a basis for self-esteem and perception of opportunity, improved decision-making skills, and specific knowledge of child development. The parents are thus taught by the AVANCE staff that they can be educators. Parents are shown concretely how to facilitate the development of their own children in classes and during monthly home visits. The AVANCE experience has fostered maternal knowledge of child development, increased hopefulness about the future, enhanced prospects in this poor community, decreased punitive approaches to child discipline, and generally improved the climate of mother-child interaction.

Positive Role Models

One special need for any adolescent is to have a positive, visible role model, a person who not only is caring but tangibly exemplifies desired attributes of adult behavior. This is particularly important for adolescents who do not have a stable family or extended kin network. Such an adult can help a young person to appraise life options constructively and develop a sense of self-esteem. One potentially important talent pool for such roles is older people, mostly past sixty years of age, although some in the fifty- to sixty-year-old group are available as well. Particularly significant would be those who have had reasonably successfully experiences as parents, grandparents, aunts, or uncles. The essential point is that real-life experience with a variety of growing children, well assimilated and a source of some gratification, can provide a useful underpinning for tackling the difficult tasks of intervention with socially disadvantaged young parents and other adolescents.

The potential contribution of young people eager to serve and also needing to earn some extra money is worth considering. College and even high school students can serve as role models for young adolescents in junior high or middle schools. It would be preferable to have students in such roles who have had extensive contact with younger children in their own families or in community experience.

Community-Based Support

Youth-serving organizations can play a significant supportive role in enhancing the education of young adolescents and in promoting healthful behaviors. In the United States, there are more than 300 adult-sponsored organizations that serve millions of children and youth. With the changing demographics and needs of young people, youth organizations have had to develop program material in areas such as substance abuse, self-awareness, parenting education, nutrition and health, child abuse prevention, building employability skills, career exploration, human sexuality, and eliminating sex-role stereotypes. For example, Girls Incorporated, whose membership is typically young adolescents, has a major program for pregnancy prevention that focuses on parent-child communication about sexuality, teaches assertiveness training, goal setting, decision making, and future planning, and bridges the gap between educational services and clinical services in the community. An evaluation of this program is currently under way.

The potential of youth agencies is great. They serve approximately thirty million young people annually and are second only to the public schools in the extent of their influence. They offer some advantages over the schools in that they are free to experiment, they reach children early in life, and they work in small groups with ten to fifteen young people at a time. Typically, youth organizations are tied to the community by virtue of their membership and voluntary leadership. Many youth agencies work in collaboration with schools or are actual providers of programs in schools. In some cases, they are providers of programs after school hours. Youth organization activities can cross age barriers and provide services to the elderly. In other cases, young people work with children as tutors or aides in playgrounds or extended day care.

Youth-serving agencies are one means of providing young adolescents with an opportunity to develop a sense of competence through mastery of life tasks in small, protected settings. Young people can begin to learn about responsibility to their community and about citizenship through church projects or under community sponsorship. Although not specifically designed to address adolescent health needs, the Early Adolescent Helper Program engages young adolescents, eleven to fourteen years old, in responsible and important work in their communities and in their schools. The purposes of this program, which is based in New York City, are to provide parents of young adolescents with a fuller understanding of the needs and potential of this age group, to help schools that serve young adolescents to develop and implement community service programs, to incorporate community service and active learning into the curriculum, and to reduce the isolation of schools from the community.

The program has been in operation since 1982. The participating students perform community service, gain understanding of their community and how neighborhoods function, and learn employability skills. The program offers an opportunity for at-risk youth, often separated from the mainstream by the conditions of their lives and environment, to move toward a constructive adult life and to relate to diverse individuals and groups. These activities tend to build self-esteem by demonstrating that the young people have something to contribute that is worthwhile. Indirectly, such activities are likely to foster health-promoting behavior during adolescence.

Opportunities for Research and Implications for the Future

What opportunities currently exist for individuals and institutions or agencies to promote healthful behaviors and prevent disease in adolescence? Do institutions need to be reshaped in order to facilitate adolescent development? Churches, schools, and community organizations can be mobilized to meet the needs of young people in ways that foster health and education.

Toward this end, institutions must be ready to support small groups that have certain characteristics: a mutual aid ethic, the ability to pool resources and foster reliable attachments and coping skills, the ability to contribute to self-esteem, and an orientation toward health or education. The institutions need to be dependable and attractive to young people. Which institutions would connect education and health in a way that would have enduring value? Are social support functions best provided as an aspect of other activities, such as prenatal care, preschool education, and the transition to junior high school?

Restructuring the Middle Schools. The middle or junior high schools play a central role in the lives of most young adolescents. The transition into early adolescence brings a greater capacity for exploration; a greater need for independence; a heightened sense of individual interests, abilities, and appearance; and a need to develop an identity through trustworthy interactions with peers and adults in addition to parents. The structure and curriculum of most American junior high and middle schools do not come close to meeting these developmental needs.

For most young adolescents, the shift from elementary to junior high or middle school means moving from a small, neighborhood school and the stability of one primary classroom to a larger, more impersonal institution, typically at a greater distance from home. In the new setting, the composition of the class will generally change as many as six or seven times a day, creating real obstacles to establishing stable peer groups, close relationships, and support from reliable adults. The sudden increase in the number of teachers and other school personnel comes at a time when young people are renegotiating their relationships with their parents.

Middle-grade education should lead children through the initial physical, intellectual, and social transformations to adulthood and equip them with capacities for thought and action that will be fully compatible with a productive adult life. In addition to making the curriculum of the middle schools challenging to each middle-grade student, and to providing each with a solid base for continued learning, a reshaping of the middle-grade school would include forming productive alliances with families, fostering constructive peer groups, and developing partnerships for youth service in the larger community.

Despite these crucial issues, the junior high and middle school institution has been largely ignored in the recent ferment of education reform. Yet these middle grades constitute an arena of educational casualties — damaging to both students and teachers as presently constituted. To address this serious gap in reports on education reform in the 1980s, the Carnegie Council on Adolescent Development established a Task Force on Education of Young Adolescents in 1986. In 1989, the task force produced a report, *Turning Points: Preparing American Youth for the 21st Century*, that delineates ways to build support for and educate young adolescents through new relationships among schools, families, and health and community institutions. The report not only seeks basic upgrading of the middle grade school, but aims to facilitate the personal development of these young people in and out of school.

Revising the Life Sciences Curriculum. There has been a significant drop in interest in science exhibited by both minority and majority students during the middle school years. This aversion to science is particularly damaging for the education of this generation of young people at a time when there is a broad consensus that an understanding of science and technology should be as fundamental in American education as reading and writing. This belief is tied not only to the concern about U.S. competitiveness in a world economy based increasingly on advances in science and technology but also to the desire to ensure effective citizenship in this country's participatory democracy, which includes the development of informed-decision-making skills.

Carnegie Corporation is supporting a project at Stanford University to create a new life sciences curriculum for early adolescence that will involve a comprehensive, interdisciplinary approach that integrates the biological sciences with the behavioral sciences. A middle-grades life sciences program should present young adolescents with a broad view of the life sciences, stressing the relationship between science and the student's own life experiences. It should be designed to give adolescents the information they need on disease prevention and health promotion in a way that is consonant with their motivation to understand the changes in their own bodies during puberty. Such a course could well serve as the main organizing principle for the junior high and middle school curriculum in general.

School-Related Health Facilities. One approach to meeting adolescents' health care needs is through the school-linked or school-based health center. Currently, there are 177 school-based and school-linked adolescent health centers in operation, with many more in the planning stages. Most school-related health facilities are located in urban areas with high concentrations of poor, medically underserved adolescents who are members of racial or ethnic minority groups. The recent increase in the number of such centers derives from concerns that adolescents' health care needs are often unmet, that the main causes of morbidity and mortality in adolescents are potentially preventable, that adolescents underuse health services in relation to their health needs, and that adolescents have special needs as a function of their developmental status. School-related health facilities are in need of further evaluation to determine the conditions under which they are likely to be widely useful.

Other Institutions That Support Adolescent Health. Although the family is still alive and its functions are still of great significance, it has been pulled out of shape throughout the world, in some places to such an extent that it has been seriously damaged. Therefore, it is necessary to think about ways in which other institutions might tend to compensate in part for family vulnerabilities. Self-help, mutual aid, and other support systems are not widely available from family or social service systems in very poor communities, although there are relatively strong institutions, such as churches, around which social support networks for children, adolescents, and young parents can be organized. Indeed, a variety of institutions may be involved in deliberate efforts to build constructive social support networks that tend to foster health and education. In particular, such social support networks can focus intensely on mastering the tasks of parental responsibility and family formation. These problems are most severe among high-risk youth in poverty-concentration areas, but they are also present throughout modern society.

Weakened families may be strengthened by cooperative efforts among relatively strong institutions such as churches, schools, and community organizations. The role of religious institutions in increasing the life chances of adolescents is important but often given too little attention. In some communities, 50 percent of adolescents attend church regularly, and church attendance correlates with a lower frequency of high-risk behaviors.

Religious institutions, of course, have traditionally provided support for youth, but their role can and should be adapted to current circumstances. Since it was first established in 1773, the black church has served as a kind of extended family, providing children with other significant adults and families with material and human resources. Since black children suffer from disproportionately high rates of school failure, drug abuse, violence, and adolescent pregnancy, and 55 percent of black families with children are headed by a single parent, this kind of community resource is needed now more than ever. The black churches are particularly strong forces to help young people in their communities. As the only institution in the black community that has traditionally been controlled by blacks, the church has great potential for addressing problems that afflict large numbers of black children and families. A variety of youth-oriented projects that are attempting to fulfill their potential are under way.

The Potential of Social Support

Social support interventions are not a panacea for adolescent problems, including health problems. There is so far only limited evidence that strengthening or developing social supports is by itself highly effective, especially for high-risk populations. Nevertheless, the promise of social supports for enabling adolescents to become productive, healthy, and caring members of society is urgently in need of exploration, especially in light of the social transformations that have seriously jeopardized the development of many contemporary adolescents. Adolescents need to be valued members of groups that provide mutual support and caring relationships; they need to become socially competent individuals with skills to cope successfully with everyday life; and they need to believe in a promising future with real opportunities.

Research is especially needed to evaluate promising interventions that provide support for behavior that is conducive to health and continuing education. The most pressing problems are those of high-risk adolescents, including racial and ethnic minorities in the United States. While research is continuing, it is crucially important not to let what we do know go to waste. It is time to apply more widely the knowledge and experience already available to prevent the spread of adolescent casualties.

In the rapid world transformation of this century, preparation for adult life increasingly involves readiness to cope with change itself. It is very difficult in the early years of life to anticipate the circumstances of adulthood—not only for children but for parents as well. Adolescence is the critical passage from being a child to becoming an adult. It is a time of fateful decisions with lifelong consequences. Its manifest difficulties in such casualties as substance abuse, school-age pregnancy, and school failure are of growing concern in many parts of the world, not only in poor communities but elsewhere. So adolescent development deserves a higher place on the agenda of research, education, and health care.

Suggested Readings

Benson, P., Williams, D., and Johnson, A. *The Quicksilver Years: The Hopes and Fears of Early Adolescence.* New York: Harper & Row, 1987.

Berkman, L. F. "The Relationship of Social Networks and Social Support to Morbidity and Mortality." In S. Cohen and S. L. Syme (eds.), *Social Support and Health.* Orlando, Fla.: Academic Press, 1985.

Bowlby, J. *Attachment.* New York: Basic Books, 1969.

Boyce, W. T. "Social Support, Family Relations, and Children." In S. Cohen and S. L. Syme (eds.), *Social Support and Health*. Orlando, Fla.: Academic Press, 1985.

Furby, L., and Beyth–Marom, R. *Risk Taking in Adolescence: A Decision-Making Perspective*. A working paper of the Carnegie Council on Adolescent Development. Washington, D.C.: Carnegie Council on Adolescent Development, 1990.

Gottlieb, B. H. "Support Interventions: A Typology and Agenda for Research." In S. W. Duck (ed.), *Handbook of Personal Relationships*. New York: Wiley, 1988.

Hamburg, B. A., and Hamburg, D. A. "Stressful Transitions of Adolescence: Endocrine and Psychosocial Aspects." In L. Levi (ed.), *Society, Stress, and Disease*. Vol. 2. London: Oxford University Press, 1975.

Hamburg, D. A. *Preparing for Life: The Critical Transition of Adolescence*. New York: Carnegie Corporation of New York, 1986.

Hamburg, D. A., Elliott, G. R., and Parron, D. L. (eds.). *Health and Behavior: Frontiers of Research in the Biobehavioral Sciences*. Washington, D.C.: National Academy Press, 1982.

Hamburg, D. A., and Sartorius, N. (eds.). *Psychosocial Perspectives on Health*. Cambridge, England: Cambridge University Press, 1989.

Hayes, C. D. (ed.). *Risking the Future: Adolescent Sexuality, Pregnancy, and Childbearing*. Washington, D.C.: National Academy Press, 1987.

House, J. S., Landis, K. R., and Umberson, D. "Social Relationships and Health." *Science*, 1988, *241*, 540–545.

Jessor, R. "Problem-Behavior Theory, Psychosocial Development, and Adolescent Problem Drinking." *British Journal of Addiction*, 1987, *82*, 435–446.

Kyle, J. E. *Children, Families, and Cities: Programs That Work at the Local Level*. Washington, D.C.: National League of Cities, 1987.

Millstein, S. G. *The Potential of School-Linked Centers to Promote Adolescent Health and Development*. A working paper of the Carnegie Council on Adolescent Development. Washington, D.C.: Carnegie Council on Adolescent Development, 1988.

Nightingale, E. O., and Wolverton, L. *Adolescent Rolelessness in Modern Society*. A working paper of the Carnegie Council on Adolescent Development. Washington, D.C.: Carnegie Council on Adolescent Development, 1988.

Price, R. H., Cioci, M., Penner, W., and Trautlein, B. *School and Community Support Programs That Enhance Adolescent Health and Education*. A working paper of the Carnegie Council on Adolescent Development. Washington, D.C.: Carnegie Council on Adolescent Development, 1990.

Rook, K. S. "Promoting Social Bonding: Strategies for Helping the Lonely and Socially Isolated." *American Psychologist*, 1984, *39*, 1389–1407.

Salzinger, S., Hammer, M., and Antrobus, J. "From Crib to College: An Overview of Studies of the Social Networks of Children, Adolescents, and College Students." In S. Salzinger, J. Antrobus, and M. Hammer (eds.), *Social Networks of Children, Adolescents, and College Students*. Hillsdale, N.J.: Erlbaum, 1988.

Schine, J. G., and Campbell, P. B. *Helping to Success: Early Adolescents and Young Children.* New York: Bruner Foundation, 1987.

Small, S. A. *Preventive Programs That Support Families with Adolescents.* A working paper of the Carnegie Council on Adolescent Development. Washington, D.C.: Carnegie Council on Adolescent Development, 1990.

Sullivan, J. F. "$6 Million Program in Jersey to Aid Troubled Teen-Agers." *New York Times,* Jan. 1, 1988, p. 26.

Turning Points: Preparing American Youth for the 21st Century. The report of the Task Force on Education of Young Adolescents of the Carnegie Council on Adolescent Development. Washington, D.C.: Carnegie Council on Adolescent Development, 1989.

Wilson, W. J. *The Truly Disadvantaged: The Inner City, the Underclass, and Public Policy.* Chicago: University of Chicago Press, 1987.

Name Index

Subject Index

A

Abortions, prevalence of, 256–257, 262–263, 265–266

Abuse. *See* Maltreatment

Academy of Pediatrics, 370

Access to health care: aspects of, 377–494; barriers to, 431–452; economic issues in, 453–467; and family disease denial, 391–394, 406; and interventions, 411–430; introduction to, 379–380; and recognizing health issues, 381–410; and utilization patterns, 431–439

Accident, concept of, 303. *See also* Injuries

ACTH, 28

Addictive behaviors, and access to care, 394–409. *See also* Substance abuse

Adolescence: antecedents of, 68–74; concepts of, 251–252; puberty distinct from, 21; turmoil posited in, 334–335

Adolescent Concern Questionnaire, 388–389

Adolescent Health Service, 464–465

Adolescent Pregnancy Program, 272–275

Adolescents: access to care for, 377–494; advocacy for, 178; assessment of, 242–247; at-risk and disadvantaged, 123–124, 531–532; behavior of, interpreting, 387, 389–390; behavioral risks of, 162–180; blamed for economic dependency, 124–126; compliance with interventions by, 468–494; as consumers, 119; control loss by, 171–174, 389–390, 398, 400; defined, 2; demand shrinking for, 120–121; denial by, 404–406; development of, normal or pathological, 387–391; disadvantaged and deprived, 123–124, 531–532; disturbed, 334–346; dysfunctional, and

maltreatment, 367; economic status of, 119–120, 454–458; education and extracurricular activities for, 139–161; family factors for, 89–180; health care needs of, 449–511; health issues for, 181–376; health of, and social environment, 529–532; hidden concerns of, 382–383, 384, 393; improving health of, 495–542; income of, 456–458; living independently, 11, 457–458; maltreatment of, 347–376; moratorium for, economic impact of, 125, 128; normal growth and development of, 17–88; parental reactions to, 111–112; as physical beings, 76–78; physical development of, 21–57; pregnancy among, 250–281; psychological development of, 58–88; responsibility by, 509; separation-individuation of, 104–110; as sexual beings, 78–81, 111; social supports for, 526–542; and societal changes, 527–528; sociodemographic trends for, 1–15; special needs of, 464–465; supervision of, 154–158; supply of, 121–124; utilization of health care by, 431–439, 503–506, 509–510; as vocational beings, 81–84; vulnerability of, 167–168, 190, 389

Adolescents, early: defined, 2; depression in, 400; development of, 390; disturbed, 336, 338; and pregnancy counseling, 279; psychological development of, 74, 76–78; sociodemographic trends for, 3, 4, 9; supervision of, 157, 158

Adolescents, late: defined, 2, 252; depression in, 400; development of, 391; identity formation in, 114; physical development of, 25; psychological development of, 74, 81–84; self-image of, 336; sociodemographic trends for, 4, 9; wealthy, 128